Principles of Emotion Change

This outstanding book is a must-read for clinicians of all orientations, offering a comprehensive and insightful synthesis for those who want to improve their skill in working with emotion. Twelve years in the making, this work combines clinical process with empirical findings in brilliant fashion, illuminating the how and why of emotional change in psychotherapy. A visionary work, this will be a main reference for clinicians and academics alike.

—**Leslie S. Greenberg, PhD,** Distinguished Research Professor Emeritus, Department of Psychology, York University, Toronto, ON, Canada

This book is an integrative masterpiece. Emotional change in psychotherapy is a jungle of theories, contradictions, and messy findings—but Antonio Pascual-Leone has expertly cleared a path to reveal what emotions to focus on, when, for what purpose, and how. This amazing synthesis will become a leading light in the field, a guiding force for psychotherapy practice, training, and research.

—**Louis G. Castonguay, PhD,** Liberal Arts Professor of Psychology, Pennsylvania State University, University Park, PA, United States

Serious EFT therapists and practitioners of related emotion-based approaches will want to read this book because it provides a solid, clearly stated scientific foundation for five key kinds of emotion change processes. The author has produced a tour de force based on a rigorous, decade-long systematic review of a wide range of applied emotion research that provides a fresh look at the key therapeutic tasks such as empty chair work, grounding them historically and in the wider field of applied emotion research.

—**Robert Elliott, PhD,** Professor Emeritus, University of Strathclyde, Glasgow, Scotland

With clarity, elegance, and precision, Antonio Pascual-Leone offers a generative new synthesis in the emotion-focused tradition. Grounded in empirical rigor and richly illustrated through clinical examples, this principle-based framework will help a new generation of therapists understand not just that emotion matters—but how it changes. At once nuanced and practical!

—**J. Christopher Muran, PhD,** Dean and Professor, Gordon F. Derner School of Psychology, Adelphi University, Garden City, NY, United States; Mount Sinai Beth Israel Psychotherapy Research Program, New York, NY; NYU Postdoctoral Program in Psychotherapy and Psychoanalysis, New York, NY

Principles of Emotion Change

What Works and When in Psychotherapy and Everyday Life

Antonio Pascual-Leone

 **AMERICAN PSYCHOLOGICAL ASSOCIATION**

Copyright © 2026 by the American Psychological Association. All rights, including for text and data mining, AI training, and similar technologies, are reserved. Except as permitted under the United States Copyright Act of 1976, no part of this publication may be reproduced or distributed in any form or by any means, including, but not limited to, the process of scanning and digitization, or stored in a database or retrieval system, without the prior written permission of the publisher.

The opinions and statements published are those of the Author, and do not necessarily represent the policies of the American Psychological Association. The information contained in this work does not constitute personalized therapeutic advice. Users seeking medical advice, diagnoses, or treatment should consult a medical professional or health care provider. The Author has worked to ensure that all information in this book is accurate at the time of publication and consistent with general mental health care standards.

Published by
American Psychological Association
750 First Street, NE
Washington, DC 20002
https://www.apa.org

Order Department
https://www.apa.org/pubs/books
order@apa.org

Typeset in Meridien and Ortodoxa by TIPS Publishing Services, Carrboro, NC

Printer: Vicks Lithograph & Printing, Yorkville, NY
Cover Designer: Gwen J. Grafft, Minneapolis, MN

Library of Congress Cataloging-in-Publication Data

Names: Pascual-Leone, Antonio author
Title: Principles of emotion change : what works and when in psychotherapy
    and everyday life / by Antonio Pascual-Leone.
Description: Washington, DC : American Psychological Association, [2026] |
    Includes bibliographical references and index.
Identifiers: LCCN 2025002629 (print) | LCCN 2025002630 (ebook) | ISBN
    9781433836602 paperback | ISBN 9781433840890 ebook
Subjects: LCSH: Emotion-focused therapy | Emotions | Psychotherapy | BISAC:
    PSYCHOLOGY / Psychotherapy / General
Classification: LCC RC489.F62 P37 2026 (print) | LCC RC489.F62 (ebook) |
    DDC 616.89/14--dc23/eng/20250512
LC record available at https://lccn.loc.gov/2025002629
LC ebook record available at https://lccn.loc.gov/2025002630

ISBN 9781433849916 (pdf)

https://doi.org/10.1037/0000460-000

Printed in the United States of America

10 9 8 7 6 5 4 3 2 1

This book is dedicated to the great women who have shaped me: First to my mother, Margarete Wolfram, psychologist, who taught me everything from statistical methods to home renovation; my inspiring grandmother Josefina Pascual, Doctor of Pharmacy in 1928; my aunt Ana Maria Pascual-Leone, endocrinologist and prize-winning researcher at the Royal Academy of Spain; my aunt Elena Pascual-Leone, a true humanist; my cousin Marta Pascual-Leone, physician and master of observation; and my stepmom, Janice Johnson, psychologist, who is a grounding force. This also goes to my lab-mate, friend, and late colleague Alberta Pos. And to senior colleagues at the University of Windsor: Sandra Paivio, Charlene Senn, and Josée Jarry—a mentor, a role model, and a confidante.

Finally, the heart of this dedication belongs to my wife, my partner and love, Megan Thomas. You gracefully balance the pragmatic expertise of an executive with a disarmingly gentle touch, warm laughter, and an unwavering commitment to seeing things through.

I am grateful to these women for their wisdom, courage, and fierce perseverance, often as trailblazers in pursuit of new frontiers.

—ANTONIO PASCUAL-LEONE

CONTENTS

Principles of Emotion Change

INTRODUCTION

Of course, the person doesn't change only because of the wisdom which the therapist tells him [or her]. The change comes through some kind of emotional digesting.
—EUGENE T. GENDLIN, *A THEORY OF PERSONALITY CHANGE*

This book is about the science of emotion change and how emotional processing happens in psychotherapy as well as in everyday life. When people talk about having successfully struggled through a personal difficulty, they often comment on some sort of emotional change. Typically, it is an offhand but conclusive remark: "I started to see things differently" or "I got used to it"; sometimes, "I just decided"; or quite often, "...well, I got over it!" When pressed, the person might observe: "It just feels different now..." Then their account usually skips quickly forward, telling a story about the consequences of their having changed—personal choices, social implications, and so on. But that is the exact moment—the remark about a transition and somehow having been internally changed or rearranged—when I lean forward and become wide-eyed: "Wait! Yes, there was a change, but how did that change happen? What was going on inside that created the change?" Often, people do not really know. It is a mystery behind the curtain, but one with great implications for the next difficulty that person will encounter. And if the answer uncovers a principle of change, then there are implications for many other people as well.

The main contribution of this book is to present a unified theory of how a difficult emotional state comes to change. It explains (a) what the different

https://doi.org/10.1037/0000460-001
Principles of Emotion Change: What Works and When in Psychotherapy and Everyday Life, by A. Pascual-Leone
Copyright © 2026 by the American Psychological Association. All rights reserved.

kinds of emotional change are, (b) what the hypothesized mechanisms of those processes are, and (c) when each type of change is most applicable. It summarizes and synthesizes existing research, sometimes offering new interpretations of previous findings. To illustrate practical implications, every chapter includes case examples from clinical practice. (All of these have been anonymized, are composite cases, or are hypothetical examples.[1]) This book is both for academic researchers and for psychotherapists who want to better understand what they are doing, and what is happening within their client, as they sit together in a therapy session.

As Kazdin (2009) notes, despite lively interest and debates about the mechanisms of therapeutic change as well as a "rather vast literature, there is little empirical research to provide an evidence-based explanation of precisely why treatment works and how the changes come about" (p. 419). Further, researchers from quite different perspectives have repeatedly called for a stronger focus on process research to determine the principles of change and to replace hackneyed debates about one or another treatment package (Elliott, 2010; L. S. Greenberg & Safran, 1987; Hoffman & Hayes, 2019; Rosen & Davidson, 2003). This book is one answer to those calls. I describe and organize the existing empirical research into a general theory of emotional change. It represents a coordination of existing theories that acknowledges their independent value but puts them in an integrated context, delineates the limits of their applicability, and resolves their contradictions. Existing theories often do not adequately address one another, so this large coordination reconciles findings from different lines of research by locating them within a larger theory, with practical implications. This is the first book of its kind, integrating findings and theories across treatment approaches to combine and delineate different forms of emotion change.

EMOTION CHANGE IS A COMMON FACTOR

Psychology has launched into an emotion revolution. From theories of personal change to advances in neuroscience to the titles of popular psychology books, the question of how and when emotion changes has taken center stage. At the same time, however, enthusiasm for emotional change has wildly outpaced the development of theory that is coherent and offers overarching explanations of how and why emotions change. The idea that therapists might help clients have some sort of corrective emotional experience is now championed as a common factor across psychotherapies (Alexander & French, 1946; A. Pascual-Leone & Kramer, 2023; Sønderland et al., 2023; Wampold & Imel, 2015).

A meta-analysis of 43 process-to-outcome studies looked at the degree to which a client's expression of emotion during psychotherapy could predict positive treatment outcomes. Although the analysis grouped together a varied assortment of constructs, it concluded that when clients were more emotionally expressive during their therapy sessions, this had a medium to large effect in the prediction of good treatment outcomes (Peluso & Freund, 2018). Another meta-analysis of 90 studies on psychological interventions with youth defined *emotion regulation* to broadly include avoidance strategies, engagement strategies, and a general lack of regulation skills. It showed this broad set of processes had a small to medium relationship with the reduction of clinical symptoms (Daros et al., 2021). A recent meta-analysis included 85 studies to consider various kinds of emotional processing and showed they have a medium to large effect in the prediction of psychotherapy outcomes (Sønderland et al., 2023). Reviews such as these are essential contributions because they help dispel an outdated Cartesian idea, and one deeply embedded in traditional medical models, which is that emotion is a messy byproduct of some other, more sterile, curative process. On the contrary, these studies consistently support working with emotion as a pan-theoretical process of change.

However, such reviews also reveal the various and discordant ways in which emotion change processes are viewed in the field of psychology. One study refers to a broad range of change processes as the term "emotion regulation," while another uses an equally wide brush but refers to the phrase "emotional expression." The studies collated in these reviews compile a wide and variegated set of measures that may or may not measure similar constructs. Moreover, the substantial overlaps between measures often is neither empirically explored nor even conceptually delineated. Meanwhile, studies may acknowledge different disparate perspectives on how emotion changes, but, having completed the lip service, they move on to present their view, making any direct comparisons or discussions from an integrative perspective impossible (A. Pascual-Leone & Kramer, 2023).

The most incisive systematic reviews have sought to group and then interpret studies based on their individual theoretical perspectives. For example, Sønderland and colleagues (2023) showed that habituation to fear (i.e., a decrease in arousal) has a medium to large effect in predicting treatment outcomes (see Chapter 3 for details) and that better experiencing (i.e., increases in emotional awareness) during treatments for depression has a medium to large effect in predicting outcomes (see Chapter 7). To these, Sønderland and colleagues also add a newer formulation of change, which is the activation of key emotion states (i.e., schemes and their sequential transformation), which had a medium effect in the prediction of outcomes (see Chapter 16). However, simply clustering studies based on the individual theories they espoused and tested still duplicates the research silos that were used. It reduces a client's true process into a single dimension of change, whatever the researcher was looking for. Empirical syntheses like this are much needed, but they are no substitute for a pantheoretical coordination that delineates the kinds of emotional change.

WHAT IS EMOTION?

While science has a new appreciation for emotion, this is not always the case for individuals. Whether struggling through everyday life or in the throes of a painful psychotherapy session, people often desperately wish they could just turn it off and feel less. A "No Fear!" bumper sticker on a pickup truck or slogan on a tight T-shirt would be another testament to the (mistaken) idea that not feeling would somehow make one tougher, perhaps invulnerable. Probably unbeknownst to the gritty owner of that pickup truck, there are indeed some people who do not feel any fear.

Urbach–Wiethe disease is a rare autosomal recessive disorder with several symptoms, one of which is that both amygdalae and surrounding parts of the medial temporal lobes get covered (bilaterally) in calcium deposits, essentially cutting them off from the rest of the brain. However, these parts of the brain are critical for generating experiences of fear. As a result, people with this condition effectively do not experience fear, and contrary to what some would guess, these fearless individuals are not particularly tough. In fact, these people are prone to folly and are relatively dysfunctional in life. They often cross the road when there is not enough time, they walk down dark alleys that would be better avoided, and when presented with a fanged and dangerous snake, they show playful curiosity and try to pet it (Feinstein et al., 2011). In very practical terms, this example illustrates what emotion is through its conspicuous absence. Above all, an emotion's meaning is embodied in its function, tacitly serving as a chief source of personal information. Emotion implicitly organizes one to interact with one's world, whether that be the external surroundings (e.g., a dangerous situation) or the internal models of one's understanding (e.g., a challenge to one's sense of identity).

Of course, emotion can be described in terms of functional states, but there are also the various ways in which emotion changes, the transitions or mechanisms of change that alter those emotion states. The rest of this section offers a brief introduction to what emotion is, highlighting its role in human functioning and the special kind of meaning embodied by these states. The section that follows outlines the chief contribution of this book, which is the elusive issue of how emotion comes to change in either intensity or quality.

Emotion as Information: Affect, Emotion, and Schemes

We navigate the world by constructing and then continually updating internal working models about ourselves in relation to others and the world. These representations help us navigate life as we know it, and this is as true for the external world of objects as it is for the internal world of our own experiences. From the perspective of a conscious organism, there are two critical kinds of information about truth. On one hand, *cognition* captures reality truths about the world we are interacting with and what it is like—the affordances and resistances it offers. On the other hand, *affect* captures vital truths, which are representations of reality that speak to survival (J. Pascual-Leone & Johnson, 2021). This distinction between the known (cognition) and the felt (affect) is one that has been emphasized by all leading emotion theorists (e.g., Damasio, 1999; Frijda 1986; L. S. Greenberg, 2021; Panksepp, 2008; Pessoa, 2013). While these are raw and unconscious facets of the lived experience, an *emotion scheme* entails the juxtaposition of reality truths with vital truths. The feeling itself embodies an implicit appraisal of the organism's state with respect to some need directly or indirectly related to survival (L. S. Greenberg & Pascual-Leone, 1995; J. Pascual-Leone & Johnson, 2021). This is the level of analysis at which we usually discuss emotion, so it is the focus of this book.

Emotion Is About Needs and Primes Us for Action
All fundamental emotional states are about needs. Positive emotions are about the pleasant experience of having one's needs met, while negative emotions are about the discomfort of one's unmet needs. The valence of an emotion also organizes our mental resources differently. Generally, positive emotions (e.g., joy, curiosity, love) facilitate further engagement and appreciation of an overall experience without getting caught up in the details, while negative emotions focus us on more urgent details without getting distracted by larger considerations. So, while positive emotions help us broaden and build on our lived experience (Fredrickson, 2001), negative emotions help us deepen and differentiate the critical meanings of a painful situation (L. S. Greenberg, 2021). These cognitive constraints and the importance of differentiating negative experience is captured in an everyday observation: Across languages, people have larger working vocabularies to describe negative emotional experiences than they have for positive or neutral experiences (Schrauf & Sanchez, 2004).

Largely because of this relationship with the vital value of needs, emotions are fundamentally procedural. They are not simply representations of meaning (e.g., the affective residue of some belief); rather, emotions are something we do. They are embodied experiences that have preverbal roots (Damasio, 1999; Panksepp, 2008; Porges, 2011). These are not cognitive meanings; they are self-organizations that orient one's attention, prepare one for action, and even shape the way one perceives reality. Polyvagal theory (Porges, 2011) describes neurophysiology that seems to support a fundamental substrate of emotional experience. The nervous system makes ongoing assessments about safety and danger and then impacts our emotions and behaviors. Although still debated (Grossman, 2023), the theory articulates how emotion regulation, social connection, and fear responses are biologically organized outside our awareness. The idea that an emotion is a procedural unit of meaning (i.e., not just a sensation with a name) and that it entails an implicit plan for engagement is essential for understanding its role in human functioning.

Emotion Can Be Either Innate or Learned
Some aspects of emotion are hardwired, inherited to some degree through the primal origins of evolution (Panksepp, 2008; Porges, 2011). For example, a baby winces with disgust at food that is unpalatable, we cry out in fear when startled by unexpected danger, and we feel frustrated when our intentions are thwarted. Typically, those are adaptive emotions. However, other aspects of emotion are learned with experience (L. S. Greenberg, 2021). Emotions learned through

unhealthy situations may ultimately be maladaptive in the person's life, even if they were functionally helpful in navigating a local, albeit dysfunctional, context. Maladaptive emotions are typically learned through unfortunate circumstances (e.g., an abusive relationship), but the fact that they were learned by no means suggests they are superficial in comparison to adaptive emotions that were part of one's biological inheritance. For better or for worse, the learned substrate of one's emotional responding shapes the brain and its emotional system (Lane & Nadel, 2020). This is the nature of emotion schemes, imperfect but functional, tailoring our pragmatic working models from interactions with reality.

Each Emotion Has Its Own Meaning

The nature of a scheme, and therefore of an emotion, is that it consists of a multimodal associative network of information. It is also highly context sensitive. Emotion schemes are inherently self-propelling in that they apply automatically as procedural tools for interpreting and managing one's reality (J. Pascual-Leone & Johnson, 2021).[2] For example, stimuli encountered in the present may resemble an earlier traumatic context and thereby reactivate experiences formed at the time of the trauma such as the feeling of fear and helplessness, related somatic experiences, or the impulse to escape danger and avoid harm, as well as beliefs about oneself and the situation (L. S. Greenberg & Safran, 1987). The activation of emotion takes place by attending to sensory and somatic aspects of an experience, which could be in the present or in a memory reconstructed from the past (A. Pascual-Leone, Paivio, et al., 2016).

In these ways, each discrete emotional experience represents a densely packaged unit of information, often implicit and so tightly packed that one might be quickly organized to engage in some way, without being fully aware of the embodied meaning at hand. Moreover, qualitatively different emotions organize the person experiencing them in specific ways (L. S. Greenberg & Paivio, 1997; Panksepp, 2008; A. Pascual-Leone, Paivio, et al., 2016; Porges, 2011). For example, the following occur on a moment-by-moment basis:

- Fear organizes one to freeze and monitor, then run, flee, and escape.

- Anger organizes one to fight and defend one's boundaries.

- Sadness organizes one to seek comfort and then to withdraw, conserving resources.

- Disgust organizes one to spit out or reject some noxious experience.

- Guilt organizes one to repair some problem or situation.

- Shame organizes one to hide from the scrutiny of others.

- Positive emotions (e.g., love, happiness, curiosity) organize one in various ways to reach out, build, share, celebrate, and explore.

The specificity of meanings embodied by a given emotion has important implications for working with emotion (L. S. Greenberg & Safran, 1987; A. Pascual-Leone, Paivio, et al., 2016).

The Meanings of Emotion Are Nested

Finally, emotion schemes can also be nested within larger social interaction and personal contexts (e.g., sociopersonal schemes) to generate higher and higher orders of functioning and self-understanding (J. Pascual-Leone & Johnson, 2021). Personal narratives and one's sense of identity are examples of these broader constructs, which are heavily influenced, bottom-up, by their constituent emotion schemes but also provide an overarching context for interpreting any newly emerging emotion. These higher order sociopersonal schemes (e.g., personal narratives that subsume emotion schemes) are frameworks of understanding deeply informed by both social and cultural variables.

Relatedly, humans have the boon of so much mental power that we can have emotions about our emotions (e.g., "I feel guilty about getting so angry"). Self-referencing and recursive feelings like these are only possible given our mental capacity, which supports the generation of additional feelings in reaction to our initial feelings or to manage these feelings (and sometimes those of others). Furthermore, because emotion has evolved as part of a signal system within the species, we sometimes use emotion instrumentally to leverage its social impact. Here again, the display rules of a given culture and one's socialization will shape both the experience and the expression of emotion. In this book, I start with ways of working with emotion in an immediate experiential moment and then build over the chapters to address increasingly complex and higher order processes of change.

Emotion Theory

Basic emotion research tends to focus on either neurobiological underpinning, evolutionary evidence, or psychometric measurement of self-reported feelings. But these do not always address the dynamic way emotions interact as one negotiates personal distress. That is the domain of clinical observation, case formulation, and the practical application of facilitating change. The puzzle of working with emotion and overcoming personal concerns has led to further understanding in terms of kinds of emotion that cuts across the discrete emotion categories (e.g., anger, happiness, sadness, fear, disgust). Distinguishing between primary and secondary emotion and between adaptive and maladaptive emotion is important for understanding the change process. The rendition of this categorization has been an important contribution of emotion-focused theory, but it clearly draws on and echoes several earlier lines of clinical theory (L. S. Greenberg & Paivio, 1997; see also Damasio, 1999; Freud, 1926). Similar categorizations also exist in several other contemporary treatment approaches, many of which are either compatible or complementary with this one.[3] What I review next are functional categories that may be empirically refutable. Nevertheless, the pragmatic utility when working through distress is what lends this typology its significance and may also explain its influence on psychotherapy at large. That said, research using interrater reliability has shown that the categories listed here can be critically examined and have construct validity in the prediction of therapeutic outcomes (Herrmann et al., 2016; J. Pascual-Leone, 2018).

Primary Adaptive Emotions

Primary and adaptive emotions include productive, meaning-laden, and idiosyncratically specific affective experiences. Here, primary emotion does not necessarily refer to natural or Darwinian emotions but to one's earliest emotional experience in response to an emerging stimulus-situation. Fear of genuine threat, sadness over an identifiable loss, and happiness about positive events are examples of primary adaptive emotions that inform a person about what is significant in their experience. (The earlier bullets on emotion as information illustrate other examples of adaptive functioning.) The adaptive value of this type of emotion is clear. Evoking such feelings mobilizes adaptive information, often embodied by some action tendency. Primary adaptive emotions are anchored in a bodily felt sensation, they embody a complex sense of preverbal meaning, and they integrate affect with perception and cognition. Some examples entail a felt experience of rich meaning, such as feeling on top of the world or all washed up (L. S. Greenberg & Paivio, 1997). When primary adaptive emotions are explored, they reveal implicit meaning, which often comes with a bodily felt release related to their newly emergent content. As a fundamental self-organization in response to reality, these feelings are also basic experiences of identity.

Primary Maladaptive Emotions

Primary and maladaptive emotions are unhealthy emotional experiences that have become fundamental forms of responding, typically developed as a person has had to contend with dysfunctional life circumstances. The learned emotional responses often had been functionally adaptive ways of responding and coping with an unfortunate history of neglect, invalidation, or abuse. Examples include learning to fear closeness because it was associated with abuse or preemptively hiding in shame to evade arbitrary rejections and humiliation. These emotions become clearly maladaptive as a person matures but continues to react to normal (i.e., potentially healthy) social interactions in the same old matter they once learned. Primary maladaptive shame, fear, guilt, and loneliness are prototypical examples of this type of emotion as observed in therapy (A. Pascual-Leone & Greenberg, 2007a). For instance, maladaptive emotion schemes are the shamebased sense of self as a failure or worthless, a sense of "bad me," or the fear-based sense of "weak me" as being fundamentally insecure and unable to cope (L. S. Greenberg & Paivio, 1997).[4] These types of emotions are often hauntingly familiar; they are thematically a painful experience of the same old story (Angus, 2012).

Secondary Emotional Responses

Some emotions are secondary in the sense that they are reactive feelings about a deeper and often more painful emotion. Whether adaptive or maladaptive, primary emotions can be hard to allow, accept, and endure. *Secondary emotions,* then, are one's internal reactions or attempts to manage the initial affects or cognitions that pertain to deeper primary experiences. Secondary symptom-based emotions are usually very salient in therapy and part of the presenting concern (e.g., hopelessness, anxiety, feeling depressed or overwhelmed, lashing out in rage). Almost any category of emotion (e.g., sadness, anger, fear) could be secondary-symptomatic in nature, depending on the individual and their circumstance. Moreover, a specific secondary emotion does not necessarily indicate or correspond to any given primary emotion (L. S. Greenberg & Paivio, 1997). A few examples of these configurations could be

- secondary anger as a defensive reaction to the primary hurt of rejection (e.g., "I resent them for not loving me"),

- collapsing into secondary sadness when making healthy assertions with primary adaptive anger gets too stressful (e.g., "I burst into tears whenever I try to stand up for myself"), or

- secondary fear (anxiety) over prospective experiences of primary maladaptive shame (e.g., "I'm anxious people will see how utterly incompetent I am").

Notice that secondary emotion occurs partly because of some deeper, more primary emotion not being adequately symbolized in awareness and thus being expressed in another form. For instance, unsymbolized anger can turn into frustrated sadness, fear into aloofness and jealousy into anger.

"Secondary emotion" is a term that has also referred to distress when it is simply too vague and undifferentiated, when there is high affective arousal but low meaningfulness (A. Pascual-Leone & Greenberg, 2007a). Here it is secondary in the sense of surface level and underdeveloped. For example, in the face of some disappointment, people may feel both angry and sad, although rather than fully experiencing each feeling on its own, people experience the feelings as fused together, creating the sense of stuckness that comes from feeling everything at once. This has often been part of psychodynamic formulations of free-floating anxiety and the notion of unformulated experience (D. B. Stern, 1997). Secondary emotion is often the first concern that someone presents and initially the most salient focus of experience.

Instrumental Emotions

Emotion has evolved both as a self-organizing system and as a social signaling system (Darwin, 1872). Therefore, authentic emotional experience may also be shaped by learned behaviors to obtain some desired effect on others. Instrumental emotions are expressions that emphasize this function, serving mostly to socially influence others (e.g., using anger to dominate an encounter, crying to elicit sympathy). Although they are real feelings, a hallmark of instrumental emotions is that they are quickly activated and, if social demands are met, may subside just as quickly. Children use instrumental emotions, particularly when they have not yet developed more mature forms of social negotiation. Among adults, instrumental emotions can remain tremendously effective in the short term but are often detrimental to relationships in the longer term. Instrumental emotions are not packages of information about working through one's internal difficulties; they are the product of operant conditioning and are primarily about acting on the external world. That social function often comes at the expense of emotion as an embodied source of personal meaning, so deeply exploring instrumental emotion typically offers relatively little adaptive information and little direction for the next course of action (L. S. Greenberg & Paivio, 1997; A. Pascual-Leone et al., 2013).

Emotions Embody Different Meanings

Working with emotion is a challenge one cannot avoid in life, particularly when working through clinical concerns. In the throes of distress, sometimes people would wish away their capacity to feel, yet emotion is not a vestigial feature of our functioning, not an evolutionary leftover that has lost its ancestral function. On the contrary, emotion is a vital source of information for our well-being, one that quickly and implicitly organizes us for feeling, thinking, and acting, often even faster than we are aware of (Damasio, 1999; Panksepp, 2008; Porges, 2011). This can be as simple as the emotional distress that comes with the pain of pinching one's finger in a door or as complex as feeling one has lost one's identity. The practical puzzle of working with emotion to resolve personal difficulties, either in psychotherapy or everyday life, also requires one to appreciate that not all emotional experiences are the same. Assessing the different functional types of emotions requires close consideration of the nuances in a person's expression, their subjective experience, and its tacit meaning. Still, identifying an emotional state is not the same as understanding the transitions between states.

HOW DOES EMOTION CHANGE?

Emotion and emotional change are often discussed as a seamless collection of processes. Unfortunately, this means there is little discrimination between emotional states as the figurative objects of experience and the operations that bear upon or manipulate those objects of experience. At the risk of using a logic metaphor, here is an example: In the game of chess, each piece on the board (e.g., pawn, rook, bishop) looks different but is also governed according to different patterns of movement (e.g., only moving in straight lines, only on diagonals). Similarly, the types of emotions (i.e., objects) signal what kind of emotional change (i.e., operations) will best apply. In short, one of the most critical issues in working with emotion is this: How emotions change depends very much on the type of presenting emotion (i.e., secondary, primary adaptive, primary maladaptive, or instrumental). Over the course of this book, I will also touch on some aspects of how emotion becomes rigid and dysfunctional, but my central aim is explaining healthy changes: What kinds of productive changes occur? How and under what circumstances are emotional disturbances absorbed?

Labeling the Problem Does Not Explain It

How does emotion change occur? In the epigraph that opened this introduction, Gendlin (1964) describes the process of emotional change as "some kind of emotional digesting" (p. 6). A few decades later, Rachman (1980) defined it as "a process whereby emotional disturbances are absorbed and decline to the extent that other experiences and behavior can proceed without disruption" (p. 51). Another several decades later, Foa and colleagues (2006) offered revisions to their theory of emotional processing, defining it as "modification of the fear structure in which pathological associations among stimuli, responses, and meaning are replaced with nonpathological associations" (p. 6). These each represent seminal papers in the field, yet for about half a century, definitions of emotional change have remained vague, essentially stating that emotional processing is what happens internally when people get better.[5] In clinical forums as much as in empirical research, terms like "emotional processing," "emotion regulation," or "corrective emotional experience" are all used as if they somehow explain what happens. However, these are no more than labels for a puzzle.[6] Beyond recognizing there is some psychological process, how it occurs remains a mystery.

Contradictions Between Theories and Within Research

Complicating matters further, the same generic labels (e.g., emotional processing) are used across the field in reference to processes that are often both conceptually and functionally distinct (e.g., compare Gendlin's account with that of Foa et al.). This has created a mixed assortment of processes all being referred to by the same name. What really is needed is a dimensional approach. Within a given treatment or research specialization, authors of the same feather use terms consistently, but these represent narrow pockets of coherence with little hope for an overarching integration. Taken together, the full body of work on emotional change is rife with theoretical contradictions and mixed empirical findings. This is because few clinical theories have fully taken stock of the fact that qualitatively different kinds of emotional change do exist. The result is that researchers and clinicians of all approaches refer to some form of emotional change without acknowledging the radically different ways in which the same notion is used by others. This has led to problems with the coherence of the field and given mixed messages to therapists working on the front line.

As a sort of ad hoc repair to manage the apparent range of ways emotion may change, some theories are expanded and then applied too broadly, as if all types of change were sufficiently accounted for by an increasingly nebulous construct. Similarly, as outlined in a special issue on the assessment of emotional change (A. Pascual-Leone & Kramer, 2023), some researchers aim to use measures that capture "a bit of everything under the emotional sky" (p. 343). Typically, such measures will be overreaching and conceptually imprecise. Because these omnibus measures are overinclusive, they struggle to adequately delineate between awareness, arousal, reflection, and the down-regulation of emotional intensity. Separating these processes is important because while sometimes they are convergent, at other times they diverge as mechanisms of change. Imprecise measurement of emotional change is often related to a fuzzy conceptualization of the change process itself. Paradoxically, as one construct is elaborated to explain away other perspectives on emotional change, it reaffirms the notion of a unitary construct, a single kind of change rather than a nuanced set of explanations. When it comes to discussing mechanisms of change or offering the kind of concrete clinical implications that therapists can apply to their interventions, we need greater specificity.

ENDNOTES

1. I duly acknowledge the brave and generous contribution of so many clients through their participation in research. Without them, books like this would be impossible. Out of respect for privacy and dignity of individuals, all examples—whether from research or clinical practice—have been anonymized through masking or the modification of identifying variables. Relatedly, any names given for clients are pseudonyms. Furthermore, examples from my own practice are anonymized composites of several cases, are hypothetical, or both.

2. Early clinical writing used the term "emotion structure" to highlight the associative network that makes up an emotion (L. S. Greenberg & Safran, 1987; see also Foa & Kozack, 1986; Rachman, 1980). Then, cognitive and behavioral theory conceptualized "emotion" as an issue of representational meaning. However, "schemes" as introduced by Piaget are psychological units, which are dynamic, self-propelling, and procedural (J. Pascual-Leone & Johnson, 2021).

3. Examples of categorizations of emotion that are convergent are found in treatments like intensive short-term dynamic psychotherapy (Abbass & Town, 2013), accelerated experiential dynamic therapy (Fosha, 2021), and dialectical behavior therapy (Linehan, 2015). A comparative discussion of emotion categorizations is not the purpose here. But throughout the book I do contrast different ways treatments understand how emotion changes.

4. It is critical to appreciate that a discrete emotion (e.g., shame, fear) may appear in several forms: adaptive or maladaptive, primary or secondary. So, although primary maladaptive shame is often observed in therapy, shame itself is not always maladaptive. For example, the feeling that goes with having betrayed one's own values or the trust of a loved one is adaptive shame; it organizes one to shield against the scrutiny of others and avoid a reoffence.

5. Clearly, some ways of engaging emotion make people worse from a health care perspective, exacerbating symptoms. In this book, I focus on the study of productive emotional change. Mechanisms of deterioration are a tangential issue.

6. In this book I refer to the general phenomenon as "emotional change," because it is broader and more impartial to existing treatment theories (as compared with "emotional processing," "emotion regulation," or "restructuring").

1

A General Theory of Emotional Change

Meaning is invisible, but the invisible is not the contradictory of the visible: the visible itself has an invisible inner framework, and the in-visible is the secret counterpart of the visible, it appears only within it.

—MERLEAU-PONTY, *THE VISIBLE AND THE INVISIBLE*

Emotional change happens. But tracing its causal determinants (i.e., how it happens) is a very different matter (Elliott, 2010). The unique effect size of a single process is probably small to medium, with several processes acting at once to generate larger effects (consider Flückiger et al., 2020; A. Pascual-Leone & Yeryomenko, 2016; Sønderland et al., 2023). Many practicing therapists understand emotional change in terms of the interventions they use, but, as this chapter will show, that is a pseudo-explanation for what really happens to the client. Similarly, in everyday life people often explain how they "got over" some event either as the result of behavioral changes, which themselves remain unexplained (e.g., "I just started doing different things"), or through the passage of time (e.g., "It gradually became less important"). Deeply coherent and generalizable explanations of how emotion changes are still lacking.

https://doi.org/10.1037/0000460-002
Principles of Emotion Change: What Works and When in Psychotherapy and Everyday Life, by A. Pascual-Leone
Copyright © 2026 by the American Psychological Association. All rights reserved.

THE PRINCESS AND THE PEA: WHY IS THIS SO HARD TO FIGURE OUT?!

Finding the mechanisms of emotional change is like the test in Hans Christian Andersen's fairy tale, "The Princess and the Pea": A princess is invited to sleep on a pile of 28 mattresses, under which is hidden a tiny but hard pea, and the test is whether she will be able to detect that pea through all the interference. The large effects of psychotherapy on symptom change are not easily traced to a single process, but that process is the pea. The princess (of course) is a psychotherapy researcher, who cannot directly observe the process itself. The many layers of reformulation that occur are each represented by a mattress in the pile, so there are different levels at which the true process of emotional change gets obscured. First, treatment theories are incomplete explanations and make sweeping claims about how they work. Second, the hands-on work of a therapist is full of real-time ambiguity. Third, clients covertly use their own agendas. And finally, but perhaps most importantly, while therapists often choose the interventions in psychotherapy, it is clients who ultimately choose the process that follows. In other words, clients selectively help themselves and even repurpose a treatment's offerings in ways that are not necessarily the treatment as prescribed.

Treatment Theories Are Incomplete Explanations

Treatment theories offer interventions accompanied by the rationale that they facilitate a target process. However, theoretical explanations may be incomplete or even inaccurate, irrespective of whether an intervention works well. As stated in the Introduction, labels are not explanations. However, part of the reason for insufficient explanations is that the lion's share of treatment research has only explored outcome (i.e., does the treatment or intervention work?). So, while we typically know whether something works, we often have only preliminary ideas about how (Kazdin, 2009). Despite what the corresponding theory says, a prescribed intervention may or may not work through the declared process. And there is often a host of undeclared processes that are also relevant since most processes are not mutually exclusive.

Existing theories of emotional change are splintered as a function of their corresponding treatment approaches, which themselves are not collectively well integrated. At the same time, emotional change is not a unitary construct. Reflecting on the current disarray in the field, A. Pascual-Leone and Kramer (2023) likened the collection of local treatment-based theories about emotional change to the parable of an elephant and six blind people. Each person gropes to examine just one part of the large animal (e.g., its side, trunk, tusk, leg, ear, or tail), and they all come to radically different conclusions about what an elephant is. Similarly, such apparent contradictions occur among various treatment-bound theories on emotional change.

Another part of this theory problem is that sometimes emotional change (or emotion regulation) is conflated with the reduced symptom distress that comes with almost all good treatment outcomes (A. Pascual-Leone & Kramer, 2023). When a client has less intense feelings after some intervention, that attenuation in arousal may indeed represent a successful outcome, but there is often much more that has occurred in terms of process, even if unmeasured. Emotional work (i.e., internal process) is not the same as reduced distress (i.e., observed performance outcome). But their conflation is common practice among researchers who pool various ways of working with emotion together under the all-encompassing rubric of "emotion regulation strategies." Relatedly, this remains a major shortcoming in using habituation as an explanation of change (Colwill et al., 2023; see Chapter 3, this volume). In some clinical writing, emotion regulation refers to everything from breathing or putting an ice pack on the back of one's neck to moments of existential meaning making to multistep planning and problem solving. But each of these processes involves dramatically different mechanisms of change on functional, psychological, and neurological levels. The true commonality among them is in their outcome, and that makes emotional regulation something of a heterogeneous catch-all. Insufficient theories of emotion change represent just the first in a series of mattresses hiding our pea.

A Therapist's Work Is Full of Ambiguity

Working real-time in session is a messy business. Most therapists report being integrative or eclectic rather than following any specific treatment approach, which sometimes means a lack of coherent framework for conceptualizing the in-session process. In any case, therapists are concerned about delivering a given treatment, which comes with tacit assumptions and allegiances to treatments or training as well as blind spots about how a classic treatment intervention might be surreptitiously repurposed by clients to some different end.

The Unbridgeable Gap

Practice unfolds faster, is more ambiguous, and is messier than the theoretical accounts of change. Just as there is an existential gap between what a speaker says and what a listener hears, there is a similar layer of inference between an intended treatment process and the process effect it has on a client. A therapist who is well attuned to this gap of ambiguity might pause to ask their client: "By your reaction, it seems like something I just said, or maybe something we were doing, was meaningful to you. Can you say what fit, or what part of this seems important?" If we are candid, most therapists will admit we do not always know what our intervention was, even if it worked.

Fat-Finger and Off-Label Interventions

The spontaneous and real-time nature of working with emotion also lends itself to what one might call "fat-finger interventions." This is a variation of the "fat-finger error," which refers to a clumsy mistake made while typing, where one unwittingly presses the wrong key. Fumbles like these can have meaningful downstream effects (e.g., typos have impacted financial markets). Here, a therapist inadvertently elicits a treatment effect that, even when it is positive, remains unknown to the therapist. When this happens, the therapist's intervention could be facilitating an unintended process, or it might facilitate several processes in parallel, rather than the specific process that was intended. So even when an intervention works, it might work for reasons other than what the therapist believes. Personal accounts of change in therapy (or parenting or mentoring) are full of examples where the helper could have almost no way of anticipating how a comment or gesture might leave a lasting or memorable impact on the client (or child or student).

Therapists also develop their artistry as facilitators of change, and they intentionally develop their own off-label uses of traditional treatment interventions. "Off-label" usually refers to the prescription of medication for a treatment concern other than that for which it was approved. For example, bupropion (i.e., Zyban) was initially developed and prescribed as an antidepressant but was later discovered to also help with smoking cessation, which then became its primary use (Wilkes, 2008). A similar phenomenon happens in psychotherapy. Whether incidental or deliberate, such off-label interventions begin as stylistic elaborations of standard manualized interventions that manifest a therapist's own beliefs, personality, or idiosyncratic theory of change. In the prediction of treatment outcomes, personal innovations of this sort contribute to therapist factors (i.e., this therapist has a special way of doing that intervention). What I refer to as off-label interventions are also a key source of treatment innovation, although at first, they are often used without the clinician really knowing how they work.[1]

Clients Have Their Own Agendas

A good therapist interprets the treatment manual and adjusts it responsively to fit their clients (Stiles, 2009). But clients have and use their own understandings of the change process: They have their own personal theories and renditions of the process. Adherence ratings in clinical trials are meant to ensure therapists are delivering the treatment as prescribed, promising more scientific rigor (Rudge et al., 2020). However, adherence to intervention is several steps upstream from the actual change process. It is no more than a proxy to the treatment being received, which has much more to do with the target process facilitated within a client. That may be a reason why a meta-analysis failed to show that adherence alone was associated with psychotherapy outcomes (N. Power et al., 2022). The *emotion stimulus critique* highlights a similar error in experiments designed to study emotion: the false confidence of using standardized stimuli (e.g., videos, evocative words) when the true target of experimental manipulation should not be the stimulus per se but rather the emotion it was intended to elicit (A. Pascual-Leone, Herpertz, & Kramer, 2016). Even when interventions (or stimuli) are identical, different clients may make use of an intervention toward very different ends. So the real treatment being received is the one that is taken up by the client.

Clients have covert and very utilitarian objectives, even though working with emotion is largely an implicit task. When it comes to a proposed treatment intervention, clients only care about two things: (a) "Does the rationale for engaging this difficult content or task make sense to me?" and (b) "Is this intervention helping me?" From that position, clients then make use of whatever they can to get better. Free of entanglements about theory, a client assumes the role of end user: They take a therapist's intervention and make their own interpretation of what is happening or should happen in treatment. Clients may not choose the intervention, but they do choose the process. Within the boundaries of what a client understands, they have a supreme veto, selecting and endorsing what to make use of and how. They also do this without giving notice to their therapist, who looks in from the outside. Irrespective of a therapist's training, intentions, or actions, the intervention is in the eye of the beholder (i.e., the client). Much of that client problem solving is implicit, a spontaneous exploration of possibilities. So clients usually do not have a clear idea of how a change occurred, having been only partly aware of the process(es).

Psychotherapy Is a Buffet of Processes, Not a Plated Service

I have outlined three reasons why a helpful intervention may be working in ways other than a treatment's declared process, which is part of why explaining emotional change is so elusive. However, even if therapists could faithfully deploy interventions as prescribed and if those interventions consistently prompted client change in precisely the way a treatment theory describes, clients would still make use of other, yet undeclared, aspects of that treatment. Ultimately, the client does not care whether the theory is true or whether their treatment is adherent; they only care about getting better.

A Buffet of Processes

Treatment manuals describe the effect an intervention is designed to deliver, but that specificity starts and ends with a therapist's effort to serve up a given process (see also Wampold & Imel, 2015). So the offerings of psychotherapy cannot be likened to a plated dinner, being served a predetermined meal of specific interventions, because treatments do not (and cannot) circumscribe which processes are available to clients. Psychotherapy is more like offering up a buffet of processes. A variety of interventions are used within an hour-long session, and clients serve themselves from the treatment buffet as they see fit. This means two clients receiving the same manualized treatment but who are drawn to different ends of the buffet could be making use of entirely different sets of processes (i.e., at the same buffet but enjoying different meals). The implication of this for understanding change is substantial, both within a treatment (as just described) but also across treatments. For instance, it puts into question the conventional understanding of what is being tested during a comparative clinical trial (see also Stiles, 2009). While the available buffet spread in Treatment A may (in principle) be distinct from what is served up in

Treatment B, clients in each treatment might be capitalizing on unique portions of (and repurposing) what is being made available to them. So, functionally, the treatment each client uses could turn out to be quite similar at the process level.

We All See the Same Clients

In most cases, clients are treated by whichever qualified therapist is available to them, irrespective of the treatment approach. Generally, this means there is nothing unique about the pool of clients who find themselves in cognitive and behavioral therapies or in a psychodynamic or humanistic treatment. In any case, most therapists take an eclectic or integrative approach. So, for example, just because a cognitive therapist may not make use of transference interpretations, this does not mean that transference never occurs during a client's session (it just means transference goes unaddressed or is not leveraged). Similarly, just because humanistic therapists invite the exploration of emotion and may encourage clients to suspend their judgments, this does not mean clients will not go home to write a list of pros and cons to think more rationally about their situation. The most enduring features of emotional change amount to forms of adult emotional development. In short, all processes of emotional change belong to clients, including processes not prescribed within a given treatment. Still, different treatments typically leverage one or another kind of change, and that marks some fundamental differences between them. However, processes described in one treatment's theory will also happen in other treatments. Clients have no treatment allegiances and are the ultimate integrationists, using any and all processes that may occur to them as potentially helpful.

Emotion Change Is a Covert Process

I have described a few issues in the tall stack of mattresses that obscure the various ways in which emotion changes. These are some of the reasons why understanding emotional change can be so difficult. Like detecting a pea hidden under a pile of mattresses, uncovering the true nature of an emotional change requires one to see through many levels and transmutations. This calls for a general theory that reaches across treatment perspectives and can coordinate them, a theory that describes the invisible inner framework mentioned in the epigraph to this chapter.

UNTANGLING THE MECHANISMS OF EMOTIONAL CHANGE

The notion that there may be separate principles of emotion change was first advocated from an integrative perspective by Les Greenberg, York University, as a deep intuition about psychotherapy process (e.g., A. Pascual-Leone & Greenberg, 2006). At the same time, the number of principles being proposed shifted somewhat over papers probably because this clinical insight still needed development and empirical scrutiny through a large comprehensive review.

A General Theory That Matters for Therapists

Making distinctions between different kinds of emotional processing is not just an academic or purely theoretical issue; it matters to therapists. For those who take a highly mechanistic (or medical) approach, one basic implication is that the clinician probably does not have as much direct influence as presumed. More importantly, conflating different kinds of emotional processes often hides the very problem that stumps therapists when they are trying to understand why a client has trouble moving forward. A systematic review and meta-analysis demonstrated the general positive effect of a therapist's competence as a predictor of outcome in adult psychotherapy (Power et al., 2022). The challenge of competently working with emotion, however, is the inherent vagueness and slippery nature of how emotion changes. Improving therapists' competence when working with emotion will thus require them to have more clarity about what kinds of emotional change are needed and when. Put simply, therapists who understand what is happening in the moment will have a clearer sense of what they need to do next.

Toward a Causal Theory of Change

Bringing out the invisible order in a person's highly subjective process, one that is only partly within their awareness, is daunting. The silos of existing treatment-based research have limited the development of general and integrative theory. This calls for a new strategy to understand emotional changes as they occur in psychotherapy and in life.

Converging Lines of Evidence

To identify the unique nature of different kinds of emotional change, I conducted a very large review. To ensure the identified kinds of emotional change were robustly supported and to retain parsimony, I made use of six separate kinds of evidence. When available, these lines of evidence were searched for convergences. The objective was to develop a framework of understanding in which there are separate kinds of productive emotional change that cut across approaches to practice and have their own functional implications for facilitating change. This discovery-oriented inquiry used a method of constant comparison as processes were continually defined alongside one another until the synthesis of theory reached saturation.

Operationally, this means almost all the chapters in this book were written in parallel to one another as emerging ideas, rather than in a traditional linear fashion. Chapters were revised, merged, disintegrated, and reordered in a dynamic process to best represent the emergence of a coherent and overarching framework. This project started in 2013 and took approximately 12 years. The six lines of evidence considered in the inquiry were as follows:

- *Phenomenological evidence.* When someone struggles to change how they feel, they usually have a sense of working at something. An important starting point for this review was simply to consider the subjective phenomenon of people implicitly working with emotion in one way or another. Although one often is not fully aware of the immediate process goal engaged in, each kind of effort comes with a qualitatively distinct subjective experience as one works to complete it. For example, finding the right words is a different subjective effort from allowing an intense bodily feeling or piecing together a feeling with one's life narrative. These subjective experiences of working with emotion are phenomenologically distinct for an individual, and that helped initially circumscribe each process.

- *Measurement.* Identifying tools that measure each form of emotional change was important to show that constructs could be concretely and reliably operationalized. Furthermore, when different measures existed for each change process, this offered partial support for the understanding that the processes were unique in nature.

- *Psychotherapy and change process research.* Each kind of emotional change had to have been identified as an observable process that predicted subsequent outcomes in health care or well-being. When available, I looked for longitudinal studies that illustrated how the process anticipated and mediated positive outcomes.

- *Basic research in psychology.* The separate processes of change should be supported within other fields of psychology (e.g., cognitive, developmental, social, personality). First, empirical evidence showing that each change process was relevant outside the clinical setting was important for establishing them as general constructs. Second, convergent theories from other areas of psychology supported coherent narratives about how relevant processes unfolded. This offered a level of analysis that was often more fundamental than what could be observed during clinical work.

- *Neurological correlates.* Functional brain imaging also offered relevant evidence in two ways. First, when the psychological accounts of emotional change were supported by neurological evidence, it helped verify them as fundamental processes. Second, when different change processes could be localized by separate (albeit interrelated) neural systems, it was further evidence that they were each quite different in nature.

- *Clinical interventions.* The existence of distinct clinical interventions to facilitate each process of emotional change verified their functional difference, particularly when those clinical interventions could be identified across treatment approaches. This line of evidence was critical in generating practical implications. If distinct processes were purposefully and reliably facilitated by the same intervention, then their differentiation (e.g., based on face value) would have little practical relevance in treatment or everyday life.

All six lines of evidence were initially explored for empirical support in what became an emerging theory or framework of understanding (i.e., the principles of emotion change).

A Review That Prioritizes Implications for Practice

While the initial search was broader, in this book I concentrate on presenting those findings with implications for practice. In other words, the aim was not to exhaustively review and present all evidence from each domain of inquiry.[2] Furthermore, I typically integrate the various lines of evidence together so as to complement one another rather than retaining domain-specific silos of evidence. I prioritized findings from applied research and clinical practice (e.g., psychotherapy, change processes, mechanisms of intervention) over those from basic research (e.g., affect, cognition, mental development) but used both. To be fair, this imbalance largely reflects the amount of available evidence about facilitating healthy change. Basic research predominantly examines the nature of emotion states rather than parameters in how those states might transition, the latter being more aligned with practical concerns about emotional change and well-being. My enduring effort is to formulate an integrated understanding that might guide people who want to change how they feel and the therapists who are looking to help.

Finally, in using these six lines of evidence to consider a range of possible mechanisms for emotional change, scientific parsimony was a critical principle. I sought to identify the minimum number of processes that could be used to explain the observed variety of emotional changes. Adding more hypothesized change processes to the list was often possible (clinical theory has no shortage of hypothetical constructs!), but expanding that list was a matter of incremental validity. If adding to the list of potential processes did not sufficiently expand both functional and clinical implications, I retained the minimum number of change principles.

The Question of Causality

Determining causality requires many steps and is rarely unequivocal, particularly when there are multiple causes that interact and in research areas where designing true experiments is challenging for practical as well as ethical reasons (Kazdin, 2009). Even so, conclusions about causality are essentially appraisals of the available evidence. For instance, a positive association between the hypothesized cause and effect is one small piece of evidence, their temporal order is another, the plausibility of the explanation is a third, and so forth— each incrementally building evidence for causality. So exploring both the strength of evidence as well as the convergence of different sorts of findings was important in building toward a causal model. This book offers a working model. It is not a conclusive explanation of how working with emotion causes personal change; that would be wildly premature for this field. Still, it brings together an array of arguments exploring and sometimes speculating on hypotheses about how emotion changes.

At the same time, discussions on emotion and the processes by which they change could range in their level of analysis from the superficial descriptions of manifest interventions to expounding on neurocognitive operations that support mentation at large. I aimed to describe mechanisms of emotional change at an intermediate level of analysis, organizing and coordinating the piecemeal collection of relevant theories. I focused squarely on clinical utility and where readers might recognize their own human experience in the processes being described.

For clinicians, this means tangible implications for working with client emotion. There are three central objectives in this book. The first is to clarify the functional differences between kinds of change, which is to map out a general and integrative theory. The second objective is to identify the unique markers of each kind of change process (i.e., the observable features that signal a change process is needed or achievable). The notion of markers is a critical issue for practice because it clarifies what to do when. Finally, I map out the available evidence for how those different kinds of processes are facilitated in various treatment perspectives. For researchers, I use this general theory to resolve contradictions in empirical literature, identify questions for future research, and suggest specific hypotheses about mechanisms and moderators that should be examined.

FIVE PRINCIPLES OF EMOTION CHANGE: AN OVERVIEW

Rather than examine different therapies as such or give instruction on how to conduct specific interventions, this book identifies functional invariants across treatment approaches. In other words, there are certain common factors with respect to the mechanisms of emotional change that cut across various approaches to therapy, despite how treatments may appear from the outside. The reason why there are invariants in processing has less to do with similarities among actual treatment and more to do with the commonalities across the clients that therapists are treating and the fundamental principles of working with human emotion. Just as classical (i.e., cognitive) problem solving is supported by general mental operations (see J. Pascual-Leone & Johnson, 2021), working with emotion represents an analogous kind of (implicit) emotional problem solving. And it too involves distinct functional operations by which emotion may change. Completing my review, I propose five major mechanisms of emotional change. The rest of this book explores the evidence for those processes.

Part I: Reduce Intensity

Down-regulating the intensity of emotional arousal (e.g., "The feeling is going away, subsiding") is the first process that I address. "Emotion regulation" is a construct applied so broadly in the literature as to be problematic, so I use Chapter 2 as an opportunity to extend this introduction by addressing those difficulties and proposing a more circumscribed definition of the process. Reducing the intensity of a feeling will be a familiar objective for many individuals when confronted with emotion (i.e., "feel less!," "turn it off!"). In Chapter 3, I explore the topic only enough to identify it as a unique way of working with emotion. The notions of habituating and learning to cope in ways that reduce distress will be change processes that are well-known to most readers, at least in general terms. Down-regulating emotion has already been discussed extensively in the literature with entire books dedicated to it. For that reason, my treatment of this topic is much briefer than other parts of the book.

Part II: Notice the Feeling

Increasing emotional awareness and engagement (e.g., "I can feel it in my body and I'm searching for the right words") is fully addressed over four chapters. Chapter 4 introduces becoming aware of the feeling as a distinct way of changing an emotional experience: defining the general process, identifying markers, and noting potential obstacles to this kind of work. Chapters 5–7 explore various aspects of this change process, explaining mechanisms of change in order of increasing complexity, starting with emotional engagement, awareness, labeling the feeling, and then ending with complex symbolizations.

Part III: Feel More, Express More

Facilitating arousal, expression, and enactments (e.g., "The feeling is in my gut, it makes me want to act, it's becoming more intense and louder!") represents another cluster of ways for productively working with emotion, addressed over five chapters. Chapter 8 introduces this as a change process, defining it, identifying markers, and acknowledging the mixed empirical findings. It then continues to address the complexity of increasing expressive arousal by identifying the contingencies that govern whether, and under what circumstances, this process is productive. Chapters 9–11 propose related mechanisms of change with increasing complexity, starting with the influence of general arousal, expressing emotion, the role of vividness, performing complex enactments, and finally with making proclamations of the self.

Part IV: Order the Sequence of Emotions

Sequential ordering of discrete emotions (e.g., "Self-compassion is the antidote to my shame, it has an undoing effect") can be used to generate categorically new emotional experiences, and it is explored over five chapters. Chapter 12 introduces this process as a unique form of emotional change, defining it and articulating the markers for when it is most useful. This kind of change is a relatively new development in theories of emotional processing. It is also inherently more complex than the processes already mentioned because it involves multiple steps that often subsume awareness and expression to some degree. Even so, as Chapter 13 illustrates, specific patterns of emotion will produce emotional transformations that are not sufficiently explained by a collection of less complex processes (i.e., awareness and expression). Chapters 14–16 elaborate how these sorts of sequential transformations unfold over various time-frames: during individual sessions, over the course of treatment, and as part of adult emotional development.

Part V: Put the Feeling in Context

Narrative framing and reflecting on emotion (e.g., "When I think of my life's purpose, my suffering today feels less upsetting") is the fifth and final kind of emotional change identified in this book. This change process is elaborated over seven chapters, addressing how it occurs in several forms and through contrasting clinical approaches. By way of introduction, Chapter 17 explains that a central axis in this way of working with emotion is the recontextualization of a feeling, which then changes its significance and meaning. The chapter also identifies markers and highlights key problematic narratives styles. Then, Chapters 18–21 propose different mechanisms of change related to narrative reflection: narrative elaboration, psychological distancing, reframing, and developing identity narratives.

As the book approaches its conclusion, Chapter 22 offers a comparative analysis of emotional awareness and personal reflection as complementary processes. Then, Chapter 23 highlights the function of existential choice. Finally, Chapter 24 gives a summary of findings and closing remarks about the future of psychotherapy.

OTHER IMPORTANT CONSIDERATIONS

Syntheses like this are always open to the criticism of not being exhaustive enough. Some readers will ask: Why only five principles? What about process *x* or *y*? While alternative groupings of emotion change are certainly conceivable, they are typically stated ad hoc without the backing of a broad and integrated review across different approaches and considering multiple lines of evidence. The science of emotion change needs to move beyond the various grab bags of pet constructs that are familiar or idiosyncratically preferred by a given group of clinicians or researchers. However, the five processes I articulate are supported by a robust conceptual differentiation at several levels of analysis and each comes with a unique set of practical implications. In more than one case, I group a set of well-known processes under a single general principle (e.g., arousal and expression, see Part III; reframing and existential choice, see Part V). Further differentiation is always conceivable depending on the discourse, but my aim was to identify a minimum number of overarching principles of change. For several additions that might be proposed, there was no evidence of distinct neurological correlates, which casts doubt on whether they are fundamentally unique and suggests they are better understood as alternative manifestations of a single overarching principle. For other possible additions, the corresponding interventions were not functionally different, so they offered few or no new implications for practice. Working with emotion in real time also demands such a list be manageable as a heuristic for the end users, so parsimony was essential to maximize clinical utility.

The Role of the Relationship

While one might debate the inclusion or exclusion of one or another process, one special exception to this is the role of the relationship. A soft division has been made between mechanisms that are interpersonal (i.e., changes in human relationships between a client and others in their lives, including the therapist) and mechanisms that are intrapersonal (i.e., working with the meaning of a client's own feelings, thoughts, and behaviors—as an information processing system). Even so, it seems impossible to fully extricate the processes of working with emotion from the influence of a warm and empathically attuned "other." Even when an individual is quite alone and productively works with emotion using these principles, the person is never cut off from a developmental history where feeling emotion has been anchored in some relational context. Yet the relational process that occurs between people is still different from the emotional digestion that occurs intrapsychically within the experiencer. A meta-analytic summary shows that the therapeutic alliance has an independent effect in the prediction of outcomes, even after adjusting for other change processes (Flückiger et al., 2020). By the same token, studies on the processes of emotional change routinely control for the role of the relationship (e.g., Auszra et al., 2013; Høglend et al., 2011; Pos et al., 2003). These are complementary and often interacting but not reducible to one another.

Interpersonal and information processing perspectives are not in opposition to one another; they represent distinct frames of references to the phenomenon of therapeutic change and personal growth. A clinician's preferred theoretical position reveals their deeper perspective on the world, but these are not contrary; they are simply relative perspectives. Contrasting one with the other is like thinking about how the earth moves around the sun or switching one's home perspective to consider that, in relative terms, the sun could also be moving around the earth.[3] In this book I focus on a person's intrapsychic process, which is where the effect must ultimately be registered for personal change to occur. This does not contest the idea that a warm and responsive relationship may sometimes also be the most efficient way of facilitating any of the five intrapsychic processes. When a relationship event is helpful in these five ways, then that represents a certain set of corrective (interpersonal) emotional experiences (see Alexander & French, 1946).[4]

Coordination, Overdetermination, and Synergy

Synergies are common, although processes are not always compatible with one another, which requires them to be uniquely represented. There are some examples of processes that work directly in opposition to one another, which explains certain contradictions between treatment-bound theories. An example of this is the down-regulation of emotion versus increasing its expressive arousal; both are helpful ways of working with emotion, yet they are logical opposites that could function at cross-purpose to one another, if one did not have a clear idea of their different targets. Another example is meaning making (e.g., through awareness and narrative identity) versus habituation or inhibition (i.e., forms of down-regulation). Hypothesized causal processes such as these are antithetical within a single intervention moment, but they are not mutually exclusive over the course of ongoing personal change. Therefore, their coordination is critical and offers a higher order explanation (e.g., see A. Pascual-Leone, Yeryomenko, et al., 2016). As I maintain throughout this book, theories of individual therapies are much narrower than what is truly happening in session. In practice, various processes described in this book likely all occur to some degree, and they each help clients change, even if they are not well recognized within a treatment's theory.

When different processes are compatible, they often overdetermine the emotional change that follows. *Overdetermination* is when a single observed effect is simultaneously produced by multiple causes, when each cause alone would have been sufficient to generate the effect (Freud, 1926; J. Pascual-Leone & Johnson, 2021). Another issue is the change processes that co-occur may act synergistically, interacting with one another to produce a combined effect, greater than the sum of each process taken separately (J. Pascual-Leone & Johnson, 2021).

Most of the ways emotion changes are tacit, often partly elicited outside awareness, but also through some deliberate efforts on the part of the individual. This combination of several kinds of processes may be declared or undeclared by a prescribed theory. A process is sometimes purposefully attended to although, at other times, cued automatically. Also, various processes may dynamically converge to interact in a single moment. Nevertheless, it is not a single event but rather the repetition of collective experiences over time that builds toward final and enduring personal change (Lane & Nadel, 2020). Still, treatment-based explanations of emotional change are fragmented, largely because there are different ways a given emotional experience might be productively worked with. This book explores the operators of emotional change and how they are best applied to problematic emotional states. It offers an integrated understanding of what emotional change really is, how it happens, and when to promote what.

ENDNOTES

1. Of course, sometimes those personal innovations are then formally developed and disseminated, which contributes to the evolution of treatment techniques. Creative applications of exposure, or of chairwork, are good examples of this, particularly when they turn out to be facilitating different processes from the original intervention.
2. An exhaustive review would be a prohibitively large endeavor, given the current contribution already cites a curated selection of close to 850 references.
3. I am grateful to Dr. Ken Critchfield, Yeshiva University, for this formulation about the relative perspectives.
4. I indicate this is "a certain set" of corrective emotional experiences because the full scope of helpful interpersonal and relational experiences reaches beyond the question of emotional change. Interpersonal relationships are also related to additional kinds of change processes that are not covered in this book.

REDUCE INTENSITY

INTRODUCTION: REDUCE INTENSITY

The reduction of symptom distress is an objective shared by all psychological treatments. However, how reducing emotional distress in the short term parlays into the distal treatment gains of reduced symptoms is often not as straightforward as it may seem. I begin Chapter 2 by exploring the notion of *emotion regulation*, which is a general term often used as a unifying umbrella to capture a variegated range of processes. Unpacking the proposed mechanisms of mindfulness helps illustrate how broad processes like these are overdetermined by a collection of more specific mechanisms. Relatedly, the operational definition of emotion regulation poses a challenge because although researchers and theorists formally define it quite broadly, the intervention objectives in clinical practice often turn out to be much narrower. One process that is well-represented under this umbrella term is the down-regulation of emotional intensity, which refers to directly reducing emotional arousal within a given moment. Down-regulation is the first principle of emotion change explored in this book and is depicted in Figure I.1 as a change in the quantity or amount of emotion that is being experienced.

Trait-like characteristics, such as a person having a low level of distress tolerance, point to one's baseline vulnerability to emotion dysregulation and the possibility of feeling overwhelmed. Both lifestyle factors and automatizing healthy emotion habits can preventively reduce one's reactivity and bolster emotional resilience (see Chapter 3). However, particularly in a moment of

FIGURE I.1. Reduce Intensity: The Principle of Down-Regulation

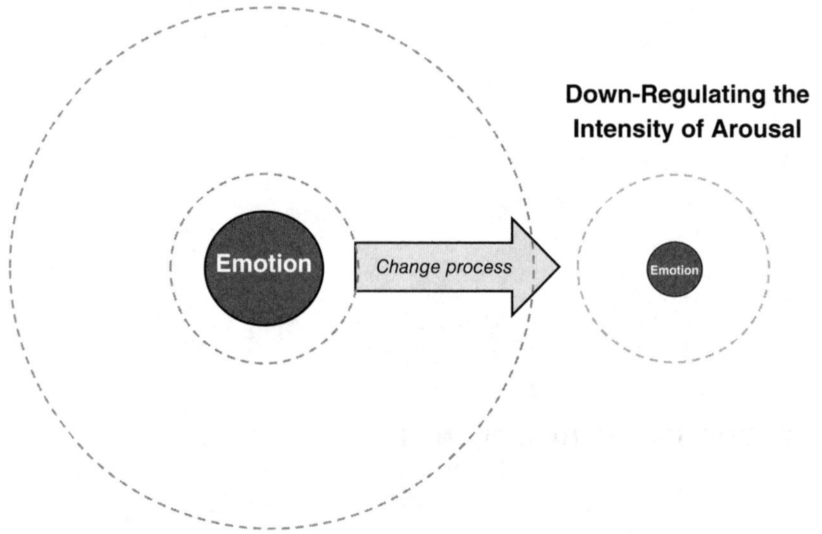

Emotion

Change process

Down-Regulating the Intensity of Arousal

Emotion

Note. Down-regulating emotion is a principle that involves reducing the amount of intensity. The process is depicted here as a feeling quantitatively shrinking in size. This is one of five categorically different processes that change emotion.

crisis, dialing back emotional arousal that has already become too intense is an essential process for returning to a safer, tolerable, and more functional range. Chapter 3 identifies key processes that facilitate the down-regulation of emotion: adaptive avoidance, desensitization, and the use of behavioral coping. These three pathways of action directly attenuate the amount of feeling one experiences in the moment.

Processes for reducing arousal have also been discussed extensively in the literature, and for that reason my treatment of this topic is briefer than for other parts of the book. That stated, most of the different processes discussed in this book pertain directly to what is sometimes included in the notion of emotion regulation at large.

2

Down-Regulating Emotional Intensity

All you need is love. But a little chocolate now and then doesn't hurt.
—CHARLES M. SCHULZ, *PEANUTS EVERY SUNDAY, VOL. 5: 1971–1975*

Sometimes people just need to feel less and reduce the intensity of their emotion. Although emotion can be a vital source of information that supports healthy functioning, there are still times—at moments of crisis, desperation, or when one simply needs a bit of reprieve—that attenuating arousal is the best way of working with emotion. At the right time and place, down-regulating emotion is an invaluable process. Yet working with emotion across situations demands more complexity than a single process. This has led to some awkward extensions and reworking of the often-cited construct "emotion regulation." At present, the term is used to refer to a seemingly inexhaustible list of processes. In this chapter, I discuss definitional challenges to understanding and using emotion regulation as a construct, then I move on to focus more narrowly on the down-regulation of emotion, which I argue is the primary emphasis in strategies for emotion regulation.

WHAT DOES EMOTION REGULATION MEAN?

Psychological theorists and researchers have come to use the term "emotion regulation" in a manner that encompasses all of the following: avoidance, distraction, habituation, behavioral activation, mindfulness, affect labeling, rumination, emotional expression, meaning making, decentering, cognitive reappraisal,

https://doi.org/10.1037/0000460-003
Principles of Emotion Change: What Works and When in Psychotherapy and Everyday Life, by A. Pascual-Leone
Copyright © 2026 by the American Psychological Association. All rights reserved.

problem solving, acceptance, self-compassion, focusing on values, and seeking social support, among other processes (Daros et al., 2021; Gross, 2015; Linehan, 2015; Muran, Teachman, et al., 2024; Renna et al., 2017). This is quite different from what regulation means in everyday usage. A more typical understanding of the term, as might be found in a dictionary, defines *regulation* as simply when some specified function is being moderated or controlled in some way, not that the function itself changes. For example, the accelerator pedal of a car up-regulates its speed, while the brake pedal down-regulates speed. Or, similarly, the dial on a stereo regulates the volume to either increase or decrease—but moderating the volume will not categorically change the content of a melody that is playing! When people successfully label an emotion, actively work through some personal problem, or generate new meaning, all these ways of working with emotion have been referred to as forms of emotion regulation. However, such processes transform the affective experience *itself*, far beyond the original function of presenting distress. They do not just change the intensity (i.e., volume); they actually change the content of experience (i.e., melody). Referring to those kinds of changes as regulation is a distortion of how the term is used in most other contexts and has led psychologists to discuss virtually any kind of emotional change (i.e., quantitative or qualitative) as emotion regulation.

Emotion Regulation Is a Catch-All Term

James Gross, a psychologist at Stanford University, spearheaded the field of emotion regulation but candidly observed that "enthusiasm for this topic continues to outstrip conceptual clarity, and there remains considerable uncertainty as to what is even meant by 'emotion regulation'" (Gross, 2015, p. 1). Another example of this line of concern comes from the American Psychological Association (APA) Advisory Steering Committee for Development of Clinical Practice Guidelines. The committee recently charged a group of clinical researchers to investigate the feasibility of developing interventions guidelines to address "emotion regulation" as a transdiagnostic change process. This new interest in emotion processes marks an important advancement from previous APA practice guidelines, which focused exclusively on the treatment of circumscribed disorders (Muran, Teachman, et al., 2024). However, the first significant challenge identified by the group was in defining the construct because, as they report, there is so much

> variability in how emotion regulation is conceptualized across non-clinical domains within psychology (e.g., affective science, neuroscience, social and developmental psychology) and even within different clinical traditions (e.g., psychoanalytic/dynamic, cognitive-behavioral, emotion focused). These conceptual distinctions are critical because they have implications for how . . . change . . . should be defined and measured. (p. 17)

Perhaps pragmatism takes the day, should one want to create very general clinical guidelines. A clear definition might not matter if the goal is simply to list interventions for working with emotion. For example, emotion regulation therapy is a treatment developed from the observation that depression and generalized anxiety (sometimes referred together as "distress disorders") are highly comorbid and have common temperamental features that entail underlying difficulties in managing emotion. The treatment is heavily informed by cognitive and behavioral interventions and, to a lesser extent, also borrows from experiential schools. It aims to target mechanisms of emotional change through exposure-based interventions, regulation skills training, and awareness skills (Renna et al., 2017). Development of this integrative approach to treating a transdiagnostic set of change processes should be applauded and is in line with the APA's initiative to develop practice guidelines to address emotion regulation at large (Muran et al., 2024). However, in this case, every intervention (no matter how different) is considered some form of emotion regulation, hence the treatment's name. And the aim of this transdiagnostic treatment is (again) emotion regulation, whether the nature of change be to the intensity of an experience (i.e., volume) or switching out the content of that experience (i.e., melody).

The amorphous nature of what gets referred to as emotion regulation sometimes borders on tautological. But, more importantly, the hazard is that an overly broad definition preempts a more sophisticated understanding of the various kinds of change that occur and how their respective mechanisms may be categorically distinct (consider, e.g., affect labeling, desensitization, meaning making, narrative framing). In short, the same term (emotion regulation) is used to refer to a very heterogeneous collection of mechanisms. The obfuscation makes both treatment interventions and training in them less precise than they should be. Whatever the case, the reason for this catch-all approach to theorizing about emotional change is ultimately related to a reductionistic understanding of emotion as an undifferentiated morass of affective experience. When discussing emotional changes, the term "emotion regulation" is often a misnomer. The term strongly favors a behavioral framework, in which emotion is understood to be symptomatic and typically something to be attenuated. The original root of that position can be traced back to a Cartesian split between mind and body, in which rational process merit scrutiny but the passions are an animal vestige that simply needs to be managed if not suppressed. Terms like "exposure" and "habituation" are similarly used in behavioral frameworks for what is often a much more complex suite of processes (see Chapter 3).

Gross (2015) presents a model of how emotion changes whereby emotion is generated through a relatively linear process. An important merit of the model is that it attempts to separate discrete process steps that are ordered in time (i.e., situation-attention-appraisal-response sequence). However, in doing so it also resembles an assembly-line production of how emotion happens rather than the organic, nonlinear, highly overdetermined, and dynamic process of construction that renders emergent experience. Furthermore, from this reductionist perspective, any change process that eventually results in a treatment outcome of reduced distress is subsequently conceptualized as having been successful "emotion regulation."

Conflating Process With Outcome

In Chapter 1, I identified a ubiquitous error in which much theory and research on "emotion regulation" conflates the process of emotional change with its manifest outcome. This critique applies in varying degrees to the treatment of specific processes such as habituation (see Colwill et al., 2023; Chapter 3) as well as broader formulations about emotion regulation (e.g., Gross, 2015). Consider the case of reappraisal, which is often referred to as a cognitive strategy for emotion regulation. Explanations of this process typically posit that the person calms down because they are able to think about their problem differently. Considered more carefully, calming down is the intervention's outcome, while thinking differently is the process by which that happened. Indeed, reappraisal (as a process) has to do with adding new and different contextual information that is the means for achieving an end (see Chapter 20). Other interventions help more directly with reducing painful emotion. For example, when someone feels overwhelmed and then decides to put some soft music on, take a hot bath, or do diaphragmatic breathing, it often calms them down (i.e., the positive effect, or event outcome). These soothing interventions aim to directly reduce physio-affective and sensory arousal (i.e., the process), which leads manifestly to a state of reduced emotional arousal (i.e., event outcome).

Both reframing and behavioral soothing help one calm down (event outcome), so both get cast under the very wide umbrella of emotion regulation. During reappraisal, however, the process of change involves introducing new information. Changing that content and the framework of one's experience impacts one's level of arousal. Indeed, reframing works because the emotion subsequently means something different. So the mechanism of cognitive reframing is to add a new or revised context of meaning to a presenting emotion (i.e., changing the framework but not directly working with the feeling per se). Still, researchers and clinicians looking to help clients calm down rarely make additional inquiries about whether the intervention added a new sense of meaning or if it helped the client better understand their experience—even though, presumably, it was some new meaning (as a process) that precipitated any reduction in arousal (the event outcome; see Chapter 20). By extension, consider an existential reframing that helps someone focus squarely on their purpose in life (see Chapter 23). People will endure great amounts of suffering simply by focusing on a higher purpose (e.g., my client who hated cleaning public toilets but did it anyway, happily knowing the extra money was for her children's education). Here the negative emotion per se was not substantially reduced (e.g., the client assured me her disgust was still there!), but those instances of negative emotion were simply given less importance as the client set her gaze on a further horizon of higher virtue.

In contrast, behavioral soothing does not change the meaning of one's emotional experience. Here, the metaphorical song remains the same, but the intervention works by turning down the volume on that same affective experience. The outcomes may be similar, but the underlying processes are qualitatively distinct.[1] Some interventions facilitate processes that are immediately, directly, and transparently related to reducing affective intensity, while others facilitate processes that are qualitatively different in nature, even if they produce functionally equivalent outcomes. This conflation of means (process) with ends (event outcomes) has significantly muddied the clinical literature on emotion regulation.

The Time Frame Is Open-Ended

Good theories about mechanisms of change demand an account of the sequential order of events that lead up to a change, as proposed in Gross's (2015) model. This is particularly true when measuring therapeutic processes and outcomes at various stages. Immediate processes and their positive within-session effects (event outcomes) contribute to the causal chain that leads to long-term symptom outcomes. However, the time frame of an immediate process and its positive effect, or event outcome (now, both serving as means), versus long-term symptom outcomes (the final ends) needs to be considered. Otherwise, anything that occurs in a successful treatment ultimately gets construed as managing and reducing emotional distress.

At the conclusion of any effective treatment, of course, people have fewer symptoms and less distress. However, the implicit argument that commonly follows is that these symptom changes are just the linear accumulation of smaller efforts at managing and controlling emotion. Symptom changes are thus presumed to mirror (and are attributed to) what were within-session event outcomes (i.e., emotion regulation). This makes sense in a learning model, whereby one understands the within-session events as a scalable change that progresses until mastery (final symptom outcome). An example of this might be when using systematic exposure to treat agoraphobia. However, the formulation overlooks other pathways to change. Paradoxically, in this framework, even increasing the intensity of one's arousal and meaning-laden emotional expressions come to be understood as a mysterious form of indirect emotion regulation. So, in some roundabout argument, heightening and expressing emotion is said to help reduce and manage arousal.

Careful considerations of the mechanism implied here are often perplexing and sometimes allude to outdated notion of catharsis (see Chapter 8). Whatever the case, in practice this is an unwieldy attempt to corral a grab bag of assorted interventions under a unifying umbrella. Lumping together dissimilar constructs under a single banner offers a quick fix for the conundrums of many research findings on working with emotion, but it creates gaping contradictions across the scientific literature. This stifles the advancement of more nuanced and diversified theories on how emotion changes.

It Is Not Just About Down-Regulation. . . . Or Is It?

Proponents of emotion regulation as a conceptual framework argue that this construct is not only about down-regulating emotion and claim that it may involve all the processes discussed in this book. Of course, in principle that is true, and emotion regulation therapy (discussed earlier) is a good case in point (Renna et al., 2017). Still, because of emotion regulation therapy's behavioral roots, reducing reactivity, inhibitory learning, and distancing oneself from emotional experience loom large as central efforts in this type of therapy. We see something similar in how dialectical behavior therapy (DBT) addresses emotion regulation (Linehan, 2015). These, and other treatments that focus on emotion regulation, typically include a range of different ways for working with emotion, but then a subtle contradiction emerges between theory and practice (i.e., the construct as formally defined vs. what clinicians are trying to do). This contradiction is borne out in the objective or intended goal of how interventions are construed and then applied.

In discussions about theories of emotion regulation (e.g., Gross, 2015), the process is defined to include both up-regulation (i.e., increasing, promoting, and elaborating emotional experience) and down-regulation (i.e., reducing, calming, and decreasing the intensity of feelings). In contrast, the emphasis in clinical practice is consistently much narrower in focus, where down-regulation and reducing the intensity of a client's feelings is often the only objective. As a case in point, cognitive reframing is typically used to curtail arousal and bring an end to an experience; it is almost never to heighten emotion.[2] Again, in the final report of the APA's working group for developing practice guidelines, emotion regulation was defined in the broadest possible terms (Muran et al., 2024). However, when it came to providing examples of the process, most illustrations described concrete instances of down-regulating emotion: for example, "such as when one actively restrains an impulse"; "such as when one shifts one's gaze away . . . to reduce arousal" or "such as when a parent seeks to calm an upset child" (p. 17). In short, perhaps the construct of emotion regulation could refer to a plurality of processing objectives, but in practice, that is rarely if ever the case.

Published research shows a similar incongruence. Researchers sometimes assert that a given process facilitates emotion regulation, which is only to say that it changes emotion. But in what way does it change—increasing or decreasing emotion, or perhaps something else? What was meant becomes clearer when the research design makes use of, for example, affect intensity ratings, revealing that the author presumed to refer more narrowly to how a reduction in emotional arousal was facilitated. So another way of understanding what emotion regulation typically means is to consider how it is measured, which offers an operational definition. The Degrees of Emotion Regulation Scale (DERS; Gratz & Roemer, 2004) is a self-report measure to assess common problems that interfere with a person's ability to regulate emotion. It has become the most widely used measure of emotion dysregulation, cited close to 5,000 times and translated into several languages. Such popularity highlights that researchers and clinicians recognize problems with emotion as a key area of interest. A meta-analysis of studies on individual therapy, for example, showed that change on the DERS has a medium to large effect in the prediction of subsequent symptom reduction for clients who presented with various anxiety disorders (Sønderland et al., 2023). Presumably this reflects some change mechanism (or a collection thereof) because it measures change as it seems to have been observed outside the treatment sessions.

However, the DERS seems not to capture as broad a conceptualization of emotion regulation as was initially intended. Firstly, while the DERS has six subscales (Gratz & Roemer, 2004), four of them measure the degree to which people can control and manage emotional distress, usually in cognitive or behavioral terms. These are (a) unwillingness to accept an emotion (e.g., "When I'm upset, I become angry at myself for feeling that way"), (b) difficulties with impulse control (e.g., "When I'm upset, I become out of control"), (c) limited strategies for feeling better (e.g., "When I'm upset, I believe there is nothing I can do to feel better"), and (d) difficulty using goal-directed cognition and behavior when distressed (e.g., "When I'm upset, I have difficulty getting work done").

Secondly, a person's ability to simply tolerate or endure distress seems central here (as opposed to working with it, making meaning, or qualitatively changing it in ways that may not modulate intensity at all). This observation is consistent with a finding that various short versions of the DERS are highly correlated with measures of poor distress tolerance (Burton et al., 2022; also discussed later in this chapter). Furthermore, that overarching theme is consistent with the finding that there is a general underlying factor in the DERS (in addition to specific factors; Hallion et al., 2018).

The other two DERS subscales (Gratz & Roemer, 2004) are (e) having a lack of emotional clarity (e.g., "I am confused about how I feel") and (f) emotional awareness (e.g., "I am attentive to my feelings"). But this relates to a third issue, suggesting that the DERS is not as comprehensive a measure as one might have hoped. Across several clinical and nonclinical samples, psychometric properties of the DERS were stronger when the Awareness subscale was omitted (e.g., Burton et al., 2022; Hallion et al., 2018). As Hallion and colleagues explain,

> the consistency of these findings, both in the present study and in the extant literature, leads us to conclude that the DERS as a whole is psychometrically stronger when the Awareness subscale is excluded. . . . Whereas the other DERS subscales aim to assess how an individual *reacts* to emotions . . . emotional awareness . . . does not appear to be the same construct (2018, pp. 7–9; emphasis in original).

In Chapter 5, I suggest such a finding is likely because emotional awareness can lead to either intensifying or reducing affect, depending on how that process was presented and engaged.[3] In any case, it turns out that the DERS may essentially be a measure of "When you get upset, how good are you at calming down?" Even so, developing a more precise measure for down-regulation as a circumscribed way of working with emotion would be very valuable. But rather than focusing deliberately and squarely on down-regulation as such, the DERS is taken as an omnibus measure of how well people work with emotion. The point here is that being able to calm down is not the only objective for emotional change (or regulation).

In summary, emotion regulation is often quite broadly defined (Gross, 2015; Muran et al., 2024), but as a framework of understanding it is also steeped in cognitive and behavioral traditions. Part of the catch here is that although emotion regulation could include many different process objectives (in theory), the behavioral framework puts a high premium on reducing arousal. It follows that the measurement and interventions for emotion regulation (as such) are overwhelmingly focused on attenuating emotional experience. But reducing arousal is not the only goal when working with emotion. Reducing symptoms, yes, but sometimes that involves feeling more fully, more richly, and more deeply (e.g., during grief, in the healthy anger of self-defense). Feeling more in these ways is not compatible with behavioral reductions in arousal. Finally, down-regulation and up-regulation are not the only two options. Working with emotion sometimes involves categorical change, such as a shift between states involving entirely different emotions. These shifts are qualitative and quite apart from the modulation of intensity.

Having offered these arguments, I now essentially sidestep the issue of emotion regulation in favor of more precise terms. The rest of this book focuses on narrower constructs that specifically describe distinct ways of working with emotion. The latter part of this chapter explores the down-regulation of emotional intensity as one of the specific kinds of change.

MINDFULNESS: AN EXERCISE IN SELF-REGULATION

Mindfulness is a 2,500-year-old approach to working with psychological suffering that originated from Buddhist practice. In both traditional and scientific accounts, it is often referred to as an overarching factor that promotes well-being. However, the treatment of mindfulness in clinical literature offers a good illustration of the complexity in understanding mechanisms of change and the massive oversimplification that comes with referring to a process as "regulation."

Despite its ancient history, only the last 50 years have seen the practice of mindfulness as a subject of numerous, independent, randomized controlled trials, confirming its positive impact. A meta-analysis of over 400 randomized controlled trials that compared mindfulness to other interventions for promoting well-being (broadly defined) found mindfulness to be one of the top interventions. Mindfulness produced a small to medium effect in improving well-being in the general population and a medium to large effect for those suffering a clinical diagnosis related to mental health (van Agteren et al., 2021;

see also Goldberg et al., 2018). This effect was also moderated by intensity of mindfulness training, so more training had a more substantial impact. Finally, benefits have been observed among adults, adolescents, and children (see also Tao et al., 2021).

Disentangling the Mechanisms of Mindfulness

The essential characteristic of mindfulness is defined as focused attention and the ability to maintain a metaperspective, yet the practice of mindfulness draws on a much more diverse set of principles. For many, the notion of sitting calmly, perhaps closing one's eyes, and attending to one's breath is a process of down-regulating the nervous system. That is the premise of mindfulness-based stress reduction (Kabat-Zinn, 2013; see also Lotan et al., 2013). A body of evidence shows that is indeed the case, but the question is how. While the practice of mindfulness may seem straightforward, it serves as a case in point to illustrate the mix of mechanisms that can be involved in a single intervention. The benefits of mindfulness practice are not contingent on any sharper clarity about change mechanisms (i.e., it's good for you—that's all that matters from a practice perspective). Only when research seeks to examine underlying mechanisms is the conceptual fuzziness quite apparent. Mindfulness has married well with cognitive and behavioral therapies, as seen in third-wave treatments (see Chapter 20). Cognitive theory points to mindfulness as helping with the de-automatization of habitual maladaptive patterns of thinking and feeling (Kang et al., 2013). Notice that language referring to "decoupling reactive habits" already suggests something more complex than just reducing negative arousal. Even within that tradition, however, there really is no clear explanation for how mindfulness works (Orsillo et al., 2004), signaling that the impact of this intervention may be highly overdetermined.

Taking stock of the many purposes for which mindfulness is used highlights the conceptual difficulties. After a review, researchers seeking to measure mindfulness described eight distinct facets of mindfulness (Bergomi et al., 2013). These were consistent with and subsumed other proposed mechanisms of action for mindfulness (i.e., Hölzel et al., 2011; Kabat-Zinn, 2013; Tao et al., 2021). Mindfulness was then explored as a (trainable) quasi-trait in the general population. No single measure of mindfulness was found to cover all facets, and instead, findings revealed four latent general factors (Bergomi et al., 2013). Factor 1, Open, Nonavoidant Orientation, refers to nonavoidance, nonidentification, and being ready to observe and attend. This essentially refers to a readiness and willingness to engage in a process as such. However, Factor 2, Present Awareness, captures the process of observing (e.g., awareness of breath, bodily sensations, mental states), which is discussed in Chapters 4 and 5 of this book as emotional engagement and awareness. Factor 2 also captures acting in awareness, which is discussed in this book as the intentionality with which someone expresses arousal and engages in enactments. These are discussed in Chapters 6, 9, 10, and 11. Factor 3, Describing Experience, is discussed in

Chapters 6 and 7 as labeling emotion and symbolization. Factor 4, Accepting, Nonreactive Insightful Orientation, refers to self-acceptance, nonjudgment, nonreactivity to experience, insightful understanding, or shift in perspective. It thus has elements that are closely related to reflection on emotion and decentering or shifting between narrative frames, which are discussed in Chapters 17, 20, and 22. These four factors in mindfulness are said to describe and putatively capture the mechanisms of its action. However, they reach so broadly as to cut across almost the full range of processes for emotional change—as I hope I have highlighted by cross-referencing various chapters within this book. This issue does not at all undermine the value of mindfulness as a clinical intervention, but it highlights the lack of specificity when mindfulness is too simply framed as a strategy of emotion regulation.

Going further than the factors extracted from self-report measures, the ritual aspects of mindfulness should not be underestimated and must not be naively separated from mindfulness practice itself (Safran, 2003; see also Wampold & Imel, 2015). Yet the distinction between a single mindfulness intervention and the ongoing practice required for it to be used effectively signals a host of additional processes that remain undeclared in the modern understanding of this ancient practice. So one might hypothesize several other factors that go beyond the four factors that were empirically identified (by Bergomi et al., 2013).[4] For instance, one might postulate a Factor 5 to be Having a Practice (see Safran, 2003). This highlights the notion of sitting and of practice, which creates a process event in itself. So, even before one begins to make use of the declared facets of mindfulness, the practice provides an opportunity, a time and place, for deliberate focus on self-functioning. This involves basic functions required for a commitment to show up and work or follow through on the elaboration of some effortful task, which is a process I discuss in Chapters 10 and 18. Mindfulness offers a palpable tool for clients to use. The explicit training creates both a sense of agency and an actual skill set to deploy in times of need (e.g., "I need to calm my mind, so I'll try doing some mindfulness"). Finally, mindfulness often entails some form of repetition or mantra, the impact of which is often overlooked but is discussed in Chapter 23.

One would also do well to consider a possible Factor 6, Identity Narratives and Tradition. Dedicating oneself to the practice of mindfulness offers the comforting existential affirmation that one is on a path toward change (Safran, 2003). On the one hand, this sense of being on a tried-and-true journey, an ancient pilgrimage, offers the reassurance of being part of a spiritual tradition. On the other hand, knowing one is dedicated to a practice offers the palpable reassurance that "no matter what happens, at the end of the day and again tomorrow morning, I will do my practice, I will feel grounded, I will have some sense of calm, and I will be back on the right path." The reassurance and stability of having routine self-care built into one's day offers tremendous security to a growing child, and it should not be surprising that having a ritualized practice for self-care serves a similar function for many adults. The narrative theme is that one is working toward a special form of psychological development, where getting better at meditation is seen as working toward a solution to one's distress. Purpose in life and existential issues are rarely cited in cognitive accounts of how mindfulness is helpful, although this is a process with deep significance as discussed in Chapters 21 and 23. Lastly, one could even argue for Factor 7, Mentorship and Solidarity. The practice of mindfulness very often involves an explicit instructor or mentor, particularly in traditional frameworks, which entail important relational processes. For dedicated practitioners, mindfulness may also involve a group identity or even community. These are also critical to change, although interpersonal processes go beyond the scope of this book.

An Example of Many Processes Overdetermining Outcome

In the end, mindfulness is not a process; it is an intervention or practice that likely draws on a loose collection of different processes. It is commonly associated with calmness and stress reduction but too often oversimplified as a strategy for down-regulating emotion, even if that may be one aspect of how it works. However, the studies that examine mindfulness alongside distress tolerance reveal these to be different predictors of symptom change. A 4-week mindfulness training for a nonclinical sample of adults helped improve their self-reported tolerance of distress, but these improvements were independent of positive changes to their skill in mindfulness (Lotan et al., 2013). A similar finding was observed in a high-risk clinical sample of individuals with borderline personality disorder (BPD) who attended 20 sessions of DBT skills and mindfulness training (Zeifman et al., 2020). There were meaningful improvements in both clients' mindfulness and their distress tolerance, but each process independently affected the relationship between treatment and psychopathology. The impact of mindfulness in reducing negative affect is overdetermined by a range of mechanisms, and they converge to produce its salutary effects.

I have detailed a diverse range of mechanisms that likely overdetermine the impact of mindfulness on improved well-being. I also offer this as an illustration, relevant to many other kinds of complex interventions in clinical literature (e.g., behavioral exposure, experiential enactments). As I indicated in Chapter 1, while the therapist chooses the intervention, only the client chooses the process. And as the end user, the client will make use of an undisclosed range of processes inspired by the intervention. The puzzle now is to disentangle the mechanisms of emotion change without reducing them to an amorphous construct of regulation. The next section begins by considering the specific process objective of reducing emotional intensity.

WHAT IS DOWN-REGULATION? WHEN IS IT IMPORTANT?

In the epigraph to this chapter, Charles Schulz, one of most influential cartoonists of all time, balances the utility of specific experiential meaning (i.e., all the complexity of love) with a basic sensory strategy for regulating emotion (i.e., eating chocolate!). The message here is that having a broad repertoire of ways for working with emotion and tailoring them to the presenting context is essential. There is an optimal occasion for each process. Relatedly, reducing emotional distress has been discussed differently from insight-oriented (psychodynamic, cognitive, experiential) and behavioral traditions (A. Pascual-Leone, Gillespie, et al., 2016).

Two Approaches to Down-Regulation: Making Meaning Versus Reducing Intensity

There are two main approaches to down-regulation, and each is championed by different treatment perspectives. First, self-soothing and reducing distress from an insight and experientially oriented approach is primarily done through the search for meaning (e.g., Frankl, 1963; Gendlin, 1996). In this approach, feelings of distress are treated as meaning laden and are elaborated. Painful emotion is alleviated through the exploration of memories and idiosyncratic meanings. By the end of that process, negative emotion is soothed by finally articulating as unmet existential need, which often then leads to the emergence of new feelings, meanings, and a change in perspective (see Chapters 13, 14, and 20). Generating new meaning about one's painful experience can be soothing and inherently calming in that it helps contain and makes sense of one's distress, but the search for new meaning also shifts one into different affective-meaning states.

However, there is a catch to this way of working with emotion. One often needs to stay with the painful experience a bit longer, momentarily increasing arousal as one stays with the feeling just a bit more, to make sense of it. Whatever the epistemological level of one's engagement (e.g., affect labeling vs. identity narratives), a search for meaning is not complete until one is able to articulate the personal and very idiosyncratic nature of what one needs to feel better (e.g., "I need that particular kind of love, the love that only a parent could give"). But if arousal is already too intense, one is pressed into the upper limit of what one can tolerate, and one may not have the room to elaborate meaning or stay with the feeling until it is complete. This is where a behavioral approach to down-regulating distress skills is helpful.

Second, reducing distress and self-soothing from a behavioral approach is about turning down the intensity (Foa & Kozak, 1986; Hofmann & Hay, 2018; Linehan, 2015). In this approach to working with distress, emotions are treated as global and reactionary symptoms that remain largely unexplored. Painful emotion is alleviated through general skills and actions. Meanwhile the feelings themselves are left largely unexplored in their experiential details and may even remain undisclosed (e.g., Therapist: "On a scale of 1 to 10, how much negative affect do you have right now?"). So, rather than elaborating new meaning, behavioral interventions are about quantitatively turning down the volume on distress. Unlike a highly personal search of one's experience, behavioral interventions offer universal tools for calming where the generic process of action is one-size-fits-all. For example, calm music and a cup of hot chocolate are generally soothing no matter who one is or what the situation (no doubt, Schulz would agree!).

Sometimes working with emotion will occur directly and can be executed relatively rapidly, as with behavioral strategies of distraction and some cognitive strategies such as reappraisals of the problematic situation. Other kinds of processing, such as experiential work, may be more time consuming and require a longer period of time to complete. Neural imaging supports the idea that cognitive and experiential strategies are supported by different patterns of brain activity and that they require differing time spans for that neural processing to be completed, whereas experiential strategies take longer (Wang et al., 2022). Yet different ways of working (e.g., the search for personal meaning, a reappraisal of the situation, turning down the volume) serve different functions when working with emotion, so they are not easily interchangeable. More importantly, the fastest solution is not always the right solution.

When to Use What? It Depends on Tolerance

How to work with client distress in each moment is an important decision for therapists (and clients themselves). Therapists who are easily alarmed by client distress may use interventions that continually shut down the client's experience through down-regulation (for more on this, see Chapter 8). But healthy individuals should have a broad set of capacities for working with emotion, and some of that will only be possible by working through one's (tolerable) distress (Kennedy-Moore & Watson, 2001). An optimal repertoire would range from using general one-size-fits-all behavioral approaches, such as listening to calm music, to using much more specific and idiosyncratic meaning making that addresses one's existential needs and personal goals (Gross, 2015; Kucharski et al., 2018).

Table 2.1 presents intervention objectives according to a client's immediate level of distress. The immediate distinction between behavioral strategies, which are generic in nature, and meaning-making strategies is whether the emotion is tolerable or not (A. Pascual-Leone, Gillespie, et al., 2016). Next, the treatment objectives for clients who chronically suffer intolerable distress (Table 2.1, top right) have sometimes been referred to as Stage I treatments (e.g., DBT), whereas treatment goals for those whose distress is usually tolerable enough to explore (bottom right) have sometimes been referred to as Stage II treatments (e.g., emotion-focused therapy). However, in practice clients can often work on both kinds of treatment goals in parallel, so the issue is a matter of emphasis as well as the pace of engagement. Table 2.1 speaks to clinical case formulations around issues related to the intensity of presenting emotion, whether and how it should be managed. However, there are other critical aspects to working with emotion. The lion's share of this book is dedicated to clarifying what approach to working with emotion is most effective for which kinds of problems.

TABLE 2.1. What to Do When It Gets Too Intense: Clinical Implication of Appraised Distress

Immediate level of distress is . . .	Short-term needs (intervention objective)	Long-term goals (treatment objective)
Not tolerable (e.g., dysregulated, dysfunctional, dangerous)	Generic strategies for down-regulation (e.g., behavioral coping, distraction, sensory soothing)	Develop a set of behavioral coping skills, desensitization, lifestyle changes to reduce dysregulation
Within tolerable limits	Specific strategies for meaning making (e.g., deeper experiencing, identifying and expressing unmet needs, insight)	Develop personal meaning, expand emotional repertoire, elaborate identity narrative and life purpose

Note. Data from Pascual-Leone, Gillespie, et al., 2016.

Distress Tolerance

Distress tolerance is the perceived degree to which someone can withstand negative emotional or physical states.[5] This is a subjective experience of being at an emotional breaking point. Although that upper limit of intensity can be reliably measured within an individual, there is a poor relationship between self-reports (e.g., "Feeling upset and frustrated is unbearable to me") and behavioral methods of measurement (e.g., measures of persistence during difficult tasks; Bernstein et al., 2011). Several meta-analyses have shown that distress tolerance has a small to medium negative relationship with psychopathology (e.g., problematic substance use, disordered eating, symptoms of posttraumatic stress disorder, BPD). Furthermore, that relationship is stronger when distress tolerance is measured by self-reports. There also seems to be no moderation by disorder, supporting this as a transdiagnostic concept (Akbari et al., 2022; Mattingley et al., 2022).

Research on BPD has further clarified the role of distress tolerance by showing that it moderates the degree to which intense negative emotion predicts psychopathology (Bornovalova et al., 2011). Consequently, a range of BPD symptoms and maladaptive behaviors such as substance use, self-harm, and social dysfunction as believed to stem from an individual's unwillingness to endure emotional distress, motivated by desperate attempts to stave off painful emotion (Linehan, 2015). The relationship between childhood trauma and psychopathology also seems to be mediated by one's tolerance of distress, such that lower tolerance means childhood trauma will predict higher psychological distress (Gaher et al., 2013; McLaughlin et al., 2020). In addition to higher psychopathology, low distress tolerance is associated with poor treatment outcomes including dropout and relapse into substance use (Bornovalova et al., 2012).

Although many processes are implicated, the tolerance of distress is a unidimensional construct (McHugh & Otto, 2012). As such, it is likely the summative expression of an individual's general capacity to work with immediate distress in a range of ways. For example, having a disposition to feel things more intensely or having lower impulse control is associated with a lower tolerance of distress. These dynamically interact with other factors that are associated with higher tolerance of distress, namely, being more emotionally aware, having mastery in a wide repertoire of self-regulation skills, and practicing mindfulness (Bernstein et al., 2011; Gaher et al., 2013; Mattingley et al., 2022; Zeifman et al., 2020). Taken together, the degree to which someone can tolerate emotional distress seems to represent an individual difference or trait-like characteristic when working with emotion. Again, this is consistent with the close association between measures of distress tolerance and difficulties in emotion regulation (Burton et al., 2022). And still, there is evidence that the relevant capacities that inform tolerance are malleable factors that can change over time. Ultimately, distress tolerance represents a capacity to endure painful or frustrating emotion even if it does not attenuate. So, while one might have more capacity to work with emotion in other ways, one must still be able to down-regulate emotion at critical moments.

When to Focus on Down-Regulating Emotion: What Are the Markers of Dysfunction?

Although negative affect is inherently unpleasant, arousal can sometimes intensify beyond what is tolerable while the problem it relates to cannot be immediately resolved. The specific moment-by-moment markers to make use of adaptive avoidance, disengagement, desensitization, and coping skills involve observations about either situation-specific responding of hyperarousal or a specific moment of crisis. On one hand, when a person is routinely triggered into hyperarousal when exposed to certain cues and then unable to function due to their overarousal, then exposure, desensitization, and coping skills are indicated. On the other hand, if people find themselves in an intolerable moment of emotional crisis, then strategic avoidance, distraction, and other coping skills are indicated. A *crisis* is a short-term and highly stressful situation that must be coped with immediately (Linehan, 2015). In short, immediately down-regulating emotion is useful (a) when a person's involvement in an emotional process carries imminent risks (e.g., harm to self or other in the present or very near future) or (b) when people feel overwhelmed and become disorganized, such that they are no longer able to adequately process information or make useful meaning (e.g., in a panic attack, sobbing uncontrollably, unchecked aggression, dissociation).

Although the foremost marker for down-regulation is the intolerable intensity of affect, there are several kinds of emotion that may be targeted by this change process. First, secondary symptomatic as well as instrumental emotions offer little informational value (see Introduction), so when they are predominant experiences and cannot be bypassed, they should be down-regulated. Second, if the arousal of primary emotion becomes too intense, the specificity of its meaning typically deteriorates, changing the experience itself and derailing effort to either use emotion as a guide or transform it. Recall, from the Introduction, that the purpose of engaging primary maladaptive emotions will be to clarify one's core concerns (see Chapter 7) and then follow with sequential transformations (see Chapter 12). However, meaning making requires a tolerable experience, beyond which momentary down-regulation will be necessary to help keep clients working within a safe and functional range. Even primary adaptive emotions may need to be down-regulated at times, if only to slow down and titrate the intensity of emotional engagement as one continues to make meaning from the core experience.

Immediately down-regulating emotion often involves disengaging in some way, and there are moments, like crisis management, where that is precisely the kind of deceleration one needs. But it is important to note there are also moments when down-regulation could be unhelpful or harmful. Detachment or reducing responsiveness to one's emotional situation will not be helpful and can become problematic when applied to everyday situations, when used habitually, or when used for extended periods of time (Daros et al., 2021; Linehan, 2015). Furthermore, down-regulating emotion will not solve significant life concerns and will be unhelpful when trying to make meaning of one's life.

OBSTACLES TO THE PROCESS OF DOWN-REGULATING EMOTION

Making use of the processes to down-regulate emotion is more difficult for some people than for others. There are at least five major obstacles to effectively containing and down-regulating emotional arousal when it becomes too intense (see also Gratz & Roemer, 2004; Hallion et al., 2018). Some of the obstacles are more challenging to address than others, but clarifying what prevents someone from calming down is an important starting point.

First, basic physiological needs can both potentiate and exacerbate affective dysregulation. Physical deprivation represents a broad set of factors any of which can create a diathesis such that people become more susceptible to emotional volatility and then also have difficulty controlling it (e.g., Chekroud et al., 2018; Kaplan et al., 2007; MacCormack & Lindquist, 2019). In this case, psychological insight is unlikely to help, and what people need are lifestyle changes. This might involve monitoring and ensuring adequate sleep and eating habits, reducing substance use (e.g., alcohol), and managing both stress and disruptions in life. Additional lifestyle change could include mindfulness-based practices and improving self-care habits.

Second, some individuals have characterological traits of impulsivity, disinhibition, affective lability, or high excitability (Bornovalova et al., 2011; Lotan et al., 2013; Mattingley et al., 2022; cf. Jones et al., 2007). Each of these can contribute to unwieldily or rapidly accelerating emotional intensity. These dispositional traits need to be managed through lifestyle changes and compensatory strategies such as mindfulness and improved self-monitoring.

Third, people may be unaware of the need to down-regulate, usually because of poor self-monitoring. This could be related to issues such as low psychological mindedness or, more broadly, poor metacognitive capacity (Dimaggio et al., 2020; Linehan, 2015; McLean et al., 2007). When clients become aware of or anticipate the need to decelerate their arousal, they can divert their attention and resources to do that (Linehan, 2015; Mackintosh et al., 2014).

Fourth, some people lack necessary skills and simply do not have an adequate repertoire of strategies to calm themselves down when needed (Neacsiu et al., 2010; A. Pascual-Leone, Gillespie, et al., 2016; Zeifman et al., 2020). For emotionally healthy people, many of the strategies they use throughout the day to modulate emotional intensity are automatized, woven into the fabric of their moment-by-moment functioning, habits, and lifestyle (Kucharski et al., 2018). However, when people have never learned healthy coping strategies or when these are not sufficiently automatized, reducing arousal at times of crisis is elusive (Lynch et al., 2006).

Fifth and finally, sometimes individuals are unable or unwilling to change cognitive-behavioral sets. At times this may be related to low metacognitive capacity (Dimaggio et al., 2020). At other times, the individual may be ambivalent about reducing their high arousal, perhaps because it serves an instrumental function (Linehan, 2015; A. Pascual-Leone et al., 2013; Peters et al., 2018). This obstacle could be addressed by increasing mindfulness and cultivating nonattachment to the issue at hand. It can also be worked with through candid self-reflection, insight, and then an existential choice to work with emotion differently (see Chapters 20 and 23).

In conclusion, feeling less remains an essential way of working with emotion, and although it does not offer a panacea, clinicians of any orientation recognize that there are critical moments when people must make use of that capacity. Although being able to reduce arousal and essentially truncating one's emotional experience is critical at times of crisis, the process will also work at cross-purpose with emotional awareness or a search for personal meaning (see Chapter 4).

MECHANISMS AT WORK: HOW DOES REDUCING EMOTION CREATE CHANGE?

A person's vulnerability to high emotional arousal and dysregulation can be addressed in several ways. One of those is preventive action, whereby lifestyle changes and skills training over the lifespan generally improve one's distress tolerance. When a specific moment of crisis or impaired functioning calls for the immediate reduction of emotional arousal, there are at least three general mechanisms: using avoidance, progressive desensitization, and applying behavioral skills. These processes are explored in the next chapter.

Subsequent parts of this book (Chapters 4–23) explore different ways of working with emotion that do not involve the immediate down-regulation of emotion but still facilitate symptom change. Over time, all ways of working with emotion independently help a person develop a general capacity for emotional resilience and self-regulation in the broadest sense.

ENDNOTES

1. There are optimal times to use one or another strategy for working with emotion, but that is not the question here. In fact, most of this book will be about sorting out what works best and under what circumstances.
2. While cognitive reframing is typically used to curtail arousal, existential interventions would be the rare exception. Such interventions are often used to create urgency around an immediate choice in one's identity narrative. For example, a therapist might highlight the larger framework of life implications and then ask, "And so, at this moment, I guess you are deciding, 'What kind of person do I want to be?'" (see Chapter 23). That, however, is quite afield from the standard cognitive interventions being used for symptom management.
3. When awareness is framed more cognitively and as a close-ended task, it reduces emotional intensity. In contrast, an open-ended and experiential approach will often increase intensity, bolstering further exploration. See Chapter 5 for an explanation of this with empirical evidence.
4. I am grateful to the late Dr. Jeremy Safran for sharing his insights on these other mechanisms of mindfulness. I credit these ideas to him, gleaned over several years of conversation.
5. *Experiential avoidance* is a related but distinct construct from distress tolerance. Distress tolerance is generally considered a broader construct, it is strength-focused, and it may be achieved sometimes through adaptive avoidance. Even so, the emphasis here is on what level of distress someone can tolerate engaging with, coping with, or otherwise manage. Another related construct is the notion of *mental toughness*, which extrapolates the notion of distress tolerance to elite performers, namely sports athletes (see Jones et al., 2007).

3

Avoidance, Desensitization, and Behavioral Coping

Keep calm and carry on.

—BRITISH MINISTRY OF INFORMATION

"Keep Calm and Carry On" was one of several public messages created in 1939 by Britain's wartime propaganda department, the Ministry of Information. The iconic motivational poster with this message was intended for mass distribution to reassure people so they would continue enduring in the event of wartime disaster. Millions of these posters were printed—but in true stoic fashion, they were mostly kept on reserve during the Second World War, in anticipation of what might be an especially tremendous crisis. Ironically, most of that stock was never used and eventually destroyed (R. M. Lewis, 2004). Nevertheless, the slogan was rediscovered by popular interest in the 2000s as an evocation of the British stiff upper lip, a great show of self-restraint against expressions of personal emotion when faced with adversity.[1] As an epigraph to this chapter, the slogan speaks to keeping up good habits, avoiding emotional engagement, enduring adversity until one eventually gets acclimatized to it, and above all, behavioral coping. All of these are forms of reducing emotion in the immediate service of practical functioning—and postponing the working through of any deeper issues until a more suitable time.

The previous chapter clarified that the term "emotion regulation" is so broadly defined in clinical writing that it is amorphous, sometimes making it a hollow construct. In contrast, the down-regulation of emotion is a more precise process with a clearer clinical objective, and that is the narrower focus of this

https://doi.org/10.1037/0000460-004

Principles of Emotion Change: What Works and When in Psychotherapy and Everyday Life, by A. Pascual-Leone
Copyright © 2026 by the American Psychological Association. All rights reserved.

chapter. In a diathesis–stress model, the intensity of emotional distress could be reduced either preemptively by using lifestyle strategies (i.e., reducing the diathesis) or by directly addressing the moment-by-moment emergence of an emotional crisis (i.e., reducing the immediate stress response) within a circumscribed situation. I address each of these in turn, beginning with three preventive lifestyle factors, followed by three immediate processes for reducing emotional intensity.

LIFESTYLE FACTORS FOR REDUCING VULNERABILITY TO DYSREGULATION

Lifestyle factors impact affective lability such that healthy habits reduce one's general vulnerability to emotional dysregulation. Many biopsychosocial factors are relevant here (and social contact is a very important one), but I mention only three pertaining to an individual's self-care, which could be modified relatively easily and quickly. While sleep, exercise, and nutrition are not processes for directly working with emotion, they underpin emotional functioning in important ways. For the most part, these are preventive measures that increase the threshold margins or lead time before extreme dysregulation. This is like lengthening the wick of a fuse. In practice, these essentially represent low-hanging fruit for moderating arousal, but when compromised, they undermine the healthy modulation of emotion.

Getting a Good Night's Sleep

Research on emotional functioning and sleep has primarily focused on how psychopathology interacts with disordered sleep and points to getting a good night's sleep as an important contributor to mental health. A review of the literature also shows that sleep deprivation makes one more sensitive to stressful stimuli and susceptible to negative affect and increases emotional arousal (Vandekerckhove & Wang, 2017). For instance, after inadequate sleep, people show an exaggerated startle response, illustrating the role of poor sleep in over-aroused emotional responding. Research also supports the commonly held understanding that emotion and sleep have a bidirectional relationship: While emotional issues can lead to restless sleep, poor sleep also makes one more emotional, and it is the latter point that is most relevant here. Good sleep hygiene reduces one's vulnerability to becoming emotionally dysregulated.

Physical Exercise

Physical exercise is a master regulator, moderating the affective system but also several other important physiological processes that individually impact emotion and its regulation. The regulatory function of physical exercise applies to (a) appetite, (b) sleep, (c) mood, (d) proprioceptive grounding (i.e., awareness of self in reality), and (e) palpable experiences of personal agency. Physical exercise is negatively associated with mental health difficulties, in both clinical and nonclinical samples.

A cross-sectional study of 1.2 million people in the United States looked at the relationship between exercise and mental health burden, as indexed by the number of days per month a person reported having poor mental health (Chekroud et al., 2018). Individuals who exercised for 45 minutes per session and 3 to 5 times per week had the fewest days of poor mental health. Exercising less (in duration or in frequency) was associated with greater mental health burden, while exercising more did not carry any considerable advantage and sometimes was associated with higher mental health burden. These patterns were remarkably consistent across a range of different exercise activities. In samples matched for key sociodemographic and physical variables, people who exercised enjoyed a 43% reduction in the number of days suffering poor mental health (i.e., 1–2 fewer days/month) compared to those who did not exercise. Specifically, among those with a previous diagnosis of depression, people who exercised enjoyed a 34% reduction in the number of days with poor mental health (i.e., 3–4 fewer days/month). These effects of exercise on mental health are large compared to that of other modifiable variables, such as education and income, even though those would also be more difficult to change. By using matched samples, the study allows one to rule out several alternative explanations for the association between exercise and better mental health. Other studies, however, have been designed to directly test causation.

Both longitudinal research and randomized controlled trials have been conducted with much smaller samples, and they confirm the role of exercise (e.g., walking, resistance training) as a probable mechanism for reducing depressive symptoms and improving mental health in older and middle-aged adults, as well as adolescents (Chekroud et al., 2018). A meta-analysis of 33 randomized control trials concluded that for people with mild to moderate depression, short workouts of resistance exercise (e.g., lifting weights for less than 45 minutes) had a large effect on reducing depression (Gordon et al., 2018). Taken together, the research suggests a dose-response effect and has very concrete behavioral implications for self-regulation and how one might hedge against, or even treat, mental illness.

When people with clinical levels of depression or anxiety were included in a partially randomized patient preference design, running therapy (45 minutes, twice a week or more) was compared to antidepressant medication, and at the end of 4 months, the two treatments had similar effects in eliminating or reducing symptoms of psychopathology (Verhoeven et al., 2023). And, of course, the side effects of exercise versus medication on physical health (i.e., stamina, weight loss, libido) are often directly opposite to one another. However, the role of self-selection and strong client preferences loom large here. Adopting a lifestyle habit is more challenging for individuals than taking a pill, and for some, committing to an exercise regimen will also be more difficult than attending talk psychotherapy.

This highlights that health researchers and clinicians should take seriously the fact that encouraging exercise is usually about neither medical evidence nor educating people: Most people already know exercise is good for them! Rather, getting people to exercise is a puzzle for psychology. There are several variables that determine whether someone will maintain an exercise regimen. Among others, these will include scheduling (i.e., Do you have specific days and times you plan to exercise?), social accountability (i.e., Is someone else expecting you to show up?), goal setting (i.e., Are you working toward some outcome?), and committed costs (i.e., Did you already pay for the class or membership? Do you already own equipment?). Some of the largest potential gains in health research might be simply finding the best ways for motivating people to exercise.

Nutrition

The experience of being irritable because one is hungry will be familiar to many people and has been studied experimentally (MacCormack & Lindquist, 2019). Although the relationship between emotion and eating has been known for some time, we now have a better understanding of the extent to which nutrition impacts emotional functioning. There is emerging evidence that poor diet, deficits in micronutrients, and inborn genetic errors in metabolism may produce vulnerability to mental disorders. The growing field of nutritional psychology focuses on the connections between nutrition, physiological processes, and psychological well-being. Randomized controlled trials and case series show that micronutrient supplements may be useful in treating emotional deficits and attenuating affective symptoms, including those related to anxiety, depression, and aggression (Kaplan et al., 2007). For example, treating mood disorders among youth and adults using supplements of broad-spectrum micronutrients is an intervention associated with a decline in psychiatric symptoms comparable to that of pharmacotherapy (Popper, 2014). There seem to be various physiological mechanisms by which nutritional deficiencies are associated with deficits in emotional functioning. Four ways that nutritional deficiencies may impair emotional functioning have been identified: the inflammation of bodily tissue, a reduction in the number of gut microbacteria, proliferation of reactive oxygen molecules, and mutations in mitochondrial DNA (Kaplan et al., 2015).

Tightly controlled experiments suggest the process by which nutritional factors impact emotional functioning in the brain, which could either undermine or bolster healthy psychological and behavioral strategies. For example, consuming high-fat foods seems to be causally related to the feelings of emotional comfort. In a study that demonstrated this, either sad or neutral feelings were induced in healthy participants using music and images of expressive faces (Van Oudenhove et al., 2011). Then, in a blind manipulation, fat was infused through a small plastic feeding tube directly into the stomachs of participants in the experimental condition, while water was infused to participants in the control condition. When participants who were sad received the infusion of fatty acids in their stomachs, it reduced their subjective experience of sadness. The fat-by-emotion interaction was observed not only behaviorally (reported changes in mood and hunger) but also at the level of neural activity using functional magnetic resonance imaging (fMRI), where brain regions associated with emotional responding were quieted. A landmark study has also shown the effect of probiotics on brain activity using fMRI (Tillisch et al., 2013). Astonishingly, eating probiotic yogurt over 4 weeks significantly modulated the activity of specific brain regions, namely the periaqueductal gray, both while attending to negative emotional states and while at rest. The observed brain patterns were characteristic of decreased emotional reactivity. It appears that some aspects of emotional functioning can be influenced using probiotics.

Moderating Arousal by Routine

When working with emotion, a substantial advantage of using behavioral routines is that they are not contingent on someone already having a well-developed capacity for emotional awareness. Consider a young computer programmer I saw in my practice for the treatment of his depression.[2] The client protested that he sometimes felt "tension" but that he never knew if it was about "something serious." For me, the comment highlighted the client's deficit in emotional awareness (see Chapter 6 for more on this, and on affect labeling). Nevertheless, one day he came to session with a solution he had invented, which he called a "subroutine" for coping with affective discomfort. He explained as follows:

> If I don't feel right, the first thing I do now is go to the bathroom. . . . Sometimes I have to go but I'm putting it off because I have work to do and don't want to lose my place. . . . But if that doesn't work, and I still feel bad, the next thing I do is go make myself a sandwich . . . maybe it's a blood sugar thing. . . . Then, if that doesn't work, I take a nap. Bathroom, sandwich, nap—and if I still feel bad after a nap, then level four: it's serious!

In this case, "serious" meant that the client wanted to work on it in our session: It would require deeper attention and effort (e.g., perhaps expanding awareness, promoting expression, sequential transformations).

A unique aspect of all behavioral strategies for working with emotion is that they allow one to regulate emotion in the context of relatively poor emotional awareness (as with my client). Although changing one's lifestyle is not always easy, these factors for moderating arousal are not contingent on insight or even psychological mindedness. Aside from other obvious benefits, having healthy lifestyle habits offers a sort of insurance policy against the full force of an unanticipated emotional crisis (e.g., risks of angry outbursts, imminent self-harm), which typically requires very rapid and strong responsiveness. To some degree, moderating arousal by routine rather than insight is central to behavioral approaches, which extends to the immediate processes that I discuss next.

Immediate Down-Regulation of Emotion: What to Do When Things Get Too Hot

The efforts one makes to reduce the intensity of what one is feeling, even if only in the very short term, is something we all do, either intentionally or not, and often in small ways, as part of navigating through life. For healthy individuals, the modulation of engagement, and therefore arousal, is largely automatized. Nevertheless, there are at least three common mechanisms by which this down-regulation of emotional arousal occurs and can be deliberately applied. In order of increasing complexity, first, with some anticipatory sense, one might strategically avoid stimuli and situations that otherwise would be too evocative. Second, a great deal of research has considered desensitization, through habituation and automatic inhibition, as another mechanism by which emotional intensity is down-regulated. Third, individuals also learn skills for behavioral coping to reduce or manage their arousal when it has become too intense.

Many authors have added a lengthy list of additional processes, but most of the other processes often subsumed under "regulation" are better and more clearly addressed as categorically different ways of working with emotion (see other chapters). A commonality of these three processes (i.e., adaptive avoidance, habituation, and coping skills) is that they do not attempt to change the inherent quality of an emergent emotion (i.e., what one is feeling) but rather aim to reduce the quantitative intensity of that feeling (i.e., how much of the feeling one experiences). Of course, other ways of working with emotion can help the individual shift laterally to another feeling, move on to the next step of a larger feeling process, or simply clarify the initial presenting feeling, but these are different processes in that they alter the qualitative experience of a feeling. Changing the qualitative experience, particularly when it is a fruitful and productive way of working with emotion, will often also impact the intensity of one's distress. But it is critical not to conflate what are inherently quantitative changes (i.e., down-regulation) with qualitative changes (i.e., alterations to personal meaning or tone of an emotion). Adaptive avoidance, desensitization, and coping skills are three processes uniquely related to the immediate down-regulation of emotion and cannot be explained by other types of emotional change.

Adaptive Avoidance: "I Need Some Time-Out!"

Excessive avoidance is the hallmark of anxiety, among other disorders (Aldao et al., 2010). When people rely on avoidance as a way to keep their emotion at bay, it entails significant hazards and has an often pathological role in their functioning.

Avoidance as Dysfunctional

If one understands anxiety as a behavioral problem, it follows that exposure becomes a staple component of treatment for anxiety disorders. This involves repeated sessions where clients are given prolonged exposure to their feared stimuli and are discouraged from using avoidance strategies. This is challenging because patterns of avoidance are notoriously resistant to extinction for several reasons (Ball & Gunaydin, 2022).

First, avoidance can be negatively reinforced (e.g., anxiety is relieved through avoidance, which then increases future avoidance behaviors). Second, avoidance also works prospectively as a defensive reaction and plays a strong role in the subsequent formation of habits, which then shape future engagements (or lack thereof). So avoidance is more than just an escape; it also involves defensive reactions as well as habit formation. This has been demonstrated through neurological functioning as well as specific molecular processes within the amygdala and other areas (LeDoux et al., 2017). A third issue in understanding the intractability of maladaptive avoidance is that these circuits (i.e., governing avoidance, defensive action, and habit) operate nonconsciously in the regulation of behavior and are different from those that generate conscious experiences of fear and anxiety. This means, for example, that when a situation no longer elicits fear, people may continue to avoid it. Measuring adaptive as opposed to maladaptive avoidance has been done objectively using indices in controlled laboratory situations (Ball & Gunaydin, 2022). But ultimately, avoidance is maladaptive when it occurs in the absence of any real threat.

Clinical research, particularly from a behaviorist perspective, has consistently held that avoidance and other disengagement strategies are maladaptive ways of coping with emotion that are highly related to psychopathology and inversely related to good treatment outcomes (Aldao et al., 2010; Daros et al., 2021). While this may sometimes be true, particularly if one examines research on working with anxiety or depression, it is an overgeneralization. On one hand, the sweeping categorization of avoidance and disengagement as being unhealthy or maladaptive forms of emotion regulation often does not adequately consider the critical role of context (A. Pascual-Leone, Gillespie, et al., 2016; Kucharski et al., 2018). On the other hand, avoidance is typically a pathological behavior when working with problematic fear, but that is not necessarily true for all emotions (Hofmann & Hay, 2018).

Avoidance as Adaptive Disengagement: When and for What?

Ideas about adaptive avoidance are less grounded in experimental research or neuroscience but follow from clinical models (Hofmann & Hay, 2018). Some researchers have clarified that disengagement skills are a unique subset of emotion regulation strategies, highlighting that they represent an adaptive strategy for dealing with crisis situations (Daros et al., 2021; Linehan, 2015). Such situations may involve avoiding exposure to a real threat, purposeful disengagement to get some reprieve from distress, or delaying a dangerous (e.g., violent) emotional expression. For example, when immediate down-regulation is called for to avert risky behavior or urges to relapse, one might productively use distraction to bide some time, such as counting all the red cars that go by on a busy road, to otherwise interrupt overwhelming distress (e.g., as in dialectical behavior therapy [DBT]; Linehan, 2015). Purposefully stepping back from painful thoughts by creating psychological distance is also a technique used in several treatments (e.g., diffusion techniques in acceptance and commitment therapy; S. C. Hayes et al., 2012).[3] Although mechanisms of bilateral stimulation in eye movement desensitization and reprocessing have been somewhat contentious, there is clear evidence to support the orienting function and dividing someone's attention as a sort of intermittent distraction to render distressing content less upsetting (Landin-Romero et al., 2018). So another adaptive function of avoidance is to titrate or pace one's level of emotional engagement.

Irrespective of the skills one could use, there are key situations where an individual may be best served by using disengagement to work with their emotion. This was neatly illustrated in a study of high-functioning varsity athletes who were asked to imagine and describe what they did to successfully negotiate their negative emotion (e.g., anxiety, self-doubt, self-criticism, sense of inadequacy) either before a competition or game, or after a defeat or loss. Before a competitive event, athletes reported relying significantly more on avoidance, disengagement, and suppression than on other strategies. However, when addressing their negative emotion after a defeat, they reported using significantly more exploratory awareness, meaning making, and self-compassion as compared to other strategies (Kucharski et al., 2018). It is important to note that this selective use of disengagement from emotion (i.e., before a competitive event) was related neither to any genuine crisis nor to these individuals having any lack of alternative strategies. This study illustrates the value of selectively using avoidance and disengagement based on the characteristics of a given situation.[4]

In functional terms, proactive avoidance may be a form of agency (Moscarello & Hartley, 2017). In practice, purposeful disengagement may also be related to mindful acceptance of reality as it is (S. C. Hayes et al., 2012; Linehan, 2015). I conducted a clinical interview with a 93-year-old man suffering issues related to bereavement but who also had astonishing existential clarity. He reported that even during periods of extreme adversity in his life, he had always been a peaceful and sound sleeper. This is uncommon for older adults and particularly for someone with a life story like his—of surviving war, oppression, and isolation. When I asked what might explain his sleeping so well every night, he replied: "Whenever I feel anxious about something going on in my life that might prevent me from falling asleep, I say to myself, 'The best thing I can do about that right now is just to have a good night's sleep.'" The anecdote is an example of how sometimes disengagement by delaying problem solving can be an effective strategy for down-regulating distress.

It should be obvious that as part of a defensive repertoire, avoidance in situations of acute danger is highly adaptive. In addition, people sometimes simply feel overwhelmed by emotion, so this protective function of avoidance might extend to shielding the person from too much intensity. Furthermore, using avoidance strategically can enhance a person's sense of control over potential threats (Ball & Gunaydin, 2022). Even in anxiety-provoking situations, using avoidance can help moderate exposure and allow people to more willingly and quickly engage with difficult situations (Hofmann & Hay, 2018).

Avoidance can also be useful when working with emotional experiences other than fear. Problematic anger and aggression are strong cases in point. Secondary anger or rage is reactive and often poorly differentiated in terms of its meaning specificity, a prime example of when self-interruption and avoidance may be the optimal process. Folk wisdom for managing these challenges often says to avoid or leave the situation as part of immediate coping. The Roman philosopher Seneca has been quoted for almost 2,000 years as saying, "The greatest remedy for anger is delay." Both folk psychology and clinical practice have many examples of this kind of time-out strategy for crisis intervention, ranging from simplistic (e.g., close your eyes and count to 10 before you reply!) to the superbly practical (e.g., if you have a history of violence and you get really angry during a conversation, you should excuse yourself and immediately leave the room; Bjureberg et al., 2023; Mackintosh et al., 2014). Of course, other ways of working through emotion (i.e., processing and making meaning) may be relevant too, but those kinds of emotional change can often happen later, when the arousal is not as intense.

There are negative as well as positive aspects of avoidance in therapeutic work. To distinguish adaptive from maladaptive avoidance, the function of a behavior is key. Behaviors that allow one to organize, pace, or purposefully slow down one's emotional engagement may not interfere but rather facilitate healthy emotional work. There is clearly a time and a place for the healthy use of disengagement and avoidance as a short-term fix (Hofmann & Hay, 2018). Persistent, rigid, or excessive use of avoidance is likely maladaptive, particularly in response to nonthreatening stimuli. The key is in using this flexibly and accurately as a strategy for the immediate down-regulation of emotional arousal that would otherwise be intolerable.

Desensitization: "I Got Used to the Feeling, so It Disappeared"

The idea that one gets used to something and becomes less sensitive over time is intuitive. This way of working with emotion is a pillar of behavioral treatments and is particularly effective for reducing symptom distress. Still, the underlying process has been elusive.

What Happens During Behavioral Exposure?

Exposure is an intervention, not a mechanism of change (Carey, 2011). Even so, many therapists and even some authors refer to exposure as if it were a change process, in what amounts to conceptual shorthand. What happens during someone's exposure to painful content is also interpreted differently (and likely is quite different) based on the treatment perspective. For example, according to behaviorist theory, telling and retelling an account of traumatic events (e.g., imagining a perpetrator, recounting the plot and characters of what happened) is a form of systematic exposure intended to facilitate desensitization to what are evocative details (Foa et al., 2007). In contrast, experiential therapies see imagining a perpetrator and elaborating on the impact of narrated events as the generation of new meaning, which is a categorically different process from the notion of desensitization (Paivio & Pascual-Leone, 2023). These represent two different ways of working with emotion, each following from somewhat similar interventions (e.g., both involve remembering evocative details of what happened) and both of which have been described as exposure (depending on the author). However, the significant underlying difference here in terms of process is highlighted by the fact that while meaning making has been shown to increase emotional arousal in the short term, repeated exposure to narrative cues decreases arousal in the longer term. Furthermore, research on expressive writing about trauma has further shown that the temporal pattern of these two distinct kinds of emotional processing is syncopated together (A. Pascual-Leone, Yeryomenko, et al., 2016; see Chapter 8).

As an intervention, behavioral exposure can be done with either imagined or real stimuli and may be done either gradually or intensely, producing a 2 × 2 matrix describing the four types of exposure therapy. On the one hand, these are (a) systematic desensitization and (b) graded in vivo exposure (i.e., imagined or real, both graded); on the other hand are (c) implosion and (d) flooding (i.e., imagined or real, both intense; Tryon, 2005).[5] As suggested, exposure could be used to several ends (e.g., engagement, desensitization, learning, an entry point to generate personal meaning; Carey, 2011). Nevertheless, all four methods of behavioral intervention aim to produce desensitization when there are no competing processes. *Desensitization* is a process of diminished responsiveness to some evocative stimuli over repeated exposures. The mechanistic formulation here is also an effort to steer clear of explanations that suggest explicit learning or complex thinking. One can become desensitized to either negative or positive stimuli, but interventions typically aim to attenuate symptom distress, particularly anxiety.

Exposure and desensitization are about down-regulating arousal. But what is the internal mechanism within an individual that results in this desensitization? Clinical applications stand to be meaningfully impacted when the mechanisms are eventually spelled out (Colwill et al., 2023). Consider, for example, that while treatment theory for prolonged exposure was well established in the 1980s (e.g., Foa & Kozak, 1986), it was another 30 years before any comprehensive review of potential mechanisms was undertaken (Cooper et al., 2017). Furthermore, proposed mechanisms of prolonged exposure therapy include an assortment of possibilities, from belief change and between-session habituation (both with a strong evidence base), to emotional engagement and inhibitory learning (with an intermediate evidence base), to narrative change and within-session habituation (a weak evidence base; Cooper et al., 2017; Foa et al., 2007).

Habituation: The Gradual Attenuation of Arousal

A broad clinical review on the possible mechanisms for exposure-based interventions observed, "the cognitive revolution in psychology occurred partly because functional statements made by behaviorists lacked causal mediating explanatory mechanisms. . . . Exposure therapy appear[s] to work but there is little agreement as to why" (Tryon, 2005, p. 69). There are several explanations for how exposure works to reduce arousal, with varying degrees of supporting evidence. However, the most robust is that, following an exposure protocol, the reduction of distress is explained by habituation. Exhaustive reviews and a series of meta-analyses on process to outcome effects in psychotherapy have examined research designed specifically to study the mechanisms of exposure-based treatments (Kazantzis et al., 2018; Sønderland et al., 2023). Analyses show that, for anxiety disorders, habituation has very robust effects for working with emotion. Although, the question remains as to what is happening and whether within-session changes and between-session changes are indeed the same kind of process (although both get referred to as habituation).

Habituation was originally thought to be different from the mental operations of learning in the associative or content-based sense; it was considered a very basic, almost homeostatic function (Colwill et al., 2023; Tryon, 2005). Whatever habituation is, it seems to capture a unique kind of emotional change, directly down-regulating arousal on an organismic level. There are other terms that should also be addressed here. Regrettably, desensitization is sometimes used to denote a treatment intervention (i.e., systematic desensitization), but at other times it refers to a process. Relatedly, desensitization as a process is often used synonymously with habituation (although distinctions exist, these are not meaningful to clinical work).[6] Also, extinction simply describes the long-term effects of habituation. Furthermore, reciprocal inhibition and counterconditioning are other process explanations put forward to explain how exposure reduces symptoms, but they also introduce a new notion of competing processes. Therefore, they are better explained as other kinds of processing (for more on this, see Chapter 12).[7]

Whatever the case, the process for attenuating arousal is now commonly referred to as habituation, but how that process occurs remains an issue of debate. Nearly 20 years after the review quoted earlier (Tryon, 2005), another review of theory and evidence again concluded,

> There are serious problems with the conventional way habituation has been measured . . . and we disagree with the commonly held views that habituation is non-associative and the simplest of all learning phenomena. Rather we see habituation as a surprisingly complicated, multi-faceted learning process that emerges from what is a very simple procedure, the repeated presentation of a stimulus. (Colwill et al., 2023, p. 8)

So part of the problem in understanding habituation has to do with the way it is typically measured. Measuring it by way of a reduction in response patterns

> blurs the important distinction between learning (an inferred change) and performance (an observed change in behavior). . . . It is important to draw a distinction between the encoding and retention of information (learning) and the subsequent expression of that knowledge through behavior (performance). (Colwill et al., 2023, pp. 2–3)

This is a major reason why theories of habituation have limitations and why its mechanisms have yet to be well articulated. Be that as it may, we know for sure that habituation works best when the stimulus being habituated to (a) is presented in spaced intervals over time rather than all at once (i.e., massed or continuous presentation) and (b) is presented with a strong intensity rather than weak. There is also good evidence that habituation may be even more effective when the intensity of a stimulus gradually increases from weak to strong (Colwill et al., 2023; Tryon, 2005). In clinical applications this may mean that the variability with which a stimulus is presented can be more important than the duration or frequency.

Returning to the mechanisms by which exposure attenuates arousal, there are short- and long-term changes that seem to result from habituation. Importantly, these changes are conceptually distinct and are likely attributable to different underlying mechanisms, and although they are related, they do not necessarily build upon one another. Furthermore, the evidence suggests that a short-term process for attenuating arousal is more specific to the internal features of the stimulus and is not context bound. Meanwhile, multiple mechanisms of associative learning may explain long-term process for attenuating arousal, which would be more context dependent (Colwill et al., 2023).[8] The best understanding to date is that habituation is explained by a combination of (a) automatic inhibitory processes and (b) new learning about expectancies. These two subprocesses work together to produce what is commonly referred to as habituation, that is, the attenuation of arousal following repeated exposure.

Automatic inhibition: The short-term change in performance. The first factor in habituation is developing a habit of not doing or ignoring. Inhibition is either effortful and deliberate (e.g., consciously trying to resist something) or automatic. Fear habituation within a session (according to client rating on subjective units of distress [SUDS]) can be thought of as this kind of short-term change. A meta-analysis (based on 11 studies) found within-session habituation to have a medium-sized effect on the reduction of target symptoms at the end of treatment (Sønderland et al., 2023).

Here, the psychological mechanism of habituation is an automatic inhibition of internal or environmental information that is not useful, in the sense that it is inconsequential. Biologically, animals instinctually have a criterion of relevance, and they attend to things that are relevant to their well-being and goals. In short, some features of reality matter while others do not. The attentional tendency becomes extinguished as stimuli are found repeatedly to be irrelevant. In this way, when the stimulus offers less consequential information, it becomes automatically inhibited, and that process is not contingent on context. This is a characteristic of the living, acting organism that allows for flexibility in one's responding and for novel ways of engaging the world to potentially introduce variation in what one attends to that may be more meaningful (J. Pascual-Leone & Johnson, 2021; Pessoa, 2013). One just gets used to it and comes to ignore it, freeing up attention. For instance, one might be initially disturbed by the sound of an alarm or machinery but then eventually get used to it, after which one no longer seems to notice it. With evocative stimuli that are cues for emotional distress, the repeated exposure to a cue without newly unfolding consequences eventually renders it meaningless. This is the essence of habituation, and it occurs for almost all behavioral responses in virtually all organisms (Colwill et al., 2023).

Responses that can be habituated could also be recovered (i.e., dishabituated), either spontaneously following some break or reprieve from the stimulus or by introducing some variation in the stimulus itself, such as changes in intensity (either up or down). Incidentally, this is one of the of the key features that show habituation to be different from various kinds of fatigue (e.g., the adaptation of sensory receptors, motor-muscle fatigue). Moreover, spontaneous recovery (or dishabituation) is not the interruption of a habituation process but rather a separate process of sensitization that is superimposed onto habituation (Colwill et al., 2023).

New learning changes expectancies: Long-term behavioral change. I have highlighted how the measurement (and definition) of habituation conflates the issues of inferred mechanism(s) with observed performance, which has hidden the fact that there are probably two processes at hand. In the *short* term, habituation as an observed moment-by-moment performance is likely a nonassociative process of inhibition, working outside one's conscious intentionality. However, the long-term changes that result from repeated exposure are believed to operate through a more involved mental process. Long-term changes alter the internal working models (i.e., cognitive-emotional schemes) one uses to understand and to know what to expect from the world (J. Pascual-Leone & Johnson, 2021). Here, reductions in observed emotional arousal (i.e., performance) reflect an underlying process of basic leaning, whereby one creates new associations between a stimulus and its context. This represents habituation as a more enduring or long-term form of down-regulation (Colwill et al., 2023). Habituation to fear between sessions of exposure (according to client SUDS ratings) can be thought of as the long-term change in exposure-based treatments for anxiety. A meta-analysis with rigorous design criteria has shown that that process was associated with a large effect in the prediction of reduced symptoms (based on 13 studies; Sønderland et al., 2023).

In this change process, someone approaches an old situation with cautiousness because of their past experiences with that situation or the circumstances surrounding it. The initial issue with a fear-inducing situation is that it was unexpected, after which novel situations of a similar kind carry a cue of threat. In other cases, the situation may have been unequivocally threatening or traumatic. But the degree to which elements of a stimulus are surprising or predictable changes over time, particularly with the experience of multiple exposures. So the anticipation of negative consequences is corrected by neutral or even slightly positive expectations through the discovery of a nonthreatening experience. Elements that are already anticipated (i.e., have been primed) receive increasingly less mental attention, meaning they are less salient and processed to a lesser degree (Colwill et al., 2023). When the world around us unfolds as expected, old stimuli no longer elicit the same alarm and orienting response as before, so navigating them becomes rote performance.

Because this takes more time to formulate than automatic inhibition, this second process has also been referred to in the literature as latent inhibition because the new learning acquired during exposure-based exercises inhibits still previously learned (maladaptive) emotions and their expression, such as the sequela of trauma. This is the new learning that has been added to theories of exposure (i.e., changes to beliefs; Cooper et al., 2017). Consistent with the idea that this is a more involved mental process, affect labeling has been shown to bolster this long-term habituation (Kircanski et al., 2012; Marks et al., 2019; see Chapter 6). This kind of learning may even be tangentially related to still more complex modeling of reality, as in personal meaning making. Although, the part here that pertains to habituation would be the degree to which certain facets of one's place in the world (i.e., narrative coherence, identity) are taken for granted as reliable and predictable (see Chapter 21).

The two subprocesses of what is referred to as habituation (i.e., short-term inhibition and long-term expectancy changes) unfold either separately or concurrently. In practice, however, they may reflect within-session and between-session aspects of habituation. I treated a middle-aged woman who had a long career as a bank manager and had suffered the misfortune of being a victim of not only one but two violent robberies within an 18-month period. The second attack involved being shot at, point-blank, through bulletproof glass, the back part of which shattered onto her and sent her to the hospital. When she came for treatment, she was having panic attacks at the sight of people wearing hooded sweatshirts and was unable to approach a cash register, even as a customer, in any store. The very brief treatment was behavioral, habituating the client to the stimuli that evoked her debilitating distress.

We looked at pictures of people wearing hoodies, we counted people wearing them in the hospital lobby, and by the end, we both wore hoodies and walked through hospital hallways with our heads covered. She habituated over short intervals to each of these exercises, suggesting automatic inhibition. Other aspects of working with this pointed toward a change in expectancies. For example, she joked and referred to the hoodie as our "therapy uniform," playfully musing, "I wonder if all these other hooded people are in therapy too?" After several weeks of behavioral homework, she stopped noticing the garment.

Graded in vivo exposure over several sessions moved her closer and closer to the hospital cafeteria's cash register. Eventually, she was able to wait in line and purchase something and even spent time imagining herself as the cashier. These exercises restored her expectations about what should happen when someone approaches a cash register and the usual, banal exchange of money that would ensue. The short treatment was almost entirely about downregulating the excessive arousal that prevented her from functioning. The pattern of reduced arousal and good outcome probably correspond to a summation of both the short- and long-term mechanisms that support habituation. The attenuation of the client's arousal over time preceded symptom reduction and was likely the result of progressive automatic inhibition (rendering certain stimuli meaningless) or the more conscious shifting of expectancies (from negative to neutral or positive).

Using Behavioral Coping Skills: "I Have a Strategy for Managing This!"

Clients often enter therapy asking for coping skills or strategies to manage their problems. Avoidance and habituation may occur implicitly and even outside the individual's conscious awareness. But another way to down-regulate emotion is by making a deliberate choice to use a behavioral strategy that one has learned and practiced in anticipation of crisis. These prescribed activities and skills may involve such things as actively choosing to avoid or delay engagement when one feels too vulnerable, actively doing things to calm oneself down (e.g., taking a hot bath, listening to soft music), or practicing mindfulness to psychologically distance oneself from the evocative content. Notice that this management of difficult emotion is a second step, one that follows the initial generation of an emotion. Skills training involves learning to respond to distressing circumstances in a prescribed way. These are often generic strategies (i.e., universal tools) intended for all clients and for a range of situations. The aim of skills training is to replace unhealthy or destructive behaviors with more skillful ones to be used when one is in the throes of intolerable distress. Ideally, skills are also practiced until they are automatized and become integrated into the fabric of one's everyday response repertoire (see top row of Table 2.1).

Is Working With Emotion a Skill?

The distinction between "skills training" and "process work" (e.g., meaning making) is sometimes used divisively between treatment approaches, but I suggest this is often more a matter of perspective and pedagogy rather than an immovable distinction between treatments. Examples of a skill-based approach are widespread in behavioral treatments (e.g., as championed in DBT; Linehan, 2015), but they also appear, albeit less often, in humanistic–experiential treatments (e.g., focusing; Gendlin, 1996). So what makes something a skill? Rather than being inherent to a treatment approach, whether working with emotion can be conceptualized as a skill seems to depend on at least two issues.

The first issue is how explicitly clients are instructed to do something and then practice it. Explicit instructions, however, cannot be taken for granted and need to be formulated as such. So the teachability of a change process necessarily has to do with how complex it is, whereby highly complex change processes (e.g., the relational experience) are neither easily manualized nor highly teachable. For what it is worth, the teachability of a change process is also related to its commodification.[9] In sum, whether something is a skill has a lot to do with whether the content has yet been distilled and adequately packaged into a textbook-like format. It is difficult to anticipate what might one day be rendered a teachable skill. Ultimately, this is about the translation of knowledge from science and technology for public consumption, which takes many iterations. Consider, for example, that Isaac Newton's theory of gravity was once three large volumes but now essentially fits into a single chapter of a high school textbook.

The second issue is that a skills-based treatment is often contingent on whether the work itself is believed to happen primarily within the session (e.g., a lived experience and insight) or between sessions (e.g., homework and practicing skills). For example, if a treatment theory posits that the client needs a corrective emotional experience, then typically the aim is to generate that experience during the therapeutic hour. And correspondingly, that same treatment also typically assigns less value to practicing skills outside the target experience (Singh et al., 2021). While clients would be developing awareness and expanding their emotional repertoire during the working through of some personal issue, it seems inappropriate to refer to that implicit learning and capacity building as skills improvement, at least not in the conventional sense of teaching, learning, and practice. In contrast, if a treatment theory posits that a client's fundamental challenge is their deficit in skills, then clients will be instructed how to use those skills out in the real world and to do homework that automatizes skills use into new habits. In this way, the bulk of client change occurs by going out between sessions to apply what they have learned (Neacsiu et al., 2010; Singh et al., 2021). Even so, as processes of change come to be better understood, what were previously elusive experiential moments within a session can sometimes be distilled into follow-up exercises, if not skills practice per se. Thus, specific homework between sessions can become a natural extension of the lived experiences that were targets of within-session work (Warwar, 2024).

Behavioral Strategies to Cope With Immediate Distress
The fact that distress tolerance may reflect shortfalls across a range of different capacities for working with (i.e., processing) emotion also suggests that improving one's distress tolerance would be supported indirectly by personal development via any of the other four principles discussed in this book. However, here I focus on learning and using skills that are applied immediately and directly for tolerating and down-regulating emotional intensity.

Universal tools for short-term relief. In DBT, clients are explicitly taught strategies for dealing with critical moments of intolerable distress. Still, distress tolerance skills are a group of behavioral strategies that are functionally related yet operationally independent (Linehan, 2015). The strategies are typically one-size-fits-all prescriptions to help people endure overly intense emotion, and they may make use of initial elements from a wide range of different kinds of processing: for example, affect labeling (Chapter 6), shaping bodily expressions (Chapters 9 and 10), self-compassion (Chapter 13), mindful acceptance (Chapter 20), and reflecting on personal meaning and existential purpose (Chapter 23). Those more complex kinds of processing are selectively borrowed from and used in a piecemeal manner for the very practical and circumscribed goal of quickly reducing arousal. Meanwhile, when such processes are fully elaborated, they prove to be categorically unique kinds of processing, with process goals that are qualitatively distinct from (or even contrary to) down-regulating arousal.

Other distress tolerance skills are, in their entirety, concrete and direct forms of managing and curtailing distress, no more and no less. These include deciding to strategically avoid evocative stimuli or delay the expression of destructive anger. Highly teachable examples include TIPS, an acronym to suggest clients use (T) temperature changes (e.g., plunge one's face in cold water), engage in (I) intense exercise to calm the body (e.g., running), or use (P) paced breathing paired with muscle relaxation (e.g., diaphragmatic breathing and progressive muscle relaxation; Linehan, 2015). One could also add the use of (S) sensory stimulation to help soothe, disengage, and down-regulate the nervous system (e.g., playing calming music, rubbing moisturizer on one's feet, lighting a scented candle).[10] Critically, these are brief, generic tools that are not tailored to any individual's specific or idiosyncratic needs. They serve only one critical purpose.

Addressing specific issues, predicting positive outcomes. Studies have suggested that shoring up someone's tolerance of emotional distress using prescribed activities and skills is a promising avenue to leverage change for specific concerns. The empirical evidence for this comes in several forms: administering behavioral strategies as a stand-alone intervention to reduce someone's distress, teaching individuals the skills to tolerate distress on their own, and providing skills training as an adjunct to more elaborate treatment packages.

As individuals with dementia suffer worsening symptoms, they can sometimes become intensely agitated for prolonged periods of time. The expression of this distress may be crying, screaming, or yelling obscenities. Sadly, people with dementia often also lose the capacity to soothe or calm themselves. Pharmacological interventions, however, do not work as well as psychological and behavioral interventions for reducing the agitation and aggression of adults with dementia. A meta-analysis of 148 studies highlighted the importance of interdisciplinary care, noting that optimal interventions entail sensorimotor soothing in the form of massage and touch therapy, which can also be combined with soothing music. These are interventions administered to assist individuals with their distress tolerance. They have a large effect and are more efficacious than medication and care as usual (J. A. Watt et al., 2019).

Regulating emotional intensity through learned skills has also garnered empirical support as a mechanism of change, particularly for clients who suffer from episodes of intense negative affect. Distress tolerance has been taught in the form of stand-alone skills training to help clients in treatment for substance abuse. In a randomized clinical trial, clients who received six sessions of skills training in distress tolerance showed greater improvements on behavioral measures of distress tolerance than clients who received an equal number of supportive counseling sessions or treatment as usual. Clients in the distress tolerance training also enjoyed larger clinical improvements than those in the other treatments (Bornovalova et al., 2012).

When skills training is integrated into a larger treatment package, behavioral strategies continue to be process predictors of outcome. A review of all available meta-analyses on change processes in cognitive behavior therapy (CBT) showed that behavioral strategies (including exposure and activation, but also activity scheduling and contingency management) have small to large positive effects specifically for anxiety disorders, panic disorders, and obsessive-compulsive disorder (Kazantzis et al., 2018). Anger management treatment is a group therapy based on CBT for which skills training is an important component. When veterans with posttraumatic stress disorder were treated using this approach, improvement specifically in their self-calming skills predicted large decreases in anger symptoms by the end of treatment, whereas gains in other kinds of regulatory skills (e.g., cognitive coping, behavioral control) did not predict a decrease in symptoms (Mackintosh et al., 2014).

The ability to behaviorally regulate emotion has also been identified as a key mechanism of change in the treatment of BPD, whether from CBT or DBT approaches (Rudge et al., 2020). Furthermore, there is reason to believe that when individuals with BPD improve in DBT, the degree to which they experience intense emotion may not change so much; rather, their improvement may be explained by having a new ability to skillfully disengage when they feel intolerably intense emotion (Lynch et al., 2006).

A study that randomized individuals to either DBT or a control treatment showed that although all participants reported using some DBT-type skills before the beginning of treatment. By the end of their respective treatments, those in DBT were using three times more skills than participants in the control treatment (Neacsiu et al., 2010). This supports the understanding that a skills-based treatment helps clients by fostering their learning and use of concrete behavioral skills for managing distress. Moreover, the study found that using skills fully mediated a client's decrease over time in suicide attempts, decrease in depression, and improvements to their anger control while partially mediating the occurrence of nonsuicidal self-injurious behavior. Of course, behavioral skills could have an impact in several ways, so research has also measured self-reported improvements in distress tolerance to explore it as a mechanism in 20 sessions of DBT skills training (Zeifman et al., 2020). Improvements in distress tolerance indirectly mediated the relationship between skills training and psychopathology, suggesting the training in skills leads to good clinical outcomes by increasing a person's tolerance of their painful emotion.

Finally, knowing one is proficient in a set of strategies, an emergency tool kit of skills, is itself likely to offer a reassurance that helps moderate distress in much the same way as having any established practice for self-care. DBT typically offers clients in a suicidal crisis the option of calling a therapist for immediate skills coaching. In taking such a call, one of the first questions a therapist would ask is, "What skills have you tried, so far?" If the client says, "None, I'm too upset!" the therapist might say, "Okay, right now while we are on the phone, I want you to go get your skills training book." In short, determining an immediate strategy to mitigate risk also entails orienting the client to the wealth of resources offered by a skills-based approach. The implicit message is clear: "You are in a program that works, so let's do the program." This narrative context is also part of what bolsters skills training.

ENDNOTES

1. Here, a trembling upper lip is taken as a sign of fear, hence stiff upper lip.
2. As stated in the Introduction, to respect the privacy and dignity of clients, all case examples in this book have been anonymized through masking or modification of identifying variables, are composites of several cases, or are hypothetical examples.
3. More complex forms of psychological distancing involve reframing and narrative sets, signaling another kind of process, which is discussed in Chapter 20. The two kinds of processes are often conflated.
4. The study also has implications for working with athletes because it highlights situations that call for exploring and expressing emotion. Cognitive and behavioral interventions that encourage athletes to control and manage their distress (i.e., reduce emotion) are easily the dominant approach in sports psychology today. However, there is a strong rationale for adding interventions that focus on working with emotion through principles (see Tamminen & Watson, 2022).
5. Sometimes the term "systematic desensitization" is used to describe "systematic exposure," which is a cause of confusion. "Desensitization" should refer to a hypothesized process of action. Meanwhile a therapist intervention (i.e., some sort of exposure) would have led to that reduced sensitivity. Regrettably, some authors have used the hypothesized process to denote the intervention protocol (e.g., as in "systematic desensitization therapy").
6. In perceptual processing of external stimuli, there may be differences at the level of neurotransmission. Desensitization does not involve input gating, which is the degree to which information is taken into working memory (Poon & Young, 2006). Desensitization is no longer noticing the input, like having a sensory firewall that filters out stimuli. By contrast, habituation is no longer attending to or making use of that input. This distinction is less useful for understanding emotional experiences, which are already internal phenomena.
7. *Reciprocal inhibition* and its longer term effect of *counterconditioning* describe the attenuation of symptom distress when exposure is done in the presence of antagonistic inhibition, meaning that the exposure stimulus is paired with some opposite kind of experience. However, this conflates the very separate constructs of (a) inhibition with (b) antagonistic processes. I address this in Chapter 12, where I argue that counterconditioning is an oversimplification and better explained in terms of a more complex process described as emotional sequences.
8. Classical theories of habituation state that it is a nonassociative learning process, although that is now debated.
9. As evidenced by efforts to trademark psychotherapy brands and skills training (e.g., Linehan's DBT). Another example of ready commodification is the packaging of various treatment facets into online training modules.
10. DBT has enumerated an accessible and comprehensive list of strategies for helping clients stop, disengage, and immediately relieve a moment of excess arousal. "TIP" is one of these skills. However, to complete the illustration, I add the use of sensory experience (i.e., the S in TIPS), which is consistent with DBT practice at large.

II

NOTICE THE FEELING

INTRODUCTION: NOTICE THE FEELING

Meaning making is the product of a moment-by-moment process in which one makes sense of one's lived experience, and it can be thought of at several epistemological levels.[1] Consider, for example, how these levels unfold as subjective moments: When you start to have a feeling, you automatically orient toward it. Then you might also choose to attend a bit more to the sensation, your attention lingers, and you allow the feeling to happen. You have now engaged the emotional experience. Of course, alternatively, you might have recoiled and taken steps to avoid the feeling rather than engage with it. Acknowledging this implicit choice highlights that engagement is not always the starting point for working with emotion. Recall (from Chapter 3) that purposeful disengagement and adaptive avoidance are also concrete operations for working with emotion—to reduce its intensity.

In any case, if you did lean into an emergent feeling, the next process moment is when you start to search for a word or label that best captures your emotion (*affect labeling*). As you elaborate on that immediate level of meaning, you start to create a more elaborate portrait of it: for example, "What's happening inside? What's it's like to be me, at this moment?" Tacitly exploring such questions renders a more complex symbolization of your lived experience. Symbolizing the feeling effectively changes it, because even a tentative model helps render a vague sensation into a more specific point of reference. All of these—engagement, affect labeling, symbolization, and deepening the experience of a feeling—are aspects of *emotional awareness,* in order of increasing complexity. These are the topics covered in Part II of this book (Chapters 4 to 7).

While phrases like "the body knows" or "trust your gut" have some value, they are mostly nonchalant simplifications that offer little in the way of instruction. Attending to one's visceral sensations is only the first step in an array of process events because, ultimately, looking inward is also about formulating a certain kind of meaning. Implicit and embodied meaning are the seed of some affective experience that still needs to be unpacked and elaborated into a specific symbolization, one that goes beyond the visceral sensations that imply it. *Emotional awareness* is a group of processes for working with emotion that includes (in order of increasing complexity) emotional engagement, then labeling emotion, and finally, meaning symbolization. So making meaning from awareness is about drawing out and explicating the tacit significance of an immediate feeling (e.g., You notice a feeling . . . but what is that about? What "flavor" is it, and what might it mean?). One can think of emotional awareness, heuristically, as clarifying the boundaries that discriminate an emergent feeling, shifting it from a blurry or fuzzy experience to a sharper delineation as depicted in Figure II.1.

FIGURE II.1. Notice the Feeling: The Principle of Emotional Awareness

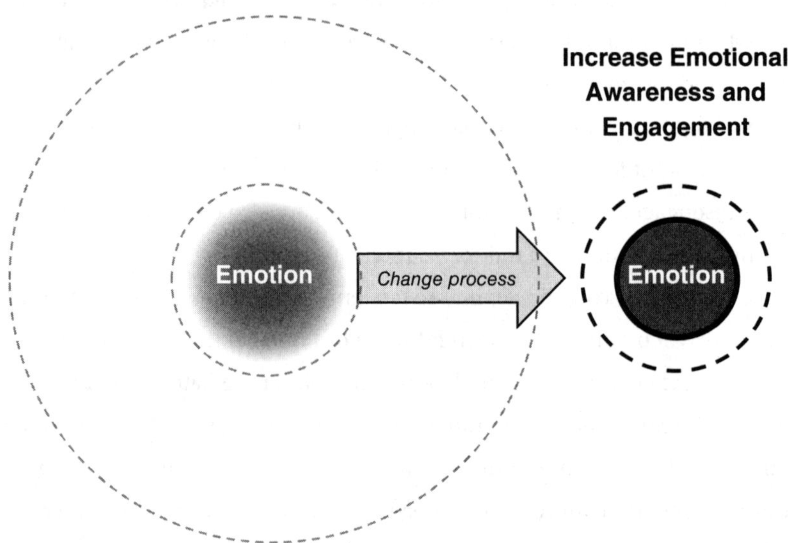

Note. Emotional awareness is a principle that involves increasing the degree to which one attends to and clarifies one's emotional experiences. The process is depicted here as the felt experience moving from blurry and out of focus, to an experience that has become clearly defined as an emotion. This is one of five categorically different processes that change emotion.

There are other processes that are relevant but not addressed in this part of the book. For example, awareness at large is contextualized within the notion of consciousness, one of the great mysteries of psychology. Basic research on consciousness, however, goes beyond the scope of this book. Meaning making also continues beyond basic emotional awareness, involving still other principles of change. For example, the arousal of emotion is a separate process, although it can certainly amplify your awareness. Still later on, pondering the experience, you might develop a plot with characters to formulate some narrative: "What happened and what does this feeling mean to me within the story of my life?" There is a slippery continuum of processes between these graded kinds of meaning making, yet they represent different moments in an overarching effort to make sense of one's felt experience.

The problem I focus on in this part of the book is the way emotional awareness, in and of itself, serves as a principle of change when working through personal difficulties. Chapter 4 begins by presenting an overview of conceptual issues related to the general construct, measurement, and the clinical relevance of emotional awareness. Chapters 5–7 give more applied descriptions, explaining the mechanisms at work. There, I piece together the evidence supporting separate pathways of action through which engaging and expanding emotional awareness leads to positive personal change. The four mechanisms to be laid out are as follows:

- Engaging emotion opens up a new source of information (see Chapter 5).

- Labeling emotion turns it into a point of reference, which can either regulate or further differentiate it (see Chapter 6).

- Deepening the experience of an emotion enriches its meaning (see Chapter 7).

- Symbolizing emotion changes the feeling and generates a sense of direction (see Chapter 7).

Over the chapters that follow, I explain each of these potential mechanisms of emotional awareness, highlighting their relevance to research on therapeutic change, and explicate some of the psychological or neurological processes that support them.

ENDNOTE

1. See also Chapters 4 and, particularly, 17 for an elaboration of how meaning making might be created at various epistemological levels.

4

Emotional Awareness

From Engagement to Symbolization

[One] has information about one's experience only to the extent that one has tended to communicate it to another or thought about it in the manner of communicative speech. Much of that which is ordinarily said to be repressed is merely unformulated.

—DONNEL B. STERN, *UNFORMULATED EXPERIENCE*

Consider for a moment how the image in a picture might be blurry, not just the background or some facet, but the entire image is blurred and out of focus. Making sense of a blurred image might serve as an analogy to navigating a personal concern using a very limited level of emotional awareness. Without a sharply delineated sense of what one is feeling, one would also have trouble labeling it. Perhaps one would describe the experience as "bad feelings and stuff like that." At a moment like this, increasing emotional awareness would serve as a moment-by-moment process of change. First, the lived experience is simply given more attention, and then it is brought into focus. In this way, the present feeling becomes clearer, rendering a sharper image of what is happening. It also becomes easier to find just the right word or image to symbolize that feeling. As a result, the feeling could also become more poignant and the "handle" one was using to label it might ring truer, affirming one's sense of what is happening here and now—and even some of what that means. This is emotional awareness in action.

Parts of this chapter are based on A. Pascual-Leone and Greenberg (2007b).

https://doi.org/10.1037/0000460-005
Principles of Emotion Change: What Works and When in Psychotherapy and Everyday Life, by A. Pascual-Leone
Copyright © 2026 by the American Psychological Association. All rights reserved.

WHAT IS AWARENESS? WHEN IS IT IMPORTANT?

As a construct, emotional awareness can be thought of as a continuum of closely related processes. The first inkling of emergent awareness is often just some acknowledgment of one's engagement, that one is having an emotional experience of some kind. Later, more extended, and deeper levels of awareness inevitably lead one to try making sense of that burgeoning experience, often capturing it in words. As one appreciates the fuller significance of what is being labeled, that symbolization may bloom into a rich portrayal of personal meaning. In any case, the essence of *emotional awareness*, as a process, is attending to and clarifying an emergent feeling at the same time as it is being experienced.

When to Focus on Increasing Awareness: What Are the Markers of Dysfunction?

Insight-oriented therapies are founded on the assumption that increasing client awareness of experience (usually the origins, meaning, and consequences of emotion) is an important change process. But specifically facilitating emotional awareness is a critical process at key moments in treatment, and identifying the need for that process is part of an ongoing moment-by-moment case formulation. In short, therapists should use interventions to deliberately promote their client's emotional awareness when the change process is at an impasse and when it becomes clear the client has a poor sense of direction, a lack of behavioral intentionality, or a lack of clarity on what they want. This is because one reason emotional difficulties may remain unresolved is a lack of awareness about the meaning behind one's uncomfortable feelings, or because emergent emotions are being suppressed or actively avoided, which often also leaves people numb and desensitized.

Provided that clients are willing to engage in feeling *more*, another key distinction that should be made early in case formulation is whether the object of distress is clearly identified. In other words, the client may feel upset but be unable to identify what specifically is upsetting them in the situation (e.g., regarding some story, the client reports just that "something about it is painful"). If the object of distress is still vague, the client should explore, deepen, and differentiate emotion. While some of this can be covert, clients who need greater clarity should also explicitly label and organize their ongoing experience out loud. The goal in performing these tasks and in increasing emotional awareness is ultimately to use emotion as means for focusing one's attention and psychological resources to moving the construction of meaning from general body-based perceptions to increasingly specific and dynamic insights about oneself in the world (i.e., emotion within some context of meaning).

Nevertheless, there are also moments in session when increasing emotional awareness is bad for treatment, and at those moments, interventions that target awareness are counterindicated. For example, if arousal is very high and emotional experience is already too intense, then facilitating further awareness will often be evocative and exacerbate a client's distress. To complicate matters, some strategies for regulating emotion are predicated on a modicum of emotional awareness, but if arousal is already intolerable and disorganizing, then some transitional regulation through distraction or suppression (i.e., the antithesis of expanding awareness) may be preferred.

Another counterindication of emotional awareness could be described as emotions in *pseudo-transformation*—when clients change too quickly from one emotion to another, which may have a somewhat dramatized quality or may simply be a shot of wishful thinking (e.g., "I say I 'deserve to be loved,' but deep down, what I feel is how desperately I yearn for it and how I wish it were true"). This kind of surface-level processing does not allow the natural wave of emotional experience to be complete (what D. N. Stern, 2010, referred to as a *vitality curve*), creating a shallow experience with little depth to explore. If this happens, clients should be encouraged to stay with the feeling before they hastily move to subsequent thoughts or feelings. While both breadth and depth are necessary, when it comes to emotional awareness, breadth must never come at the expense of depth. Finally, inauthentic emotional experiences, often involving manipulative interpersonal objectives, should not be engaged as targets of deeper emotional awareness. As discussed in the Introduction, instrumental emotions are inauthentic or feigned emotions, but they often still have elements of genuine experience. Nonetheless, these are counterindications for deepening emotional awareness because doing so encourages clients to invest more heavily in expressions that do not directly tap into deeper intrapersonal meaning.[1]

First, Get in Touch; Second, Find the Words

There is an affective tone to every conscious moment (Wundt, 1897/1998). However, the depth with which one explores that emotion is a critical issue that has long been discussed in psychodynamic and humanistic therapies alike, and while this has not been discussed explicitly in cognitive therapies, it is clearly a valued process related to rational insights (Samoilov & Goldfried, 2000). As Gendlin (1996) discussed it, the critical issue about new awareness is that it is on the edge of the client's emerging experience, what he called the *leading edge*. The key point is that activated emotion is always on the frontier of emerging experience. This is due to the orienting function of emotion. Nobody gets emotional about things that are not important to them. So, whenever there is emotion, it points to something of significance, even if at first one is unsure why it may be significant. (Of course, not everything on the leading edge of experience is necessarily emotionally activated; there also may be rational insights, associations, etc.) However, one of the advantages of exploring emotion is that affect provides a sort of divining rod (or compass), orienting clients toward critically relevant content and helping attuned therapists identify where to deepen or focus the exploration process. In this way, emotion can be used as a marker or signpost, one that says, "look over here!" Following that thread, the poignancy with which content is delivered is the most direct way to determine what the core issues of treatment should be. Emotion is a means to an even more profound end: some newly unfolding experience and better understanding oneself or one's situation.

Awareness does not involve just thinking about a feeling but rather consciously feeling the feeling and accepting it as part of an emergent experience.[2] In fact, a study comparing therapists in interpersonal therapy and cognitive behavior therapy of depression concluded that essentially two factors described therapists' style of engagement in these treatments: "collaborative emotional exploration" and "educative/directive process" (Coombs et al., 2002). Collaborative emotional exploration related positively to outcome in both forms of therapy, whereas educative/directive process had no relationship to outcome (which puts into question whether it was really valuable learning). These findings point toward exploration of emotion as centrally important to good therapy regardless of theoretical orientation. Similarly, emotional awareness does not necessarily involve an elaboration of contextual information on the origins, meanings, or consequences of the target emotion (something that is indeed valuable but better captured by another process called reflection on emotion; see Chapter 17).

Stages of Awareness

There are two categorically distinct stages to facilitating this deeper emotional awareness-in-feeling, and these offer a working definition of emotional awareness. The first stage of awareness is getting in touch with emotion, which refers to the initial discovery of feeling and an affective impulse. This stage of awareness is sometimes referred to as *emotional engagement.* (Sometimes heightening arousal can also help here, but that would be a synergistic blending of different processes; I address arousal in the next section and expound upon it fully in Chapter 9.) Gestalt therapy captures this with the notion of making contact between the boundaries of one's internal and external worlds and gauging one's relationship to an emergent experience as either "too close" or "too far" (i.e., the presence of feeling as too intense, too evocative, or too immersive vs. disconnected, disembodied, or even disavowed). Furthermore, when exploring new feelings and memories, a person's attention is naturally drawn to personally meaningful and affectively charged material (i.e., the *internally lived story*), not simply behaviors or events (i.e., just *plot and characters*). We can think of this as a definition of getting in touch with emotion, and it is a requirement for incipient to moderate levels of emotional awareness. In short, it is the deliberate act of affective engagement.

The second stage of awareness is finding the right words, and it involves labeling emotion and the richer *symbolization of meaning.* Sometimes, this second stage has been inadequately thought of as (external) *exposure* to new information, but that understanding overlooks the deeper aspect of what psychological engagement really means, which is the (internal) *generation* of new information. After initial engagement, this second stage of awareness involves producing deliberate and creative descriptions of one's immediate experience. So, initially, awareness consists of deliberately searching inward to access memories, images, beliefs, feelings, desires, values, and bodily sensations, but in the second stage, formulating and symbolizing these facets of experience into words is essential. In short, on one hand, *experiencing* is the process of attending to the ongoing but unverbalized visceral flow, while on the other hand, it involves using that stream of lived experience as a referent against which one checks tentative symbolizations of meaning. This reciprocal process leads to the recursive discovery (i.e., generation) of meanings about what one is feeling and its significance (Gendlin, 1996). Tentatively symbolizing these experiences is what allows them to be integrated into one's existing perspectives and is what moves the process of change forward.

The Forward Shift

There is a dialectical relationship between the two stages of emerging experience and the symbolization of that previously tacit experience. Creating awareness is the process of accepting, capturing, and progressively articulating "that which is there." Rogers (1959) described a *forward shift* in awareness as having as a productive process and having four qualities:

> (1) It is not a thinking about something, it is an experience of something at this instant in the relationship. (2) It is consciously feeling as much as one feels, without holding back and without exaggeration. (3) This is the first time it has been experienced completely. (4) The experience is welcomed and acceptable to the client. (pp. 52–53)

A therapeutic shift of this kind captures the newness of awareness as an experience-near insight. Thus, I refer to *awareness* as the emerging symbolization of meaning from an ongoing flow of experience.

Awareness Versus Arousal: Entwined Processes

In either clinical writing or process research, aroused "expression" is all too often used as a proxy or conceptual shorthand when moment-by-moment symbolic representation is the sharper issue at hand. While increasing arousal can help boost emotional awareness, it is important not to conflate these change processes, as they require different interventions and will be used for different treatment purposes. The meaning making involved in emotional awareness is not the same as the core process in emotional expression, which may or may not involve a well-differentiated symbolic representation. Awareness is about exploring emerging experience, while arousal is about energy and action.

To complicate matters further, increasing awareness often requires some minimum degree of arousal and immersion into bad feelings, whereby one actually contacts the emotional pain and is accepting of that experience. Again, these conditions are fundamental to the effectiveness of exposure-based procedures. This is also the assumption underlying the posited change processes of emotional insight and challenging "hot cognitions" (Coombs et al., 2002).

Nevertheless, although the importance of emotional awareness is acknowledged by varying approaches to psychotherapy, emotions associated with psychological distress are frequently suppressed or avoided such that clients feel flat or numb, which poses an obstacle to emotional awareness. In these instances, deliberately increasing arousal is productive, not for cathartic purposes but rather to activate the emotion and thereby increase awareness of the information associated with that experience (for more on this, see Chapter 9). However, intentional engagement with "feeling bad" is difficult for clients. Moreover, when a client's arousal increases in a session, therapists who have not been explicitly trained to engage affective arousal can similarly become anxious and abandon the task of expanding emotional awareness. In turn, the truncation of an emerging awareness is sometimes perceived by clients as invalidating and may reinforce their avoidance.

In contrast, therapy that focuses on building a client's capacity for emotional awareness helps a client approach, tolerate, and accept emotions instead of avoiding them (L. S. Greenberg, 2021). Therapists model approaching and valuing emotion by empathically attuning to client's experience and avoiding theoretical talk and external narratives. The client learns that emotion is important and acceptable and starts to attend more inwardly to experience.

EMOTIONAL EXPLORATION IN CONCRETE TERMS

While many clinicians will have a sense of what Rogers (1959) was trying to describe as "consciously feeling as much as one feels," it still begs some concretization in operational terms. How does one know when a client is becoming fully emotionally aware? What does that mean in terms of content? Answering this requires one to consider the nature of emotion. Affective events are encoded as a multimodal network of information (i.e., a scheme or structure), and experiencing emotion entails activating the scheme to deliberately explore its components. When a client definitively states that he feels a certain way (e.g., "Well, it's just embarrassing, nothing else"), many therapists who are learning to work with emotion have difficulty knowing how to explore the issue further. So the therapy process gets stuck or becomes redundant. Therapist and client are sometimes at a loss about where else to go (e.g., After all, the client already said how he feels, so what else is there left to explore?). However, labeling emotion is only one part of the awareness process. This is because most of the elements in an emotional experience are tacit, and the unpacking or elaborating of such tacit information, or meaning, is an integral part of a client fully experiencing their emotion and its significance.

Five Facets of an Emotional Experience

To describe the components of an emotional experience in response to a given situation, researchers (L. S. Greenberg & Korman, 1993; Pos et al., 2003) focused on segments in therapy when clients disclosed past or present emotional experiences. Although this was initially intended as a research strategy, being familiar with the essential components of these kinds of moments can provide direction for therapists intending to explore a client's feelings beyond simply labeling them. Accordingly, when a client refers to a particular feeling (e.g., sad, happy, afraid, embarrassed), the given emotion usually entails five elements or facets of experience, each of which might be a point for further exploration in session: (a) situation or interpersonal context, (b) action tendency, (c) somatic component, (d) unmet existential or interpersonal needs, and (e) concern regarding the self (or self in relation to other).

Situation or Interpersonal Context

The situation or interpersonal context is some stimulus or circumstances of the emotion (e.g., Client: "I failed in my marriage" or "My mother left me alone"). What has triggered or released the generation of the emergent state is typically an external cue (e.g., Client: "the smell in the hospital waiting room"), a facet of some event, the evocative aspect of an interpersonal encounter (e.g., Client: "the way he sneered when he said goodbye"), or an associated fragment of meaning. In some cases, emotion appears to emerge without the client's understanding of the situation or context; in other cases the situation is salient, while the person has only a vague sense of the feeling that has started to organize them.

Action Tendency

Since one of the purposes of emotion, evolutionarily speaking, is to organize one for some response or behavior, emotional experiences are almost always accompanied by some kind of action, an impetus toward action. In fact, sometimes clients first present an action tendency (e.g., Client: "I wanted to crawl into bed and pull the covers over my head").

Somatic Component

Emotions are "embodied" (Damasio, 1999), and working with the somatic component of emotion is particularly elaborated in focusing, gestalt, and experiential body-based therapies. Unlike action tendencies, these somatic elements are not usually indicative of particular goal-oriented behavior. Rather, as described by Gendlin (1996), these represent a preverbal aspect of meaning that can be captured in metaphors or images (e.g., Client: "I have butterflies in my stomach" or "I feel warm inside, imagining her beside me"). "Focusing" (Gendlin, 1996) is a technique that can be especially useful for elaborating affective meanings via the somatic component of an experience.

Unmet Existential or Interpersonal Needs

When emotions are differentiated enough, they organize us for action toward some implicit goal. Thus, therapists need to be attuned to core existential and often interpersonal needs that drive affective and cognitive goal-oriented behavior. The verbal symbolization of existential and/or interpersonal needs is pivotal in the full elaboration of the meaning of these experiences (e.g., Client: "I needed love, affection, even just some acknowledgment that I was there!" or "I was not put here to be mistreated. I have a right, and I must, be who I am!"). While the unmet need is a common focus in emotion-focused therapy, a similar notion is captured by the unfulfilled *wish* described in many psychodynamic therapies.

Concern Regarding the Self (or Self in Relation to Other)

The articulation of self-related difficulties (e.g., feelings of insecurity, worthlessness, or harsh self-criticism) usually emerges as the client explores the effects that difficult experiences have had on personal identity, hopefulness, and relatedness to others (e.g., Client: "Maybe I'm just an angry person; I wish I weren't that way" or "I just don't bring enough to the table"). In many cases, at a deeper level this is essentially the core dysfunctional belief that is the focus of many cognitive behavioral interventions. Concerns about the self are usually relatively easy to access in clients who are already emotionally aroused (Nardone et al., 2022). Sometimes it is sufficient to guide a client from the circumstances of the situation to focusing more on the personal ramifications it may have (e.g., Client: "She just stood there and watched him beat the crap out of me!" Therapist: "So, somehow that says something about both of you—the fact that she didn't intervene?"; as cited in A. Pascual-Leone, Paivio, & Harrington, 2016, p. 171).

Talking Points for Therapists

Awareness of these five aspects of an emotion can be a useful framework for therapists in deciding where and how to explore further when the process gets stuck and clients present their feelings as deceivingly straightforward. At the most basic level, these are essentially talking points for therapists, different avenues to explore, rather than repeatedly asking clients "What do you feel?" Furthermore, because these elements of an emotion scheme are linked together in a network, elaborating one such facet of experience can lead to each of the others. So one might also think of each of these elements as different doorways or access points for entering and activating an emotional experience. Addressing each of these facets presents a potential avenue for further emotional awareness.

What Is Deep Emotional Experiencing?

Experiencing first came to be recognized as a salient factor in therapy within the context of client-centered and focusing-oriented psychotherapies. Initially, Rogers (1959) brought up the concept of "experiencing" in describing the client's active exploration of their perceptual field. Several years later, he defined the goal of successful therapy as helping the client reach optimal personality functioning by becoming open to experience as it constantly changes during the process of living. In describing the therapeutic transitions of the client from being closed to opening, or from rigid to fluid, Rogers highlighted the need for *deeper* experiencing that entailed increased awareness, acceptance of feelings, and use of emotional information for further exploration. Pathology was understood as being associated with low levels of experiencing, while growth and change was associated with increased experiencing.

Gendlin, who was a student of Rogers, approached psychotherapy sessions as an in-the-moment source of phenomenological processes (Gendlin, 1981). He observed his client's use of the session as a space to reflect on incipient (often preverbal) thoughts and gut feelings as they emerged during the interaction and how clients used this new understanding to create further meaning about themselves and their world. His major observation was that it was not only the content of discussion but also the *manner* of experiencing that content that was significant (i.e., highlighting experience rather than conceptual knowledge). Thus, *depth of experiencing* defines the degree to which clients engage and explore their feelings moment by moment as part of the process of personal meaning making (Gendlin, 1996).

Over the past 60 years, a sizable amount of research has examined the relationship between "experiential depth" and therapeutic outcome. This in-session process emerges moment by moment and describes the degree of a *client's involvement in the exploration of new feelings and meanings* in relation to the self (L. S. Greenberg & Safran, 1987; Hendricks, 2009). Several measures have been used to help define this intrapersonal process, although the most widely used has been the Client Experiencing Scale first manualized in 1969 (Klein et al., 1986). This tool has been instrumental in defining and operationalizing the concept of experiential awareness. Clinicians well versed in this observational measure are able to appraise their client's depth of experiencing in vivo during a session, and thus it has also found its way into the appendices of several treatment manuals for humanistic–experiential therapies. Furthermore, this specific measure has been used to study a diverse range of treatment approaches, reaching well beyond humanistic–experiential therapies, and it is the single most widely used measure of good in-session process. Indeed, given the narrative reviews and conclusive summaries that appear in a number of psychotherapy handbooks, the depth of client experiencing has been regarded by process researchers as the gold standard of good psychotherapy process.

The shallow end of the scale (i.e., lower ratings) captures unengaged levels of experiencing, wherein clients recount external events in a removed and neutral manner. Thus, at low levels of experiencing, the speaker refers primarily to "plot and characters" (the external narrative of events), and disclosure of *subjective* experience is conspicuously absent. For example, Level 1: "My dad was the kind of person who yelled a lot," or Level 2: "Someone in my shoes wouldn't be too happy."

In contrast, middle levels of the experiencing scale include a reference to the self or to one's internal experiences such as behavioral reactions, feelings, or emotion.

- Level 3 represents an *initial emotional awareness* and may have an unelaborated reference to feeling: for example, "I feel like kicking something" or "When I got the letter, I just felt really sad, that's all."

- Level 4 tends to reflect a more *elaborated emotional awareness*, a rich portrait of the client's internal world: for example, "I feel resentful about the feedback, it's unfair, and it leaves me with a bitter taste in my mouth" or "I've never been so hurt. . . . When I think of her, it feels like broken glass inside."

At deeper levels (i.e., high ratings), clients become more introspective as they begin to question, formulate, and process newly emerging experiences to create fresh meanings in the moment (Klein et al., 1986). The deeper levels of experiencing go beyond simple narration of events and do not stop at vague or general references to inner experience. Instead, clients are actively engaged in the experiential process, using present tense while they search to formulate a newly emergent meaning. Longer pauses and using metaphors to describe one's experience are an increasingly common part of this deep experiencing:

- Level 5: "I proposed we get married but then when my partner started talking about actual dates, I got this lump in my throat . . . like noticing the tip of an iceberg, an iceberg of fear. It's weird, I thought I wasn't affected by my history but now . . . I wonder if it'll haunt me?"

- Level 6: "I've usually put myself second because I always played 'helper' in my family. I would have this embarrassing sense sometimes that somehow the whole family would fall apart if I didn't take care of my parents. Mom and Dad seemed so incompetent that I always ended up holding the bag."

  Another example is the following: "Actually, since we are talking about it that way, I feel a kind of spark coming up inside, like a little voice that says, 'Hey, wait a minute! I'm not putting up with this!' It's just like these gentle sparks, but it's a *good* feeling."

- Level 7: "Looking back, it's kind of bittersweet. It's sad I had to live through that. . . . At the same time, I'm different now, so I know I can handle most situations."

Research on observational ratings using this scale has shown that the deeper half of the client experiencing scale (e.g., Levels 4 to 7) is increasingly predictive of successful treatment outcome. However, as descriptions of this ordinal scale suggest, the levels represent *qualitative* differences. Generally, shallower (i.e., lower rated) levels of client experiencing reflect a process of approaching, exploring, and tolerating emerging emotional experience. Deeper (higher rated) levels of client experiencing seem to reflect meaning making, pondering, and formulating new emotional experiences within some framework. This refinement in understanding the experiencing scale comes from qualitative appraisals made by clinical researchers in the literature and is backed by empirical support (Pos et al., 2017; Watson & Bedard, 2006).[3] Indeed, the experiencing scale was originally developed as a broad measure of how preverbal experiential meaning might be productively attended to, engaged, and symbolized (Gendlin, 1996). However, specifically in relation to emotion, different parts of the scale seem to speak to distinct subtypes of emotional processing: from *emotional awareness* (i.e., Levels 3 and 4, as discussed in this chapter) to *reflecting on emotion's* latent meaning and the significance of one's immediately emergent experience (i.e., Levels 5–7). Thus, the full range of the measure bridges more than one subtype of emotional processing (A. Pascual-Leone & Yeryomenko, 2016).

Finally, it is important to note that, although the construct of client experiencing and its corresponding scale originated from a humanistic–experiential tradition, process ratings of this kind seem to apply equally well to sessions of either cognitive behavioral or psychodynamic psychotherapies. Moreover, examining a wide range of therapies (e.g., humanistic–experiential, cognitive-behavioral, psychodynamic, interpersonal), a meta-analysis that showed client's depth of experiencing was a predictor of outcome also concluded that this relationship held, irrespective of the therapy approach being used (A. Pascual-Leone & Yeryomenko, 2016).

AWARENESS VERSUS META-AWARENESS

Awareness is a fundamental and basic perceptual process. However, as the content of awareness becomes more abstract, the process itself becomes less perceptual and more conceptual or "reflective." This becomes what one might refer to as *meta-awareness*, the awareness of one's emerging perspective (A. Pascual-Leone & Greenberg, 2007b). Meta-awareness describes a special awareness of how one perceives things or how one processes information to construct one's own experience. Thus, some types of experience-near insight involve *awareness* of discovering something new (e.g., "I experience feeling sad about a loss"). Other types of insight involve meta-awareness, the gaining of a new perspective in vivo (e.g., "I realize I put up a wall to avoid closeness") or the awareness of one's awarenesses (e.g., "I notice that I'm always attentive to any hint of abandonment"). This higher level of awareness speaks to constructs such as metacognitive functioning and mentalization, both of which refer to someone's capacity to reflect upon their own emotional experience.

Metacognition

Higher order levels of emotional awareness (e.g., meta-awareness) can also be thought of in terms of much broader mental faculties, such as metacognition, and one's general ability to reflect on or contemplate emotion. *Metacognitive functioning,* as it applies to working with emotion, entails reflecting on one's emerging process while considering the broader context of needs, personal resources, and intentions (Dimaggio et al., 2020). This way of understanding emotional awareness considers the local process within the ongoing management of mental resources and intentions, which are the operational context of "noticing a feeling in the here and now." Emotional awareness has been conceptualized in the literature at different levels of abstraction (e.g., awareness, meta-awareness, metacognition), but these constructs should be thought of as nested within one another, creating a graded continuum in how we understand the subjective experience of working with emotion.

Reflection on Emotion

Because one can construe a continuum, concepts like *mentalization* (Bateman & Fonagy, 2013) are sometimes defined so broadly as to include what I am referring to as "awareness" and "reflecting on that awareness" and even the implicit strategies for "regulating the arousal entailed during awareness"—all under a single rubric. *Reflective functioning* has been offered as an operationalization of the mentalization construct (Bateman, & Fonagy, 2013; for a critical synthesis, see also Solbakken et al., 2011). However, criticism of the mentalization construct is that it is too broad (e.g., Semerari et al., 2007). While related, "emotional awareness" and "reflection on emotion" are psychogenetically distinct operations that can each be somewhat independently applied to emotion for therapeutic effect.

Neurological evidence does seem to support the notion that "emotional awareness" and "reflection on emotion" are distinct subtypes of emotional processing. In a revealing study on the amygdala's role in emotional memory, researchers presented pictures that were either emotionally neutral or highly arousing to participants who had lesions to the medial temporal lobe including the amygdala (Adolphs, Tranel, et al., 2005). Participants were asked questions about the main gist of complex pictures (e.g., Who were the central characters? What was happening?) or about specific background details of the pictures (e.g., What did the clouds look like? What were the characters wearing?). Those with amygdala damage had impairments in memory for the gist of complex and emotion-laden pictures, but not for their details. This is consistent with the idea that the amygdala picks up on the essential characteristics of salient information (Pessoa, 2013). Furthermore, different patterns of neural activation were found for the details versus gist, and this differential effect was enhanced when the context for memory encoding was emotional. This suggests that the details of reflecting on emotion have a different neurological substrate from the main gist or relevance, which is principally related to emotional awareness. The study concluded that the amygdala focuses processing on the gist of complex stimuli, and this is true for emotional stimuli in particular, making the amygdala a key anatomical structure in emotional awareness. Finally, the different patterns of neural activation that were observed for the emotional memory of details versus gist highlights a distinction between "emotional awareness" and "reflection on emotion" as distinct subprocesses. Additional research has now also shown how different psychotherapy interventions facilitate these distinct kinds of processing at the neurological level (Wang et al., 2022). According to this perspective, both top-down and bottom-up processes are important in the process of meaning making, contributing synergistically to a client's search for meaning in a dialectical process.

Treatment interventions that target the moment-by-moment experience of emotional awareness are "experience-near," emotionally evocative; they do not necessarily involve any logical, rational, or conceptual connecting. In short, emotional awareness is primarily a bottom-up approach to the construction of new meaning (see also Chapter 17). From an experiential perspective, meaning is constructed by exploring specific personal situations in depth in order to discover what one is in fact experiencing (L. S. Greenberg, 2021). Clients are better able to "taste" their immediate experience by exploring a single experience in depth and subsequently make use of inherent, spontaneous, and adaptive self-organizing processes to promote survival and growth (L. S. Greenberg, 2021). Of course, the potential drawback of such a bottom-up approach is that clients might find it difficult to discern a pattern or theme in their lives across situations without the benefit of an external bird's-eye view. This is where the other forms of emotional processing, such as reflection on emotion, highlight the roles of reframing, decentering, and narrative reconstruction. These provide a counterpoint to the moment-by-moment process (those processes are covered in Chapters 17–23).

OBSTACLES TO THE AWARENESS PROCESS: FORMULATING THE PROBLEM

As a process in treatment, emotional awareness is sometimes taken for granted. It is so easily overlooked, until it is conspicuously missing. Furthermore, unlike regulating or reflecting on emotion, awareness is not often thought of as deliberate or effortful (although it can be). For these reasons, it is useful to consider obstacles in the development of emotional awareness, which are common. In Dickens's (1843) story *A Christmas Carol,* character Ebenezer Scrooge offers one such example when he is confronted with a ghost from his past, and then attributes his disturbing mental experience to a malfunction of his own body. He refers to this emotional experience as "a slight disorder of the stomach" and says to the ghost, "You may be an undigested bit of beef, a blot of mustard, a crumb of cheese, a fragment of underdone potato. There's more of gravy than of grave about you, whatever you are!" (p. 13). The initial confusion of indigestion with emergent emotion is a funny but classic example of poor emotional awareness, and reference to the gut–affect connection is on point. The second part of the statement ("There's more of gravy than of grave about you. . .!") also suggests the willful denial or blocking of experience, which is another obstacle to emergent emotion. These hinder emotional awareness in its function as a mechanism of therapeutic change.

Therapists should be mindful of several obstacles to facilitating awareness: (a) shallow levels of affective processing, (b) overly cognitive processing, (c) affect dysregulation, (d) suppression or avoidance of negative feelings, and (e) inauthentic experiences. Given the fundamental role of awareness, these obstacles often also interfere with other subtypes of emotional processing discussed in subsequent chapters (e.g., on expressive arousal, transformation, or reflection). In any case, when clients seem to have stifled emotional awareness, therapists can consider these issues to troubleshoot the process as they work with emotion.

Shallow Levels of Affective Processing

The shallow processing of experience reflects a limit in capacity, precluding deeper awareness, and this manifests itself in several ways. In Chapter 6, I will discuss alexithymia as the antithesis of emotional awareness, an inability to identify and symbolize emotional experience. This trait poses an individual difference in people's basic capacity, limiting their ability to engage in awareness. As such, it is not usually amenable to rapid intervention, although therapists should be reassured by studies that show poor emotional awareness (i.e., alexithymia) is not entirely intractable and seems to change as an outcome of experientially oriented therapies.

Another related reason for shallow emotional awareness is that the client may have a basic lack of interest or curiosity about their emotional life. Thus, an issue that should be clarified early on in case formulation is whether a client is interested in having a richer or more nuanced emotional life. Some clients show signs of poor emotional awareness, or they simply may not be "psychologically minded." Often, they have sociopersonal histories (related to culture, family style, general upbringing, or gender-specific socializations) that have not fostered the exploration of deeper feelings or meanings and consequentially, simply have less interest in developing that dimension of their life experience (Levant et al., 2009; Lo, 2014; McLean et al., 2007). Some of these people with limited practice in differentiating their feelings may actively dismiss their emotional experience and then report feeling numb. Consider the common example of men in psychotherapy who become visibly distressed and then begin the session by saying, "I'm tired"—when in actuality they feel "sad." Similarly, case studies describing individuals with more neurotic personality styles (Davanloo, 2005) have observed that such clients are often unable to differentiate between anxiety and anger when confronted by emotionally difficult content.

When this difficulty is very pervasive over one's lifetime, such clients may reveal they also have a thin sense of identity: "I don't know. It's not that I'm unhappy, it's just that I don't really have strong feelings either way. It's always sort of like that for me. I'm like plastic wrap." said a young client of mine. Further describing how he gropes for ephemeral emotional experiences, he continued, "There seems to be something . . . but I don't know what it is. It's like I'm trying to grab at the wind. As soon as I think I'm onto something, it's gone." These clients do not have mountains and valleys in their emotional landscape, but they do have bumps and little dents. It will be part of the therapist's work to notice the divots in a client's emotional life, bring attention to them by mirroring this texture of experience, and then magnify it for the client so the experience becomes increasingly palpable.

Thus, the challenge for psychotherapy becomes how to "work with emotion" when treating people who have little inclination, or otherwise have had little interpersonal support, for labeling and exploring their emotional experience until now (perhaps initially missing in the relational experience with attachment figures, caregivers, then partners, close friends). Some authors (e.g., Watson & Greenberg, 2017) have even referred to the lack of interest or exploration of one's inner experience as "self-neglect," stressing the downstream implications of not attending to one's inner life. Therapists can both model and foster curiosity in discovering one's visceral emotional experience but should also be mindful that some highly externally oriented individuals simply are less intrigued by the nuances of their inner experience and expanding their emotional repertoire. The remedy in these cases is often to use the leverage of the other kinds of emotional change discussed in this book, either in synergy or as alternative routes to change.

Overly Cognitive Processing

Stylistically, there are also manners of processing that interfere with emotional awareness. An overly cognitive emphasis actively constricts feeling. Research from a variety of theoretical perspectives has indicated that a cognitive emphasis is counterproductive to emotional processing of trauma memories. For example, a systematic review concluded that when exposure therapy was "augmented" with other cognitive interventions, the combination can decrease the effectiveness of treatment with respect to emotional awareness and its subsequent processing (Foa et al., 2003). This suggests that a cognitive emphasis can impede working through difficult emotion, perhaps because it serves as a distraction from affect.

Therapists should also be mindful that when clients ruminate, it is different from holding their emergent experience as a focus of awareness. Research has argued that the rumination most characteristic of worry is distinct from and antithetical to the "working through" necessary for emotional processing (Borkovec et al., 2004). Worry is understood by these researchers as a "cognitive control strategy": a response that orients individuals to a threat while insulating them from the immediacy of emotional experience, thereby allowing one to avoid the deeper pain and more primary emotional experience. Furthermore, this role of highly cognitive-verbal processing also maintains ruminative forms of depression (Fresco et al, 2002; Nolen-Hoeksema, 1991; Watkins & Baracaia, 2001).

The unhealthy and defensive process of worry and rumination paradoxically allows some clients to be highly active yet only superficially engaged in the deeper pain of their emotional experience. Like skipping flat stones along the water, the client keeps busy in this way and insulates themself against being submerged in deeper and more complex feelings. The cognitive, verbal-linguistic behavior of anxious or depressive rumination suppresses potentially evocative imagery, underlying meanings, and even somatic activity. In this way, rumination, worry, or brooding melancholy can block the natural course of experiential processing. The consequence of rumination blocking healthy engagement is that it seems to extend the duration of depressive episodes (Nolen-Hoeksema, 1991). So effective interventions direct clients to explore core emotions that underlie anxious and depression symptoms (e.g., a sense of self as inadequate, fragile, flawed).

A focus on feelings is not only central to exploring affect and its significance but also essential to the task of recalling painful memories themselves. As one might expect, individuals diagnosed with Cluster C personality disorders (i.e., characteristically anxious and worried) report higher rates of worry as compared to controls. However, this shallow and verbal form of worry has also been shown to mediate the relationship between Cluster C personality disorders and the specificity observed in their autobiographical memories (Spinhoven et al., 2009).

Other clients may use intellectual (and seemingly accurate) descriptions of emotion, although these elaborations may remain somewhat shallow or hypothetical as talking about feelings takes the place of deeper lived experiences. These intellectual descriptions are captured by what some authors have called *pseudomentalizing*, whereby the bodily experience of emotion, as information, is ignored or discarded (Bateman & Fonagy, 2013; Fonagy et al., 2002). Each of these stylistically cognitive emphases contrasts with the here-and-now affective and perceptual components in emotional awareness, which is generated bottom-up. In short, habitually using an abstract style of processing or engaging in worry and rumination seem to be modes of cognitive processing that engender generic and overly general meanings, limiting the exploration of specific and idiosyncratic ones.

Affect Dysregulation

Dysregulated emotional experience often derails awareness because, when arousal is too intense, it becomes disorienting and overwhelming. In the extreme, emotional awareness is abruptly aborted by dissociative breaks from distressing content. Some of the mechanisms of this interference are well known. For instance, hormones released by the neuroendocrine system are critical to how emotional memories are stored, recalled, and hence explored (Haas et al., 2008; Talmi, 2013). Lane and colleagues (2015) have summarized that stress activates the hypothalamic–pituitary–adrenal axis, which results in stress hormones accumulating and influencing brain regions important for emotional memory (i.e., the hippocampus, prefrontal cortex, and amygdala). Sustained exposure to elevated stress hormones interferes with both proper encoding and the subsequent consolidation of emotional memories. Therefore, when highly dysregulated and under stressful conditions, people can have impaired and less accurate emotional memories and undermined awareness of their experience both in the present and in the recalled experience itself. Therapists should make note that expanding awareness of an underregulated emotion can exacerbate symptoms.

Furthermore, even when clients have some awareness, unchecked arousal is infamous for hijacking the meaning-making or transformational processes. The problem with dysregulated emotion as it interferes with awareness (or reflection on emotion) is captured by the example of someone going on an angry tirade before admitting, "I've lost track of what I'm fighting for . . . but I'm still angry!" (A. Pascual-Leone et al., 2013). Here, awareness, emotional insight, and making use of those emergent meanings are derailed by overly intense arousal. At moments when emotion is too intense and becomes dysregulated (e.g., a client begins to sob uncontrollably), the therapeutic effort to expand awareness becomes derailed and prevents progress within that subprocess. Essentially, when emotion is experienced as inconsolable (i.e., a sense of shame become unbearable), a client's implicit goal abruptly changes to containing and protecting the self (e.g., seeking distractions, self-soothing) rather than exploration of meanings related to that target emotion (e.g., identifying unmet needs). However, the intensity of secondary emotion (e.g., rage) can likewise eclipse deeper and more central experiences, such that a more central experience of, say, sadness or shame is forced out of awareness.

Similarly, restricted arousal also often quashes emergent awareness by rendering experience too shallow for adequate exploration. Thus, *over*regulation can present another obstacle, which is when clients are too restrained or inhibited to feel and make functional use of their emotions as a potential source of insight. In more severe cases of personality disorders, particularly in association with histories of interpersonal trauma, both overregulation and underregulation of emotional experiences may be present in the same client depending on the content and area of functioning (Paivio & Pascual-Leone, 2023). Individuals with such complex difficulties in dysregulation often switch between a mode of restricted emotional processing and feeling overwhelmed by their poorly integrated emotional state, making emotional awareness a punctuated and haphazard effort.

Avoidance and Suppression of Negative Feelings

Shallow and overly cognitive ways of engaging, as well as suffering dysregulated affect, can often be thought of as functional dispositions or enduring processing styles that are a priori hindrances to emotional awareness. In contrast, avoidance and suppression are more episodic or context-sensitive impediments to deepening awareness, which may be momentary events or could become acquired and entrenched coping styles themselves. Behavioral approaches have led the way in recognizing the importance of overcoming behavioral as well as emotional avoidance (e.g., Barlow et al., 2004; Foa et al., 2007), which prevents the processing of upsetting experiences. Emotional awareness can be circumnavigated by clients (either deliberately or unwittingly) through physically avoiding evocative cues (e.g., taking alternate routes, averting one's gaze) or through the more subtle psychological avoidance of changing topics and using humor to systematically deflect genuine engagement.

Both classical psychodynamic and contemporary experiential therapies have highlighted the roles of interrupting, suppressing, or repressing emotional experiences. In dynamic formulations this is commonly discussed as a client's "resistance" to emotional awareness and engagement. And while self-imposed injunctions on emotion are real obstacles (e.g., boys don't cry; anger is forbidden), other obstacles to processing are better understood as sacrifices clients make in some (dysfunctional) effort to manage their painful experiences. Thus, experiential therapies sometimes refer to disowned, disclaimed, split-off, or disembodied emotions as sequestered from awareness and therefore not amenable to change. Essentially, these short-term strategies are the result of an incipient emotion being deemed unacceptable.

Emotions that are interrupted, disowned, denied, or suppressed could be either inherently adaptive or maladaptive. A client's ambivalence about engaging painful and maladaptive experiences of themself as intrinsically shameful or defenseless presents natural triggers for emotional avoidance. However, the issue is that at a given moment, the client may be unable to fully engage or tolerate the painful experience, so it is driven from awareness, even if it is adaptive. For example, one of my clients was a young woman who had given birth to her first child at a time when she was also caring for her suddenly ailing husband, the breadwinner of their family. Tragically, the husband died of cancer only 2 months after the birth of their child. Mourning the loss of her husband and the life they had hoped for was necessary and would have been an adaptive process, but the grief of this new mother was precipitously interrupted and "put on hold" (suppressed) as she attended to her newborn and was forced to negotiate survival as an underemployed single mother. Awareness and experience of an otherwise adaptive emotion was interrupted and postponed until several years later, the time it took mother and infant to gain some security in health and housing. Staving off emotion created a mounting sense of core pain for her, until the client came for help and was in a position to grapple with the totality of her loss.

Avoidance and various forms of suppression assume some initial engagement or awareness that the client then reacts to. However, another obstacle to emotional awareness is what D. B. Stern (1997) called "unformulated experience." The notion here is that when people are genuinely unaware, their emotional distress is not actually resisted so much as it was not palpably existent in the first place. As Stern already posits in the epigraph to this chapter, much of what is commonly said to be repressed is actually just unformulated. Thus, if repressed experience is captured by the statement, "I'm not going there!" then unformulated experience is more like, "I haven't really gotten around to exploring it." When this happens, one may have the preverbal *felt-sense* (to use language from Gendlin, 1996) that there are pieces with some potential for synthesized meaning but one has not yet put them together and does not fully appreciate their personal significance. Leaving experience unformulated, when one has these tendrils of poorly defined thoughts and feelings, is something that could be understood as a mini-dissociative moment, one that preempts having an emotional experience at all. Of course, substantive episodes of dissociation or depersonalization are also about truncating one's presenting experience but are usually a reaction to more explicit and intolerable contents of awareness (Laoide et al., 2017). Finally, avoidance, suppression, and trying not to formulate one's experience are each obstacles to awareness, but they also interfere with other forms of emotional processing such as arousal, expression, and reflection, which all usually require the emotion to be at least minimally within one's awareness.

Inauthentic Experiences

The final obstacle to genuine emotional awareness covered in this chapter is that of inauthentic experiences, which are present more often when working with people who suffer from personality disorders. To some degree, inauthentic experiences may be a result of shallow emotional processing, but they are also often related to placing particular emphasis on the interpersonal impact of one's expressed emotional experience (Kramer & Pascual-Leone, 2018). Crying "crocodile tears" or raising one's voice in anger as ways of influencing others are classic examples of what has been discussed in the Introduction as *instrumental* emotion (L. S. Greenberg & Paivio, 1997).

However, instrumental emotions are not necessarily hollow theatrics; they can entail very real affective experiences with genuine arousal, and in many instances, individuals may be unaware of the way they are *using* emotion. For example, a man with a history of having angry outbursts when his demands are not met as a customer is likely to be having genuine experiences of anger and frustration. At the same time, the fact that his outbursts usually result in him getting his way in commercial transactions provides repeated reinforcement for his angry behavior (A. Pascual-Leone et al., 2013). These types of emotions need to be changed, and while reflecting on the interpersonal function is useful (see Chapter 23), it is not useful to engage in deepening the experience itself. For example, efforts to help the angry customer (mentioned earlier) to attend to and symbolize the deeper personal meanings of his anger are not likely to be as fruitful as reflecting on the social impact of that expressed emotion. So, when clients present inauthentic experiences as their focus in session, this is an obstacle to productive emotional processing. Indeed, research has shown that the more "interpersonal maneuvers" clients show during an intake session, the less likely they are to enjoy symptom relief at the end of an insight-oriented psychodynamic therapy (Kramer & Sachse, 2013). The reason why inauthentic experience is an obstacle to expanding awareness is likely that the attentional focus of a client who engages in interpersonal maneuvers is generally external (i.e., on social interaction and interpersonal objectives) and, consequentially, any information that the emotional experience has to offer as an internal process is overlooked (Kramer & Pascual-Leone, 2018). In short, inauthentic experiences and instrumental emotions are not appropriate targets for awareness.

MECHANISMS AT WORK: HOW DOES EMOTIONAL AWARENESS CREATE CHANGE?

In practice, emotional awareness is often both tacit and multifaceted, making the hypothesized mechanism of change difficult to isolate and identify. However, from a practice-based review of the field, I suggest there are several distinct aspects of emotional awareness that explicate it as a general mechanism of therapeutic change. To start, engagement is understood here as the initial step for increasing emotional awareness: First, one "gets in touch," and then one "finds the right words." Engaging emotion subsequently opens a new source of personally relevant information, which itself represents emotional change. However, once engaged, a person can articulate their experience into symbols, paving the way for more elaborate aspects of emotional awareness. These downstream mechanisms of emotional awareness entail refining and developing the lived emotional experience during ongoing engagement. Furthermore, the deeper one's experiential awareness of emotion, the clearer one's sense of direction becomes, which also speaks to emotional awareness as a subtle form of meaning construction.

ENDNOTES

1. In Chapters 4–7, I am generally referring to awareness of internal affective material. However, one could also refer to the awareness of external material, such as interpersonal problems and patterns that make up the context of meaning in relation to moment-by-moment emotions. The narrative and interpersonal context of emotion is explored in Chapters 17–23.
2. Thinking about a feeling is a distinct process and plays its own role in emotional processing, but one that is unique from the lived experience of feeling. See Chapter 17 for conceptual clarifications on this and on its implications for meaning making.
3. For example, one finding related to the Client Experiencing Scale is that the relationship is stronger between expressed arousal and lower levels (i.e., 1–4) of client experiencing, as opposed to the deeper levels (i.e., 5–7). This fits with the clinical observation that initially approaching and exploring emotion seems to be facilitated by moderate levels of arousal, but this is not usually the case for deeper reflective levels (Pos et al., 2017).

5

Emotional Engagement

Getting in Touch With What's There

And the day came when the risk to remain closed in a bud became more painful than the risk it took to blossom.

—ELIZABETH APPELL[1]

The previous chapter introduced the construct of emotional awareness as a unique form of emotional processing, identified common obstacles to emotional awareness, and outlined pathways of action through which this process promotes change. However, the first proposed mechanism (of four) for emotional awareness is simply "getting in touch" with one's affective life, which is the focus of this chapter. The process of *emotional engagement* (i.e., orienting to emergent awareness) is the initial step in explicitly working with emotion. It begins with an openness to some experience that, until this moment, has remained tacit and unexplored.

ENGAGING EMOTION OPENS A NEW SOURCE OF INFORMATION

One of the puzzles for explaining emotional engagement is this: How does noticing the feeling lead to change? Although clients (and therapists) are often ambivalent about engaging emotion, one typically must fully "arrive" in a feeling before one can leave the feeling behind (L. S. Greenberg, 2021). Knowing what one feels allows one to access vital information about needs and goals, as well as action tendencies for meeting them. Usually, approaching and engaging

https://doi.org/10.1037/0000460-006
Principles of Emotion Change: What Works and When in Psychotherapy and Everyday Life, by A. Pascual-Leone
Copyright © 2026 by the American Psychological Association. All rights reserved.

emotion is a prerequisite for emotional work. From an experiential perspective, the new source of information that comes from emotional engagement is the lived meaning and direction, which is implicit in each emotional experience. Experiential meaning is also different for each client and different within each instance of change. In the example from humanistic–experiential therapy that follows, a client has become aware of some previously unexplored aspect of their experience, and she elaborates on what it is like to have a moment of emotional awareness:

CLIENT: I'm not sure how I get to that sad feeling. [*she wipe tears from her face*]

THERAPIST: Uh huh . . . and right now . . . where do you feel that in your body? . . . Can you describe it?

CLIENT: It's there. But I think that's the first time I've ever felt it. I mean, I knew it was there. Such a big empty space [*she points to the center of her chest*] . . . the only way I've been able to explain it to people is as a lack of direction, an emotional void . . .

THERAPIST: . . . longing for something more tangible, more solid . . .

CLIENT: Yeah, more meaningful. (A. Pascual-Leone, Paivio, & Harrington, 2016, p. 155)

This lived experiential meaning is somewhat different from the new source of information as typically understood from an exposure-based perspective. Behaviorally, new information is taken to be the realization that previously avoided emotion is not as threatening or unwieldy as one had anticipated. However, one's engagement with evocative content needs to be contrasted with other processes that follow it, namely, deeper and more meaningful awareness or the other mechanisms underlying behavioral exposure.

Furthermore, the nature of engagement differs on some undeclared variables, which I suggest have to do with the way a given internal stimulus or referent is engaged. For example, initially exposing oneself to feelings involves being open to experiencing that feeling and, in some sense, curious about making sense of it. This is already a challenge for some people. For example, a meta-analysis on borderline personality disorder has shown that the inability to tolerate emotion in the present moment may be another core feature of that disorder, one that is distinct from emotional dysregulation (Cavicchioli et al., 2015). So accepting emotion is part of this challenge too, but although the mindfulness approach is to accept the reality (i.e., not suppress, interrupt, or repress emotion), that does not necessarily involve pursuing or changing it more directly. In short, increasing emotional awareness is not the same as the acceptance of one's presenting reality, although it does presume the individual accepts the presenting emotion as part of an ongoing process, allowing it to be felt in an authentic experience. Finally, even when an experience is allowed, the optimal levels of engagement will still be constrained by an individual's processing style.

Engagement is the initial step in allowing experience and emotional awareness. Sometimes a client is ambivalent about entering into some emotional content, for example, "I know it's there, but I don't want to go there." When this happens, a client may only be aware of an emotion tacitly, essentially disavowing and resisting the experience (either consciously or unconsciously). For instance, while commenting on the video of their session, one client disclosed what it was like for them to be on the threshold of emotional engagement: "She [the therapist] is trying to provoke some emotion to illustrate what I was feeling at that moment. . . . I was reluctant because I don't want to open it up, or else it will all just come flooding out, and I will have no control" (Watson & Rennie, 1994, p. 504). In contrast to this example, *engagement* is the (a) willing exploration and (b) ability to tolerate or endure discomfort without losing one's focus, as one persists in the exploration of an emotion.

DIFFERENT OBJECTIVES IN EMOTIONAL ENGAGEMENT

Engagement is often a starting point for working with emotion, but to what end? It turns out that different treatment perspectives use engagement for quite contrasting process objectives. *Exposure* has long since been discussed as an intervention in relation to emotional processing, although often conflated with the notion of emotional engagement. Nonetheless, exposure is an intervention while engagement is a process. While early theory held the position that exposure led directly to habituation, it is now recognized that there is more than one mechanism by which exposure may facilitate emotional change. Moreover, these mechanisms may be ordered sequentially (Carey, 2011; Colwill et al., 2023; Kramer, Pascual-Leone, et al., 2018; A. Pascual-Leone, Yeryomenko, et al., 2016).

The Role of Agency in One's Engagement

Using exposure as an intervention requires that a client be emotionally engaged (i.e., willing and able to persist; see Chapter 3). This is essentially the same as what experiential and contemporary dynamic theorists have discussed as a critical initial step for emotional change. Humanistic theorists, however, shy away from using the term "exposure" because it connotes a relatively passive client (i.e., "patient") who is subjected to interventions, while the term "engagement" is more descriptive of a client's agentic role in the process.

Historically, different therapeutic emphases have played a part in how one's personal agency is framed when a client engages emotional work: Behavior therapists expose their patients to outside stimuli, whereas experiential therapists help their clients attend to internal experiences. Still, notice that by its very nature, "interoceptive exposure," activating and attending to often fear-inducing visceral experiences such as feeling dizzy or a rapid heart rate, inherently requires that clients be actively engaged in the process, willingly attending to their internal somatic experiences. Furthermore, with the rapprochement of contemporary and more integrative perspectives, this distinction has all but dissolved, and many behavior theorists now also regard internal affective experience as a stimulus to which clients may be exposed (e.g., "exposure to feared affect" or supposed "habituation to shame," Orsillo et al., 2004). The agentic involvement of clients is even more apparent when they are asked to creatively recall or imagine some fearful situation, such as the inside of an aircraft when one has a fear of flying.

A client's creative involvement further increases as one moves beyond simple exposure to more complex and meaning-laden tasks in experiential therapy, for example, when a client recalls and vividly imagines the angry grimace of an abusive parent (Paivio & Pascual-Leone, 2023). In the middle ground are contemporary hybrid therapies, such as the treatment of "affect phobia" (McCullough et al.'s, 2003, dynamic-behavioral approach). These approaches have explicitly extended the behavioral notion beyond physiological experience to describe emotional engagement as a sort of exposure task, whereby clients learn to tolerate and negotiate psychologically painful experiences.

Engagement for Exploration? . . . or for Habituation?

Part of the conceptual puzzle in understanding emotional engagement is that there are often undeclared processes from either perspective: Behavioral exposure often involves more than the declared change mechanism of habituation or inhibition, while an experiential account of evoking emotion and making meaning often similarly overlooks the fact that basic exposure and desensitization is probably also an implicit process, particularly in the initial steps of an enactment task. Whatever the case, behaviorist and experiential therapists will agree that if a client is not engaged with personal and evocative content (stimuli), then the subsequent change process will not unfold as prescribed. One aim of this book is to discuss ways of changing emotion that occur in psychotherapy irrespective of whether a treatment approach explicitly acknowledges the substeps involved.

First, the process of emotional engagement is a common process in working with emotion. Next, explicitly acknowledging and *labeling the feeling* (i.e., creating a referent) has also been shown to help regulate arousal (Paivio & Laurent, 2001; Torre & Lieberman, 2018). However, in the processes that follow, experiential and classical behavioral approaches make use of this initial "labeling" in quite different ways. This is where an increasing disparity emerges in how different treatment perspectives contemplate engagement and emotional awareness. From a behaviorist perspective, the purpose of engaging some emotionally evocative context over a certain period of time is that it leads to the attenuation of arousal, the mechanism of which was understood in early literature as desensitization and habituation (although more recent studies point to inhibition and change in expectancies; Chapter 3). Thus, in this second step of the behavioral sequence, a therapist's style or framework of intervention emphasizes identifying, containing, and eventually attenuating high emotional arousal.

In contrast, from an experiential–humanistic perspective, engagement is important first and foremost because it opens the possibility of symbolizing personally relevant meaning. In other words, once a client is emotionally engaged, a network of associated meanings (and other feelings) is co-activated. This activation is often described in experiential and dynamic literatures as gaining "access to feelings." A moderate level of arousal allows the client to attend to and articulate these emotional experiences: expanding emotional awareness. Thus, this second step of the experiential sequence, initial emotional engagement, is in the service of symbolizing and articulating newly emerging affective meanings. Emotional engagement, where a client willingly enters an experience, is the first step to deeper awareness of internally felt meanings. Taken together, this means that although emotional engagement may be a common starting point, it can be embarked on as a process to different ends, depending on the treatment approach.

OBSERVING FROM OUTSIDE VERSUS EXPERIENCING FROM WITHIN

Emotional engagement is touted as a key process in seemingly contradictory mechanisms of change (e.g., exposure and habituation/inhibition vs. the deepening of personal meaning making). Even so, little attention has been given to the nuance of how emotion is being presented by a therapist or regarded by the client, and what happens next depends largely on this manner of engagement.

Demand Characteristics in the Task of Engagement

The vantage point from which one explores their feelings changes the process that will ensue (Libby & Eibach, 2011). This means that a person about to work with emotion takes much of their direction or instruction on what kind of process to engage in from how that task is being presented or set up. Meanwhile, a therapist (or experimenter) may not be fully cognizant of their influence in this; it is conveyed through demand characteristic of the task and their implicit expectations on what is being solicited from the client. In this case, the task expectations might be presented formally through instructions or informally through ongoing dialogue (e.g., "Yes, that is the kind of answer I was looking for, keep going!" or "Hmm, that's not what I was expecting, maybe I can help, let's try again"). Therefore, the way a given emotional experience is regarded and engaged is a hidden, yet fundamentally defining, feature of the clinical intervention that ultimately unfolds. In short, how a client or therapist engages emotion (e.g., their curiosity, tentativeness, and the task objective they have) matters so much that it shapes the treatment approach as a whole.

The issue is that an emotion can be initially engaged in two markedly different ways, which essentially reflect the vantage point or working distance one adopts in relation to one's feelings (also see "decentering," Chapter 20). The way one engages and contemplates emotional experience will emphasize either a more empiricist or a more phenomenological understanding of the feeling. Fundamentally, this has to do with the basic set of assumptions one has about working with emotion, which treatment models, therapists, and clients themselves bring to the problem of emerging awareness. As a result, emotion comes to be regarded as either a more static or a more dynamic process, and this key distinction alters the way one's framework of meaning will subsequently be elaborated.

On one hand, an individual can contemplate and engage one's own emotion from an *observer's perspective*. In this approach, one takes a working distance from the feeling, as if it was somewhat external to the self (e.g., me in relation to that feeling). Engaging emotion "from the outside" lends itself to representing and experiencing the feeling as relatively more static. Once an emotion is labeled, then the task is essentially complete; emotion is known and contained. While this is very helpful for organizing and down-regulating clients, engendering an observer's perspective also implies a conclusiveness to the experience, as if to say, "Is that your final answer?" So even the pace and phrasing of a therapist's response can create a momentary sense of closure for (and curtail) emergent feeling: "Ah, so that's it. Well, now we know what you feel!"

On the other hand, as Gendlin highlighted from a phenomenological perspective, "Nothing that feels bad is ever the last step" (1981, p. 26). So an alternative kind of engagement is to regard one's emotion as the *subjective experiencer*, working from within an immersed or *embedded perspective* (e.g., right now, this is what "being me" feels like; J. Pascual-Leone et al., 2015). Engaging emotion from within the feeling lends itself to a different trajectory of intervention, one that might not immediately reduce arousal. From this perspective, the static representations of affect labeling are typically obsolete as soon as they are uttered because the feeling is ongoing. The emotion is regarded as a *dynamic process*, continually undergoing revision and inherently in flux. Gendlin's (1981, 1996) "felt shift" describes the subjective visceral experience that goes with a change or development in personal meaning. Sometimes this "experienced shift" is about the further differentiation in meaning within the same feeling, while at other times the felt shift comes with a palpable transformation in a discrete emotional tone, which goes with that meaning. This is a phenomenological account of one's internal covert experience as one gropes through some affective-meaning process.

When one is actively engaged in experiential meaning making, the discovery-oriented manner of emotional engagement conjures up *meaning as a dynamic stimulus*, one that sparks periodic increases in arousal each time the issues of personal significance are elaborated in new ways. This is the eager and curious pursuit of meanings that lay within. Thus, as a client explores personal meaning, the stimulus itself continually shifts, taking new directions, and feelings freshly emerge anew. While the generated meaning will eventually be consolidated, these active moments of engagement in a constructive process of searching are emotionally evocative, precipitating bursts of increased arousal as one deliberately enters into and grapples with the significance of one's presenting distress. For example, in experiential interventions that seek to deepen awareness and generate new meaning, clients are encouraged to "stay with that feeling, and just notice whatever comes up. . . . If the feeling shifts, follow that. . . . What's the worst part of it? . . . What does it need?" (see Gendlin, 1996). This manner of engagement regards meaning as dynamically unfolding, and it likely provides an evolving stimulus, which is the focus of awareness. Incidentally, this manner of engagement also often stokes arousal during the task itself, which is antithetical to the down-regulation of emotion (A. Pascual-Leone, Yeryomenko, et al., 2016). Although certain therapy tasks seem to frame one's working with static versus dynamic stimuli, the theoretical distinction I make here is ultimately in the mind of the client and is contingent on the kind of process they intend on engaging in. While the client ultimately chooses which process to embark on, their therapist shapes that process by pointing toward a particular objective (see Chapter 1).

Is the Meaning Static or Dynamic?

How one frames the task of engagement determines whether the meaning one subsequently constructs will be regarded as either static and definitive or dynamic and constantly shifting. Ultimately these are two epistemologically different ways of contemplating and working with one's experience (i.e., empiricist or phenomenological), and they correspond to the therapy approaches that encourage each of these frames of engagement. While the distinct ways of addressing experience are often highly polarizing for therapists of different approaches, the reality is one can engage and negotiate negative emotional experiences from each of these two very different stances based on the manner or style of engagement one uses. They have different merits, but they are not simultaneously compatible (Chapter 22). The issue of observing emotion as an objective external observer versus a subjective experiencer from within is critical for fully appreciating the difference in emotional awareness tasks from cognitive-behavioral versus experiential approaches. The issue is related to whether an intervention precipitates a change in either increasing or decreasing arousal (A. Pascual-Leone, Yeryomenko, et al., 2016; see Chapter 8, this volume). Indeed, the initial phase of experiential work typically intensifies negative emotion as compared to cognitive strategies that reduce arousal. Furthermore, each of these approaches to working with emotion (i.e., experiential or cognitive) relies on the activation of different brain regions (Wang et al., 2022).

Implications for Facilitating Emotion Work

Based on my reading of the literature, the process of habituation/inhibition will occur most effectively with exposure to *meaning as a static stimulus*, one that does not require continual reappraisal and readjustment and instead allows the participant to become familiar and habituated to its presence. Although a static stimulus may initially trigger emotional arousal, its relatively stable and predictable nature provides good conditions for the eventual down-regulation or inhibition of negative affect, even in the continued presence of evocative content (Colwill et al., 2023; see Chapter 3, this volume). For example, in the behavioral interventions of exposure and response prevention, or during prolonged exposure, patients are presented with emotionally evocative stimuli, but the intervention style of a behavioral approach encourages that stimulus to be taken at face value, a knowable and known stimuli (i.e., a static phenomenon). Incidentally, while the link is not usually explicit, I suggest this is part of why mindfulness has been so highly compatible with cognitive behavioral approaches. Observing one's experience from a place of detachment, just acknowledging it without further involvement, is an essential aspect of traditional mindfulness. As such, despite some initial similarity, the notion of mindfulness contrasts starkly with the ongoing effort to explore deeper experiential meaning (see Chapter 22).

The distinction I raise between these two modes of engagement is elusive in practice, precisely because they are based on both the moment-by-moment perspective of one's experience as well as the covert intention one has in working with emotion. However, laboratory experiments on the impact of affect labeling offer empirical evidence to support this idea (see Torre & Lieberman, 2018). Experiments on "affect labeling" typically prompt participants to label their emotions using one of two distinct procedures. One methodological approach has people spontaneously generate emotion words to describe their subjective experience as it occurs: essentially, using a first-person perspective to create a bottom-up formulation of one's experience from within. In contrast, the alternative research strategy has been to externally structure the affect labeling task, for example, using a computer screen that prompts participants with a menu of choices, from which they select a suitable emotion word. In other words, this strategy uses a third-person or outside-observer perspective to consider and choose from a set of provided labels to best approximate one's experience. In these kinds of experiments, labeling one's affective experience has been shown to have a measurable effect, reducing physiological arousal either immediately or with longer term delayed effect. Intriguingly, however, which of the two paradigms a study uses to prompt participants in labeling their affect seems to anticipate their different findings. Specifically, the kind of prompt one uses may influence how long it takes for the affect labeling process to attenuate arousal. A review of this research observes the following:

> Nearly all studies reporting only delayed effects required participants to self-generate the affect labels themselves rather than have them provided . . . while none of the studies reporting immediate decreases did. In fact, the only reported case where affect labeling significantly *increased* self-reported affect or autonomic arousal during the initial exposure [i.e., emotional engagement] also required participants to self-generate and verbalize their emotional experiences. . . . But the reason for this dichotomy remains unknown. (Torre & Lieberman, 2018, p. 121; emphasis in original)

In sum, while choosing suitable labels from a menu had the immediate effect of down-regulating arousal, finding one's own words to describe emotion created the same effect but only after a delay (and on occasion it may precipitate a brief increase!). I suggest the explanation for this puzzling dichotomy is in the distinction I have made here, such that the manner with which one regards and engages one's emotional experience is a critical variable that moderates the impact of this early step in emotional awareness. Indeed, Torre and Lieberman (2018) go on to make conjectures in support of my formulation:

> It could be that being provided labels is simply easier, reducing need for introspection. . . . It may also be that while self-generating labels may be more difficult and less effective in the immediate situation, those labels are ultimately more relevant to the individual generating them and lead to longer lasting effects as seen in expressive writing paradigms. (p. 121)

A clinical implication is that the way a therapist makes empathic reflections of their client's emotion will shape the impact that finding the right words has, either decreasing or increasing arousal at a given moment in session. For example, when clients are overwhelmed and becoming dysregulated, therapists should provide more circumscribed and conclusive statements to help clients find labels for their feelings (e.g., as more typically encouraged in cognitive and behavioral therapies). Doing so is likely to help with a more immediate down-regulation of distress, containing the experience and closing the task (Marks et al., 2019; Torre & Lieberman, 2018). For example, a therapist might offer options to choose from: "So, right now, is this more about feeling ashamed and bad? Or is this more about feeling sadness, like about the loss? . . . Oh okay, that sounds like shame. Is that right?"—a query that is relatively instructive, closed-ended, and conclusive. (Writing the client's answer down on a pad of paper would bring the search to an even more definitive end!)

In contrast, when clients are emotional but nevertheless able to tolerate their distress, clinical practice could call for an evocative approach to finding the right words. Here the reflection would deliberately be exploratory, open-ended, and tentative (e.g., as practiced in experiential therapies). The poignancy in such empathic reflections potentiates a momentary increase in arousal, to further differentiate the symbolization not only of emotion but of the visceral experience itself. For example, a therapist might conjecture: "So painful . . . I see you close your eyes, and I guess it's something about feeling . . . 'inadequate'? Or . . . ? Stay with the feeling, let the words come. . ." Although keeping the exploratory task open a bit longer could delay the alleviation of distress, it also has the longer term benefit of providing a rich insight (Gendlin, 1996; A. Pascual-Leone & Greenberg, 2007b; Watson & Rennie, 1994).

A HEALTHY DOSE OF QUALITY ENGAGEMENT

Emotion awareness and engagement is not simply knowing what one feels or talking about emotion, but also feeling it. For many people, deepening their emotional engagement in this way feels risky. So, as one might expect, engagement is contingent upon several conditions. A study of psychodynamic therapy collected clients' self-reports session-by-session on their emotional engagement, asking them to retrospectively report on a scale from 0, *In today's session I was disconnected from my feelings,* to 7, *I was emotionally involved, and I fully and vividly experienced my emotions* (Fisher et al., 2016, p. 108). The study also collected session data on the quality of each client's relationship with their therapist and their reported level of clinical functioning. This allowed researchers to examine the association between the three variables and the directionality of their possible influence to explore the chain of events. Overall, the quality of relationship between therapist and client in a session predicted the client's emotional engagement in the next session, which in turn predicted better client functioning in the session after that. Furthermore, while temporal associations revealed that a good relationship precedes (and seems to facilitate) deeper emotional experience, the inverse was not true. So, in this psychodynamic therapy, a client's emotional engagement did not seem to subsequently strengthen the relationship, at least not by itself. This highlights a critical issue that has not yet been mentioned: A good treatment relationship is often a precondition for a client's deeper emotional engagement.

In contrast, the association between a client's emotional engagement and their level of functioning has been repeatedly shown to be reciprocal, such that each is a meaningful predictor of the other in the following session (Fisher et al., 2016). Evidence for this reciprocal relationship between emotional engagement and clinical improvement comes from psychodynamic therapy (described earlier) but has since been replicated in the study of emotion-focused and cognitive-behavioral therapies (Pinheiro et al., 2021). Taken together, there is strong evidence for the direction of change (i.e., a good relationship potentiates engagement). Furthermore, research points at multiple contributors to a healthy dose of emotional engagement (i.e., both the relationship and ongoing symptom improvement anticipate further engagement).

What Is Optimal Emotional Engagement?

Providing the conditions for people to engage with their emotion does not necessarily mean the ensuing process will be productive. It is clear people sometimes can get overwhelmed because they are overengaged with emotion, while at other times they remain disconnected and out of touch with their feelings. As one decides how deeply to wade into a feeling, the practical question is: What does good engagement look like? There is a paucity of research on what characterizes a healthy dose of emotional engagement, although benchmarks have been developed in clinical practice. Behavioral approaches have systematically assessed client engagement in emotion work by asking clients to rate their immediate experience of somatic marker distress: for example, "How anxious or distressed are you right now on a scale of 1 to 10?"; 1 being *It doesn't affect me* and 10 being *I've never felt worse.* Specifically, in exposure-based tasks, the clinical guidelines are that optimal engagement is usually about a rating of 8.

Despite some initial psychometric critiques, using these ratings of Subjective Units of Distress (SUDS) has proven to be an extremely practical and effective way of monitoring client process within session (Tanner, 2012; Wolpe, 1958). While often used as a measure of anxiety, it seems the SUDS (which does not require one to label the affective experience) appeals to and measures undifferentiated distress. SUDS ratings do not distinguish between states of arousal that have little cognitive involvement and aroused states that entail substantial cognitive processing of emotional material. In other words, for better or worse, this well-practiced method of measurement equates emotional arousal with emotional engagement. However, upon closer consideration, "heightening arousal" (for an eventual habituation; Chapter 3) and "expanding awareness" are each distinct ways of working with emotion. And collapsing these concepts (i.e., arousal, engagement, and awareness) precludes other facets of the process when assessing what makes for optimal engagement, although if habituation is the only objective (as opposed to the elaboration of meaning), then a single criterion will seem sufficient.

Fortunately, some efforts have also been made to operationalize engagement in a way that goes beyond asking clients to rate their own emotional engagement. As therapists know, there tends to be a lot of variability in the quality of a client's engagement. So, for treatment approaches interested in considering the quality of engagement beyond the straight amount of arousal, the issue of whether clients are sufficiently engaged has been a critical one. A key study on this topic (Paivio et al., 2001) has developed observational criteria for this in a Level of Engagement Scale to describe the quality of engagement that seems to predict treatment outcomes. Clinicians should look for the process in terms of three dimensions, and consider a client's

- involvement in the process (e.g., willingness, spontaneous involvement, enactment),

- expression and exploration of emotion (i.e., admitting feelings, arousal), and

- psychological contact with the object of emotion (i.e., vividness, using "I" and "you" language rather than speaking in third person, making eye contact with an imagined person, part of the self, therapist).

This complex measure of engagement captures the client's openness to explore, feel, and make sense out of arousal, which turns out to have little or no association with simple ratings of distress using the SUDS (Chagigiorgis, 2010). Yet, when Paivio and colleagues (2001) used the measure to study emotion-focused therapy (EFT) for complex trauma, their observation of a client's engagement, particularly during the first time a client did an empty chair task (i.e., imagining a conversation with one's perpetrator), it was prognostic of treatment success. This single observation about engagement from the early phase of therapy (i.e., session 4) predicted symptom outcome at 6 months posttreatment.

Another study using the same treatment sample showed that, as one might hope, observer ratings on a therapist's level of empathic response predicted a client's subsequent emotional engagement (Mlotek, 2013). That moment-by-moment observation converges with research (cited earlier) suggesting that quality of the therapeutic relationship is a precondition for client engagement. However, in this study of EFT, the impact of therapist empathy on eventual treatment success was also mediated by client emotional engagement (Mlotek, 2013). These studies point to emotional engagement as one causal determinant of change.

How Much to Emotionally Engage and How Often?

The initial level of engagement when working with emotion seems to set a benchmark for similar enactment interventions that follow, because engagement tended to be stable across these EFT interventions: Some clients were consistently highly engaged, while others were less so (Paivio et al., 2001). However, when it comes to participating in emotionally evocative experiential tasks such as chairwork, the quality of engagement turns out to be independent of the frequency of participation. In short, *dosage* (i.e., quality of process multiplied by frequency of engagement) was an independent predictor of outcome in EFT, and more important than either quality or frequency of engagement alone (Paivio et al., 2001). The clinical implication is that clients whose engagement is more limited during emotionally evocative tasks can make up for this shortfall by being encouraged to participate in such tasks more frequently, thereby receiving the same benefit as others who were able to engage more fully or easily.

Interestingly, this formulation of emotional engagement in terms of dosage (i.e., quality multiplied by frequency) as a key variable in reducing trauma symptoms is consistent with behavioral research that has examined the impact of exposure-based interventions (Foa et al., 2007; Tanner, 2012). This practical definition (i.e., some interaction) of what kind of engagement really matters echoes an age-old debate in exposure-based therapy. On the one hand, some have argued that the number of exposure trials is the primary determinant of desensitization and extinction (Rescorla & Wagner, 1972), while others have concluded that the decisive issue is the cumulative exposure time (Gallistel & Gibbon, 2000). Experiments based on the exposure paradigm have suggested that the number of exposures (i.e., engagements) a client has with fear-inducing stimuli is the primary factor (Golkar et al., 2013). However, when a clinical task is couched in less behavioral terms, such as in the elaboration of personal meaning, that will also take more time than confrontation with feared circumstances. For these reasons, the dosage of engagement as described by Paivio and colleagues seems most incisive in the discussion of how clients concretely cultivate their emotional awareness.

Findings like this indicate that emotional engagement during chairwork, and likely other evocative interventions, is one possible mechanism of change

(Paivio et al., 2001). A practical implication of this research is the importance, early in therapy, of facilitating clients' emotional engagement with painful memories. For example, studies of recovery patterns in sexual and nonsexual assault victims found that, in general, long-term recovery was impeded if the indispensable emotional engagement with traumatic material in therapy was delayed (Gilboa-Schechtman & Foa, 2001). Good client engagement, early in therapy, is particularly important because it sets the course for therapy and allows maximum time to explore and process emotion related to personal concerns such as traumatic memories (Paivio et al., 2001).

Finally, as hinted at the top of this section, it is also possible for clients to overengage in emotional awareness. When clients have difficulty disengaging or periodically shielding themselves from the raw awareness of painful emotion, then arousal may escalate unchecked. This may be more characteristic of certain psychopathologies whereby clients are chronically overengaged in either secondary emotion (e.g., symptomatic anxiety) or primary maladaptive emotion (e.g., feeling shameful and worthless). Panic disorder is a related example of this, in which individuals are excessively attuned to their bodily sensations, even if they are accurate. So overengagement can also be a challenge to other processes, such as the down-regulation of emotion (as discussed in Chapter 3).

NEUROBIOLOGICAL CORRELATES OF EMOTIONAL ENGAGEMENT

There are several specific brain regions involving the awareness, activation, and general regulation of emotion including the amygdala, insula, orbital prefrontal cortex, and subgenual cingulate cortex (Abbass et al., 2014; Craig, 2009; Lane & Nadel, 2020; Pessoa, 2013). The polyvagal theory has also postulated pathways for how several affective systems regulate socio-affective engagement (Porges, 2011). Whatever the case, these brain areas are all implicated in the implicit goal-directed behavior of engaging emotion.

Detecting Emotional Relevance

Although many parts of the brain are involved in working with emotion, the amygdala seems to have a unique role in sparking up engagement. Simply put, research on what activates the amygdala has shown it to essentially be a "novelty detector" and a "relevance detector." Although this brain region is not exclusive to emotional processing, the amygdala is associated with emotion because emotion itself is a psychobiological response to personally relevant content (Pessoa, 2013). By detecting what is novel or relevant to one's implicit goals, the amygdala provides an emotion-orienting function, and this is part of what helps clients spontaneously engage.

In one study of a well-known neurological case, a woman who lost functioning in both amygdalae was unable to spontaneously notice and orient to salient cues related to emotion and fear, in particular (Adolphs, Gosselin, et al., 2005). However, when she was verbally instructed to attend to specific features of a stimulus (e.g., examine the eyes of a frightened face), then her perceptual processing of emotion was entirely normal. This underscores that one of the many functions of the amygdala is to automatically orient one to facets of emotion. So clients who can respond to emotional stimuli and then make use of emerging emotion in psychotherapy will do this effortlessly and tacitly because the amygdala offers an emotional orienting function. Furthermore, that function ushers in opportunities for sustained engagement with emotion. However, the case study cited earlier also suggests that when clients are not adequately orienting to their affective experience, or when they are ambivalent, then therapists can help by offering more structure or explicit direction to get things started.

Bodily Feelings Inform Awareness

While orienting to relevant stimuli is an initial part of emotional engagement, in healthy functioning this is quickly followed by some implicitly adaptive self-organization. One of the proposed neural mechanisms for this is that somatic markers tacitly guide an individual's behavior. This phenomenon has been systematically studied in the context of decision making, where individuals who have impaired bodily awareness are found to make poorer choices than those who experience such somatic cues (Bechara, 2004). In an experiment known as the Iowa gambling task, participants are given no information except to choose from several decks of cards with the aim of maximizing their profits, when unbeknownst to them certain decks are biased as either risky or conservative "bets." Meanwhile, participants' anticipatory responses are measured before they draw each card using skin conductance (e.g., sweaty hands as a measure of anxiety). After only a short amount of playing time, the physiological reactivity of healthy participants spiked in anticipation of choosing from "risky decks," but this was several rounds before participants later reported having "discovered" that some decks were particularly risky. Furthermore, when patients with lesions of the ventromedial sector and orbitofrontal regions from the prefrontal cortex played this game, their anticipatory response failed to generate the anxiety-related skin conductance as they picked up risky cards, and it also took them longer to realize the decks were loaded differently (Bechara, 2004). Studies like this support the *somatic marker hypothesis*, which states that bodily changes are generated subconsciously and reflect an emerging awareness about emotionally significant events, one that precedes any explicit knowledge people use for decision-making.

The Mysterious Feelings in Your Gut

Very different parts of the nervous system have also been implicated in the initial emergence of affective experience. In a comical anecdote, I gave a client the age-old advice, "Trust your gut." To which my client quipped, ". . . but I have gastritis!" The playful exchange refers to difficulties in identifying and labeling emotion but also to the long-held belief that there is a connection between the gut and tacit affective experience. Interestingly, research now supports this physiological–neurological connection, although the details remain unclear.

The enteric nervous system, in the wall of the human gut, is composed of about five times as many neurons as the brain of a rat (Mayer, 2016). Knowing how much psychological research on cognition, memory, and motivation is based on the study of rats should give anyone pause, to appreciate the neural capacity the human gut seems to have for working with complex information. While this system is primarily concerned with controlling digestion and sensing "environmental threats," researchers have argued that this system, which "feels" our internal world, is much too complicated to have evolved for managing digestion alone. The *enteric nervous system* is made up of various types of neurons, has its own version of the blood–brain barrier, and produces hormones, as well as about 40 neurotransmitters of the same class as those found in the brain (Mayer, 2016).

Neurons in the gut are thought to produce as much dopamine as is produced in one's brain, and most of the serotonin present in the body at any one time is found in the enteric nervous system. This "second brain" can function independently but also influences the brain. In fact, 90% of the signals passing along the vagus nerve up to the brain come from this part of the gastrointestinal tract—not the other way around (Powley & Philips, 2002). Thus, it seems that the gastrointestinal–immunological system for detecting threats "in here" may be more closely related to the psychological system for detecting threats "out there" than previously imagined.

This now has clinical implication for treating mental illness. For example, stimulation of the vagus nerve coming from the gut has been shown to be an effective treatment for chronic depression that has otherwise been treatment-resistant (Corcoran et al., 2006). In Chapter 3, As previously mentioned, consuming probiotic yogurt for several weeks altered brain activity in healthy women, particularly in regions that integrate sensory and emotional information to coordinate threat responses. These changes were specific to situations involving negative emotional states and were not observed in a control group (Tillisch et al., 2013).

Clearly, this second neural system informs our emotional experience in ways that are still quite obscure, although "butterflies in one's stomach" are a common example of a stress response coming from the gut that signals some form of emotional engagement. However, based on physiological research, some have argued that our everyday emotional experience is likely influenced on an ongoing basis by the nerves that originate in our gut (Mayer, 2016). These discoveries are consistent with the somatic marker hypothesis (Bechara, 2004), which proposes that peripheral mechanisms (e.g., the vagus nerve, spinal cord, endocrine route) contribute to emotional involvement and guide subsequent cognitive-emotional processing and behavior.

Attending to Sensations, Emotions, or Both?

In an experiment on individual differences and the neural substrates of awareness, researchers examined the relationship between emotional and visceral bodily awareness through a simple task of introspective accuracy: Healthy participants were asked to determine if an audible pulse was (or was not) in synchrony with their own heartbeat (Critchley et al., 2004). Four participants turned out to be exceptionally accurate (and confident!) in determining, every time, whether a pulse was synchronous or asynchronous with their heartbeat. In contrast, two participants seemed to have no sense of whether the audible pulse was in or out of synchrony and were apparently guessing at random. The rest of the participants fell in the middle range in terms of their sensitivity to internal bodily activity. Moreover, variation in how sensitive, or body-aware, people were corresponded to the emotional intensity they reported feeling in everyday life, such that people with more visceral awareness also generally felt emotions more strongly.

In the same study, brain imaging (fMRI) was also used to simultaneously measure neural patterns during the task and showed enhanced activity in the insular, somatomotor, and cingulate cortices (Critchley et al., 2004). Brain activity in the right anterior insula predicted both participants' accuracy in the heartbeat detection task as well as the intensity of their reported emotional experience. Together, these results support the idea that visceral bodily awareness is closely intertwined with emotional awareness and that the right anterior insula is a brain region that supports the representation of these subjective feelings. Finally, just as importantly, this study highlights that there are vast individual differences among people in their levels of introspective awareness and their sensitivity to internal feelings. I will return to the issue of individual differences in the next chapter when I discuss alexithymia and how some people seem to be better than others at not just noticing but also labeling their emotional experience.

Nevertheless, it is also important to remember that individual differences are often quite hard to distinguish from developmental differences, and this is particularly apparent in observations about emotional processing. For example, a study using a similar task of heartbeat perception accuracy assigned participants to 3 months of contemplative mental training or a control condition (Bornemann & Singer, 2017). The accuracy of participants' heartbeat perception and level of emotional awareness (i.e., using the Toronto Alexithymia Scale) was assessed at regular intervals during the training. Participants' ability to accurately perceive their own heartbeats increased steadily over the 3-month training and beyond, with small to medium effect sizes emerging after 6- and 9-month follow-ups. Furthermore, the changes in their interoceptive accuracy, as well as attending to and engaging physical experience, were predictive of concomitant changes in emotional awareness.

The significance of research like this is that it illustrates how visceral self-awareness plays some palpable role in the emergence of emotional awareness. In short, there is a process by which individuals engage and then become aware of their affective experiences. As the next chapter will show, research on alexithymia also tells us a lot about the absence of emotional awareness.

ENDNOTE

1. This poem is often misattributed to Anaïs Nin: https://readelizabeth.com/2012/12/anais-nin-and-i-are-in-lock-step/

6

Labeling Emotion

Finding Just the Right Words

"Les mots juste" is a French expression, highlighting the critical nature of finding, "just the right, exact, or most appropriate words."

—ORIGINALLY ATTRIBUTED TO THE FRENCH NOVELIST GUSTAVE FLAUBERT

Emotional awareness is a complex and often implicit process. However, from the perspective of a clinician working in session, emotional awareness should be understood as entailing two distinct and major efforts for intervention. As explored in the previous chapter, the first major effort is helping clients get in touch with what's there, which essentially refers to perceptual awareness and deliberate emotional engagement. The current chapter picks up with the second part of what completes the process of emotional awareness, which is finding the right words to tentatively capture that experience. In contrast to "feeling something inside" as a simple perceptual experience, the addition of this second part, symbolization, is what makes emotional awareness a unique form of emotional processing in and of itself.

The effect of emotional awareness can be understood by considering it either as an active process or through its conspicuous absence. First, once one is engaged, emotional awareness involves continuing to attend to and then label the presenting feeling. When emotion itself is used as the point of reference, it becomes a target for intervention. Finding the right words is more than just a verbalization of preexistent meaning; it is the search and refinement of a meaning that has not yet been fully formulated. Of course, certain impairments (i.e.,

https://doi.org/10.1037/0000460-007
Principles of Emotion Change: What Works and When in Psychotherapy and Everyday Life, by
A. Pascual-Leone
Copyright © 2026 by the American Psychological Association. All rights reserved.

alexithymia) can interfere with that process, and such difficulties essentially represent the antithesis of emotional awareness. So, a second part of explaining emotional awareness comes from understanding what happens when people cannot find the words for their feelings. Each of these topics is now addressed.

LABELING EMOTION TURNS IT INTO A POINT OF REFERENCE

Experiential schools following the work of Gendlin emphasized the experiencing process and focusing on the bodily felt sense (tacit somatic meanings) to carry forward emerging experience. So, rather than classic notions of insight and new understandings being produced by an act of conceptually linking elements together, insight is seen as the product of explicating and creating new meaning in an ongoing process of awareness (Gendlin, 1996). Gendlin (1964) explains the role of attending to and symbolizing experience through awareness as contrasted with a conceptual understanding of insight:

> We often discuss self-exploration as if it were purely a logical inquiry in search of conceptual answers. However, in psychotherapy (and in one's private self-exploration as well) the logical contents and insights are secondary. Process has primacy. We must attend and symbolize in order to carry forward the process and thereby reconstitute it in certain new aspects. *Only then,* as new contents come to function implicitly in feeling, can we symbolize them. (p. 158; emphasis in original)

Thus, symbolizing an emerging affective experience objectifies it, and attending to it further refines the experience, which expands one's emotional awareness.

Understanding the neural underpinnings of experiential awareness helps one appreciate just how different the processing of implicit emotional knowledge is from the often-explicit knowledge of hard logical reasoning. Functions are generally organized such that structures in the right side of the brain are mostly responsible for processing nonverbal, bodily sensations and lower order information about emotion (e.g., right insula; Farb et al., 2007). Neuronal wiring is also more local in the right hemisphere, facilitating the awareness of concrete experiences. Because emotion is largely driven by automatized cues, this kind of wiring makes the cue function richer and broader in the right hemisphere. For example, this right-sided lateralization has sometimes been associated with increased emotional and nonverbal artistic sensibilities such as visual arts and music (Q. Chen et al., 2019; Lindell, 2014). In contrast, the left side of the brain is responsible for some of the higher order cognitive processes involved in emotional awareness, such as verbally labeling one's feelings and working further with emotional information (Q. Chen et al., 2019; Farb et al., 2007). So, although the quote earlier, from Gendlin, describes the felt sense from a phenomenological perspective, generating that kind of embodied knowledge also corresponds to certain aspects of how the brain functions. In short, emotional awareness can be broadly thought of as emerging bottom-up from this right-hemispheric activity, which eventually is connected to the left-brain processes of finding the right words to symbolize that experience.

The Process of Finding the Right Words

After engaging an experience, beginning to symbolize emotional experience often entails finding some label to describe the feeling. The creation of a well-crafted visual image or a poetic metaphor allows one to capture or symbolize an essential meaning. The symbolization (broadly defined) of meaning through some medium allows one to subsequently use it as a touchstone that one might return to and build upon, rather than continually reinventing or reexperiencing the same ephemeral truth about the self, world, or other. This process is what Gendlin (1981) aptly described as "getting a handle" on a felt sense. To appreciate the distinction between expression and symbolization of meaning, it is worth noting that some forms of artistic expression essentially allow for more precise articulation of meaning than others. While dance, for example, may better allow for other subprocesses, such as arousal and expression, it does not lend itself as well to the same articulation of meaning as when one finds the right words. Arguably the potential for more precision in meaning-making increases from dance to visual art, to poetry, to conversational prose, which affords the highest level of potential for developing awareness in the sense of articulation (for some discussion of this regarding instrumental music, see Esteves & Conceição, 2022). Bear in mind that emerging expressiveness is a separate process.

If *awareness* is understood as the process of representing some internally felt experience, its content is perceived concretely and in the given moment. Focusing, for example, is an intervention that seeks to accomplish this result (Gendlin, 1981, 1996). Thus, when a client comes to a realization and then labels a feeling (e.g., "I'm scared"), it is the generation of meaning (i.e., a mini-insight) through a bottom-up process. In doing this, clients are synthesizing various aspects of their immediate psychophysical experience with their linguistic-based understanding and find themselves suddenly able to adequately capture an aspect of their own subjective world. Gestalt therapy also provides a wealth of awareness exercises (Perls et al., 1951; Stevens, 1971). Sometimes this involves "reowning" sequestered aspects of one's conscious experience. At other times it is simply managing to symbolize something that has hitherto previously not been articulated (A. Pascual-Leone & Greenberg, 2007b). The notion of awareness was elaborated in Gestalt psychotherapy as the forming of a new figure against the background of one's ongoing experience (Perls et al., 1951). Thus, the concept of bringing aspects of oneself or one's experience into awareness requires an experience, in vivo, but does not necessarily require connecting or linking to already established self-understandings (A. Pascual-Leone & Greenberg, 2007b; also see Chapter 17, this volume). In emotion-focused therapy (EFT), for example, naming or labeling a feeling is the simplest form of new awareness (L. S. Greenberg, 2021). Notice, the line between perception and emotional awareness begins to blur in this context, suggesting a continuum.

Labeling a Feeling Can Contain and Regulate It

Affect labeling is one aspect of emotional awareness; it refers uniquely to the simple act of finding just the right word. While it may be an entry point, affect labeling itself does not refer to more complex symbolizations of meaning such as actively exploring the deeper meaning of an experience or elaborating a narrative framework of that understanding. However, affect labeling, as a circumscribed process unto itself, can serve as a type of incidental emotion regulation. In short, without either consciously monitoring one's distress or explicitly intending to down-regulate arousal, finding the right words is inherently calming. It alters emotion by moderating its intensity, even as the experience itself unfolds (Gendlin, 1981, 1996; L. S. Greenberg, 2021; Paivio & Laurent, 2001; Torre & Lieberman, 2018).

The impact of simply labeling one's emotion has been intrinsic to processes described in humanistic–experiential psychotherapies since the work of Rogers (1959) and was discussed at length by Gendlin in the 1980s. However, seemingly unaware of these origins, practitioners have recently rediscovered the same process within cognitive behavioral theory, using more mechanistic terminology (hence, affect labeling; Marks et al., 2019). Still, it has not been until the last decade that the immediate impact of simply describing one's emotional experience has been systematically studied in a laboratory setting (for a review, see Torre & Lieberman, 2018).

Affect Labeling Immediately Reduces Autonomic Responses

When individuals are confronted with an emotionally evocative stimulus and then encouraged to verbalize their subjective emotional state, it helps reduce the physiological intensity of their emotional reaction. Furthermore, this attenuation of emotion is larger than when people are given a control task in which they are instructed to focus externally and make labels that describe the evoking stimulus itself (Torre & Lieberman, 2018). This has implications for even the most dispassionate and incidental assessment of someone's momentary emotion (e.g., So, what are you feeling right now?), because asking for a self-report is itself a measurable manipulation. In fact, after the induction of anger, asking people to simply label their feelings by rating them on an analogue scale has been shown to reduce the autonomic correlates of emotional reactivity, such as heart rate, cardiac rhythm, and peripheral resistance (Kassam & Mendes, 2013).[1] At the same time, individuals tend to be unaware of the impact that affect labeling has on their emotional arousal. It is a subtle, interactive, and very dynamic process, yet labeling one's experience has measurable impacts downstream. Even so, and somewhat ironically, affect labeling is often palpably experienced as an effortful and cognitively demanding process, particularly when one is in the throes of distress.

In a study of exposure therapy, participants were asked to approach a live tarantula as it sat in a box (Kircanski et al., 2012). Participants started by standing 5 feet away and then followed a series of graded steps, where the last step was attempting to actually touch the spider. The study compared four separate conditions: Participants in the affect labeling group were instructed to make a statement that included a negative word to describe the spider and their emotional response (e.g., "I am scared the gross spider will bite me!"). Those in a reappraisal group used only neutral words to describe the spider, reappraising their initial reaction as more benign. Meanwhile, a distraction group made statements about furniture in the room, and, finally, those in a traditional exposure group made no verbalized statements at all. Results showed that affect labeling was more effective than any other condition (i.e., reappraisal, distraction, or exposure alone) in decreasing skin conductance, a physiological measure of distress and anxiety. The advantage of labeling one's emotion in the face of distress was apparent not only in the immediate moment but also even a week later, when participants were again exposed to the spider. Furthermore, the more anxiety and fear words that participants spontaneously verbalized when approaching the spider, the greater the attenuation of their affective response, and the closer they were willing to approach the spider in the last step of the task, as well as when they attempted it for the second time a week later (Kircanski et al., 2012).

This phenomenon has also been explored in the context of self-critical processes, which illustrates the role of affect labeling in more complex internal appraisals. Participants delivered 10 one-minute speeches in front of a small audience (Niles et al., 2015). However, in the 30-second interval between each speech, participants were systematically prompted by a computer to do either affect labeling or a control task. Those in the affect labeling condition were asked to select from a menu the word that best described their emotional experience and then to also describe their feared outcomes (e.g., I feel . . . "afraid"; The audience will . . . "think I'm stupid"). Compared to those in a traditional exposure condition, participants who were regularly prompted to label their affect during the exposure had a faster reduction in their physiological fear response during exposures (i.e., as measured using moment-by-moment heart rate and skin conductance). Furthermore, participants who initially had difficulty labeling their affect were also eventually the ones who gained the most from adding such verbalization to standard exposure procedures. Participants returned several days later and were confronted with the same feared task. Again, those who had previously used more anxiety-related labels during the first exposure session also enjoyed more pronounced benefits, evidenced by a lower fear response, than those who had described other aspects of the experience. This final part of the study shows that the impact of affect labeling not only was immediate but could also be sustained after a delay of several days (Niles et al., 2015).

Studies like these demonstrate that following instructions to label one's emotional experience can be inherently calming, attenuating the physical reactivity of one's distress. Interestingly, although affect labeling immediately lowers one's physiological reactivity, it does not typically reduce the amount of subjectively reported feeling.[2] In any case, affect labeling is now recommended to enhance the effectiveness of exposure and desensitization-based interventions. The suggestion here is that it bolsters the mechanisms of inhibitory learning (described in Chapter 3, this volume; Marks et al., 2019; Torre & Lieberman, 2018). While affect labeling as a technical improvement is an instant and valuable contribution to practice, the theoretical formulation here is unfortunate. By assuming that affect labeling is simply facilitating better inhibitory learning, one overlooks the qualitative distinctiveness of affect labeling (i.e., finding the right words) in contrast to down-regulation (i.e., reducing intensity). Thinking of these both as ways of managing (i.e., attenuating) emotional arousal precludes the understanding that they are separate kinds of emotional processing, operating either in tandem or synergistically.

Mechanisms of Affect Labeling

Affect labeling has been shown to reduce negative emotions both immediately and with delay. Based on the evidence, it seems that neither distraction nor self-reflection is a mechanism by which affect labeling reduces emotional intensity. It is more likely that finding the right words to label one's emotion reduces the uncertainty of that emerging experience—especially for feelings of fear and anxiety (Torre & Lieberman, 2018). The initial phase of experiential awareness recruits areas of the brain typically involved in somatosensory processing. Then, top-down cognitive processes work with emotion by activating brain areas to control and allocate mental attention (Wang et al., 2022). This means symbolizing an evocative stimulus using labels notifies the prefrontal cortex that the perceived "threat" has been responded to through categorization, which decreases the necessity for increased activation in the amygdala. This explanation is consistent with the fact that the amygdala responds to the uncertainty of stimuli (Pessoa, 2013). Furthermore, the significance of managing uncertainty also plays out developmentally. When adolescents were followed over 6 months, their intolerance of uncertainty anticipated difficulties in emotional processing, more than the other way around (Lauriola et al., 2023).

Reducing uncertainty also entails an increased confidence in a specific emotional trajectory. This is because emotion is not only representational (i.e., something you feel); it is also inherently procedural (i.e., something you do). Labeling affect is a constructive process, whereby the feeling also involves a set of action tendencies, unmet needs, and implicitly goal-directed behaviors. As it becomes clearer what one is feeling, one is simultaneously increasing the degree to which one is committed and engaged in a given emotional trajectory. Thus, affect labeling dispels uncertainty but also creates momentum in an emergent direction.

Relatedly, affect labeling also likely works through the *symbolization of experience*. As discussed in Chapter 5, however, the way one engages experience (e.g., as an outside observer or exploring it subjectively from within) probably moderates whether symbolization will increase or decrease emotional arousal. For instance, symbolizing a stimulus using more abstract labels also increases one's psychological distance from that stimulus, dampening arousal (Trope & Liberman, 2010). At the same time, while finding the right words for one's immediate experience may attenuate the physiological intensity of that feeling, the subjective experience is still carried forward in symbolic formulation as something that has personal meaning for negotiating the presenting events. This would be where the label one gives to an emerging emotion might develop into a more complex sense of awareness, and perhaps even narrative elaboration.

Finally, the impact of affect labeling may also be moderated by the kind of emotion one is symbolizing. Some authors (e.g., Kassam & Mendes, 2013) have suggested that self-referential emotions (e.g., shame, as opposed to anger) might be less influenced by affect labeling. However, I suggest an alternative explanation, which is that affect labeling may be more useful in immediately attenuating *secondary* emotions (e.g., defensive anger and general frustration as in the study by Kassam & Mendes), whereas attenuating *primary* emotions (e.g., shame and disappointment over one's performance) requires additional work, and labeling it is only the beginning.

Neurological Correlates of Affect Labeling

Several studies have also examined neurological activity during the exact moments in which someone finds the right word to describe what they are feeling. A meta-analysis of 385 studies on amygdala activity during various tasks that presented people with evocative stimuli concluded that amygdala activation decreased significantly when people were instructed to label emotions they observed, as compared to passively viewing the stimuli (Costafreda et al., 2008). Furthermore, there is strong evidence that the ventrolateral prefrontal cortex (VLPFC) and the amygdala are in closed communication during the process of labeling emotion. More specifically, the VLPFC's role in semantic meaning-making seems to attenuate arousal of the amygdala (Torre & Lieberman, 2018). Individual differences also matter because some people have more capacity for this process. Being inclined to simply notice and identify the ebb and flow of one's feelings is reflected, in part, by trait levels of mindfulness. Indeed, functional magnetic resonance imaging (fMRI) research has shown that when individuals with higher trait levels of mindfulness were asked to complete an affect labeling task, they showed stronger and more robust neural activations than those who were low in mindfulness (i.e., increased VLPFC as well as dorsolateral PFC activity and decreased amygdala activity; Creswell et al., 2007).

Affect labeling is a momentary process, but while working through difficult life circumstances, it is a process one will repeatedly engage in. For example, myriad instances of emerging awareness are embedded within the ongoing elaboration of one's personal narrative, and that cumulative process eventually impacts symptom change. In another study of individual differences, fMRI was used to measure participants' neurocognitive activity while they responded to a visual task, in which they were asked to label the emotions being expressed in stock images (Memarian et al., 2017). Although this task reflects the perception and recognition of emotion in others (i.e., externally focused affect labeling), it arguably offers a proxy for how easily people can connect verbal labels to their own interoceptive experiences (i.e., internally focused affect labeling).

Indeed, when the same participants were then asked to write for several sessions about a difficult emotional experience from their lives (i.e., expressive writing), the neural responses during their externally focused affect labeling predicted their improved depressive, anxiety, and life satisfaction outcomes resulting from the expressive writing task. Specifically, better outcomes due to expressive writing correlated with increased activity in the right VLPFC and lower activation in the left amygdala (Memarian et al., 2017).

In summary, within conscious awareness, there is no such thing as the passive perception of emotion. Findings suggest that the act of labeling one's emotional reaction recruits activation of the prefrontal cortex and correspondingly decreases activity in the amygdala. Labeling turns the emotion into a point of reference, and once one finds the right words, there are some quite different avenues for emotional processing downstream. One may use the initial symbolization of one's feelings to contain the experiencing, which typically helps soothe and down-regulate distress. Alternatively, one may continue to elaborate the emergent emotional experience, which typically involves ongoing activation (perhaps even spikes) of emotional arousal, which is the process discussed next.

UNPACKING AN EXPERIENCE CREATES A NEW HORIZON

Initially finding the right words and labeling one's feelings can offer some reprieve as one gets a handle on emotion, and that may be the interim goal. However, at other times, delving into emotional experience will point to a more elaborate form of emotional awareness. Symbolizing complex and freshly emerging experience with images or words is a truly novel moment in processing one's experience. When therapists who use focusing ask their clients to "check inside" or Gestalt therapists ask their clients to "experiment and try it on, see if those words fit," they are encouraging their clients to verify and test out the viability of a novel way of representing (and therefore experiencing) the presenting feeling. When emotional awareness introduces a new trajectory of self-organization in the client—a new way of perceiving and engaging the self, world, or other—it is an example of emotional processing. For instance, in a study of systematically facilitating a client's emerging awareness, one client recalled:

> I wasn't sure exactly what it was that I wanted to say. . . . She [the therapist] started something and I went a little bit further and I managed to come to the work "mindless," which was what I had wanted to say but I didn't quite know that's what it was. (Watson & Rennie, 1994, p. 503)

Or, as another client in the same study summed up, "It put a label on it and made it clear. The word fit perfectly" (p. 503).

New Ways of Perceiving the Internal World

For a person who is striving to engage the self, world, or other in increasingly productive ways, the newly represented experience, or new way of perceiving one's internal world, eventually proves to be either useful or not useful. To that end, some of the new ways of perceiving one's internal world improve the representational repertoire one has to articulate and grapple with that presenting experience. So a novel way to symbolize one's experience will only be retained if it enhances one's repertoire for working with the object of awareness. This process of expanding awareness occurs by engaging, labeling, and then continuing to symbolize one's experience into a horizon of meaning. To the extent that they capture the resistances of one's internal reality through an evolving psychological construction, these small advancements in emotional awareness are functional and adaptive events, therapeutic changes that further the client's personal development (A. Pascual-Leone & Greenberg, 2007b). Accordingly, when an attentive listener helps someone explore and deepen their experience, it facilitates emotional change.

As emotion is actively engaged and regarded as an increasingly dynamic process, the way one labels that experience also becomes increasingly complex. When the process initially is less exploratory, it may begin and end with finding the right words (e.g., "It's 'fear.' Yup, that's the feeling I have."). But eventually, describing the emerging experience as it unfolds in the moment can itself be a dynamic process of exploration (e.g., "Well it's a bit of fear . . . but as I say that, I also get this heavy feeling. I mean there is regret, as well. There is something really sad about having to accept things as they are. It's not just scary but sad and unfair . . ."). A critical issue here is the degree to which these processes rely on deeper levels of emotional awareness (beyond labeling), which also contrasts behavioral versus experiential frameworks of intervention (see Chapter 5).

Clarity and Discrimination

One of the perennial puzzles is how to measure the level of discrimination someone has in their own emotional awareness: Is emotion being experienced in black and white, with a limited color palette, or is it richly differentiated and in full color? Self-reports on one's own emotional clarity are inherently limited by their method. In fact, making an appraisal on one's own emotional clarity is sometimes more about an individual's use of goal-directed efforts when trying to cope with emotion, which is a different issue. For instance, "How clearly do you know what you want to do about the fact that you are emotional?" is not quite the same question as "Can you clarify the exact flavor of your emotional experience?" (See discussion of the Degrees of Emotion Regulation Scale in Chapter 2, this volume; Hallion et al., 2018.)

Whatever the case, a more direct and incisive approach to measuring someone's "skill" at differentiating their emotional experience is to use standardized tasks in what amounts to laboratory-based assessments of someone's performance (A. Pascual-Leone & Kramer, 2023). This approach measures an individual's trait-like capacity for emotional awareness, and it contrasts with the dynamic assessments of someone's observed performance within a session (e.g., the client experiencing scale; see Chapters 4 and 7). Still, the notion of emotional awareness as a capacity or facet of emotional intelligence will be familiar to most clinicians. One example of research on the degree to which people differentiate their own emotional experience involves presenting participants with several sliding scales to represent discrete emotions so they can use the collective set of scale ratings to best describe their immediate emotional experience. Over a number of trials, an index of emotional differentiation can then be calculated based on the degree to which ratings are highly correlated or contrasted (Nook et al., 2018). This is an intriguing approach, if only for the fact that it seems to make the individual's internal process remarkably more transparent.

Using this method, research has shown a U-shaped pattern in the lifespan development of emotional differentiation, where adolescence is a particularly murky period in one's emotional life (Nook et al., 2018). Children (5- to 10-year-olds) typically have high levels of emotional differentiation, and this is because they are more likely to only experience isolated emotions that are exclusive of one another (e.g., feeling either afraid or sad). Adolescents develop the mental capacity to coexperience multiple emotions at once, and with this influx of emotional depth comes much more ambivalence. Particularly as adolescents are still learning to disentangle various aspects of their experience, they lose ground in terms of their ability to emotionally differentiate. So the U-shaped developmental curve bottoms out at about age 15 to 17. Recall that intolerance of uncertainty during adolescence predicts trouble with emotional processing several months later (Lauriola et al., 2023). Nevertheless, as people move into their early to mid-20s, their ability to differentiate emotions from one another returns in a more sophisticated way (Nook et al., 2018). Although individual differences in this will range quite a bit, healthy adults are more or less able to articulate a complex mix of feelings with nuance and precision.

The Levels of Emotional Awareness Scale (LEAS; Lane, 2020; Lane et al., 1987) is another laboratory-based measure of emotional awareness, and it uses short, fictional, emotionally charged vignettes about situations involving the reader and another person. After reading the vignette, the participant is asked to write an open-ended response to the following questions: "How would you feel?" and "How would [the other person] feel?" Participant responses are then rated in terms of their complexity in their use of emotionally evocative language. When measured this way, one's level of emotional awareness is positively correlated with attending to one's feelings and the use of sophisticated emotional language (Lumley et al., 2005). Better emotional awareness (according to this measure) is also related to increased activity in the anterior cingulate gyrus (Lane et al., 1998).

Implications for Treatment

Some research has been conducted on how labeling one's emotional experience relates to intervention and treatment outcomes. For clients who experience panic attacks, for example, without any apparent precipitating event, the capacity to identify and label affective experience as such is critical. In a randomized clinical trial of psychodynamic psychotherapy versus cognitive behavior therapy (CBT) plus exposure therapy as treatments for severe panic disorder, emotional awareness was measured at intake using the LEAS (Beutel et al., 2013). While both brief treatment models were quite successful, researchers discovered that a client's level of emotional awareness was a strong moderator of treatment effectiveness, irrespective of the therapy approach. Because clients' initial levels of emotional awareness had such a strong effect on the success of treatment, one clinical implication is that assessing emotional awareness might help with identifying those most suitable for short-term psychotherapy. With respect to research, stratifying clients by their initial level of emotional awareness may be a fruitful strategy for future trials (Beutel et al., 2013).

The fact that labeling one's emotion is so relevant to markedly different treatment approaches (e.g., psychodynamic, CBT) begs some deeper consideration about the latent processes at work and whether finding the right words is truly operating in the same way across treatments. In this section, I have argued that naming one's emotion can help one access and unpack the subjective meaning of that experience, which is more typical of psychodynamic and humanistic discourses. However, as discussed in Chapter 5, emotion can be engaged from two quite distinct vantage points. One can regard the presenting emotion either from a first-person perspective as the experiencer from within or from a third-person perspective as an outside observer who is noticing the feeling. So, aside from the fact that symbolization in vivo helps develop one's moment-by-moment awareness and elaborate meaning, the very act of labeling could alternatively help assuage or regulate negative affect. The latter function is more in line with CBT interventions, where finding the right words is used to help anchor and contain a distressing experience. In other words, if one takes the observer's perspective, then once a feeling is suitably labeled, the process is considered complete, which helps down-regulate arousal. In the end, labeling emotion probably acts in both of these ways in any given therapy, sometimes even within the same session—although they are not compatible within the same moment. This represents a deeper level of process analysis, in which we understand treatment interventions as framing and potentiating certain corresponding processes, but ultimately the client's immediate intentions and motivations are the primary determinants that shape the emergent process (see Chapter 1).

POOR EMOTIONAL AWARENESS REVEALS A KEY COMPONENT IN EMOTIONAL PROCESSING

A common issue in psychotherapy is that some clients have marked difficulties accessing and elaborating their emotional experience. *Alexithymia* is a term derived from the Greek which literally means "lacking words for feelings." Its current conceptualization describes an individual's limited capacity to symbolize and elaborate emotional experience (Lane, 2020; Taylor & Bagby, 2013). Thus, people with alexithymia are said to have cognitive and affective deficits in processing emotion.

Foremost, people with alexithymia are typically vague or uncertain when asked how they are feeling (e.g., ". . . I don't know"). Then, when they do identify an emotion they have difficulty verbalizing those feelings ("It doesn't feel good, it's just confusing"). A revealing point is that they may have difficulty differentiating their emotional feelings from purely physical sensations. In a quirky example, a troubled client of mine whose girlfriend was leaving him inadvertently captured this with a play on words, musing: "Is this what heartbreak feels like?! . . . or is it just heartburn?" Finally, they have a cognitive style characterized by its operative thinking. They tend to focus on external events (i.e., plot and characters), referring to behaviors rather than any accompanying internal experience ("I just wanted to push him out of the way"). This cognitive style also includes a restricted fantasy life, poor imagination, and dreaming less at night (Lumley et al., 2005; Samur et al., 2013). To date, there are over 6,000 papers on alexithymia,[3] which on account of its general stability over time, is widely discussed as a personality trait.

Alexithymia and Deficits in Emotional Awareness

Alexithymia can be thought of as the antithesis of emotional awareness.[4] Indeed, self-report measures of alexithymia (i.e., using the Toronto Alexithymia Scale; Bagby et al., 1994) have been repeatedly shown to have a moderate to large inverse relationship with general measures of emotional intelligence (Lumley et al., 2005). However, it seems important to highlight that while emotional awareness is a clinically intuitive and relatively coherent notion, the various measures that relate to that specific type of emotional processing have been developed and validated largely in isolation of one another. For example, implicit measures of emotional awareness (e.g., the LEAS) seem to have a low to negligible relationship with explicit self-reports on alexithymia (e.g., the Toronto Alexithymia Scale). Nevertheless, there is still general agreement that these, and other measures, speak to perhaps distinct facets, or levels of complexity, in emotional awareness as either a process or capacity (or both).

There is also an ongoing debate as to whether there are subtypes of alexithymia based on the observed overarching dimensions of cognitive deficits (i.e., difficulty identifying and verbalizing emotion) versus affective deficits (i.e., lower arousal, lower fantasy; Lane, 2020). Some neurological evidence supports this formulation by relating these two dimensions of alexithymia to different neuroanatomical profiles of activation (Goerlich-Dobre et al., 2015). If this were the case, an important issue for clinical consideration would be that cognitive versus affective dimensions of alexithymia, and hence poor emotional awareness, may have different developmental pathways toward psychopathology (Lane, 2020; Moormann et al., 2008). However, the evidence based on self-reports still supports a unidimensional view of alexithymia, where identifying and verbalizing emotional experience are the main factors (Watters et al., 2016). One way these perspectives might be reconciled is to consider that as one's degree of emotional awareness increases, it categorically shifts the way one dynamically engages with one's internal or external world. Increases from one level of complexity to the next produce a qualitative continuum, one that reflects distinct ways of interacting with an emotional experience (A. Pascual-Leone & Greenberg, 2007b; Watson & Bedard, 2006). Whatever the case, the construct of alexithymia elaborates our understanding of emotional awareness and its role in health.

Base Rates and Variation in the General Population

The rate of alexithymia in the general population is estimated to be 10% (Taylor et al., 1997) with variation across cultures (Le et al., 2002; Ryder et al., 2018). A handful of studies show that people with East Asian backgrounds (e.g., Chinese, Malaysian, Chinese American, Asian Canadian) score a bit higher on measures of alexithymia as compared to European Americans or non-Asian Canadians.[5] However, the issue of emotional awareness and cross-cultural measurement is complex. The construct of alexithymia itself comes with Western cultural values. Cultural differences in psychological mindedness are also associated with the impact of social values, education, birth cohort, and parenting styles (Ryder et al., 2018). Mediators help begin to explain these effects. First, the influences of culture and gender on alexithymia are mediated by the socialization of emotion offered by one's parents (Le et al., 2002). That process, of teaching children to understand and navigate emotion through their parenting (i.e., emotion socialization), has also been successfully manipulated in experimental interventions (Peterson et al., 1999). Second, the effect of culture was also mediated by social values, for Canadians of Asian as well as non-Asian heritage. Those who valued purity from desire and respect for social order were a bit more alexithymic, perhaps because they were less likely to reflect on internal experiences that were "impure" or socially disruptive. In contrast, people who valued trustworthiness, patience, and kindness were a bit less alexithymic (Lo, 2014).

Rates of alexithymia are universally higher among clinical samples. However, some other groups, such as athletes in high-risk sports (e.g., rock climbing, scuba diving, skydiving), also have rates of alexithymia that are higher than the general population, up to 30% in some cases. This has led some researchers to test what I will call the *ignorance is bliss* hypothesis: the idea that poor emotional awareness might be advantageous to people who engage in anxiety-producing tasks (Proença Lopes et al., 2022). That idea also appears in folk theories of psychology (e.g., just don't think about it!). However, a meta-analysis of alexithymia and symptomatology among athletes in different sports failed to support this. As with the general population, higher alexithymia among athletes is related to elevated anxiety, depression, addiction, burnout, and risky behavior (irrespective of preferred sport). In short, apparently being oblivious to one's own emotional distress offers no immunity to its effects.

Functional and Clinical Correlates of Poor Emotional Awareness

Individuals with alexithymia may express aroused emotion (e.g., weeping, having an outburst of rage) but often in a nondifferentiated way, consistent with what has been clinically described as *global distress* (i.e., low meaning despite high arousal; A. Pascual-Leone, 2018). Furthermore, when these individuals are questioned in detail about their experience, they are often unable to connect these expressions to either memories or specific situations. In fact, experiments show that when people high in alexithymia are presented with emotion-soliciting scenarios, like those discussed in therapy, the scenarios do not prime or elicit emotion words as they do for the general population (Suslow & Junghanns, 2002). As most psychotherapists can attest, this does not bode well for working with emotion.

Moreover, this clearly goes beyond the simple issue of vocabulary. The deficit is related to what seems to be a pervasive pattern of processing differences. Alexithymia is linked with impairments in the recognition of emotional faces (Grynberg et al., 2012) and in processing the melody of speech (i.e., prosody) that typically goes with emotional content (Goerlich-Dobre et al., 2014). People with severe alexithymia essentially have difficulty conceptualizing emotion in general, with less semantic differentiation and presumably less differentiation in the experience of emotion itself (Wotschack & Klann-Delius, 2013). One candid example comes from a study of fathers in treatment for intimate partner violence, being interviewed about parenting. One participant stated:

> I don't like talking about feelings [. . .] What you can grasp and hold and feel in your hand—that is OK [. . .] I know that feelings [. . .] I am not good at dealing with this in relation to the kids. (Mohaupt et al., 2019, p. 866)

Far from emotion being reducible to the sum of its physiological experiences, these observations exemplify the critical aspect of emotion as an experience that carries embodied meaning with a lived narrative-significance. And those are the targets of healthy emotional awareness.

A host of studies have now shown that when individuals have higher levels of alexithymia, it predicts increased psychopathology in a range of anxiety, mood, body image, and substance use disorders. It also predicts specific difficulties such as interpersonal problems, lack of empathy, shame, and borderline symptoms, and it is even predictive of psychophysiological disorders such as hypertension and chronic pain (Franzoni et al., 2013; Gaher et al., 2013; Lumley et al., 2005; Ogrodniczuk et al., 2012; Salsman & Linehan, 2012). While these associations are mounting, their directionality remains to be fully explained. To that end, a recent study has shown that the link between alexithymia and having a personality disorder is at least partially independent from its symptoms. Even when their symptom distress is low, people with personality disorders have specific difficulties with focusing on their internal experience (De Panfilis et al., 2015). Findings like this have important treatment implications because, if impaired emotional awareness were fully attributable to symptom severity, treatment would only call for more vigorous efforts at decreasing psychological distress. However, the observed degree of independence suggests that bolstering internal emotional awareness should also be a unique treatment focus.

Neurological Underpinnings of Alexithymia

A study used fMRI to compare men with and without alexithymia in their response to intense emotional pictures. Researchers concluded that the medial prefrontal and specifically the anterior cingulate cortex is involved in the capacity for reflective awareness of emotional experience. Individuals with alexithymia appear to have the same regions activate as those with normal brain functioning, just to a lesser extent (Berthoz et al., 2002). Interestingly, alexithymia has also been associated with structural differences in the white matter of the brain. By examining brain regions of interest, one study found the corpus callosum was larger in people high in alexithymia. Because emotional perception (right brain) and verbal labeling (left brain) are generally lateralized to different hemispheres, researchers interpreted the larger number of pathways between the two sides of the brain as reflecting their inefficient communication and poorer integration between hemispheres in people with alexithymia (Goerlich-Dobre et al., 2015).

Although there is still a widely held belief that almost all forms of emotional processing are ultimately related to regulating the arousal of emotion (see Chapter 2), such a course view overlooks the relative interdependence of other emotional subprocesses (e.g., emotional awareness, in this case). An incisive study using fMRI has similarly questioned that position by evaluating the neural correlates of emotion regulation as a function of levels in alexithymia (van der Velde et al., 2015). In short, while alexithymia was related to distinct patterns of brain activation, particularly during the perception of emotion, it did not influence areas related to either emotion regulation or its arousal. These results indicate that difficulty finding the right words to describe emotional experience is related to a shortfall at an early processing step, where the perception and awareness of emotion is initially generated. In contrast, alexithymia was not related to circuits in the frontal lobe where higher order forms of emotion regulation and reflection occur (van der Velde et al., 2015).

This is important because demonstrating that the neural substrates for emotional awareness are distinct from those involved in reflecting on emotion supports the view that mentalizing about affect is not represented by any single capacity. Rather, mentalizing is a heterogeneous mix of processes and the product of several distinct operations. These qualitatively different processes can be ordered in terms of their increasing complexity, and they sometimes are both active, or people might toggle between them (see Chapter 22). This gives the impression of a seamless processing continuum, much like a car that automatically shifts smoothly from lower to higher gears. In short, neurological evidence supports the conceptualization of emotional awareness as a unique subprocess under the broader rubric of emotional processing, one that is distinct from both the down-regulation of emotion and from the higher order reflection on emotion.

EMOTIONAL AWARENESS OVER TIME: DEVELOPMENTAL AND CLINICAL CHANGE

Finding the right words is a specific way of working with emotion; it is a process that unfolds moment by moment as one attends to internal experience and then unpacks its meaning. As discussed above, some people have deficits in emotional awareness, which is associated with clinical impairments. But understanding the role of this process within a causal chain requires a longitudinal perspective of development over the lifespan and of the impact that treatment may have over time.

Developmental Implications of Problems With Emotional Awareness

While some have pointed to alexithymia as either an obstacle or an additional target for insight-oriented treatments, others suggest that it has a causal role in the generation of symptom distress (Samur et al., 2013). A longitudinal study on a sample of adolescents highlighted how important the differentiation of negative emotion is (Starr et al., 2020). In the context of naturalistic stressors in a teenager's life, having a low level of differentiation of one's negative emotions seemed to amplify the relationship between everyday hassles or stressors and receiving a diagnosis of depression 18 months later. Concretely, simple statements that one feels bad or upset are vague and global expressions of distress, and it is precisely that lack of differentiation that predicted a teenager's vulnerability to depression. Meanwhile, those that used words with more specificity (e.g., feeling annoyed, hurt, bitter) were less susceptible. In short, adolescents who were better at describing their negative emotions in nuanced and precise ways were also more able to stave off depression, as compared to peers who were less articulate (Starr et al., 2020). The discussion of neurobiological correlates (see Chapter 5) and alexithymia at large (discussed earlier this chapter) suggests that this variation in emotional awareness may represent individual differences in cognitive-affective processing style. However, another line of research has also linked poorer emotional awareness to the hardships that some people have endured earlier in their lives.

The Role of Early Trauma

Accumulating evidence now shows childhood maltreatment is connected to somatic complaints subsequently reported in adulthood. A handful of studies with large samples have illuminated how this tragic cascade might occur. In a sample of adult psychiatric outpatients, alexithymia mediated the relationship between childhood abuse and somatic complaints (Ogrodniczuk et al., 2014). Similarly, two other studies show that alexithymia in college students explained the relationship between their childhood trauma and self-injurious behaviors or other symptoms of borderline personality disorder (Gaher et al., 2013; Paivio & McCulloch, 2004). In short, the mechanism of harm seems to be that if people suffer abuse during their childhood, those who have poor emotional awareness (i.e., difficulty identifying and describing emotion) are unable to adequately process the traumatic experience, which then produces somatic clinical symptoms. In other terms, the treatment implication is that better emotional awareness seems to protect people against certain kinds of psychological harm.

Because alexithymia is such a general and pervasive deficit, the temporal order of events by which it leads to psychological symptoms is a process that unfolds over several years. That makes it difficult for researchers to capture the causal connections within a narrow window of time. However, one could also look for converging evidence from a related phenomenon that is more specific and occurs in circumscribed situations. *Depersonalization* is usually understood as a defensive reaction where one feels detached from one's emotions, thoughts, and behaviors. So, while alexithymia manifests as a general processing style, depersonalization can occur as a discrete and identifiable event. Depersonalization and feeling unreal is obviously an obstacle to well-grounded emotional awareness, precisely because it is a (dysfunctional) way of coping with distress by avoiding engagement with (and awareness of) one's experience. Like the studies on alexithymia, research on a large sample of young adults has shown that moments of depersonalization mediate the relationship between one's childhood history of abuse and subsequent symptoms of psychological distress (Laoide et al., 2017). In short, someone with a history of emotional maltreatment suffers distress as an adult if they also use depersonalization as a way of avoiding emotional experience.

The Social Influence in Neglecting One's Emotion

In addition to the biological correlates discussed earlier, social learning theory offers the explanation that developing awareness of emotion, and learning to adequately communicate it, is something that is socially fostered and encouraged (or not) during one's upbringing. This formulation has also inspired the *normative male alexithymia hypothesis*, which states that traditionally reared men have a pattern of restrictive emotionality because of gender stereotypes (e.g., boys don't cry, men don't talk about their feelings). Indeed, a meta-analysis confirmed that, on average, men tend to have slightly higher levels of alexithymia than women, and this small gender effect does not seem to be a function of clinical versus nonclinical samples (Levant et al., 2009). A cross-cultural study of college students showed that the gender difference is explained by the socialization of emotion by one's parents (Le et al., 2002). Within a clinical population, women report more somatic symptoms compared to men. Moreover, women who have more difficulty in identifying their feelings (alexithymia) are also more likely to have pain interfere with their activities. In contrast, alexithymia among men did not seem to impact the relationship between pain and their daily functioning (Ogrodniczuk et al., 2018)—perhaps because of clinical base rates or social norms.

The Double Injury

An explanation of how alexithymia and trauma may relate to one another helps further elaborate the clinical-developmental portrait. Having alexithymia is essentially an emotional processing deficit that poses a vulnerability to one's health. Of course, this individual difference can exist quite independently from suffering any trauma. However, when abuse does occur during a critical period in a child's development, it likely entails a double injury. The adverse experience of childhood trauma is inherently harmful, and moreover, the developmental context in which abuse occurs often does not actively nurture a child's capacity for emotional awareness. Further to this point, childhood neglect has been found to have more adverse psychological effects than physical abuse on its own, and one of those effects is alexithymia (Gauthier et al., 1996). This compounds the initial injury by crippling the degree to which one might subsequently process a psychological trauma.

Going forward, when people who have difficulty identifying their feeling are activated by other affective stimuli in their lives, they focus on the accompanying somatic sensations rather than the nature or emotional meaning of those feelings. The fact that studies have found alexithymia mediates the impact of childhood maltreatment irrespective of whether it was physical abuse, sexual abuse, or neglect supports this interpretation about emotional development. Of course, without having tracked symptom change over time, one cannot conclusively determine the role of alexithymia in producing somatic or psychological symptoms.

Furthermore, a study of undergraduate students showed that while a history of childhood neglect or abuse covaried with having lacked healthy socialization of emotion as one grew up, these early experiences were jointly mediated by alexithymia in the prediction of later having insecure attachments in one's adult relationships (Mlotek, 2018). This adds yet another layer to the role emotional awareness plays in healthy development. An early history of neglect can make it difficult to develop healthy relationships later in life, perhaps even with a therapist. And then the quality of those relationships will still depend on a client's ability to talk about their feelings. So, beyond early childhood maltreatment and then poor socialization of emotion—a double injury that may contribute to alexithymia—that configuration also makes it harder to benefit from healthy relationships, which are often the means to remediate or shore up against alexithymia.

Treating People Who Have Difficulty With Emotional Awareness

While not mutually exclusive, another possible harmful impact of alexithymia is that it may hinder the degree to which people can make use of certain interventions (or otherwise curative processes). Experimental research offers some insight into this. Making personal disclosures, by either journaling or talking, has a small but very well-established impact in reducing a range of clinical and subclinical difficulties (Frattaroli, 2006; van Agteren et al., 2021). A handful of controlled experiments that used this simple psychological intervention to treat chronic somatic concerns (e.g., arthritis, chronic pain, headaches, gastrointestinal and other somatic symptoms) have also shown that the benefit was mediated by alexithymia. Although these studies examined nonpsychiatric populations, they suggest that the degree to which someone benefits from talking or writing about personal problems depends on their initial capacity for identifying and articulating emotional experience (Lumley, 2004).

Baseline Alexithymia Moderates Treatment

It should not be surprising that psychotherapy clients who are high in alexithymia often overlook and do not make use of emotional experiences while working in session. Indeed, alexithymia is related to poor treatment outcomes in both traditional psychodynamic and supportive psychotherapies, irrespective of individual or group format (Ogrodniczuk et al., 2011). Research also revealed that a client's level of alexithymia has surprisingly little influence on the treatment approach they may prefer (Ogrodniczuk et al., 2011).

Nevertheless, some have suggested that cognitive or behavioral therapies may be better suited to these clients because these treatments are thought to be less emotion oriented (Kennedy & Franklin, 2002; Lumley, 2004). The argument is that cognitive and behavioral interventions allow one to either bypass the deficit in emotion processing or for clients to receive a more gradual introduction to working with emotion. While this remains speculative, there seems to be some support for the idea from a study of group-based CBT for panic disorder, where baseline levels of alexithymia did not impact the success of final treatment outcomes (Rufer et al., 2010). As we have already seen, however, when using other measures of low emotional awareness (e.g., LEAS), it predicted poorer outcomes in the treatment of individuals with panic, whether the client was using CBT or psychodynamic therapy (Beutel et al., 2013). The deeper issue may be that contrasting treatments use a more affective versus more cognitive emphasis when negotiating a client's low level of emotional awareness. That hypothesis was supported by observations during the treatment of depression, in which client statements in sessions of CBT revealed that they were more distant and disengaged from their emotional experience as compared to clients in EFT (Watson & Bedard, 2006).

Treatment's Effect on Alexithymia

Network analyses assume that alexithymia is causally interrelated with the symptoms of psychopathology (rather than being caused by some broader underlying or latent disorder). Research using this method has highlighted the most central aspects of alexithymia that treatment interventions should prioritize, such as increasing a client's awareness of affect while also reducing externally oriented thinking (Watters et al., 2016). But despite alexithymia's known relationship to psychopathology, research on how treatments might impact alexithymia (i.e., as either a target complaint or a comorbidity) remains surprisingly sparse (Samur et al., 2013).

Some researchers have focused on a training approach and proposed that the use of more frequent practice opportunities for personal disclosure, along with more explicit guidance, might serve as an intervention to help people who are high in alexithymia (e.g., Lumley, 2004). Additional didactic efforts to directly reduce alexithymia could include training in emotion, vocabulary, and psychoeducation. However, while there is little doubt that creating more opportunity for working with emotion would be useful, skills-based approaches seem to require an intensity that is comparable to that of psychotherapy itself (Kennedy & Franklin, 2002). In short, this kind of emotional development ultimately requires attentive moment-by-moment scaffolding by an emotion coach—and an empathic therapist might be in the best position to offer that (L. S. Greenberg, 2021). A review of changes in alexithymia suggests that this deficit in emotional processing is partly modifiable, particularly when the intervention is specifically intended to address alexithymia (Cameron et al., 2014).

Alexithymia is not usually the primary target of treatment, although it may be identified as a comorbidity. There are only a handful of controlled studies on the changes in alexithymia that occur during psychotherapy, and all these studies used short-term treatments (i.e., 20 sessions or fewer) despite the fact that the emotional shallowness of alexithymia has often been regarded as a personality trait (Taylor & Bagby, 2013). Given the connection between alexithymia and somatic problems such as hypertension, the first of these studies specifically sought to reduce alexithymia among patients who had recently suffered heart attacks (Beresnevaite, 2000). Results showed that short-term group psychotherapy (using techniques from Gestalt therapy, supportive therapy, and behavioral training in expression and relaxation) decreased the level of alexithymia for these patients by design, but that was not the case for those in a psychoeducation group. Changes were maintained at a two-year follow-up, where decreases in alexithymia also predicted fewer cardiac events.

The impact of psychotherapy in reducing alexithymia over the course of treating a presenting psychiatric concern is important to quantify for understanding emotional awareness as a mechanism of change, and early research examining that suggests it is favorable. A study of EFT for complex relational trauma (i.e., adult survivors of childhood abuse) found a 68% decrease from pre- to posttreatment in the number of clients that met criteria for alexithymia (Ralston, 2006, as cited in Paivio & Pascual-Leone, 2023). Because the aim of an experiential therapy is to deepen experiencing, one interpretation of the incidental reduction observed in alexithymia is that it occurred on account of therapists' closely facilitating their clients' moment-by-moment process in exploring and symbolizing emotion.

Emotion coaching of this kind unfolds as a therapist continually orients toward the client's affective experience. The collaborative process is illustrated in the vignette of a woman who was concerned about her romantic relationship but habitually distanced herself from difficult content and interrupted her emotional process (Paivio & Pascual-Leone, 2023, p. 118). In session, she touches on how this also leaves her feeling uneasy:

THERAPIST: That sounds like a very important relationship to you . . . wanting to spend as much time as possible with him.

CLIENT: When I start thinking about it, I start sweating again.

THERAPIST: What is that sweat telling you?

CLIENT: That I don't want to talk about it; it makes me unhappy, scared?

THERAPIST: Okay, scared, so don't think about it; push it away, push it away, keep it all inside.

CLIENT: Yes, keep it all to the side.

THERAPIST: Keep it all to the side. But somehow, it keeps intruding, interfering with your ability to concentrate, intruding on your life. It's hard to keep it compartmentalized.

CLIENT: Yes, it is affecting my life.

THERAPIST: So, this is a big deal, this relationship. You care a lot about him. But something is not right?

CLIENT: It's a very big deal. . . .

The client then disclosed her sense that the relationship is not reciprocal, a fear that she is giving more than she is getting.

THERAPIST: So, you are settling for whatever he will give?

CLIENT: Yes. [*eyes well up in tears*]

THERAPIST: I see that makes you feel sad. You are not getting what you want, but are you getting enough?

CLIENT: No, I am not getting enough. . . . I feel used. . . . I feel like I'm just a joyride.

THERAPIST: A joyride—that doesn't feel good! You must resent being used like that.

Here, the therapist helps refine the embodied meaning with successive conjectures, which remain exploratory rather than prescriptive (i.e., meaning is construed as dynamic rather than static; see Chapter 5). Through this process, the client gains a sense of emotional clarity.

There can be little doubt that using EFT to treat adults who suffered childhood abuse must represent a very different kind of treatment process from a

CBT approach to group work and skills training. Even so, a CBT group treatment for panic disorder has also been shown to reduce clients' presenting levels of alexithymia from pre- to posttreatment (Rufer et al., 2010). Adding to this, two forms of psychodynamically informed therapy were also related to reductions in alexithymia during the treatment of a general psychiatric population, a positive effect that was maintained at a 6-month follow-up (Ogrodniczuk et al., 2013). A special merit of this last study is that using a randomized trial allowed researchers to examine whether alexithymia was differentially affected by a more supportive or more interpretive approach to conducting treatment. The supportive-dynamic treatment, which focused on more externally oriented perspectives and was more cognitive in nature, offered a small advantage in reducing alexithymia. In contrast, the more interpretive-dynamic approach may have been overwhelming or too demanding of clients' capacities for emotional introspection (Ogrodniczuk et al., 2013). Finally, while poor emotional clarity seems to contribute to symptoms of borderline personality disorder (Salsman & Linehan, 2012), evidence also supports increasing the clarity of one's emotional awareness as a mechanism of change in dialectical behavior therapy (McMain et al., 2013).

A Possible Mechanism of Change

Taken together, the impact of baseline alexithymia on treatment success suggests that assessing and having some sense of a client's capacity for emotional awareness may be helpful in tailoring treatment appropriately. Evidence also suggests that psychotherapy may be an opportunity to correct alexithymia and essentially increase emotional intelligence over the course of a relatively brief treatment. Notice that these observed changes to alexithymia can be interpreted in several ways. From one perspective, improved emotional awareness is a collateral benefit, gained en route to the successful treatment of other target complaints. Another, more provocative and more likely perspective, is that reducing alexithymia is part of the emotional development needed to address psychological symptoms that often represent more poignant clinical concerns. When treatment changes occur through emotional awareness, psychotherapy may be more about developing someone's emotional functioning rather than solving specific personal problems per se. Then, with an expanded ability to navigate and make use of emotion, some presenting concerns may essentially resolve themselves.

This chapter has explored the role of emotional awareness by considering both what happens when someone is able to successfully label their emotions and also when someone consistently has difficulty in finding words for their experience. Another aspect of emotional awareness is the *depth of client experiencing,* which captures how personal meaning unfolds moment by moment. That depth is sometimes regarded as a gold standard for good psychotherapy process, and I explore it in the next and final chapter of Part II.

ENDNOTES

1. While this finding that labeling one's feelings reduces emotional reactivity is a compelling example of affect labeling as a singular change process, the authors of that study (Kassam & Mendes, 2013) are more focused on the problem of using self-reports to measure emotional experience. (For more on the measurement problem, see A. Pascual-Leone, Herpertz, et al., 2016; A. Pascual-Leone & Kramer, 2023.)

2. For a possible explanation of why affect labeling lowers one's physiological reactivity but does not typically reduce the amount of subjectively reported feeling, refer to Chapter 5: "Observations about emotion from outside" versus "experiencing emotion from within."

3. "Alexithymia" is listed in a title or abstract of 6,187 papers in the PsycInfo database (February 15, 2025). Interestingly, most of this work is in the areas of either personality or industrial–organizational psychology.

4. As mentioned, there seems to be a cognitive component of alexithymia as well, which involves having a more operative thinking style. That makes alexithymia a broader construct than someone simply having trouble labeling their feelings (Lane, 2020; Moormann et al., 2008). Even so, rather than suggesting alexithymia is somehow a different process, I believe the observation helps fill out some of the functional implications related to someone having deficits in emotional awareness.

5. This effect size regarding cross-cultural differences in measures of alexithymia is small, cautioning against any exaggerated interpretations or cultural stereotyping.

7
Deepening Emotion Through Symbolization

[A bridge can] bind territories that remain disparate, albeit joined . . . through transformations, semantic abstractions, and the multiple associations of the relations into which it is bundled. . . . Each bridge, in offering a new solution, creates a new problem.
—THOMAS HARRISON, *OF BRIDGES: A POETIC AND PHILOSOPHICAL ACCOUNT*

Nothing that feels bad is ever the last step.
—EUGENE T. GENDLIN, *FOCUSING*

Deepening the experience of emotion enriches its meaning. As we have seen, research on alexithymia tells us how a deficit in emotional awareness is associated with, but not fully attributable to, poor mental (and physical) health. The fact that a person's capacity for attending to and articulating emotion can be improved over the course of psychotherapy is encouraging. However, therapists seeking to address specific mental illnesses and help reduce their clients' symptoms are still left asking what process to facilitate within the session: "Will working on emotional awareness during psychotherapy improve my client's final symptom outcomes?" Research on the trait-like deficits in emotional awareness (i.e., alexithymia) also informs our understanding of what moderates health care outcomes, but finding out whether the in-session process is actually part of what makes psychotherapy work requires a performance-based measure so emotional change can be observed in action.

https://doi.org/10.1037/0000460-008
Principles of Emotion Change: What Works and When in Psychotherapy and Everyday Life, by A. Pascual-Leone
Copyright © 2026 by the American Psychological Association. All rights reserved.

DEPTH OF EXPERIENCING: THE FEELING HOLDS SIGNIFICANCE

The concept of *depth of experiencing*, as introduced in Chapter 4, is a process dimension that essentially expresses the antithesis of alexithymia. Although poor emotional awareness can be thought of as a baseline characteristic (i.e., alexithymia), it is also amenable to change through effortful practice. Measuring a client's moment-by-moment depth of experiencing as they work in therapy has helped dramatically in elaborating our understanding of what that experiential awareness is. Unlike self-report methods that ask clients about what they usually do or to retroactively recall some process of what happened, the experiencing scale is applied by a third party trained observer (i.e., it is based neither on client nor therapist reports).

Recall from Chapter 4 that this observational measure organizes qualitatively different stages of processing onto an ordinal scale (Klein et al., 1986). As a result, when one considers the application of this scale specifically to emotional experiences, the measure cuts across several subprocesses related to working with emotion (e.g., while lower levels 1–4 speak to emotional awareness, level 5 refers to reflection on emotion, and level 6 suggests a sequential transformation). So, upon closer consideration, the client experiencing scale is best thought of as an amalgam of several other more specific and narrowly definable facets of emotional processing (A. Pascual-Leone & Yeryomenko, 2016; Pos et al., 2017; Watson & Bedard, 2006). Notice that this implicit amalgamation of constructs is probably one of the reasons why the client experiencing scale often subsumes large portions of explained variance when it competes with other process measures used jointly in the prediction of treatment outcomes.

Even so, there are two reasons for focusing on process-to-outcome research that uses the experiencing scale, specifically in this chapter on emotional awareness. First, despite the full range of the scale, a review of research that applied the experiencing scale to psychotherapy has indicated that, in actual practice, client in-session process is largely captured by lower level ratings (e.g., levels 2–4, with an average mode rating of around 3, and an average peak of around 4; based on my estimates that combine recent studies with those in A. Pascual-Leone & Yeryomenko, 2016). Second, as I have argued, the lower half of this scale captures the specific processes of emerging awareness about emotion and its associated perceptual meanings. The implication here is that most of the available data collected on depth of experiencing during psychotherapy bears most substantively on the specific client process that I am referring to as emotional awareness (i.e., the engagement, labeling, and complex symbolization of emerging personal experience).

Symbolizing Experience Predicts Good Psychotherapy Outcomes

It is now widely accepted that client experience is predictive of good outcome, and that deeper process leads to better health care outcomes (Hendricks, 2009; Sønderland et al., 2023). Antonio Pascual-Leone and Yeryomenko (2016) conducted a meta-analysis on the relationship between client experiencing and subsequent treatment outcomes based on 10 published and unpublished studies of clinical populations, which included primarily individual but also couples therapy.[1] About half of these studies examined experiential treatments although several significant data sets were also included from cognitive behavior, psychodynamic, and interpersonal treatments. When client experiencing was measured during the middle portion (i.e., working phase) of therapy it predicted improvements in symptom of depression, general psychopathology, interpersonal difficulties, and bolstered self-esteem by the end of treatment. The authors reported several effect sizes estimating this process had a small to medium effect. To put that into perspective, the range of effect this process has on psychotherapy outcomes is likely to be in the same vicinity as the impact of the therapeutic relationship. A later meta-analysis included 13 published studies on individual therapy and concluded that client experiencing had a large effect on treatment outcomes (Sønderland et al., 2023). It is worth noting that these two meta-analyses each included treatment studies that addressed a variety of mental health problems, although major depression was by far the most frequently treated concern.

According to both meta-analyses, the effect of client experiencing seems to hold across treatment approaches, whether they were humanistic–experiential or not (e.g., cognitive behavior, interpersonal, psychodynamic). Moreover, an additional study that compared long-term psychoanalytic, psychodynamic, and cognitive behavioral therapies found that for all three approaches, client experiencing in the middle phase of treatment could predict reduced depressive symptoms as much as 3 years after treatment had ended (Klug et al., 2022). So, while further studies are needed, client experiencing seems promising as a common factor in psychotherapy. For instance, while interventions such as problem solving or setting goals based on one's personal values provide therapists with explicit tasks, deepening client experience is typically an implicit and microtask, one that transcends a host of manifest interventions.

This area of research has mostly focused on individual psychotherapy with adults, although several studies also highlight the importance of this process when working with couples. Nevertheless, a recent multi-site study has now also looked at client experiencing among 13- to 15-year-old adolescents who were in school-based humanistic counseling (Geyer et al., 2024). It showed that when depth of experience was measured in the middle of treatment, the process had a large effect in predicting the symptom outcomes of young people. Taken together, there is robust evidence that clients who are internally focused, engage in deeper exploration, refer to their emotions, and who reflect on their experience to create new meaning, have measurably better treatment outcomes than those that do not engage with their experiences in an affectively meaningful way.

Baseline Ability Versus Improvement in Processing

Despite the relevance of clients' baseline capacities in alexithymia or emotional awareness, the initial advantage some clients bring to therapy is a separate issue from the client's development or subsequent improvement in this kind of processing. The latter issue represents a treatment-related change process. To understand what happens during psychotherapy, one needs to consider the degree to which client experiencing might improve over the course of their treatment. Narrative reviews on a diverse sample of clinical and nonclinical studies have concluded this is indeed the case for client process: People can learn to deepen their capacity for the awareness and symbolization of their internal experiences (Hendricks, 2009).

A study on the treatment of depression carefully considered this issue. Researchers (Pos et al., 2009) used the experiencing scale to study only those therapy segments during which clients discussed emotional content, a procedure which effectively yields a precise measure of emotional experiencing (i.e., emotional awareness and symbolization). As one would expect from the research on alexithymia, they found when a client's individual capacity for this kind of deep emotional processing was observed early in therapy it predicted better outcome at the end of treatment. However, they also discovered an increase in one's emotional awareness and symbolization from early to mid (or early to late) phases of treatment was an even stronger predictor of outcome than a client's initial levels of experiencing. In fact, that growth in capacity was also a stronger predictor than the quality of the early therapy relationship. Interestingly, this means that even when clients have an initial capacity for emotional awareness and symbolization, it does not necessarily promise good outcomes down the road. On the flipside, when a client does not have this capacity, it should not be taken to mean that working at experiencing and awareness is futile. While an advantage, having an initial baseline ability in emotional awareness and symbolization appears not to be as critical as the ability to acquire or increase that depth of one's emotional experiencing over the course of therapy (Pos et al., 2009).

As it turns out, the degree to which clients improve in their use of this process may highlight the most critical issue in how depth of client experiencing predicts outcome. In individual psychotherapy, a client's average modal score on the experiencing scale changes by about 14%, and this happens between the early and middle (i.e., working) phases of treatment (based on my estimates that combine recent studies with those already in A. Pascual-Leone & Yeryomenko, 2016).[2] After that increase during the middle phase, some process studies showed a plateau (Pos et al., 2009; Watson & Bedard, 2006), although another study with more time points suggests process gains continue steadily from the beginning to the end of treatment (Pinheiro et al., 2021). In either case, clients' depth of experiencing (i.e., level of emotional awareness and meaning) can improve during treatment, and the resultant level of processing predicts outcome. This presents an opportunity for interventions to maximize the process, during either individual or couples therapy (Kailanko et al., 2022; A. Pascual-Leone & Yeryomenko, 2016; Pinheiro et al., 2021).

Generally, research that examines what process works best for whom helps therapists know whether they should build on their client's processing strengths, or if they should shore up against a client's shortcomings (i.e., improve capacity). A study of emotion-focused therapy (EFT) for complex trauma did this by first assessing both the therapeutic relationship and a client's depth of experiencing early in therapy. Then researchers looked at the same clients later, in the middle phase of therapy, to see which of those two processes subsequently emerged as the best predictor of outcome (Harrington et al., 2021). For clients who initially had difficulty engaging in deeper experiencing at the beginning of treatment, their depth of experiencing during the middle phase of therapy was the best predictor of outcome (assuming an adequate relationship[3]). However, for clients who were already good at deep emotional experiencing early in treatment, any growth in that capacity was unimportant as contrasted with growth in other variables such as developing the quality of their relationship with the therapist. More research is needed, but this suggests that when deficits are observed in emotional awareness, shoring up on that should be a treatment goal. The early to middle phases likely represents an important time for helping clients to deepen awareness and symbolize their experience (A. Pascual-Leone & Yeryomenko, 2016). Whether or not the depth of experiencing typically levels off in late treatment, other processes (e.g., expressive arousal, narrative identity) likely come more into play as one approaches the end of therapy.

The Chicken or the Egg?

As people engage in treatment processes, client symptoms start to improve over the course of their work in psychotherapy: process and outcome are both unfolding over time. This poses a challenge if one wants to determine what came first: deeper experiencing or symptom change—which one is the chicken, and which is the egg? Longitudinal mediation is a method that allows one to consider the temporal interaction of ordered events. A comparative treatment study on depression has examined these week-by-week patterns of prediction (Pinheiro et al., 2021). Higher levels of client experiencing anticipated symptom decreases in the next session, but this also worked the other way around, in which symptom intensity then anticipated deeper emotional processing. In short, process and outcome predicted each other in an interdependent way. Furthermore, that intertwined relationship was observed in EFT as well as in cognitive behavior therapy (Pinheiro et al., 2021). The same pattern has also been observed in psychodynamic therapy, where a client's previously reported level of experiencing predicted subsequent changes to functioning, as well as the other way around, unfolding reciprocally session by session (Fisher et al., 2016).

These observations point to a cycle by which the capacity for good processing contributes to positive symptom change, but where the intensity of symptoms also impacts a client's ability to work with emotion, either constraining or facilitating their meaningful engagement and creating either vicious or virtuous cycles (Pinheiro et al., 2021). This adds new complexity to the hypothesized causal relationship between process and outcome. A finer grained level of inquiry is needed here, one that looks at specific moments when experiencing is helpful instead of analyses that aggregate the total amount of processing within a session. Causal models need to consider what kind of emotion was being explored to identify the best markers for when therapists should try to help clients deepen their experience.

How Do Treatments Compare at Deepening Experience?

Looking for a clinical edge, several authors have conjectured on whether a given approach to treatment can mediate the deepening of clients' experiencing over the course of treatment. For example, clinical theory suggests that because an experiential approach to treatment focuses on a client's moment-by-moment emerging experience, perhaps it would best promote the exploration, awareness, and deepening of client experiencing. A conclusive answer to this question is not yet possible. Although a handful of studies, all of which looked at the treatment of depression, have now compared various treatments across time.

Two studies compared client depth of experiencing in EFT to that of cognitive behavior therapy across the course of treatment (Pinheiro et al., 2021; Watson & Bedard, 2006). Findings suggested treatment approach did not have a meaningful impact on the pattern of change over time: Clients in both treatments demonstrated the same sized increase in their depth of experiencing. However, in both studies, EFT had higher process ratings indicating that, by a small but consistent margin, clients were more deeply exploring and elaborating their experience. Another study showed the level of client experiencing was higher in sessions from the working phase of psychoanalytic psychotherapy as compared to the working phase of cognitive behavior therapy (Klug et al., 2022). These modest differences in process between treatments likely reflects a matter of emphasis and the kind of work being engaged in and is not a difference in the degree to which clients grow in their capacity for this process (i.e., in statistical terms, this is a difference in intercept, not in slope). For example, when therapists take a more directive and pragmatic stance (e.g., as in traditional cognitive and behavior therapy), that can make it difficult for clients to fully explore their emotional experiences. Meanwhile therapists who value their client's deep engagement in affective experiences will try to enhance the process (Klug et al., 2022).

Finally, an unpublished study (Hakim, 2010) pooled several studies to create a large process research sample and examine the depth of client experiencing in a three-way comparison of cognitive behavior, interpersonal, and emotion-focused psychotherapies. Again, although there were absolute differences between the three treatments, the magnitude of those differences was relatively constant. So, when considering the initial level of process early in therapy, treatment approach had no further effect on the depth of client process that was demonstrated later. In sum, while all three treatment groups increased in their awareness and symbolization of experience from early to middle phases, they did so in parallel. The average depth of experiencing for each of the three treatments remained measurably spaced from one another by a small amount, with EFT scoring relatively higher, cognitive behavior therapy relatively lower, and interpersonal therapy in the middle range.

This finding on the absolute levels of client experiencing by treatment approach are consistent with findings from published studies that compared EFT with cognitive behavior therapy (Pinheiro et al., 2021; Watson & Bedard, 2006) or compared cognitive behavior therapy to psychodynamic and psychoanalytic psychotherapy (Klug et al., 2022; Rudkin et al., 2007). In my estimates, based on available research, the magnitude by which a client's level of experiencing may differ early in one or another of these treatments, is about the same magnitude by which that client would subsequently improve in their level of processing over the course of psychotherapy. For example, one study showed that at the conclusion of a cognitive behavior treatment the modal level of client experiencing was quite similar to that of clients who were just starting in a course of EFT (Watson & Bedard, 2006). Despite possible differences across treatments in the baseline degree to which they presumably facilitate client experiencing, the predictive power of experiencing on treatment outcome does not seem to differ by treatment (A. Pascual-Leone & Yeryomenko, 2016).

Intervention Facilitates Deeper Client Experiencing

Although client experiencing plays an important role in therapy and changes in this process anticipate better treatment outcomes, the argument that awareness and symbolization of internal experience is a causal mechanism requires additional kinds of evidence. For example, one should not take for granted that therapist interventions will directly facilitate deeper client experiencing. Determining this is tricky since the empathic reflections that facilitate awareness and deepen experience are often microinterventions that unfold from one talk-turn to another.

Three studies using different psychotherapy samples have each demonstrated that therapists have a medium to large effect in directly influencing their client's experiencing on a moment-by-moment level of talk turns (e.g., Adams, 2010; Hitz, 1994; A. Pascual-Leone et al., 2025). For example, when therapist interventions are couched in a manner that deliberately points the client toward a deeper level of experiencing, clients were found to be nine times more likely to immediately follow suit and deepen their own process as compared to when therapist interventions simply matched a client's prior level of experiencing (Adams, 2010). Of course, clients' internal processes cannot be directly manipulated (i.e., clients are not puppets) but the issue is more one of influence, where strategic prompts make it more likely that clients go deep (A. Pascual-Leone & Yeryomenko, 2016).

Furthermore, a process analysis of EFT for depression suggested a therapist's ability to deepen client experiencing is one of the pathways of influence on treatment outcomes (Adams, 2010). Exploring this further, an experiment with students suffering trauma used different instructions to invite participants to write about their distressing experience, to influence the depth of their emotional experiencing. Even in the absence of a therapist, a change in written instructions promoted deeper (or more shallow) emotional awareness. After three writing sessions of this kind, the corresponding process predicted a reduction in anxiety symptoms four weeks after the experimental intervention (Harrington et al., 2018). Meanwhile, research on successful sessions of EFT showed that a therapist's effort to deepen client experiencing is mediated by the client being in key emotional states (A. Pascual-Leone et al., 2025). Specifically, primary adaptive emotions (e.g., healthy anger or grief) can serve as markers indicating when therapists will more likely be able to successfully deepen their client's experience. Findings like these promise that therapists might leverage a client's use of awareness and symbolization to deepen their experience.

Conclusions About Client Experiencing

Experiencing is among the most systematically and well researched measures of emotional change in psychotherapy (Sønderland et al., 2023). Summing up, several conclusions can be drawn from this research. First, experiencing is a common factor. Deeper within-session client experiencing predicts better treatment outcomes, irrespective of treatment approach (e.g., humanistic–experiential, psychodynamic, cognitive behavior therapies) or modality (e.g., working with individuals or couples).

Second, experiencing is important for working with depression. While client experiencing is championed as a benchmark of good processing, the empirical support for that comes primarily from the treatment of clients suffering depressive symptoms, if not major depression. This observation, and my own reading of the various effects of experiencing by types of outcomes (i.e., measures of depressive versus general or other symptomatology), has led me to the hypothesis that although experiencing often impacts several kinds of outcomes, it might be more closely related to changes in depressive symptoms (see also Klug et al., 2022). To what extent this process is best suited to facilitating change in depression as compared to other presenting concerns is a research question with important implications.

Third, treatments may differ in their use of client experiencing. As reviewed earlier, five studies have compared the level of client experiencing between various treatments for depression, and they reveal consistent differences by treatment (Hakim, 2010; Klug et al., 2022; Pinheiro et al., 2021; Rudkin et al., 2007; Watson & Bedard, 2006). Experiential therapies seem to facilitate more of this process, as shown by a baseline difference observable from the very beginning of therapy and onwards, and this edge seems to be followed by psychodynamic, psychoanalytic, and then cognitive behavior treatments. However, these are complex observations based on a small number of studies. As such, they should be interpreted with caution and used to guide future inquiry. Furthermore, the average difference observed between any two treatments is small in absolute terms, and particularly compared to the large variation one sees between individuals.

Fourth, clients improve in their depth of experiencing. Irrespective of treatment approach, clients seem to improve over the course of therapy in the degree to which they make use of this process. Further, improvement in processing (as contrasted with baseline ability) is what matters most when predicting treatment gains. Furthermore, evidence suggests the magnitude of those positive changes in processing (i.e., the amount of deepening, in relative terms) is the same, irrespective of treatment approach. Although research remains limited to date, there is no evidence to suggest that depth of experiencing is a better outcome predictor in one or another approach to therapy. Researchers looking to further study client experiencing as a predictor of outcome should consider using a client's change score (i.e., from early to working phase), rather than the absolute level of a client's depth of experiencing (e.g., Pinheiro et al., 2021; Pos et al., 2009).

The bottom line for intervention seems to be that the total benefit an average client will gain from deepening and symbolizing experiential awareness ultimately depends on the general emphasis a given approach puts on facilitating that kind of process. To make sense of this in the broader context of psychotherapy research, it is important to remember that if a treatment approach has more of some key process, one cannot make the simplistic assumption that such a treatment will have better outcomes than another approach. Although the benefit leveraged by a specific process (e.g., experiencing) can be compared between clients within the same treatment, such a comparison does not hold across treatments. This is because distinct approaches to intervention will differentially leverage distinct kinds of processing. Otherwise stated, even though the same kinds of processing (i.e., experiencing) may be observable across treatments, they are being utilized to varying degrees. In Chapter 1, I introduced the metaphor of psychotherapy as offering a buffet, and despite the overlap in offerings across approaches, clients make use of functionally different parts of that buffet, even if they are within the same treatment. While experiential therapies may champion the common factor of deepening emotional awareness and symbolization, other treatments probably facilitate emotional change through other forms of emotional processing.

Fifth, therapist interventions matter. Several studies provide evidence that therapists directly shape their client's depth of experiencing through the nature of their moment-by-moment empathic reflections (Adams, 2010; Hitz, 1994; A. Pascual-Leone et al., 2025). When all these findings on client depth of experiencing are taken together, they begin to describe a mechanism of change (Kazdin, 2009) that therapists can use to directly influence in session.

NEUROLOGICAL CORRELATES OF REPRESENTING EMOTIONAL EXPERIENCE

Evidence from research on the impact of brain lesions, as well as positron emission tomography and functional magnetic resonance imaging studies seem to converge on the conclusion that the amygdala along with the insular cortex, ventromedial, and dorsolateral prefrontal cortices with a few other brain regions function together as part of an emotional circuit (Davidson & Irwin, 1999). Regarding emotional awareness, regions of the prefrontal cortex are related to symbolizing and more finely articulating emotional experiences. For instance, when neurologically normal participants were asked to identify and label emotional faces, activation increased in the right ventrolateral prefrontal cortex (Lieberman et al., 2007). Furthermore, that area is connected to the amygdala through the medial prefrontal cortex, which others have also found to be a key structure for labeling emotional experience (Berthoz et al., 2002). As an aside, activation in the right ventrolateral prefrontal cortex was inversely related to the magnitude of activation in the amygdala, which speaks to the process of labeling emotion as playing a potentially regulatory role (something already discussed in Chapter 6). In any case, the general finding is consistent with other neurological findings, supporting the idea that the process of engagement and initial awareness is a precondition to being able to reflect on emotion (Holzel et al., 2011).

Regarding areas specifically implicated in emotional awareness, which was discussed in the previous chapter, emotional engagement is the most basic or preliminary form of this kind of process and is supported by the amygdala. Later, the ventromedial part of the prefrontal cortex is directly involved in the representation of basic positive and negative emotion states, whereas the dorsolateral is involved in the representation of goal states, towards which basic emotions are directed (Davidson, 2000). Notice that as one elaborates the psychological process of emotional awareness from orienting and engagement, to initially labeling emotion, and then to symbolizing complex and dynamic internal experiences—brain activation comes to recruit from limbic to increasingly more frontal cortical areas. Both the representation of emotion and knowledge of their importance are part of the emotional awareness process, speaking to different facets of the dialectic between engagement and the elaborate reflection on emotion and its implications. Finally, identifying and then differentiating one emotion from another requires symbolic representation and finer articulation that is supported particularly by the insular cortex as well as the ventromedial prefrontal cortex (Bernhardt & Singer, 2012; Craig, 2009; Davidson & Irwin, 1999).

SYMBOLIZING AN EMOTION ACTUALLY CHANGES IT!

Thus far, after engagement (see Chapter 5), I have described labeling and symbolizing emotional experience as key facets of emotional awareness. Labeling emotion makes it a point of reference to work with (see Chapter 6), while deepening one's experience of emotion is a way of elaborating its continually unfolding meaning (this chapter). The review of research up to this point provides some converging evidence for these facets of emotional awareness, although in practice they are almost seamlessly intertwined. Illustrating this, May (1969) gives a case example in which engagement and awareness essentially afford a new experience, fostering change:

> But one day, he came in reporting that he had made a surprising discovery. When an acute attack of loneliness was beginning, it occurred to him not to try to fight it off—running had never helped anyway. Why not accept it, breathe with it, turn toward it and not away? Amazingly, the loneliness did not overwhelm him when he confronted it directly. Then it seemed even to diminish. Emboldened, he began to invite it by imagining situations in the past when he was acutely lonely. . . . But strangely enough, the loneliness had lost its power. (p. 151)

Taken as a whole, emotional awareness represents a probable process of change in psychotherapy. However, the argument for a mechanism of change also requires some narrative explanation of the basic psychological process by which identifying and symbolizing emotion can alter what one is feeling, or how one construes the meaning of one's experience, and ultimately spark new directions in action. This final section focuses on describing the process of awareness and how it precipitates therapeutic psychological change.

Differentiation and Integrations: The Two Prongs of Development

Explicating what is significant about one's affective experience will change the very feeling of an emotion. This is a profound reflection of the recursive process by which meaning is constructed. Once emotion is initially labeled, differentiating that experience is the central effort of increasing awareness. Even so, one needs to explain how refining the symbolization of experience leads to an eventual shift in the totality of that experience, rather than it simply leading to a tangle of disparate (or even incoherent) fragments. A phenomenological account helps to illuminate this. The differentiation of emotional experience usually begins with global and more general states, and then works toward more refined and specific states of affect and meaning. However, as the feeling of an emotion and its implied meanings are increasingly elaborated rather than simply being a more focused version of itself (i.e., in linear quantitative terms), the emotion being differentiated often actually comes to be qualitatively changed (see also Chapter 18).[4] For example, as a client explores and elaborates some feeling of global distress it may entail free flowing anxiety, but when differentiated, that anxiety could come to focus the client's experience on core shame, which in turn can be differentiated until it reveals a deep and unmet need. Even when that need is elaborated, the newly emergent meaning eventually also reorients the client toward assertion, and so forth. In this way, through a progressive search for increasingly articulate representations of one's immediate emotional experience, the process of emotional differentiation produces successive qualitative (rather than simply quantitative) shifts.

This is a fundamental and explicitly recognized process of change in classical person-centered therapy, where Rogerian empathic reflections aim to facilitate it (Paivio et al., 2016; A. Pascual-Leone, 2016). Nevertheless, this is a client process and as such it will also be implicit across other approaches to psychotherapy (to varying degrees, depending on the therapist's responsiveness). Even so, while some therapists may be decidedly focused on encouraging clients to explore and differentiate their feelings moment by moment, there is a complementary process that clients also simultaneously make use of, one that is automatic, less effortful, and much more tacit.

The radically different construal and self-organization that can be produced through the process of differentiation is in part because differentiation always occurs hand in hand with some form of integration. While clients effortfully differentiate their experience, an ongoing, tacit integration serves to assemble newly emerging and complementary facets of affect and meaning into a new generation of coherent states of emotional meaning (i.e., schemes). In fact, there is a dialectical complementarity between differentiation and integration; they are essentially the two prongs of development, observed in various forms of psychological, as much in biological growth (Maturana & Varela, 1980). In short, at the same time as facets of experience become differentiated and increasingly refined, those experiential details are always being simultaneously subjected to another process that seeks to organize and coordinate them into an experiential gestalt. The microintegration of emerging disparities is a hidden process within the client that creates continuity, coherence, and essentially makes sense of experience. This integrative synthesis is what bridges the islands of emotional meaning.

The tension between differentiation and integration as opposing forces is a fundamental dialectic in the growth of all complex systems (Maturana & Varela, 1980). Together they create functional constraints on a system (in this case, a framework of meaning), so that it becomes efficient, coherent, and as adaptive as possible for the organism (J. Pascual-Leone & Johnson, 2021). That dialectic implicitly guides construals that are constantly being made through expanding awareness as a microprocess. In a more explicit manner, the same dialectic shapes how personal narratives unfold, as a macroprocess (for more on that, see Chapter 22).

Finally, in the messy tumble of working with emotion, the process of awareness is not usually a stand-alone process. Rather than operating in isolation, it will interact with the other major forms of emotional processing. For example, awareness may be indirectly supported by arousal, shaped by the context of narrative reflection, and it may precipitate a sequential cascade of transformative emotions. Nevertheless, emotional awareness represents a unique operation unto itself, largely because of the ongoing tacit dialectic between differentiation and integration.

Emotional Awareness Is a Dynamic Creation of Meaning

Emerging emotion is a form of information about the self that must be first differentiated and then integrated into both one's representational repertoire (i.e., What am I feeling? What does this mean?) and one's functional repertoire (i.e., What does this make me want to do? How do I usually respond to this?).[5] When emotional information is integrated into one's experiential repertoire, it can be thought of as an emotion scheme (i.e., a psychological unit of lived meaning that has both representational and functional properties for helping people tacitly interpret and navigate their world; see Introduction). Some client problems arise when an aspect of this emotion-as-information essentially goes unrecognized or is restricted, such that it is not available to inform and adaptively organize the individual (L. S. Greenberg, 2021; L. S. Greenberg & Safran, 1987).

New Awareness Is Not Discovery, It Is Creation

In psychogenetic terms, *emotional awareness* is the creation of new emotion schemes (i.e., new psychological units of meaning action) in one's repertoire of functioning. In a strict sense, a client's emerging emotional awareness is not actually about discovery per se, but rather it is the dynamic creation of meaning. Moreover, this emergence of meaning is achieved through a unique process of accommodation.

In the study of how sensory perception is refined, Gibson introduced an understanding of accommodation distinct from that of Piaget (Gibson, 1950; A. Pascual-Leone & Greenberg, 2007b). This new sort of accommodation aptly describes the impact of interventions that aim to track and elaborate client's moment-by-moment experience (J. Pascual-Leone, personal communication, September 15, 2002).[6] In an experiential approach to therapy, the aim of treatment is to help clients explore, elaborate, and expand their experience (assimilating into the existing experiential scheme), until that unit of experience (the scheme) spontaneously splits into multiple schemes. In other words, the representation of one's initial experience precipitously differentiates into several new and unique schematic units of personal meaning and relevance (J. Pascual-Leone & Johnson, 2021). Thus, the essence of experiential awareness is to explore the individual instances of an experience right to its edges, incorporating sensory images, episodic memory, and symbolic significances (L. S. Greenberg, 2021). This is in lieu of linking elements or finding patterns that may exist across situations. When therapists take an exploratory, non-content directive approach, it helps clients elaborate aspects of their emotional experience in the moment such as their sadness, hurt, or frustration.

Gibson (1950) first introduced his understanding of how awareness develops in a description of sensory and perceptual experiences. In short, he believed we become aware of experiential objects by perceiving reliable relational patterns (i.e., invariant relationships) among figural objects and their perceptual and emotional background, which provides a rich experiential landscape. Consequentially, the focal aspects of one's ongoing experiential activity are progressively differentiated relative to one another. In conveying this concept, it is useful to draw an analogy between the experiential process in therapy and a strictly sensory venture, such as wine tasting. To the uninitiated, all red wines taste more or less the same, perhaps only slightly distinguishable from white wines. As one goes about in blind faith tasting different wines, gradually and with time, distinct features of flavor come to one's attention. With more exposure the original monolithic gustatory experience of red wine develops into a variety of more subtly differentiated experiences of flavor that, for the individual, simply did not exist before.

In this analogy, all the original flavors of wine are now slightly changed by virtue of their being more refined, and the same process holds true for the experiential flavors of affect and meaning (J. Pascual-Leone & Johnson, 2021). A change in one's experiential landscape happens simply by virtue of it having been explored (Rennie, 1998; Gendlin, 1981). Thus, in a session,

> if the listener's responsiveness makes it possible, the individual finds [themself] moving from one referent movement and unfolding to another and another. Each time the inward scene changes, new felt meanings are there for [them]. The cycles of [focusing] set into motion an overall feeling process. This feeling process has a very striking, concretely felt, self-propelled quality. (Gendlin, 1964, p. 151)

Notice this is not so much exploring to discover what was dormant or patiently awaiting, but rather it is a process of exploring to create by extending the horizon of experience. In this way, one may continually return to explore a client's presenting feelings anew, making use of their expanding panoply of meanings.

Experiencing the deeper meaning of one's feelings through a discovery-oriented process is exemplified by the following excerpt from a client who had become estranged from his family and most recently had a falling out with his sister. He says to the therapist:

CLIENT: Well, I'm really angry. I'm angry enough that I don't want to see her. And I would, ah, be very happy not to see her ever again. [*He frowns*]

THERAPIST: What happens inside you when you say that?

CLIENT: [*Sighs*] Oh, I don't know, just a feeling of sadness. [*He shakes his head, sighs deeply*]

THERAPIST: Sadness.

CLIENT: Yeah, because we have been, since 2006 . . .

THERAPIST: Speak from there . . . something about the sadness.

CLIENT: Well, it just is, uh . . . . [*long pause*] It means we won't ever get together again, to have a swim, to have a BBQ, to . . . talk . . .

THERAPIST: So it's like, "I'm sad about losing her."

CLIENT: [*Tears well up in his eyes*] Yes. I'm very sad about losing her [*Nodding slowly, he is deeply moved. He closes his eyes*] I, I, ahh . . . Oh! [*He sighs deeply, opens his eyes, looks at therapist*] . . . she more than anybody. (A. Pascual-Leone & Greenberg, 2007b, pp. 39–40).

A new emotional awareness such as this occurs from the exploration of a single situation and is formulated at a relatively low level of abstraction. Even so, clients often experience the newness felt in such an emerging experience as a tangible moment of meaning or insight.

A Cascade of Unfolding Experience

Each round of symbolization shapes the lived experience, which then asks to be symbolized in a new and increasingly sophisticated way. The progressive unfolding of experience described here is well known to client-centered and experiential therapists (A. Pascual-Leone & Greenberg, 2007b; Rennie, 1998; Rogers, 1951). In this approach, client feelings are addressed and readdressed, and in doing so they metamorphose, becoming more and more personally significant and tangible. The metamorphosis of that meaning structure occurs through the splintering of general units (i.e., schemes) of emotion into more specific subunits (i.e., subschemes). The result is the creation of a nested hierarchy of affective meanings, collectively capturing more meaning and deeper feeling (J. Pascual-Leone & Johnson, 2021).

To understand how the simple process of increasing emotional awareness precipitates clinical change, one needs to appreciate the subtlety in this dynamic creation of meaning. The newness in this experiential awareness is neither the product of associative linking nor the uncovering of meaning but rather the progressive cocreation of meaning in a single moment as a therapist facilitates the elaboration of a client's own ongoing experience. For example, L. S. Greenberg and Pascual-Leone (2006) describe a client who feels generally anxious about some impending interpersonal encounter. When the anxiety is first aroused, the therapist encourages them to describe in the moment how they notice that nervousness inside their body and any thoughts or images it may be related to. In doing this task of elaboration the client begins to describe and experience the nervousness in slightly different ways. Describing the feeling changes it, and it becomes somewhat shame-based for this client. As the bad feeling unfolds, the client continually symbolizes it in words:

> I'm tense. I guess . . . it's a bit of fear, but a bit of shame too. I feel somehow that I screwed up and I wish I hadn't. I'm afraid and embarrassed that I'll never be able to wash that stain clean. (L. S. Greenberg & Pascual-Leone, 2006, p. 47)

In this example, coming to symbolize new and more differentiated meaning is, in and of itself, an insight from emerging emotional experience. This type of learning is Gibsonian accommodation in action.

Expanding Awareness Leads to a Meaning Bridge

The clinical work in emotional awareness is about engaging, exploring, and effortfully differentiating, but the result is an experiential whole. One essentially unpacks and differentiates until there is a need to synthesize the experience and make it coherent at some higher level. As discussed, differentiation and integration are the two prongs of development, and the dialectical synthesis of these basic processes is exemplified by what some authors have referred to as a meaning bridge (Rice & Saperia, 1984). This result may occur gradually as a dawn of realization, or it may occur quite suddenly in a eureka moment, in either the case it is the Aha! experience described in early Gestalt psychology (Bühler, 1965).

When people label separate aspects of their experience, those facets come together in a bottom-up process as they connect the dots. A *meaning bridge* refers to the realization that, when taken together, the collected facets of emotional awareness renders a higher order of meaning. That sort of discovery is what happens, for example, in a connect-the-dots puzzle from a children's coloring book. The immediate task in that case is just to draw a line from one dot connecting it to the next, based on some sequence (e.g., numbers, letters), which creates a jagged line drawing around the page. But at a certain moment, one suddenly perceives the larger picture: when the series of dots are understood as interrelated, forming the outline of some larger picture! Seeing the constellation, rather than just isolated dots, is the meaning bridge. When working with emotion, it is the moment when islands of experiential meaning (schematic facets of emotion) come to be connected through a larger and overarching scheme that bridges them together.

The Culmination of Expanding Awareness

On one hand, a meaning bridge provides a link between one's emotion, behaviors, and the external environment. As suggested in an epigraph to this chapter, a bridge connects two vantage points or two passages, introducing new meaning to the overall experience through their linking. We see this aspect of bridging both materially and metaphorically: the architectural bridge, the musical bridge, and in thought bridges such as this, which were originally described by Nietzsche and Heidegger (Harrison, 2021). In terms of concretely working with emotion, this is the connecting experience between different facets of emotion (i.e., emotion label, action tendency, somatic experience, situational context, and a need or implication for the self—as described in Chapter 4). So the meaning bridge is an instance of integrative coherence in one's experience. Another way of considering this is that a problematic experience (i.e., problematic voices) become assimilated into a person's larger field of understanding (i.e., the community of voices) by building meaning bridges to disparate facets of experience (i.e., other voices). In practice, a meaning bridge could be a single word or phrase, a story, image, or expressive gesture that has the same meaning for each of the voices it connects, forming a common understanding (Brinegar et al., 2006).

On the other hand, the meaning bridge also serves as a working hypothesis, because it is a tentative effort to represent the full horizon of one's experience regarding some concern. Clients determine the fit and accuracy of that hypothesis by exploring the different aspects of emotional experience for their coherence and tracking the origins of covert feelings and behaviors to their perceptual cues (Rice & Saperia, 1984; Watson & Rennie, 1994). The further implication is that a meaning bridge allows the various (interconnected) aspects of experience to serve as resources in buttressing a trajectory of change.

Often, the meaning bridge couches emergent aspects of emotional awareness into a broader narrative context. In some sense, this is the culmination of emotional awareness: a bottom-up experience that gains coherence and is demystified as it is increasingly interconnected to part of a larger personal theme. It is critical to note, however, that reaching an overarching or connective synthesis is not imposed top-down. Rather, it emerges through exploring the concrete nuances of feelings and meaning as they are activated and imminently organizing the individual, as part of an embodied and consciously owned experience. Noticing one's bodily reaction to the world, making sense of it, and reacting to that ongoing experience, creates a lived understanding, what Damasio (1999) aptly referred to as "the feeling of what happens."

Competing Formulations Within a Systematic Exploration

Up to this point, much of the discussion in previous chapters has referred to aspects of emotional awareness (i.e., engaging, labeling, and symbolizing emotional experience) as a seemingly linear process. While the image of emergent awareness accurately describes the progression of clarity, the moment-by-moment process of developing this working hypothesis often involves an unrelenting back and forth. This is a veritable battle between formulations for some dominant or stable set of meaning perspectives. From a narrative perspective, this has also been described as competing plotlines (Angus et al., 2015; see Chapter 18). Researchers who painstakingly tracked this dynamic unfolding utterance by utterance in cases of experiential–humanistic therapy, explain how a search for meaning is mounted bottom-up, constructed both within and across sessions:

> The process of building this meaning bridge—of reaching this understanding in therapy seemed well described as a sequence of gradually slowing cross-triggering between two opposing internal voices. At first, each [of the client's opposing positions in meaning] was quick to interrupt and contradict the other, but gradually each voice learned to recognize and more fully understand the other's words, and thus became increasingly effective at conveying the experience of each voice to the other. (Brinegar et al., 2006, p. 175)

The conclusion of this work will be familiar to both therapists and clients as a particularly satisfying experience, and it is the product of purposefully elaborating emotional awareness.

From this perspective, a meaning bridge describes the transition between a clarification or statement of some problem and the eventual sense of understanding or insight that helps resolve the internal puzzle or discord in meaning. Because elaborating emotional awareness is a pervasive and somewhat nebulous task in psychotherapy, it is useful for research to identify in-session moments (problem markers) that specifically call for the elaboration of emotional meaning associated with that problematic experience. Most therapists will be able to recall a situation where their client reports feeling puzzled or troubled by their own emotional reaction to some event. That perplexity expressed by a client is the marker for an (often implicit) task that will ensue (L. S. Greenberg, 2021). For example, a client in my practice was surprised by her sudden feelings of loneliness when she received an impromptu dinner invitation from her boyfriend's family. Her reaction signals some underlying significance, but it remains outside her awareness.

Using task analysis, researchers studying humanistic–experiential therapy developed a causal model of how a client's problematic reaction like this, is typically resolved through a process of systematic emotional exploration during a therapy session (Rice & Saperia, 1984). I illustrate this using the example previously mentioned of my client who was puzzled by her loneliness. The model begins with (a) explicitly identifying the marker as a puzzling personal reaction to some event and something worth exploring (Therapist: So, this pang of loneliness just came up for you? Hmm, yeah, I can hear you saying it's so counterintuitive. That seems important . . .). Then (b), the session focuses on deliberately evoking the marker situation, using concrete and imagistic language to vividly describe the situation and scene (Therapist: Ok, so . . . take me there: You are in the doorway, still with your coat on . . . and you're about to leave, and . . . ? What else was going on? How did his mother say it?). Research suggests that clients who do this most effectively often describe the events in detail, like a movie playing in their mind's eye (Client: Well, she said, "Or you could stay and have some dinner with us, if you like." And the way she said it, she just kind of cheerfully threw it out at me from inside the house. I was turning away to go but . . . it's how free and easy she said it . . .). Then (c) clients identify sensory perceptions or salient images from the situation being recalled, to elaborate their subjective impact and explore them as triggers of the affective response (Client: I felt the cold air coming in as stood in the doorway and it was . . . so warm of them. Her voice was like "It's just an option, it's no trouble! Stay!" like someone throwing a bone out but without even knowing it . . .).

When clients explore the details of how they construed the event and its specific stimuli, it helps further differentiate their emotional reactions and symbolize them with increasing accuracy (Client: I guess it reminded me that I didn't really have anywhere else to go, not really. Leftover pasta at my apartment . . .). In this way, (d) the exploratory process broadens and deepens the client's awareness of what the personal impact was. The client gains a better understanding of the links between triggering events and their subjective meanings (Client: So, it was sweet of them, but maybe also pity? Really, they probably had no idea that I had nowhere else to go, but I knew it . . . and it was such a contrast). This last step has been referred to as a meaning bridge because it yields a changed understanding of the original difficulty, which lends the client a sense of direction and agency (Client: It's wonderful but it's so foreign for me. . . . I guess, one day, I hope I have a family like his, but I don't. And I wouldn't know where to start. [pause] We'll see . . .).

Making New Realizations: Experiencing a Bridge

In a qualitative inquiry that explored this notion of evocative unfolding, clients reviewed a video recording of their recent session and were asked to identify significant moments during which they had been trying to explore a puzzling or problematic personal experience (Watson & Rennie, 1994). Their subjective accounts revealed that after symbolizing and introspectively examining the experience, clients often reported that it culminated in "making new realizations." This came with what was described as a "sense of [personal] significance" or "triumph," where clients felt "elevated" to a new perspective. As they developed the new meaning bridge, clients also reported "revisioning the self," where they secured an "internal locus of control" and often a "decision to change," or "decision to act" (p. 509). For example, when one client came to realize that they were often silent out of fear of being exposed, they commented:

> The self-protection acts as a self-defense mechanism for me, and I think [within that moment of the session] I was starting to realize that . . . If I learn to deal with the self-protectiveness, it will help me be more expressive, which is my aim in therapy. (Watson & Rennie, 1994, p. 504)

Similarly, another client who became aware of how their social anxiety was driven by shame and personal inadequacy, simply observed: "It seems like a moment I could change. I had the option to project an alternative . . ." (p. 504). In short, expanding emotional awareness means creating a richer understanding of the needs, values, and goals that shape one's feelings and actions.

While the formulation of a meaning bridge given above comes from experiential therapy, there are other treatment strategies for generating self-knowledge. A core technique of psychodynamic therapy is when a therapist verbally delivers an interpretation to the client about relationship patterns. While the intervention is purported to facilitate insight, the client meets this with a growing level of emotional awareness, which ideally influences the timing of such interpretations. Research using a large sample of psychodynamic therapy has shown that insight or cognitive restructuring alone are not enough for therapeutic change (Høglend & Hagtvet, 2019). Rather, the success of treatment was mediated via both emotional awareness (i.e., defined as the ability to experience, differentiate, and express affect) and cognitive insight (i.e., understanding the dynamics of one's inner conflicts, patterns, and their connection to the past). Over the course of treatment, both these processes were observed to increase, while symptoms continued to decrease. Furthermore, the direct effect that insight had in predicting outcome was significantly attenuated, on account of the indirect effect exerted by affective awareness. After testing several competing mediation models, the researchers concluded, "What is ultimately required is the forging of affective conviction to cognitive insight" (Høglend & Hagtvet, 2019, p. 339).

I have primarily referred to the meaning bridge as a bottom-up construction of insight, one that emerges as emotional awareness dawns over the client. A meaning bridge is partly the symbolized of implicit meaning and another part inference, and it leads to a cognitive insight.[7] But the overarching process of personal change is recursive, and there are also other pathways to change. In turn, that insight may very well evoke a new round of feelings associated with another (higher) level of awareness. Tracking this circular chicken-and-egg relationship between processes will depend on the relative emphasis a treatment puts on emotional experience versus insight. That relative emphasis is also born through the methods used by researchers holding one or another treatment perspective (for examples using cognitive behavior or psychodynamic frameworks, see A. M. Hayes et al., 2007, or Høglend & Hagtvet, 2019, respectively).

EMOTIONAL CLARITY DIRECTS ONE TO USE IT OR CHANGE IT

In conclusion, a meaning bridge is when being aware comes together with feeling moved. However, when it becomes so pregnant with meaning, what does one do with that burgeoning feeling? Chapter 4 on emotional engagement already highlighted how expanding one's emotional awareness is not the same as the simple acceptance of emotion. During this chapter, that point was shown particularly in the way awareness does not stop at acknowledging a presenting reality but rather it involves a direct and purposeful pursuit for an emotion's underlying meaning. Early steps in noticing the feeling have an affinity to mindfulness and acceptance-based approaches, but the aim of acceptance is neither to pursue nor change emotion per se. This is a critical issue for the fruition of awareness as a form of emotional processing because once differentiated and symbolized, there is usually still work to be done. Several experiential approaches offer prescriptions for therapists to guide the change process after reaching what seems to be the core or primary emotion of concern. EFT, for example, continues to focus specifically on the trajectory of feeling itself, using client expressions of a primary emotion as a marker for intervention to either subsequently use the emotion or change the emotion (L. S. Greenberg, 2021).

On one hand, if the presenting emotion is adaptive, it is accepted and then used as a guide, as a motivator for change. In contrast, although mindfulness- and acceptance-based strategies for working with emotion try to welcome the feeling as such, they do not purposefully engage emotion or adopt it as a valuable source of information and impetus (see Chapter 20). So, according to emotion focused theory, the kind of processing called for by primary adaptive emotions is to heighten the expressive arousal of that emotion and to make use of its momentum, carrying it forward (L. S. Greenberg, 2021). Activating and using adaptive emotion as a guide is a topic that is explored next, in Part III of this book, on expressive arousal.

On the other hand, if the presenting emotion is maladaptive, EFT prescribes that the subsequent process should be to transform it (L. S. Greenberg, 2021). This can seem at odds with mindfulness and acceptance theories because it seems to suggest maladaptive emotions are not accepted. Ultimately, what must be accepted is the reality of that suffering, the process of having maladaptive emotion, and the totality of the person. Approaches like dialectical behavior therapy that espouse mindfulness and acceptance interventions, straddle this position with the much more goal directed agenda of behavior therapy by referring to this initial contradiction as a dialectic between acceptance versus pushing for change (Linehan, 2015; see also acceptance and commitment therapy, S. C. Hayes et al., 2012). So, when emotional awareness leads one to symbolize what turns out to be a primary maladaptive emotion, then it becomes a target for clinical change. Transforming maladaptive emotion is a topic that is discussed further on, in Part IV of this book.

ENDNOTES

1. This section is based on data from A. Pascual-Leone and Yeryomenko (2016).
2. Based on data in available studies, the average client increases their modal level of experiencing by about 0.4 on the 7-point scale from early to working phase of treatment. The given psychotherapy studies collectively report an average mode rating of 3 and a peak of 4. Although the experiencing scale is an ordinal scale, this may still give some reference as to the margin of change across cases. The average peak (i.e., maximum) score seems to have a slightly larger margin of change, increasing by about 0.5 over the course of treatments. This upper limit in someone's level of processing may be important for understanding how a process is leveraged. Again, these estimates are based on my own calculations, considering recent studies on individual therapy in addition to those already included in A. Pascual-Leone and Yeryomenko (2016).
3. The quality of the relationship is often a precondition for deep emotional exploration. For example, a study of psychodynamic therapy showed a stronger therapeutic alliance at the end of the first session predicted the client having greater emotional experiencing in the next session, but not the other way around (Fisher et al., 2016).
4. Chapter 18, in particular, see "Narrative Process Goes Beyond the Elaboration of Content."
5. Parts of this section are adapted from "Insight and Awareness in Experiential Therapy," by A. Pascual-Leone & L. S. Greenberg, in L. G. Castonguay and C. E. Hill (Eds.), *Insight in Psychotherapy* (pp. 31–56), 2007b, American Psychological Association (https://doi.org/10.1037/11532-002). Copyright 2007 by the American Psychological Association.
6. Acknowledgement for this insight about accommodation in the domain of experience goes to Juan Pascual-Leone, who first clarified this issue after his work on cognitive-development with Piaget.
7. While that inference might be deductive, emotional insights are most often the product of abductive inferences. *Abductive reasoning* is often referred to as making an inference to the best explanation, such as when one makes the best prediction based on incomplete observations. For more on this see Chapter 17, specifically, "Meaning Can Be Made Either Top-Down or Bottom-Up."

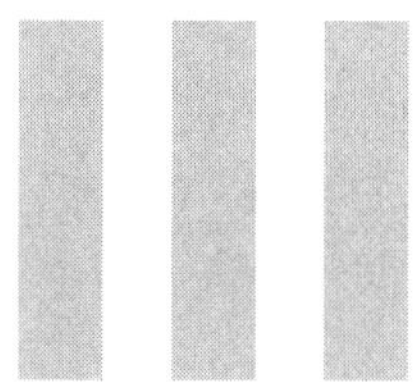

FEEL MORE, EXPRESS MORE

INTRODUCTION: FEEL MORE, EXPRESS MORE

Part III of this book discusses activating and expressing emotion as a unique subtype of emotional processing, which can be deliberately and purposefully facilitated. Facets of this kind of processing include (in order of increasing complexity) heightening affective arousal, using vividness, the expression of emotion, and finally, the use of either live or imagined therapeutic enactments. Because increasing expressive arousal in these ways is a form of processing that has been particularly elusive, Chapter 8 gives a conceptual overview, describing key features that define the target process.

On their own, terms such as "activation" or "expression" are not enough to denote this process. This is because the covert activations of emotion, whether subjectively reported or physiologically measured, are not strong independent predictors of positive change. Furthermore, expression needs to be channeled through meaning for it to be productive, and that often calls for more than finding the right words (which was already covered in Part II). Rather, this change process involves following through on the observable expression of arousal, from allowing the visceral experience of arousal, to outwardly expressing it, to exploring the meaning and implications of that ongoing bodily experience. For these reasons, I introduce the term "expressive arousal" to more precisely capture the facets of change discussed in this part of the book. Heuristically, one can think of this process as expanding and increasing the salience of a feeling-in-action and its associated meanings, such that the presenting feeling shifts to a more prominent and expansive expression, as depicted in Figure III.1.

Chapter 8 offers criteria for researchers and clinicians seeking to focus on the features of expressive arousal. In Chapters 9, 10, and 11, I propose there are at least five distinct pathways of action by which expressive arousal acts as a mechanism of emotional change in psychotherapy and in everyday life. What follows is an outline of the hypothesized mechanisms explained over subsequent chapters:

- Physiological and emotional arousal provides a general impetus for emerging affective experience (see Chapter 9).

- Going through the behavioral motions of an emotional expression can incite and generate internal experience (see Chapter 9).

- Increasing expressive arousal magnifies and explicates experience, bolstering emotional awareness (see Chapter 9).

- Enactments facilitate the exploration and creation of meaning (see Chapter 10).

- Aroused expression is an affirmation that strengthens one's sense of self (see Chapter 11).

FIGURE III.1. Feel More, Express More: The Principle of Expressive Arousal

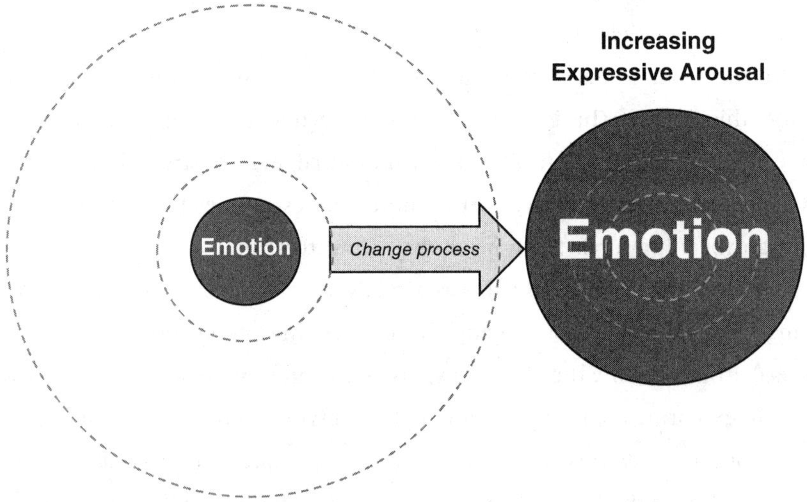

Note. Expressive arousal is a principle that involves heightening arousal, amplifying vividness, increasing expression, and the enactment of emotion. The process is depicted here as the feeling quantitatively growing in size. This is one of five categorically different processes that change emotion.

These five explanations are nonexclusive, and each one has various levels of theoretical as well as empirical support that I will review. Furthermore, it is understood that these mechanisms would usually operate in synergy with other known forms of emotional processing.

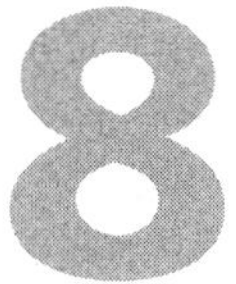

Heightening Arousal, Vividness, Expression, and Enactments

If you're going through hell, keep going.

—WINSTON CHURCHILL (ATTRIBUTED)

WHAT IS EXPRESSIVE AROUSAL? WHEN IS IT IMPORTANT?

One of the most salient aspects of emotional processing is the physical arousal of emotion and the expression of feeling. In the 4th century B.C.E., Aristotle (ca. 330 B.C.E./1996) described heightened emotional arousal as a cathartic experience that occurred while people watched the unfolding of tragic theatrical dramas in a public amphitheater. His understanding of the evocative process was that watching these vivid enactments aroused a spectator's emotion (specifically feelings of fear and pity). It was typical for emotion to be freely and openly expressed in these public events, which according to Aristotle, allowed spectators to purge some aspect of their own suffering that had been captured by the drama. This idea that the arousal and expression of emotion offers a curative or healing process was incorporated by Breuer and Freud (1895) into early theories about the mechanisms of psychotherapy.

Though aroused expression remains a core principle of modern psychotherapy, it is also the focus of much debate. From facilitating physical enactments, to working with hot cognitions, to the use of vivid imaginative re-entry into past experiences, the need for emotion to be activated in some way for it to be fully

https://doi.org/10.1037/0000460-009
Principles of Emotion Change: What Works and When in Psychotherapy and Everyday Life, by A. Pascual-Leone
Copyright © 2026 by the American Psychological Association. All rights reserved.

processed is entertained quite differently across approaches to psychotherapy. However, there is consensus that emotional processing cannot be limited to detached awareness, thinking about, or simply inhibiting and down-regulating emotion. On the contrary, at some point feelings need to be viscerally felt. Certainly, if one considers the etymology of the word "emotion" (*e-* "out" + *movere* "to move"), it would be difficult to imagine complete emotional processing in the absence of some active experience. Although somewhat tautological, the term "emotion mobilization" has even been used in some psychodynamic literature (e.g., Davanloo, 2005). Terminology like this highlights both the imperative that a true change process entails arousal, expression, and action as well as the fact that such a process cannot be taken for granted or presumed during clinical practice. The word "emotion" (i.e., to be outwardly moved) underscores the importance of both arousal and expression together.

Aroused emotional expression is defined as observable verbal and nonverbal behavior that could symbolize or communicate one's emotional experience (Kennedy-Moore & Watson, 2001). While an expression may or may not be fully within the scope of one's awareness, it must involve the observable activation of emotion through heightened arousal, vividness, expression, or enactments. In what is a counterpoint to suppression or inhibition (Chapter 3), expressive arousal is about the judicious up-regulation of emotion. This arousal of emotion sometimes works synergistically with other processes; for example, it may focus, orient, and heighten awareness. At other times it also works as an independent process by creating impetus and capturing some embodied meanings.

The relationship between the physical body and working with emotion is conveyed by many evocative yet cryptic phrases like "the body knows," "somatic memory," or "body processing." This idea is also tied to observations that physical pathology can sometimes be the embodiment of emotional distress. That formulation has been made popular through self-help and nontraditional approaches to yoga or mindfulness; as captured by statements like "Our issues are carried in our tissues." Even so, Reich's (1973) very early discussions of "body armor" may be at the origin of such observations regarding emotion and physical pathology (Sletvold, 2011; see Chapter 9, this volume). Nevertheless, van der Kolk's (2014) book *The Body Keeps the Score* argues convincingly for the scientific support of this basic idea. Chapter 6 has also already highlighted the relationship between a person's limited capacity to label their emotional experience and the severity of their somatic symptoms.

Finally, the aroused expression of emotion can also serve an important function in affirming the self. As one overcomes fearful inhibition, as covert feelings become manifest, and as one reclaims previously disowned emotion, the experience of an agentic and unique self becomes salient. In sum, this process is not about venting or habituating to secondary emotional distress (as discussed in Chapter 3). Rather, the key feature of expressive arousal as a way of working with emotion is boosting the activation of primary emotion to use it productively.

It is important to acknowledge that from a broader perspective, the control or modulation of arousal entails both down-regulation (as discussed in Chapter 2) and up-regulation (discussed in this current chapter), which has led some authors to conceptualize emotion regulation as an overarching principal that encompasses both. However, the difference between heightening versus inhibiting arousal is ultimately related to their underlying processes. To use a metaphor from Chapter 2, consider how the accelerator pedal and the brake pedal in a car represent two distinct mechanisms, not one.[1] Making matters more complicated, increasing arousal in exposure-based interventions is also an issue that needs to be set apart. In short, the function of increasing arousal is markedly different if it is for clarifying or activating emotional meaning (i.e., the process of arousal and expression discussed in this section) or if, in contrast, the purpose of increasing arousal is ultimately a habituation to one's emotional experience (i.e., down-regulation and emotional inhibition; see Chapter 2). Furthermore, the targets or indications for facilitating such processes are also quite distinct. So, while the clinical process of arousal seems common, in the case of enactment and mobilization, the target of arousal is primary emotion and it is in the service of promulgating and carrying the feeling forward (e.g., feeling more). In contrast, the target of arousal in exposure-based interventions is usually secondary emotion and it entails heightening arousal only for some interim in the service of regulation and reducing responsiveness of some feeling (e.g., ultimately, feeling less).

WHEN TO FOCUS ON EXPRESSIVE AROUSAL: WHAT ARE THE MARKERS OF DYSFUNCTION?

There are key moments in working with emotion where expressive arousal is most called for. There are also broader considerations that will relate to case formulation and treatment planning. Finally, considering the concrete instances where expressive arousal is contraindicated helps further clarify the mixed literature on this process.

Markers for Using Expressive Arousal

Facilitating emotional arousal and its expression is a critical process when the core source of dysfunction is described as feeling stuck, blocked, numb, or distant. It is also indicated when a client demonstrates a lack of agency, having either a poor sense of direction or of what they need. Focusing on expressive arousal is particularly appropriate for presenting problems characterized by suppressed emotion and depleted energy. Especially when clients have the notion that their feelings are taboo or are forbidden, therapists should invite the client to both experience and express those covert emotions. This kind of therapist response gives permission to clients by encouraging them to allow their own aroused emotion. Similarly, another marker for when it is helpful to heighten arousal is when clients are ambivalent about activating some nascent emotional experience but still clearly indicate they want help in accessing or engaging that experience. This ambivalence and the either implicit or explicit request for help to work with emotion is common in psychotherapy, and therapists should embrace it as a marker to facilitate expressive arousal in the client.

Considerations for Case Formulation

A key distinction that should be made early in case formulation is first whether the client typically has other emotional experiences that are activated and in awareness. If a presenting client generally does not seem to feel much, case formulations should consider the possible reasons for the client's flattened affect: Does the client have low reactivity, or passive insensitivity, or an easygoing and mellow character? Or does it seem like the client is actively self-interrupting and preemptively avoiding the full formulation of experiences that would otherwise be difficult or painful? Other personal and idiosyncratic factors will influence the way heightening arousal may be most useful for a client, and all of these should be part of an ongoing moment-by-moment case formulation. For example, if past experiences have led a client to expect the absence of an attentive and receptive listener, or if the client has anticipatory shame of being judged (shame anxiety), the process and experience of expressive arousal will interact with the therapeutic relationship in important ways.

To facilitate this kind of emotional processing, therapists will begin by communicating their intention to make space for and attend to a client's emerging feelings. Then a therapist needs to approach, evoke, and explicitly acknowledge the arousal. Finally, the client would actively engage and express emotional experiences as they unfold with a therapist's support. The goal of doing this is to use emotion to orient toward whatever seems most painful, poignant, or in need of attention. There is also some reason to believe that when a client's presenting symptoms are somatic rather than cognitive or verbal in nature, therapeutic approaches that are body oriented and use movement to facilitate expressive arousal are preferable in therapy over those that focus on talking. In fact, the specific emotional processes of expressive arousal and therapeutic enactment have been found to positively impact somatic–affective symptoms. This has been found across quite different approaches to treatment, including emotion-focused therapy (Stiegler, Molde, & Schanche, 2018), intensive short-term dynamic psychotherapy (Abbass et al., 2012; Davanloo, 2005), dance movement therapy (Bräuninger, 2014), as well as psychological treatments for pain disorders (Lumley et al., 2011, 2017).

Contraindications: When Not to Promote Expressive Arousal

It should come as no surprise that at other moments in session, heightening emotional arousal is bad for treatment, and at those moments, interventions that target expression are contraindicated. Some of these contraindications have to do with protecting the client against feeling overwhelmed or (re)traumatized by too much intensity. Clearly, when clients already feel overwhelmed in a given moment or are too aroused to function, down-regulation and emotional inhibition should be the only clinical objective. Thus, encouraging further expressions and enactments of vivid emotion at such a time are contraindicated and may even be harmful.

However, other reasons for pulling back may be to avoid working at cross-purposes to other forms of emotional processing. For example, if the client is engaged in a meaningful reflection on emotional experience and does not need more arousal to highlight the experience as a focus of attention, further increasing arousal can make it difficult to focus on the meaning construction at hand. For therapists managing this, it requires a delicate moment-by-moment tracking of client affect as well as the titration of one process against another. For instance, activating and arousing emotion can sometimes initially offer a client broad strokes of meaning. But later, refining the details and relating those tendrils of meaning to a broader life narrative will require a less intense and more reflective process.

While arousal puts one in the feeling, deeper reflection requires one to be slightly outside it (albeit still present and in touch with experience). Thus, the nonverbal raw perceptual experience of arousal versus rationally thinking about one's feelings represent two poles of a continuum.[2] (See Chapter 17 for a figure and full elaboration of this continuum.) So, the more searching reflection one is engaged in, from a decentered or observer's perspective, the more likely that heightening and evoking arousal risks disrupting that process. If reflection on emotion is productive within a given moment, heightening arousal at the same time could create interference (see Chapter 22). The question of whether to facilitate arousal or to focus on narrative reflections should be based on what seems most useful at that point in time and in relation to the case formulation.

As one explores the implications for case formulation, it is important to clarify that these indications and contraindications to heightening emotional arousal are based on both an assessment of the client's capacity as much as the client's moment-by-moment processing needs. While a certain diagnosis may offer some insight into the client's capacity to tolerate and make use of expressive arousal, information on that predisposition should inform the parameters of intensity that a therapist seeks to facilitate. The issue is more complex than a one-to-one correspondence or any assumption that people with certain disorders (e.g., borderline processes, anxiety, depression) will or will not benefit from arousing emotion. Rather, even for clients who are susceptible to hyperarousal (e.g., those with trauma or a history of self-harm), one may have reason to stimulate expressive arousal at a given moment in time—yet perhaps only to stimulate arousal up to a certain level of intensity, or not in the second half of a treatment session, and so on. As with all forms of emotional processing, the call for increased arousal and expression is based on a moment-by-moment assessment of what is happening within the session (i.e., marker-driven interventions). Meanwhile, case formulation about a client's general capacity for working with emotion should guide the parameters with which one makes use of expressive arousal.

Research Evidence: Emotional Arousal Predicts Outcome

When working with emotion, increasing someone's arousal is a very salient kind of emotional processing, but this process has been a point of confusion with respect to empirical findings (when available) and a point of contention with respect to clinical theory (and opinions). There are indeed a certain number of process-to-outcome research reviews that caution against increasing arousal in therapy without careful consideration (Kennedy-Moore & Watson, 2001; Nichols & Zax, 1977; Rosner, 1996). Both psychotherapy analogue studies (Bohart, 1977, 1980) as well as controlled experimental designs show that simply venting, purging, or discharging emotion is not effective in reducing distress and may even exacerbate target symptoms (Bushman, 2002). Cutting-edge observational studies in psychotherapy research have similarly concluded that raw arousal on its own is an oversimplification of the more complex processes needed to facilitate change (L. S. Greenberg et al., 2007).

Arousal and Expression Are Helpful

Despite all the complexity, a body of research is converging on the affirmation that judiciously facilitating arousal and expression is helpful. Behavioral interventions for anxiety have found a clear association between heightened arousal in session and positive treatment outcomes (Borkovec & Sides, 1979; Jaycox et al., 1998; Lang et al., 1970). A meta-analysis looked at 13 studies on exposure-based treatments for anxiety disorders and showed that the initial within-session arousal of fear was a significant positive in the prediction of symptom reduction (Sønderland et al., 2023). Similarly, when treating depression, cognitive, experiential, and self-directed interventions have all shown emotional arousal and expression to predict various kinds of symptom improvement (Beutler et al., 1991; Carryer & Greenberg, 2010; Mohr et al., 1991; Pos et al., 2017). Furthermore, in emotion-focused therapy, the degree with which a client engages full emotional arousal predicts emotional improvements with respect to interpersonal emotional injuries and complex trauma (L. S. Greenberg & Malcolm 2002; Paivio et al., 2010; Paivio & Nieuwenhuis, 2001).

A meta-analysis based on 42 studies shows various kinds of within-session client emotional expression (very broadly defined) had a large effect in the prediction of good treatment outcomes that followed (Peluso & Freund, 2018). Moreover, moderator analyses suggested the effect of emotional expression was the same irrespective of client diagnosis, psychotherapeutic orientation, use of a treatment manual, or even the treatment outcome being considered. When a subsequent meta-analysis defined emotional arousal more narrowly, according to the individual frameworks of respective treatment models, arousal seemed to have a moderate overall effect in the prediction of symptom reduction, although there was wide variation based on how the intensity of client arousal was measured (see Sønderland et al., 2023).

Finally, the salubrious impact of emotional arousal and expression on somatic concerns is also noteworthy. Lumley and colleagues have developed a program focused on awareness and expression as the two central processes in a treatment for stress-related pain among a mostly non-psychiatric population (for a review, see Lumley et al., 2011).[3] For example, a large randomized clinical trial with a 6-month follow-up showed using emotional awareness and expressive therapy to treat fibromyalgia was more effective than psychoeducation and surpassed cognitive behavior therapy in the reduction of pain (Lumley et al., 2017). For patients with breast cancer, experiencing and expressing emotion was a unique process that predicted psychological improvement, physical health status, and even fewer medical appointments (Stanton et al., 2000).

In the context of experimental research, a meta-analysis of 146 studies on expressive disclosures showed an astonishingly wide array of psychiatric, non-psychiatric, and medical populations (Frattaroli, 2006; see also van Agteren et al., 2021). In this paradigm, participants are typically asked to write expressively about an upsetting topic or to write without emotion on some neutral topic and to do this for three to five sessions of 15–20 minutes each. The conclusion was that the expressive writing task has a small but reliably positive effect on mental and physical health, and given the simplicity of the intervention, that effect is quite noteworthy.

In summary, the research suggests arousal and expression predicts successful adjustment to both intra- and interpersonal difficulties, even if the findings tend to be highly context dependent. Moreover, studies across treatment domains have carefully accounted for either the role of the therapeutic relationship or of social support in general, demonstrating that expressiveness is a unique aspect of emotional processing.

Natural Skepticism

In truth, the effect size may not be the issue. A clinician's wariness about encouraging their client's arousal in psychotherapy is only partly related to the mixed evidence. General skepticism about the benefits of emotional arousal probably is not based on a careful reading of the literature but rather is anchored in the uneasiness people have about emotional distress in general.[4] First, humans also have a primal tendency to avoid arousing and expressing painful emotion. The implication is that when clients sense their distress emerging on the horizon of experience, they instinctively want to suppress or avoid that expressive arousal—much less risk exacerbating the pain!

Second, the potential benefit of emotional arousal and expression is counterintuitive. It essentially rests on the supposition that when it comes to emotional pain that it gets worse before it gets better, and this seems like an inherently risky undertaking. No surprise, clients so often ask, "Isn't there any other way to do this?" referring to something other than exploring the fear, confronting the other person, or talking about the past. Yet, the events that clients themselves identify as most helpful in emotion-focused therapy also tend to be higher in emotional arousal than other instances in the therapeutic process (Holowaty & Paivio, 2012). This ambivalence extends to therapists as well who find it unnerving to encourage something that is aversive to one's client, to watch it happen, and to risk losing control of the session, all based on a rationale that is largely counterintuitive. We see this again in the everyday life of parents, who are often apprehensive about exploring and facilitating painful emotion in their children even when it may be adaptive. Shutting down or minimizing the painful experience is an all-too-common reaction, and the simple reason is that intense negative emotion can be unwieldy and downright alarming.

Third, emotional expression as a change process is sometimes mistaken as a sign of poor outcomes. This superficial conflation of process and outcome was discussed in Chapter 2. Concretely, sometimes people begin to express more negative emotion when interventions and treatment are working well. For example, research on psychodynamic group therapy has shown depression has an attenuating effect on the expression of negative affect (D. W. Cox et al., 2019, 2020). People who were more depressed were less likely to be emotionally expressive or to overtly communicate their distress to others. However, over the course of successful treatment these same individuals became more forthcoming and willing to express their distress. So, the alleviation of depression was accompanied by a stronger and more self-evident relationship between a client's covert intensity of negative feeling and their overt expression.

We also see micro-examples of this at the turn-by-turn interactional level, such as in the process of forgiveness between couples in emotion-focused therapy. When an injured partner discloses their pain about a transgression and that is well received by their partner who is nondefensive, the next moment typically involves an escalation in negative emotional expression by the injured party (e.g., "Oh! So, you admit what happened and are willing to hear how much it hurt me? Okay! Well then, now let me really tell you what it was like!"). Analyses showed this intensification of negative emotion in a couple's interaction is common despite the initial round of positive interaction. Next, whether the accused partner can continue to respond nondefensively and accept their injured partner's expression (rather than shut down or counterattack) is a decisive moment, one that anticipates forgiveness (Meneses & Greenberg, 2011). Similarly, when children in distress (or vulnerable adults) are not forthcoming but then are met with tenderness and compassion, a floodgate of tears often bursts open. In these examples of healing and good outcomes (at both levels of intervention and treatment), increases in emotional expression are part of the working through, a healthy reflection of internal congruence, yet the client feeling more can be misunderstood as a regression or fumbled outcome.

The Need for Clarifications and Caveats

Reviews by several forward-thinking authors have concluded that the bad reputation of aroused emotional expression (as a process) is related to a global distress and even self-deprecation being conflated with other forms of emotional experience that are actually productive and agentic (Austenfeld & Stanton, 2004; Kennedy-Moore & Watson, 2001). Furthermore, when a concern needs attention, the emotional experience may be either under-regulated (in which case soothing, suppression, etc. are called for) or the experience may be over-regulated, in which case its activation and expression are called for (L. S. Greenberg & Watson, 2005; Kennedy-Moore & Watson, 2001). So, the specific kind of emotion being worked with needs to be carefully considered when evaluating the benefits (or risks) of a process. Following an experiment on processing dysphoria, Hunt (1998) concluded that "under certain conditions, 'having a good cry' may be a more effective way of coping than trying to 'get your mind off your troubles' or 'rolling up your sleeves and getting to work'" (pp. 380–381). However, what those conditions are is a critical issue. To assuage the skepticism of therapists and clients, as well as to sharpen future research, several clarifications are needed before championing expressive arousal as a form of emotional processing. That is the aim of the next section.

PRODUCTIVE EMOTIONAL AROUSAL: WHAT MATTERS, HOW MUCH, AND WHEN?

A complete understanding of expressive arousal must articulate the contingencies and parameters that would make increasing emotional arousal and its expression a therapeutic experience. For fear of exacerbating a client's clinical issues, arousal alone has sometimes become a singular focus of critical attention. As a result, therapists, clients, and researchers alike have sometimes overlooked key factors that are concomitant and are either embedded in or contextualize the arousal. The chief objective in this section is to articulate what type of emotion should be aroused and expressed, in what way it should be activated, and when increasing arousal will be most helpful. In this section, the apparent inconsistencies in clinical and research literature are explained and resolved by considering five points of clarification.

Caveat #1: Only Specific Kinds of Emotion Benefit From Expressive Arousal

An incisive clinical insight made by Kennedy-Moore and Watson (2001) was their observation that emotional arousal can be either a sign of raw, untempered distress or a sign of working through the distress. The clinical implication of this is that the indiscriminate arousal of emotion is not going to helpful in any consistent way. Furthering this, L. S. Greenberg, Auszra, and Herrman

(2007) argue there has been a lack of differentiation in what emotions should be targeted with this process of change and that although harnessing arousal may be a powerful part of positive change, other potential targets of arousal are going to be irrelevant or even hindering.

As a rule, the targets of expressive arousal should be deeper and underlying emotional experience (e.g., primary emotion) rather than secondary or symptomatic emotion.[5] A common example of the latter is arousal in the form of whining and complaining, which essentially is a crude blend of anger and sadness. It conveys an undifferentiated experience, such as "I am frustrated about the sad hopelessness of my situations, I feel overwhelmed and un-agentic, and I secretly hope someone or something will take my frustration away if only my distress and protest is heard." Arousal in this case is a sign of global distress, and interventions that heighten this secondary emotion will not be productive. In contrast, arousal may signal a more articulate emotional experience where the client is working through distress. Consider this statement as an example: "I am full of grief and have an acute sense about the sadness of the loss I have suffered, while also having a sense of my boundaries and what I will or will not accept. I accept my loss as it is, but I will not compromise my values." Heightening arousal in this second case would help give momentum and strength to the sentiment of a primary emotion.

As L. S. Greenberg and colleagues (2007) highlight, therapists should focus on arousing primary emotion (whether adaptive or maladaptive) as an ongoing target of exploration for personal meaning and direction. In the case of primary adaptive emotion, arousal will also help one mobilize and capitalize on a given healthy direction. This means that adaptive emotion is the most important target of arousal as a change process. Poorly articulated and symptomatic experiences of secondary or instrumental emotion do not benefit from increased arousal. In fact, they are irrelevant to or may even exacerbate the problem. So, as discussed, the expressive arousal is not about creating habituation to symptomatic (i.e., secondary) emotion.

Caveat #2: There Is an Optimal Range for Productive Arousal

In a seminal paper that addresses the underlying nature of mixed findings that are so common in process-to-outcome research, Stiles (1996) reminds us that "more of good thing is better," but only when one does not already have enough (p. 915). In other words, just as offering more food is not helpful to someone who is already very well fed, the usefulness of a given treatment process is entirely contingent on what the client needs at that moment. This is never more true than when it comes to increasing arousal.

A range of treatment perspectives converge on the idea that a middle level of arousal is optimal for performance and emotional processing. In that optimal range of arousal, clients are energized, emotion is both salient and easily accessible, and both learning and performance are improved. This curvilinear relationship between emotional arousal and performance has been described in early research as the Yerkes–Dodson law (Broadhurst, 1957). The pattern represents an inverted U such that when arousal is too low, clients are under aroused, are not sufficiently engaged, and experience relatively flat affect. Sometimes clients with low arousal appear to be focused on external events, intellectualizing, or simply distant (see Chapter 6 on alexithymia and shallow levels of experiencing).

On the other side of this curve, clients who are over aroused will be cognitively disorganized by the intensity of their experience (Linehan, 2015; see also Chapter 2 on markers for the need to down-regulate). Clients themselves are often aware of this as it happens. Even within a humanistic approach, a few clients have reported that the enactment of, for example, their self-critical process, was too intense for it to be a useful exercise (Stiegler, Binder, et al., 2018). At this excessive level of anxious distress, a client's attention and cognition become increasingly impaired, and they have difficulty focusing or making meaning out of what they are feeling. From a behavioral perspective, another risk of having an overwhelming emotional experience is that it tends to confirm a client's fears about approaching emotion (e.g., retraumatization). Then, from a psychodynamic perspective, this can subsequently lead to a client redoubling their defensive efforts in disconnecting from their own affective experiences (McCullough et al., 2003; Strachey, 1943).

The Window of Tolerance

Psychiatrist Daniel Siegel (1999) aptly referred to the functional middle range of the arousal curve as a client's window of tolerance for emotional intensity, and it represents the place where treatment is arguably most productive. The issue of optimal arousal is important to several fundamentally different treatment perspectives. For example, cognitive and behavior therapies find high anxiety acceptable, particularly in exposure-based interventions, but only up to a point. Meanwhile, on the other side of the curve, cognitions still need to be hot to be meaningfully worked with (Samoilov & Goldfried, 2000). Authors from experiential, body-based, and sensorimotor approaches to psychotherapy have discussed how clients need help modulating arousal either up or down depending on what they must process (e.g., Ogden & Fisher, 2015; Paivio & Pascual-Leone, 2023). Gendlin (1981) used the phrase "working distance" to capture this zone in which one can productively feel and explore experience.

While the intervention goal is to reach but not exceed the client's window of tolerance, the practical challenge to a therapist working in session is determining whether one's client is in that optimal zone of emotional arousal. Treatments rooted in a person-centered approach rely largely on assurance that the client takes the lead or is in the driver's seat (L. S. Greenberg, 2021). However, the more directive an experiential treatment is, the more critical it becomes to assess a client's moment-by-moment tolerance. Davanloo (2005; Abbass & Town, 2013) has proposed that one can appraise client's tolerance for increased arousal based largely on dynamic observations about how a client holds and expresses anxious distress. This evaluation considers (a) tension in the voluntary, striated muscle (i.e., hand clenching, sighing); (b) somatic symptoms related to involuntary tension in smooth muscles of the viscera (i.e., migraines, hypertension, irritable bowel syndrome); and (c) the clarity of a client's cognitive–perceptual experiences (i.e., visual blurring, mental confusion). Davanloo argues that while voluntary physical tension is an indication for appropriate increases in arousal, the perturbations or impairment of cognitive or perceptual functioning as well as somatization of tension in the viscera are indications that heightening arousal is probably not appropriate. While these moment-by-moment psychodiagnostic criteria have not yet been fully subjected to empirical scrutiny, they play an important role in the practice of short-term dynamic psychotherapy. Proposed observable criteria like these offer a starting point to address what kinds of client presentations may or may not signal that it is appropriate to increase emotional arousal.

The broader experiential perspective is that this will also be a highly interpersonal process in which therapists will monitor and even act dyadically as coregulators of in-session emotion. So, in the practice of working with emotion in psychotherapy, there is a delicate balance as therapists monitor their clients moment by moment: not too hot, not too cold, just right.[6] Although it does not speak to intensity, research on the linguistic patterns during expressive writing offers some evidence of this curvilinear relationship in the amount of attention that should be given to emotion. When people included a moderate number of negative words (e.g., bad, upset) in their expressive writing content, it predicted positive health outcomes. More specifically, relative to a normally distributed sample, when a person's absolute count of negative words was in the middle range, it was related to the greatest subsequent drop in anxiety 3 months later, according to one study (Niles et al., 2016); or a drop in subsequent physician visits, according to another study (Pennebaker & Chung, 2007). In the latter study, those who used either more or fewer negative emotion words in their writing were the most likely to remain sick after the expressive writing task. Moreover, this pattern was specific to negative (and not positive) emotion words. Although Yerkes and Dodson (1908) introduced the seed for this idea over a century ago and clinicians often refer to this premise, it is surprising how little the issue of intensity has been studied in psychotherapy.

The Yerkes–Dodson Law: Hidden From View?

In a psychotherapy study that brings exceptional clarity to understanding arousal as a mechanism in experiential therapy, Pos and colleagues (2017) showed that levels of emotional arousal increased significantly across the phases of therapy, all the while remaining positively related to clinical improvement. However, they observed that while the measure of clients' expressive arousal involved ratings on a 7-point scale (Warwar & Greenberg 1999), generally only a third of the scale's range was used when applying it to psychotherapy sessions (i.e., trained observers never gave ratings of 5, 6, or 7). So, while arousal was found to successfully predict good treatment outcomes, very high levels of arousal were not part of that prediction. Nevertheless, Pos and colleagues also found some evidence of a very subtle curvilinear relationship (the inverted U) between arousal in sessions and outcome, as predicted by the Yerkes–Dodson law.

This issue of a limited range in the data is particularly important because it speaks to something that clinicians may already know from their practice, but that research has had some trouble in verifying. While the inverted U makes strong clinical sense, a true curvilinear relationship is often hidden from psychotherapy researchers at large through sampling biases that do not capture the full possible range of emotional arousal. As Pos and colleagues (2017) point out, psychotherapy data on arousal tends to present a restricted range on arousal scales, and there are several reasons for this. First, the very low range of arousal is sometimes truncated by the fact that clients in psychotherapy are suffering and necessarily present with some level of symptomatology and aroused distress. Second, the very high range of arousal is similarly truncated by the fact that psychotherapy research (e.g., on depression) often excludes clients who are highly disorganized by their distress, actively suicidal, and so on. Interestingly, in the study of highly dysregulated clients (i.e., with panic or borderline processes), the client selection may be biased in the opposite way, such that studies are truncate only at the lower range. Finally, I would add that whatever the selection bias, attentive therapists are continually working to dyadically regulate their clients, deescalate, or rechannel excessive arousal within a session (see Stiles, 2009). So, in most data sets, the reason arousal is limited to some middle range (i.e., not too hot and not too cold) is essentially the delivery of good treatment by responsive clinicians.

In summary, although the Yerkes–Dodson law seems to have some evidence across contexts, it may not be so easily observable in psychotherapy studies that examine group averages. The implication for researchers is that they will more likely find linear (often positive) relationships between the intensity of arousal and outcome, when in fact the wider picture (not available to them) is that they are looking at only one side of the hill in the inverted U. Moreover, depending on the client population being studied (e.g., having problems being either under- or overregulated), the linear relationships one finds would be either positive or negative, representing the two sides of the hill.

Heightening Arousal: For How Long and How Often?

While the first question clinicians have about productive arousal is often about how much intensity, another question is, how frequently should one dip into that level of intensity, and for how long? Here, the risk of excessive arousal is not just one of raw intensity but rather of excessively prolonged or too much repeated engagement with high arousal over time. One preliminarily study showed that within a large outpatient psychiatric sample, clients who reported crying less frequently (one to two times per month) also reported having greater emotional benefit than those that cried more frequently (four or more times per month; Bauer et al., 2008).

An observational process-to-outcome study showed that in an experiential treatment for depression, having moderate bursts of high arousal is a strong positive predictor of change, but as expected, the size of the serving is a critical issue (Carryer & Greenberg, 2010). Specifically, researchers focused on therapy sessions that were already identified as among the most emotionally intense for clients and then examined the amount of time those clients spent at different levels of expressive arousal. The aim was to get a clearer portrait of what an intense session looked like when it predicted good outcomes. The conclusion was that if, during a particularly intense session, a client spent 25% of the treatment session in a state of intense emotional activation, then it was a strong predictor of good treatment outcomes (i.e., predicting 16% of treatment variance over and above any impact of the therapeutic relationship). The duration of this intense activation also showed an inverted U in relation to good outcome: In short, about 12.5 minutes of a 50-minute session (25%) provided the strongest prediction, while shorter or longer bursts of arousal each seemed to be less helpful for outcome. One cannot necessarily generalize this finding beyond treatment approaches that deliberately foster the activation of emotion to generate personal meaning.

A critical point for therapists to note is that when arousal was only slightly above everyday baseline, it was a decidedly negative predictor of outcomes (Carryer & Greenberg, 2010). For example, if a client was about to cry but then held back, or a burgeoning feeling was left unacknowledged by a client or unpursued by their therapist, that missed opportunity seemed to signal something that was harmful to the process of change. This last point highlights the subtlety involved in activating emotion. In much more practical terms, it also speaks to the need for clients to overtly express (rather than covertly experience) their arousal. Finally, therapists who hope to work with emotion in this way will need experiential training in how to identify and foster the completion of these emotional experiences.

Caveat #3: Arousal Must Be Expressed, Not Just Experienced

An interesting point of distinction I made in the definition of this process is that for the arousal to be productive in psychotherapy, it seems it needs to be externally expressed and observable. We know this because the various efforts to get more valid measurements of covert client experiences of emotional arousal have not been as useful as one might expect. For example, to parse out the subjectivity from reports on arousal, physiological measures have been explored as alternative observational indices. However, it is now well documented that physiological measures of sympathetic arousal are not tightly related to subjective reports on the experience of arousal, let alone its expression, which is further layered by personal, social, and cultural meanings. The measurement of treatment related arousal can vary by method, and self-reports do not cleanly correlate with physiological, neurobiological, or behavioral observer-rated assessments (Mauss & Robinson, 2009). This lack of convergence has created findings in the field that are difficult to interpret.

Self-Reports Do Not Capture the Target Process

The most obvious way to begin measuring client arousal is to simply ask people about how strong their feelings are. Because arousal is essentially an internal phenomenon, subjective reports presumably offer an index that an observing researcher just does not have direct access to. Physiological measures offer another possibility, but as suggested, these indices seem to be capturing different aspects of the phenomenon. Consider, for instance, a meta-analysis on arousal as a predictor of outcome of exposure-based treatments for anxiety disorders (Sønderland et al., 2023). Findings demonstrated that higher physiological arousal measured within sessions had a large effect in the prediction of better final symptom outcomes at the end of treatment. In contrast, client self-reports (e.g., using the Subjective Units of Distress scale) showed no significant association with final symptoms. It seems that self-reports on the initial intensity of arousal (i.e., at a given moment) do not capture the mechanism of change associated with treatment gains. (The dynamic process of habituation is a separate issue; see Chapter 3.[7]) Relatedly, in Chapter 6 I highlighted that labeling one's emotional experience can immediately reduce one's physiological response, but the reduced physical arousal is not reflected in self-reports about that subjective emotional experience (Torre & Lieberman, 2018). These inconsistencies between the explanatory power of self-reports versus biological measures of arousal might be explained by the inherent ambiguity of physiological reactivity, especially in the context of personal change, where meaning is central.

Arguably a client's subjective report reflects experienced arousal while an observer report will reflect expressed arousal. Again, one might presume these two indices to be closely related, but the issue turns out not to be so straightforward. For example, shame is a critical experience for people suffering from borderline personality disorder, and it is a predictor of self-inflicted injury in the following weeks. However, observer ratings of shame based on nonverbal facial expressions were a better predictor of self-injury than participants' self-reports on their shame experience (Brown et al., 2009). One explanation for the discrepancy between methods seems to be that self-reports conflate various emotions (e.g., combining fear and shame when rating shame). Another part of the meta-analysis cited earlier (Sønderland et al., 2023) looked at five studies of emotion-focused and experiential therapies that trained observers to code both the verbal and nonverbal content of clients' emotional arousal during psychotherapy from video recordings. A summary effect across studies showed these observations of expressed arousal were moderately associated with symptom outcomes at the end of treatment, where observer ratings of higher arousal predicted better treatment outcomes.

Inquiry into how clients report their arousal reveals some of the challenges in simply asking them about their emotion. When clients' subjective reports on their internal affective experiences were collected immediately after a session of with watching recordings of that same session, it revealed dramatic discrepancies (Warwar et al., 2003). For instance, one client reported the private experience of very intense emotional pain during her session (rating her own arousal as an 8.5 out of 10) while her expressed arousal, according to trained raters, was independently judged to be quite low based on the video. The critical point being that, in the experiential treatment of depression, it was the observation-based ratings of expressed arousal that were better outcome predictors than clients' own subjective reports about what they were feeling. Similarly, in a formal comparison of these methods of measurement in a group of clients suffering from complex interpersonal trauma and treated in emotion-focused therapy, the overt expression of emotion was a more critical process variable than self-reported internal experience (Chagigioris, 2010).[8]

Finally, while a broad meta-analysis found client-expressed emotional arousal has a large effect in the prediction of psychotherapy outcomes, the use of third-party observer ratings was the only significant moderator of that effect (Peluso & Freund, 2018). When emotional expression was observed by researchers from video recordings or transcripts, it was a markedly stronger predictor of treatment benefits as compared to when it was measured by the self-reports of clients themselves. This moderation across available studies in the literature gives a summary effect supporting to the idea that for arousal to be productive, it must be observably expressed and not just covertly experienced. The most central issue here is that self-reports, specifically on emotional arousal, are poor predictors of symptom outcome, and that has been noted across treatment approaches.

There are several reasons why this disparity in predictive power might occur. It is possible that clients are simply not good judges of what was a productive emotional experience. In one anecdote from research (L. S. Greenberg, personal communication, October 4, 2005; Warwar et al., 2003), when a therapy client was asked if their intense emotion had also been productive, the client responded, "Well, of course it wasn't! I was crying my eyes out, it felt terrible, and I practically ran out of tissues!" Part of the issue is that clients tend to focus on the immediate or short-term impacts of aroused emotion, and the cumulative impact and benefits to treatment outcomes may only be evident many months later (e.g., Ellison et al., 2009). Indeed, perhaps the observer is the best judge on whether it is a good cry after all.

However, a more profound part of this is that the very act of outward expression further informs and helps develop one's lived experience. This means freely expressed arousal likely also impacts several other change processes (e.g., finding the right words, sequences of emotional unfolding, formulating a narrative, the quality of the therapeutic relationship). In short, it is not that an observing researcher or therapist is necessarily a better judge of the client's arousal than the client themselves; rather, observable expressions of arousal probably capture a more complex process than the subjective intensity of arousal on its own.

Cultural and Social Values in Expression

The fact that arousal needs to be outwardly expressed to be productive introduces the issue of individual differences, as well as social and cultural variables that shape the expression of emotion. For example, the range in people's expressiveness and their approach to coping reflects personality style, social expectations, and cultural beliefs. These factors are the framework by which someone construes both the value and implications of heightened arousal. Examining samples cross-culturally has shown that people report more improvement after crying when they are from countries that are wealthier, that have more gender equality, where crying is more common, and where shame about crying is relatively low (Becht & Vingerhoets, 2002). Meanwhile, experimental research suggests that the impact of an evocative intervention is moderated by the individual's disposition toward emotional expressiveness (Niles et al., 2013). The treatment implication is that a one-size-fits-all approach to heightening arousal is ill-advised and a therapist's intervention will need to be matched within some margin to a client's natural inclination toward expressiveness.

Caveat #4: Arousal Alone Is Usually Not Enough (Despite What It May Seem)

Arousal and expression on their own are insufficient in reliably producing therapeutic change. Magnitude is not enough; other factors matter. So, while impetus, momentum, and the energy of one's expression do potentiate change, the direction, meaning, and context of that expressive arousal are all critical in completing this vector of emotional processing. This may seem obvious in retrospect, yet significant efforts in research and theory continue to focus on arousal at the expense of a more nuanced understanding. In personal as well as clinical anecdotes on change, the salience of arousal often eclipses other concomitant processes. Hypothesis testing can similarly limit the scope of questions being asked by researchers when they examine the role of expressive arousal in producing change.

Expressive arousal is the black box of emotional processing in that it only describes external behaviors rather than internal processes, so there is usually more going on than is accounted for. The impact of arousal will vary dramatically depending on what is accompanied internally. Consequentially, the relationship between arousal and treatment outcomes entails many third factor variables that are either concomitant, or contingent on, heightened arousal and expression. While expressive arousal plays a key role, the true complexity of this change process is often hidden in plain sight. This issue is illustrated in the case of a bricklayer who came to my office as a client. He prided himself on his calloused hands and emotional toughness, playfully describing himself as a man of stone. Nevertheless, he became extremely distressed shortly after the sudden and unexpected death of his hunting dog who was his only longtime companion. The man was caught so unaware that he found himself reduced to tears at the slightest reference to his dog, sometimes crying on the construction site.

He called me, weeping, on the phone, looking for counsel: "What's happening to me? I'm a mess! Is there any quick fix, Doc?" Unfortunately, there are no quick fixes for grief. Later, during a subsequent session, he reported, "It's better now, I'm holding it together. I think I just cried myself dry! Simple: get it out. That's all I needed!" When I asked further about this change experience, his explanation inadvertently revealed a much more tacit set of processes that remain entirely undeclared but go well beyond the venting of arousal:

> I couldn't stop crying, so I packed some gear and went for a really long drive by myself. I drove most of the night to our old hunting spot. She loved it there [*referring to his dog*]. I would shoot, and she would chase down the ducks. So, I sat there at our spot and had a good cry that morning. Then, instead of shooting, I spent a loaf and a half of bread just feeding the ducks. Yeah, I decided that I'm going to spread some of her ashes there, next time I go up. So, that's it, Doc! I cried myself out, packed my gear, and drove home. Now, I'm just going to throw myself into work, sweat out any more tears I might have left in me. [*A sigh of relief, and then a nod*] I'm going to be fine.

In this account, arousal is the most overt process, and as commonly occurs in personal renditions of change, the process explanation is reduced to venting or purging emotion (e.g., "I just cried myself dry!"). Nevertheless, on closer examination, the story points to awareness, reflection, self-soothing, existential needs, and meaning making as all being covert and undeclared processes of change, and this complexity is not part of the client's self-understanding.

"Catharsis" Is a Misnomer

It is a fallacy to think of emotional catharsis as a stand-alone process. The concept originates from Greek, meaning "to cleanse," and in 330 B.C.E., Aristotle (ca. 330 B.C.E./1996) introduced the term as a purging of emotion by spectators while they watched the unfolding plots of tragic theater.[9] While this was obviously much more than purging, Breuer and Freud (1895) took the notion of catharsis and applied it to the understanding psychotherapy, arguing that the intense experience of arousal was a critical part of treatment. Freud later abandoned this idea as he developed the psychoanalytic method and put more emphasis on awareness and verbalizing an insight, while arousal came to be seen as a concomitant sense of relief (e.g., an abreaction).[10]

However, the value of expressive arousal as a primary process was picked up again in the 1960s by new treatment approaches that focused on emotive experiences and unfettered feeling. Established examples of these include primal therapy, which involves intense expressions of primal (i.e., preverbal) screaming, enduring extended periods of isolation, as well as daily therapy sessions that continue consecutively for several weeks (Janov, 1970; Karle et al., 1973).[11] Examples from folk psychology describe a similar process of purging, as suggested in titles like *Cure by Crying* (Stone, 1997). Interestingly, venting emotion also usually requires a cue or topic and referring to childhood trauma often provides an easy target for this, which may be why such treatment perspectives often hold that virtually all distress stems from repressed childhood pain. Unfortunately, in those approaches, "emotional memories continue to be thought of as foreign bodies lodged in the human psyche and requiring purgation" (Nichols & Efran, 1985, p. 46).

While certain psychodynamic and emotive theories of psychotherapy have usually sought to expand and reinterpret the definition of emotional catharsis, it is ultimately a metaphor that refers specifically to the purging of waste.[12] The point to be taken here is that there is nothing in the proper meaning of emotional catharsis that refers to meaning making, awareness, insight, finding closure, and so on. Attributing these other processes to the term involves an overly generous imputation of meaning, and rather than making a long addendum to an outdated definition, it is more fruitful to directly address the underlying complexity that relates to productive expressive arousal.

Other formulations based on catharsis have downplayed the purging of emotion in favor of putting emphasis on the idea of release from inhibition. Inhibition–confrontation theory puts forward that actively withholding distressing thoughts, emotions, and behaviors creates a state of chronic stress on the body and increases one's vulnerability to illness, whereas the subsequent expression and release (i.e., cathartic experience) reduces this stress. Inspired by Freud's early ideas, this was the initial explanation for why emotional disclosures about trauma led to salubrious effects (Pennebaker & Chung, 2007). The idea remains quite alive in popular understandings of how emotional processing occurs, although the consensus among researchers has been that more is involved than this theory suggests. For example, it was not supported by a meta-analysis of mediators in the impact of expressive writing; disclosing trauma for the first time or by more emotionally inhibited people (e.g., men) had no effect (Frattaroli, 2006).

In short, there is little to no empirical support for catharsis or the venting of arousal as a stand-alone process and yet the notion persists in popular culture. The reasons why this hydraulic understanding of anger or sadness as venting continues to persist is due to misinformed health care practitioners, mass media, and advice columns based on pop psychology—rather than science (Bushman, 2002). Indeed, the simplicity (and sensationalism) of a quick fix is appealing, and various forms of "destructotherapy"[13] produce a brief experience, even if it is superficial and short-lived. Nevertheless, the role of expressive arousal is not just a gross misunderstanding.

This misunderstanding stems from the fact that ideas about the impact of confronting, engaging, and expressing one's feelings rapidly become conflated and entangled with other, empirically well-founded, processes of elaborating awareness, elaborating new meaning, and activating a sequential transformation. As one examines the literature, it becomes clearer that in anecdotes where people describe the benefits of catharsis (or venting, etc.), they are often using such terms as a conceptual shorthand to refer to a range of much more complicated processes that remain undeclared. As one article's title bluntly states, "Which catharsis do they mean?" (Meisiek, 2004, p. 797). Terms like "catharsis" perpetuate the oversimplified myth that passive and undiscerning surrender to feelings or following one's impulse is healthy or productive. The opposite is true: Eliciting tears, laughter, aggression, or screams should not become an end in itself (Nichols & Efran, 1985).

Arousal Acts in Synergy

When arousal works, it is in synergy with other processes. Under certain conditions it can produce a unique and critical contribution to emotional processing and productive change. First and foremost, what arousal means or signifies to the client who experiences it is an issue of chief importance and cannot be separated out from the question of whether arousal is productive. This formulation was conclusively supported by a large experiment on venting anger by Bushman (2002), in which participants were led to feel angry and then invited to hit a punching bag, as is in keeping with catharsis-based interventions (e.g., punching a pillow, using a foam bat to act out a revenge fantasy). However, while one group was instructed to think about the person who had angered them, another group was instructed to think about becoming physically fit. Following the intervention, those who thought about fitness had become less angry, while those in the rumination group had become markedly more angry. This finding has crystalized the conclusion of therapy analogue studies examining catharsis, which was that expressive arousal works best when combined with other kinds of cognitive processing (Bohart, 1977, 1980).

This synergetic effect at any given instance in psychotherapy is a difficult process to track, although one line of research has demonstrated that when the moment-by-moment processes of emotional tone and cognitive reflection become synchronized, that periodic co-occurrence in therapy represented a special kind of event, one that is predictive of good over poor treatment outcomes (Mergenthaler, 1996). In short, when emotional processing is achieved through aroused expression, it is typically in the context of meaningfully articulating one's emotional experience (L. S. Greenberg, 2021). Put simply, when one has well-articulated needs, the integration of cognition with aroused affect is the mobilization of emotion (A. Pascual-Leone et al., 2013). That mobilization can be very much in the service of problem solving. So, among other things, the function of arousal depends very much on what one is thinking about.

A key function of arousal and expression as contributors to emotional processing is their ability to boost raw emotional activity, which subsequently allows these processes to work synergistically with other subprocesses. This means that expressive arousal is not about content development. Rather, the expression of emotion is often a jumping off point to mobilize the process of some subsequent emotion transformation, but the process is not usually enough in isolation. The implication of this for researchers is that they need to measure other processes as mediators or moderators when exploring the impact of emotional expression and arousal. For clinicians, the implication is they should not take arousal at face value but should rather think of it as a magnifier or catalyst when facilitating other key processes.

Moreover, there is some evidence to believe that upon activating emotional arousal, time is of the essence, and unnecessary delays may be harmful. Research on attachment-based family therapy for suicidal adolescents showed that while engaging and activating global distress (i.e., a state of high emotional arousal but low meaningfulness) was, of course, a signal of distress, but it could also be the starting point of a curative process.[14] However, when the initial episode of global distress was prolonged, it predicted poorer final treatment outcomes (Lifshitz et al., 2021). That finding is reminiscent of a trend that was unexpectedly observed in another study on the progressive pattern of emotional advancements during sessions of depressed clients in emotion-focused therapy (A. Pascual-Leone, 2009). It showed that less productive sessions did not only have more moment-by-moment emotional collapses compared with productive sessions, but also those collapses into global distress seemed to get successively longer as a session wore on. This suggests an initial spike in arousal is a window of opportunity, but holding the window open for too long is related to client deterioration. That point becomes particularly crucial in the study of distress related to suicidality (Lifshitz et al., 2021). Studies like these tell us something about the risks of having clients flounder in unproductive emotion for too long and in not subsequently activating other synergistic meaning-making processes shortly after the initial arousal of distress.

Based on explanations of desensitization or catharsis, when clients engage in emotionally expressive tasks, it should have immanent and relatively linear effects. However, this is not always the case. For example, when trauma survivors expressed intense emotion during an enactment in early sessions of emotion-focused therapy, it had no measurable impact on the end of a 16-session treatment. Yet, the same expressive event emerged as a significant predictor of outcome at a 6-month follow-up (Paivio et al., 2001). This delayed effect suggests the expressive event was more important than it seemed at first and clients continue to process such experiences even well after the termination of treatment.

The conclusion to be taken here is that in many ways, although the outward nature of expressive arousal is highly salient, it is a fallacy to think of catharsis as a stand-alone process. Inside this black box of emotional processing is substantial complexity. While emotional arousal is an important ingredient in productive emotion, arousal alone has not proven to be a strong predictor of good versus poor treatment outcomes (L. S. Greenberg et al., 2007). In short, arousal works in synergy with other processes that are often more subtle and less immediately salient. Carefully dissecting emotional productivity based on detailed video observation has led research to operationalize it into a measurable variable that combines most of the other processes discussed in this book. These include awareness (e.g., attending, symbolization, congruence), regulation (e.g., maintaining optimal levels of activation), transformation (e.g., acceptance, differentiation, agency) and, finally, expressive arousal (L. S. Greenberg et al., 2007). When emotional productivity was considered as an overarching variable that encompassed expressive arousal, it even mediated the impact that a therapeutic alliance has on treatment outcome (Auszra et al., 2013). Productive emotional processing clearly goes beyond the degree to which clients confront, feel, and express their emotion.

Treatment Perspectives on Arousal Versus Meaning

The importance of ensuring optimal arousal is a recurring theme across treatments (for a cogent review on arousal as a common process, see Lane & Nadel, 2020). However, where one finds disparity is in the various concomitant processes that different therapies emphasize. For example, consider the activation of arousal from a behavioral perspective: Exposure is emphasized as the principal intervention strategy for evoking intense emotion, but it is no longer considered sufficient on its own to produce change. Even so, the need to also add new information to the exposure experience is a critical caveat, one that gets much less theoretical elaboration (Foa et al., 2006). Moreover, behavioral theory presumes that emotional processing itself is not the creative generation of that new information, only the absorption and integration of it. This perspective on change also suggests that the requisite corrective information is somehow already latent, contained within a situational context, awaiting its deployment. For example, consider these statements: "Emotional processing requires information that disconfirms erroneous elements" and "Even when disconfirmatory information is present, during the evocative experience, emotional processing only occurs when [that information] is encoded and incorporated into existing knowledge" (Foa et al., 2006, p. 7).

However, in theories of experiential therapy the inverse is true: The role of exposure in imaginal enactments such as chairwork is usually only briefly acknowledged (if at all), with the primary emphasis being put on the subsequent steps of elaborating the meaning of a new experience (see "imaginal confrontation" in Paivio & Pascual-Leone, 2023). In experiential therapies the evocativeness of the therapist and of the meaning confrontation itself take the theoretical focus, and yet the role of exposure (in a behavioral sense) is inseparable from the engagement. So, the processes that support and act in synergy with expressive arousal as a curative process are not only complex but the way they are explained are also subject to different a priori perspectives on what treatments are trying to do.

Caveat #5: Expressive Arousal Needs to Be Seen Through to Completion

Acts of expressive arousal, including enactments, have a trajectory of experience. These are organic temporal events and as such they need to be seen through to the end if they are to be completed as experiences. However, emotional expression is routinely suppressed in everyday life and in many social encounters, that is the default. While that management of emotion does have a place in healthy functioning, when it is time for expressing emotion, completing the process means riding out the length of that experience and this often takes the time it takes. For example, an imperative to feel faster is both nonsensical and often counterproductive. Emotion is representational (e.g., it entails meaning about one's relation to the world), but just as importantly, it is also procedural (e.g., it comes with an action tendency, behaviors, it sits in a contextual sequence). So, for expressive arousal to be a productive part of emotional processing, those emotive procedures cannot be truncated or interrupted, which are common impediments to full processing (e.g., biting one's lip, choking back tears, stopping oneself mid-action). Indeed, sometimes completing the emotional experience is itself a new experience.

Allowing Emotion and Its Expression

For adaptive emotions, expressive arousal is certainly an essential piece of emotional processing. This is especially the case if that feeling has been hereto stifled, cut short, or not allowed. Acknowledging that there is a temporal pattern in the rise, peak, and decay of an emotional expression implies that feeling will unfold as part of an organic, time-based process. It is a procedure, and not reducible to a representational snapshot of meaning. An example from my clinical practice shows how clients may even be explicitly ambivalent about interrupting their emotion. The client reflected,

> I chose to terminate my pregnancy, so I don't know if I get to be sad about it. I don't regret my decision; the circumstances were so bad. But do I get to grieve it, even if I don't regret it?

In this example, the client interrupts her primary adaptive emotion and does so with full awareness. Her dilemma is about whether it can be allowed at all or if it should be completed. While examples of truncated emotion are typically much less obvious, being only on the periphery of someone's awareness, the process for working through and resolving these stuck primary emotions is the same.

Honoring the vector or trajectory of a primary emotional experience is a commitment to a short journey (e.g., often a few minutes, perhaps most of a session). However, it is a journey where sometimes, "it gets worse before it gets better" (A. Pascual-Leone, Yeryomenko, et al., 2016, p. 336; Wang et al., 2022). An illustration of this issue comes from a clinical paper in which clients wore heart rate monitors during psychotherapy, tracking their arousal beat by beat as dialogue unfolded in session (Bridges, 2006). While clients are working through past interpersonal injuries in a humanistic–experiential therapy, the contrasting vignettes that follow illustrate sympathetic nervous activity that underlies a productive experience versus the self-interruption of an emotional expression.

Allowing emotion: An example of optimal process. In one vignette (from Bridges, 2006), during the first session, a 41-year-old woman explores unresolved feeling related to her divorce, which followed the discovery that her husband was having an affair with one of her best friends. For most of the session, her heart rate is stable at around 60 beats per minute (bpm), a normal resting heart rate. As the client becomes more aware and symbolizes her fear and sadness about romantic difficulties, she feels deeply, and there are several small corresponding bumps in cardiovascular activity.

Then abruptly, starting at 61 bpm, there is a burst of high arousal where her heart rate shoots up and literally doubles in speed to a peak of 129 bpm. She seems caught off guard by having touched her sadness but then freely engages with it. She sobs bitterly, stopping only to find the words for what she is going through. At one moment she is unable to speak, but the wave of feeling is peppered with reflections on what the significance of her grief means to her: "[*long pause*] I'm so out of my head that it's hard to find the words, but it's like, 'Go slowly, tread lightly, be careful.' . . . It's not 'Don't love,' it's 'Be careful'" (Bridges, 2006, p. 563). This entire affective experience passes within 4 minutes, after which the client's heart rate dips to 53 and then returns once again to a stable baseline of about 60 bpm.

Looking at the dramatic physiological reaction and its rapid recovery, it begs for a closer examination of process. Indeed, video shows the client started experiencing an adaptive emotion (grief) that was also outwardly observed by raters as moderate to high expressive arousal. Her therapist met this by facilitating the natural course of her emotional experience: empathically focusing on emerging content, staying with and deepening client experience, and helping to symbolize the feeling in a moment-by-moment creation of new meaning. In short, there is an unhesitating and purposeful exploration of the client's feelings in the here and now, which are allowed and freely attended to until those feelings begin the shift through the very meaning they impart (recall Gendlin's, 1981, felt shift).

Interrupting emotion: A contrasting example. The same paper gives a contrasting vignette with similar narrative circumstances and demographics as the example mentioned previously (Bridges, 2006). In this case, a 51-year-old divorced woman struggles with a betrayal, in which her fiancé had a romantic affair with her younger sister. The vignette takes place during the second session, where the client is tense, talks quickly, and gives lots of detail. While ruminating on what led up to the affair and how she might have prevented it, her heart rate is about 90 bpm (i.e., within a normal resting range). Then, at some point in the session, the client becomes emotional, because she stumbles upon the poignancy of how supportive she had been of her sister over the years, which added to her pain about the betrayal: "And that she could look into my eyes and with that reality going on. . . . It's really shaken my whole . . . ." She trails off, perhaps interrupting herself, but the therapist picks up with a deep empathic reflection: "It sounds like it really shattered your whole view of yourself and those around you" (Bridges, 2006 p. 558). The client silently nods, and then wells up with tears as her heart rate jumps from 81 to 114 bpm, a sudden acceleration during the quiet pause as client and therapist sit on the brink of this poignancy. This opens the door to what might have been a deeply emotional exploration of meaning. But, for whatever reason, the therapist does not direct the client to stay with the feeling, nor does he comment on her tears; still, the client's heart rate holds at 114 bpm.

Then, after a brief pause, the therapist asks for more historical information, implicitly directing the client to an external narrative about plot and characters: "You [were also] talking about exactly how you found out about the affair?"

The client dabs her eye with a tissue as her heart rate lowers only slightly to 111 bpm. Then she obliges, covering up despite the strong internal activation of her sympathetic nervous system:

> Oh! I got distracted, didn't I? I got off on something else, didn't I? Well, he picked me up and then we went to pick his son up. And I had just moved to a new apartment. His son was in the backseat, and he was kind of chattering and asking how my move was. And he said something about a model I had made of the floor plan. (Bridges, 2006, p. 559)

When confronted with the emerging intensity of the client's arousal, the therapist seems to have hesitated and then changed the topic, shifting the conversation away from immediately presenting emotion. This diversion may have even been welcomed by the client, an opportunity to turn away from the sharp focus of painful emotion. However, all the while during the journalistic account that follows, her heart rate monitor reveals the enduring strong affective arousal that is otherwise hidden from both her therapist and the video camera. She talks about everything except what is happening inside. Meanwhile, the slow recovery from her peak arousal persists. Covertly, her heart is still pounding, lingering in a slow linear decline that takes more than 10 minutes before returning to her baseline heart rate.

Ignoring Arousal Does Not Stop It

In the two vignettes presented here, there are similar opportunities for engaging and directly exploring emotional arousal. In the first example, the client was encouraged to stay with her feeling and make sense of the aroused emotion, a difficult and distressing experience that took a total of only 4 minutes. In the second example, the flow of client emotional expression was interrupted by an initially unresponsive therapist and then a change in topic. On the surface, derailing emotional exploration in that second example seems to have worked because it avoided any further overt signs of distress. In short, the client stops expressing emotion. Yet, the client's internal and covert experience of distress took 10 minutes to dissipate, more than twice as long as the 4 minutes of full emotional expression that occurred in the first vignette.

The implication for therapists working in session is that although truncating a client's emotional expression might outwardly seem helpful in reducing distress (e.g., tidy, contained, no awkwardness, no mess), the client's experience will likely continue to covertly smolder. Not only does interrupting someone's emotional expression hide it from view, but it also precludes an opportunity for exploring and making sense out of a painful experience. Ignoring or interrupting emergent emotion signals to the client that it should be stifled and essentially takes it off the table, rendering it no longer discussable. The negotiation is subtle, but it is too common that therapists and clients are complicit with one another in avoiding or curtailing a client's emotional expression.

The boundaries on what intensity of emotion is acceptable or appropriate in therapy are established very early in treatment, often within the first one to two exchanges around an expressive event. If a therapist does not explicitly acknowledge a client's initial expressiveness (e.g., a client's flush, a break in conversation as tears well up), then the client quickly gleans a meta-message from their therapist's hesitance (e.g., "Please, try not to go there, it's not part of what we want to do here"). The catch is that to allow emotional expression is to venture into the seemingly wild and unknown. So, embarking on this brief process requires some confidence in the notion that there is indeed a natural wave or curved pattern to a specific emotional experience, one that will eventually come to pass (and not lead to an endless abyss).

Productive Arousal Has a Natural Wave

Sometimes clients themselves can retrospectively identify having had productive experiences of working through intense emotion that led to some completion or fruition. When interviewed about the emotionally evocative experience of an enactment task in emotion-focused therapy, one client candidly stated, "It was heavy and intense, but also very . . . somewhat horrendous. And very nice, actually. Because I learned a lot about myself" (Stiegler, Binder, et al., 2018, p. 247). Similarly, clients overcome avoidance by approaching and tolerating emotions in small steps in the safety of therapy. The experience of not having been consumed by the feeling is sometimes also a new emotional experience. The line of evidence that supports enduring exposure to previously avoided feelings, eventually to better regulate them (e.g., Foa & Jaycox, 1999), is distinct and was discussed in Chapter 3 in terms of learning that changes one's expectancies. However, exploration that leads to habituation still converges with the idea being presented here on the need for completing an emotional expression. Whatever one's approach, the general premise for clinical work here recalls a quote cited in the epigraph of this chapter and often attributed to Winston Churchill: "If you are going through hell, keep going!"

The two vignettes (Bridges, 2006) convey isolated instances of the expression versus interruption of aroused emotional expression. However, in treatments where it is valued, heightened moments of arousal will spark up throughout a session, often spurring it onward and giving impetus to a cascade of emotion (see Fosha, 2021). In a case study of intensive short-term dynamic psychotherapy, heart rate, vagal tone, and breathing patterns were all used to capture in-session variations in emotional activation during the treatment of a client suffering from panic disorder (Fleury et al., 2016). The success of each intervention in moving the client through an experiential process of change was closely related to the pattern in moments of heightened emotional arousal, such that each transition corresponded to a distinct physiological shift. This detailed examination of different passages within the same treatment session illustrates the ongoing role of arousal in the activation of distinct emotional changes regarding a target concern.

The research on trajectories of emotional arousal in psychotherapy is scattered, but there is some support for the idea that when successful emotional processing involves heightening arousal, it is an experiential process that needs to be seen through to completion for it to be useful. A small body of literature has described productive patterns of aroused engagement in psychotherapy as an expressive wave or an arousal spike within session, which are predictive of good outcomes. For example, single sessions in psychodynamic interpersonal therapy showed a wavelike pattern of arousal. This intensity curve over a productive session begins with low initial arousal, then high arousal at mid-session, then low arousal again near the end (Mackay et al., 2002). A study on cognitive exposure therapy for depression has documented productive arousal across multiple sessions, where transient states of symptom worsening (depression spikes, i.e., the inverse of a sudden gain) were nonetheless associated with good processes and positive treatment outcomes (A. M. Hayes et al., 2007). Furthermore, research on a range of treatment approaches has described saw-toothed, up-and-down patterns of moment-by-moment change in meaning making, highlighting that those within-session patterns of working through difficult experiences are also characteristically associated with corresponding changes in arousal and valence (A. Pascual-Leone, 2009, 2018; Stiles et al., 2004). Studies like these suggest there is a natural curve by which localized micro-patterns of increased arousal are sometimes part of healthy emotional processing.

It Could Get Worse Before It Gets Better

Activating and expressing emotion can be productive. However, there is a veritable conundrum here, one that cuts to the core of skepticism about promoting arousal and the expression of emotion.[15] In short, how can feeling more emotion, or even feeling worse, lead to feeling better?[16] As an aside, it is critical to appreciate this question is about a moment-by-moment process within some emotion event (i.e., feeling bad, in the sense of feeling negative emotion more intensely); it does not refer to the worsening of clinical symptomatology over days or weeks. Nonlinear patterns in symptom change do exist but reflect a different phenomenon (consider Owen et al., 2015).[17] Whatever the case, an answer to the question about intense emotional arousal is difficult to cleanly discern from psychotherapy sessions because client arousal is so closely intertwined with therapist responsiveness (Stiles, 2009). Responsiveness itself is embedded in preconceived treatment models about whether increasing arousal is helpful and what that should look like. This makes it difficult (if not impossible) to assess what a temporal pattern of arousal would have been if the client had not been subject to the guiding influence of moment-by-moment therapist interventions.

Even so, one strategy for teasing this apart is to examine patterns of arousal in experiments, which use either mood induction or expressive disclosure, thereby removing the confounding influences of therapists as well as treatment frameworks (A. Pascual-Leone, Yeryomenko, et al., 2016). The aim of this kind of research is to explore the organic temporal pattern of emotionally expressive arousal and how that relates to outcome. For example, a quasi-experiment that examined the temporal impact of crying after a mood induction showed that although participants felt worse than baseline 20 minutes after crying, when this was followed up 90 minutes later, their mood was enhanced above baseline (Gracanin et al., 2015).

In a more elaborate design, researchers used multiple sessions of expressive writing to investigate patterns of emotional arousal simultaneously across two different frames of times: within-session change (i.e., 15-minute micro-patterns), and between-session change (24-hour macro-patterns; A. Pascual-Leone, Yeryomenko, et al., 2016). In this study, a large sample of undergraduate students who reported distress related to a personal traumatic or upsetting event were randomized to either an emotionally expressive writing condition or a control. Then, they rated their arousal of negative emotion before and after each session over a series of three sessions. The overarching pattern in negative emotion showed a significant decrease across the three sessions of intervention taken together, representing overall improvement. However, within individual sessions, when participants engaged their emotional difficulty, the ratings also showed a locally significant increase or spike in arousal. Furthermore, before and after each session, saliva samples were taken from participants to track their cortisol changes (i.e., a dynamic hormonal marker of stress), and these biological measures of distress confirmed the pattern found in self-reports (A. Pascual-Leone et al., 2012).

Figure 8.1 shows these two separate patterns of change in negative emotion. Although each of the two patterns point in opposite directions, they combine in a syncopated manner, through an alternating zigzag pattern. A particularly unique contribution of this study was an analysis that confirmed the saw-toothed pattern over time. In other words, the study empirically demonstrated how micro-patterns of increased arousal can coexist within a macro-pattern of decreased distress (A. Pascual-Leone, Yeryomenko, et al., 2016). Concretely, this is the way feeling worse leads to feeling better.

The observation of this type of pattern in arousal was also supported in a study on the brief treatment of borderline personality disorder. Clients were engaged in the enactment of self-critical dialogues as part of a dynamic process assessment both pre- and posttherapy. Researchers then examined arousal changes within each process-assessment session, as well as over the entire 3-month treatment, using both client's self-reports and functional magnetic resonance imaging (fMRI) observations of their brain activation (Kramer, Kolly, et al., 2018). Both subjective and neurobiological indices of emotional activation over time supported the described saw-toothed pattern. In short, arousal increased by a small to medium amount within each session of chairwork, but the time between sessions showed large decreases in arousal. These changes were also associated with symptom reduction. The researchers also hypothesized that this pattern represents the natural oscillation of productive arousal when people are working through core issues (Kramer, Kolly, et al., 2018).

Returning to Figure 8.1, it is worth noting that the increases during each session start with low arousal and then progressively increase until the end of that expressive writing session, apparently ending with higher levels of arousal (i.e., see shorter within-session arrows). These increases in arousal are not easily explained by exposure-based theories of emotional change: Theories of habituation and inhibition would predict that sessions start with high arousal (i.e., high arousal upon initial exposure), followed by a within-session decline or attenuation of arousal (as discussed in Chapter 3). In other words, as participants get used to the process of working on their trauma, the prediction by classic theories of exposure and habituation would be that the three within-session arrows should point downwards in Figure 8.1. Clearly, there is more going on here. This point, the direction of arousal's within-session change, is something that highlights the role of increasing arousal as a unique mechanism of change and one that is distinct from habituation or inhibition.

FIGURE 8.1. Productive Patterns in the Intensity of Emotion: Short-Term Increases With Longer-Term Decreases

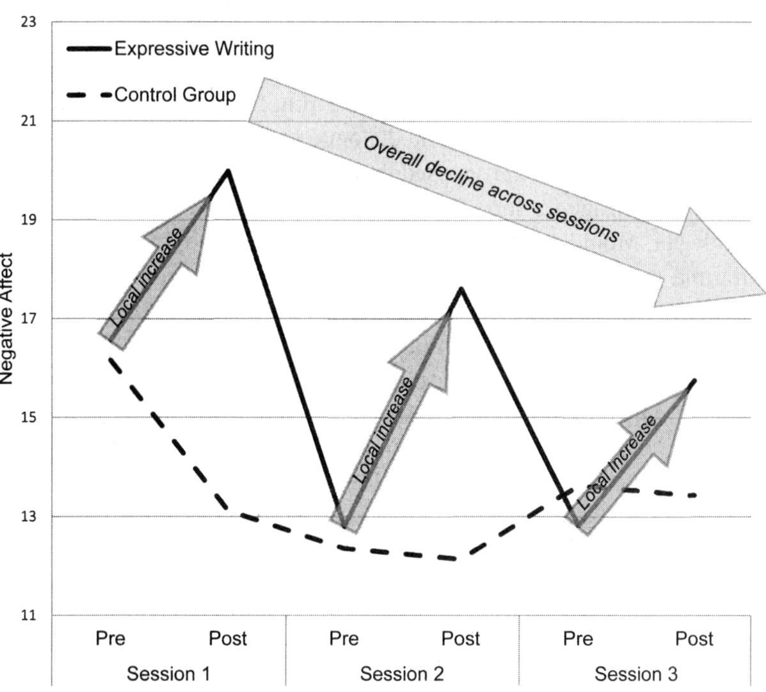

Note. From "Does Feeling Bad, Lead to Feeling Good? Arousal Patterns During Expressive Writing," by A. Pascual-Leone, N. Yeryomenko, O.-P. Morrison, R. Arnold, and U. Kramer, 2016, *Review of General Psychology, 20*(3), p. 341 (https://doi.org/10.1037/gpr0000083). Copyright 2016 by Sage Publications. Reprinted with permission.

MECHANISMS AT WORK: HOW DOES EXPRESSIVE AROUSAL CREATE CHANGE?

When considering the broader temporal frame of an entire treatment, all approaches agree that good treatment outcomes result in less pathological arousal.[18] However, upon closer consideration, different treatment perspectives on the role of arousal are typically formulating change using different mechanisms. For the most part, a treatment's theory of change provides a lens, focused on explaining isolated aspects of a client's in-session patterns of arousal.

On one hand, an exposure-based theory of change hypothesizes the gradual attenuation of arousal during a given session. According to this theory, that emotional work is believed to produce a steady decrease in arousal over the course of the session, or what Rachman (1980) described as the "absorption" of emotional distress. Over time, the incremental contribution of this decreasing arousal or reactivity contributes to either habituation or suppression, producing the larger, emergent treatment outcome of successful symptom relief. That process was discussed in Chapter 3 (see also Foa & Rothbaum, 1998; Jaycox et al., 1998).

On the other hand, experiential approaches of either humanistic or psychodynamic ilk stress the search for personal meaning, which is a categorically different process from habituation. These treatments also see increased arousal as a key process, but one that precipitates and is punctuated by vital moments of meaning making. In fact, for clients suffering from depression or anxiety, when the enactment of a self-critical dialogue (i.e., two-chair task) is not productive, research on emotion-focused therapy suggests one reason may be that clients did not engage for long enough to fully benefit or complete the enactment (Stiegler, Molde, et al., 2018). Similarly, when using chairwork for complex trauma (e.g., imagining a dialogue with one's perpetrator), where client engagement is more frequent or deeper, then the enactment tasks become stronger predictors of reduced symptoms (Paivio et al., 2001). In other words, if it gets worse before it gets better, then one would need to pass through some threshold of difficult emotional arousal before completing the experience.

So, in an ideal session of experiential therapy (broadly defined), even if emotion is not highly aroused at the beginning, the ongoing construction of new meaning is itself evocative and periodically elicits bursts of increased arousal. The repeated short-term increases of arousal (within-session microchanges) shown in Figure 8.1 reflect that ongoing meaning making, where an individual becomes aware of new aspects of experience while in the very process of their engagement (A. Pascual-Leone, Yeryomenko, et al., 2016). Again, the contribution of arousal to this dynamic and self-generated meaning making is contradictory to the notions of habituation or emotional inhibition, which are contingent on exposure to a stimulus that is relatively static (e.g., an objective representation of meaning; see Chapter 4). So, behavioral and experiential perspectives agree that increasing arousal will (in some way) be an important part of the process contributing to longer term positive outcomes. However, the nuance of what increased arousal is hypothesized to facilitate plays out quite differently.[19]

The unique contribution of expressive arousal has been demonstrated in process-outcome research. As suggested by the five caveats to productive emotional arousal and its expression, the role of this kind of process is usually synergistic. This means it depends very much on what the arousal is about and how it is used. For expressive arousal to be a mechanism of positive change in psychotherapy, it needs to be accepted, tolerated, and engaged, which also means seeing it through to completion. Expressive arousal sometimes acts independently as a productive process. Otherwise, it is perhaps more often a mediating factor that interacts in important ways with other forms of emotional processing. Moreover, the theoretical nuance in how heightened arousal works differently in exposure-based versus experiential therapies is important to whether one actively facilitates emotion, fanning the flames of emotional arousal and expression.

Increasing or up-regulating the activation of emotion through expression, arousal, or behavioral enactment represents a distinct form of emotional processing, one that is not reducible to catharsis and is a unique predictor of positive treatment outcomes. This client process is cited in several treatment approaches, albeit with several caveats for defining it as productive. Even so, describing those parameters of productive expressive arousal does not yet explain the causal role of this general change process. Indeed, particularly if one accepts that there is no substantial evidence for either catharsis or inhibition–confrontation as explanations of change, then new hypotheses about how this process might produce change are needed. Over the next three chapters, I propose several distinct pathways of action by which expressive arousal acts as a mechanism of emotional change in psychotherapy and in everyday life.

ENDNOTES

1. While there is an affinity, the two sides of regulation include, but go far beyond, the sympathetic versus parasympathetic systems as different parts of one's central nervous system. The complexity of what has been referred to in the existing literature as emotion regulation is, of course, much broader. That was discussed in Chapter 2, where I suggest the term is also used in a somewhat misleading way.
2. Labeling and symbolizing the meaning as one speaks from the feeling (i.e., facets of emerging emotional awareness) will be along that continuum.
3. Whether just these two processes are sufficient for all forms of emotional processing could be debated, particularly as one examines other populations in need of psychotherapy. For more on this issue, see Chapter 14, which discusses the additional need for sequential transformations to work with psychiatric populations. Whatever the case, Lumley has made a strong case for the centrality of emotional expression as a key and independent process.
4. The basic apprehension over feeling intense negative emotions is much more compelling than any rational arguments offered by Aristotle or Freud on the curative role of catharsis!
5. There are a few exceptions: One exception is when emotional expression is done for the first time and where being witnessed as someone in distress is permission giving and a novel relational experience. Another example is when arousal is used as a generic proxy to stimulate some overall process, which would subsequently engage more meaningful emotion. These are discussed in Chapter 9, but their commonality is to use arousal as point of entry.
6. Echoing Goldilocks, from *The Three Bears* (Southey, 1837).
7. To be clear, the self-reported intensity of arousal discussed here represents a single measure or central tendency, which is different from habituation according to self-reports, the latter being a relative decrease in arousal over time; see Chapter 3.

8. The fact that ratings by a trained expert might be a stronger predictor of change than the subjective ratings by clients themselves is not to be taken as obvious. It certainly is not true for all process predictors. For instance, client ratings of the interpersonal relationship they share with their therapist are better predictors than ratings made by the attending therapist.

9. To better understand what Aristotle was referring to as "catharsis," it is worth noticing that his description of expressive arousal was of a person's response to theatrical drama, which involved personally identifying with larger-than-life characters, bringing the meaning of those narratives into one's awareness, and then resonating with its human significance as that tragedy unfolded in real time. Moreover, all of this was happening in a public setting, where spectators often participated in vocal exchanges, calling out and expressing their fear, pity, and grief directly to the actors on stage, as well as in more private conversations among those they sat with during the show (Arnott, 1959). The fact that there are these various other, undeclared processes is reminiscent of the bricklayer's explanation from my clinical practice about how venting was more than simply getting it out.

10. *Abreaction* was a new term used by Freud (1910; first introduced by Breuer & Freud, 1895). It refers to the release of affect that can occur when one brings a given moment or problem into focus (which could also be thought of as a synergistic process of awareness plus arousal). Arguably, for Freud, elaborating awareness was essentially the method, whereas abreaction describes the sudden experience of this awareness, culminating in intense arousal.

11. Although I stress that emotional arousal is so salient as a process and therefore an easy explanation for change, studies that have examined this process bring further attention to arousal when they ask participants to consent to elaborate physiological measurements. I suggest the use of complex and sometimes invasive physiological measures also creates a strong placebo effect, bringing participants' attention to their affective arousal. While sometimes necessary, the invasiveness of these measures in research may include fitting the client with chest straps and electronic devices. In the early research of Karle and colleagues (1973), it even involved using a rectal thermometer, which no doubt had clients convinced about how seriously researchers were taking the physiological experience!

12. The fact that "cathartic experience" is only used as a metaphor in psychology has become almost entirely overlooked. In medicine, the literal meaning of "cathartic" refers to a substance that accelerates defecation (as compared to easing, which is done by laxatives).

13. Venues in various countries offer customers the opportunity to destroy a room using a baseball bat, golf club, or other weapon. A headline in *Time Magazine* reads: "Go Ahead, Smash Everything in the Room. It's Therapy" (*Time*, May 12, 2012), while a mainstream national news outlet confirmed, "The Best Way to Relieve Aggression: The Rage Room" (CBC-Life, October 28, 2016). Moreover, this is an international phenomenon with a very long history. In China, corporations encourage employees to hit a Bobo doll or destroy cars to release frustration (Bhaghat et al., 2012).

14. The issue of how sequences of discrete emotional states lead to outcome is discussed later in Chapters 12 and 13 on transformational sequences.

15. This section is based on data from A. Pascual-Leone, Yeryomenko, et al. (2016).

16. A complete answer to this question requires an exploration of both mediators and moderators. With the intent of better defining when expressive arousal is helpful, this chapter spells out the parameters for therapeutic change (i.e., its moderating conditions). The question of why expressive arousal may cause emotional change at all (i.e., mediating factors) will be explored in chapters that follow (Chapters 9–11).

17. Research on a very large naturalistic sample followed the trajectories of symptom change over the course of brief psychotherapy (Owen et al., 2015). It showed that for a small subset of clients (5.5%), their symptoms effectively do initially get worse,

and they experience deterioration in the first three to four sessions of treatment. This is then followed by a subsequent and relatively rapid alleviation of symptoms, ending the brief treatments by about session 11 with meaningful clinical change. However, one cannot presume that the role of expressive arousal while working with emotion is closely related to clinical symptom distress.

18. Although taking this sweeping observation in isolation is what has led some well-known authors to the gross overgeneralization that emotion regulation ultimately subsumes all forms of emotional processing or working with emotion, which it does not. Examples of emotion regulation are certainly important for healthy functioning, and they can all be thought of as part of emotional processing. However, the inverse is not true: Not all forms of working with emotion can be explained by emotional regulation (and much less its down-regulation, which is typically what regulation is more truly referring to; see Chapter 2).

19. As posited in Chapter 1, meaning making and gradual habituation or inhibition will work at cross-purpose with one another within a single moment, but they are not mutually exclusive and can be coordinated together over time (A. Pascual-Leone, Yeryomenko, et al., 2016).

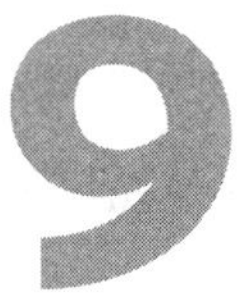

Getting Physical

Working From the Outside In

When you are young, you have the face your parents gave you. After you are 40, you have the face you deserve.

—EDWIN M. STANTON, *RECOLLECTIONS OF PRESIDENT LINCOLN AND HIS ADMINISTRATION*[1]

The heart has its reasons that reason itself doesn't know.

—BLAISE PASCAL, *PENSÉES*

The most general manner by which emotional arousal can facilitate change is that, even when it is ill-defined, physiological and affective stimulation provides a generic impetus, some general activation or bodily action (if not expression), that can subsequently be channeled into the service of emotional change. This chapter explores how generic arousal and outward physical expression can energize tangential emotional meanings. So, working from the outside in, prescribed activation can get captured by personal meaning and then boost emotion.

AROUSAL AS A GENERAL ACTIVATOR OF EMOTION: GETTING CAUGHT UP IN THE MOMENT

Although raw bodily arousal often has an impact on emotion, this specific kind of emotional leverage is not cited very often in theories of psychotherapy. Still, the process will be familiar to readers because it is amply used in advertising

https://doi.org/10.1037/0000460-010
Principles of Emotion Change: What Works and When in Psychotherapy and Everyday Life, by A. Pascual-Leone
Copyright © 2026 by the American Psychological Association. All rights reserved.

and entertainment industries. The reason for overlooking it in psychotherapy theory may be because of its crudeness. Yet, having the experiencer get caught up in the moment is ubiquitous in emotional processing. The roles of borrowed arousal and associative hype underscore the inherent dynamic and overdetermined nature of any emotional experience.

Using physical and emotional arousal as a general activator does little in terms of specificity, but it can create an initial boost in trajectory for the experience of emotion, even if that is yet to be fully shaped. This is about having action before clear direction, it potentiates changes by warming up the emotional engine. Arousal is channeled by the lens through which it is being interpreted, even as it occurs in the moment. (As an aside, narrative reflections occur after the fact and are a separate process; see Chapters 17–22.) So, the effect of arousal is mediated by the meaning one brings to it top down, whether that be a preconceived expectation, a situational cue, or even the visual imagery one assigns to the activation mounting inside. In other words, arousal generally leads one to get caught up in the moment, and that serves as a general activator of change.

Consider, for example, cold water showers or plunges, which have been proposed to potentially bolster mood and well-being. Whether or not this is useful for treating mental health problems, there are certainly biological reasons to expect an impact on the nervous system.[2] Still, immersion in cold water has been explored as an intervention for people with mild depression and anxiety (Shevchuk, 2008; see also Burlingham et al., 2022). A feasibility trial of this showed decreases in psychological symptoms over eight sessions of swimming in cold, open sea water, with most improvements maintained at a 3-month follow-up. However, without a comparison group, symptom changes could be attributable to any number of factors.

In fact, narrative accounts collected from participants offered some insights on what seems useful here. Qualitative analyses identified key themes cited by participants to explain how swimming in cold water benefited their mental health. The three themes were confronting challenges, becoming a community, and appreciating the moment (Burlingham et al., 2022). These themes reach well beyond the temperature of sea water, but they still point to the happening of some vigorous physical event.[3] Activation-based interventions such as this are mainly about generating impetus, starting up some physiological process, which includes finding the courage to act or dive in. Then, the immediate effects of arousal have longer lasting psychological impacts through what are downstream processes. Of course, while the physiological response serves as a catalyst, more is not always better, so explaining the role of arousal as a source of impetus is essential for making the best use of this process.

The Role of Visceral Arousal in Emotional Change

A body of research has examined this process in laboratory experiments. In the most famous of these, social psychologists Schachter and Singer (1962) deceived participants by telling them they were getting a vitamin injection to see how it influenced vision, when in fact those participants were being injected with a shot of adrenalin in their bloodstream or a placebo. Some participants were told the injection could have side effects related to increased arousal, while others were given bogus information about possible headaches and then asked to wait a short while in a room where there was another person. Also unbeknownst to participants, the other person in the waiting room was a confederate working for the researcher who followed a script that involved displays of either frustration and anger or being happy and playful.

This study produced two key findings. First, when participants were given information that allowed them to expect and interpret the physical arousal, it helped explain away that feeling, allowing participants to disregard it, and they were subsequently less impacted by the confederate's behavior. However, for participants who were physiologically aroused without having any known reason for it, they used the cues around them to interpret their emergent feelings as genuine emotion. Second, the study showed that when arousal was chemically induced, body-based experiences differentiated into specific emotions of anger or happiness, depending on what the situational cues around them were (e.g., what a confederate was expressing in the waiting room; Schachter & Singer, 1962).

A large body of literature has since developed on misattribution effects. People have been induced to explain away the naturally occurring arousal of emotional experiences by attributing it to injections, pills, or irritating noises, among other neutral causes. While other research designs have led people to make attributions that reallocate or augment their arousal to existing emotional experiences (Laird & Lacasse, 2014).

The counterpoint to increasing emotional experience by augmenting arousal through some artificial means (e.g., by injecting adrenalin), might be to dampen emotional experience by curtailing the arousal someone feels. One way of doing that is to take beta blockers, which are medications that interfere with adrenaline and arousal. These drugs may be useful for managing situational anxiety, as in a phobia of public speaking. However, the implications of indirectly changing emotion by using arousal-reducing medication is not only an academic issue; it tuns out to have palpable clinical risks. For example, depression is a possible side effect to taking beta blockers. Artificially lowering bodily arousal is associated with more intense feelings of sadness and is implicated in a heightened risk of suicide among those suffering from depression (Sørensen et al., 2001). Generally, reducing physiological cues of arousal will dull emotions that are usually high arousal experiences (e.g., fear). However, for emotions such as sadness, that typically already are low arousal experiences, further reducing arousal augments the feeling (Laird & Lacasse, 2014).

The basic premise of this idea, about the attribution of arousal (or lack thereof), has been studied in several ways. First, as discussed earlier, studies have used chemical stimulation (or suppression) of visceral experiences. That approach offers a test with good internal validity, but the invasiveness is fairly removed from what happens in psychotherapy. Second, the attribution of arousal has also been studied using evocative situations. An often-cited research example of this is a hypothesis about men walking over a rickety narrow bridge, which is anxiety provoking, who are then likely to misattribute their generally nervous arousal as a physical attraction toward a female stranger (Dutton & Aron, 1974). Although findings like these are not always easily replicated, the contextual and incidental factors are numerous, and a large body of evidence generally supports formulations of this kind (Laird & Lacasse, 2014).

Third, the findings most relevant to clinical intervention are from research studies that manipulate endogenously generated physical arousal in ways that influenced emotional feelings. This brings the issue of pure arousal as a generator of emotion closer to the practice of psychotherapy. One example of this is a study where young men vigorously ran on the spot and then, after the exercise, were shown a video of an attractive female confederate. When researchers minimized the salience of exercise as such but increased the salience of the female confederate (by creating the expectation of meeting her after the video), participants were most likely to misattribute their physical arousal. Under these circumstances, arousal generated through bodily exertion was construed as romantic attraction toward the woman in the video (White & Kight, 1984).

Overall, the evidence shows that visceral arousal can be an initiator of emotional feeling, although manipulating arousal does not seem to affect all emotions equally. When arousal is boosted by some other means, it is more likely to potentiate emotions characterized by high physiological activation such as fear, anger, and romantic attraction. So, sadness and other emotions characterized by low physiological activation are not expected to be affected as dramatically, in that manipulating arousal is not likely to generate more intense feelings of sadness (Laird & Lacasse, 2014). Even so, the experience of physical exertion can also have some affinity to emotional vulnerability. For example, I have had two separate clients (one male, one female) who anecdotally reported that during periods of significant romantic loss or divorce, each had trouble with spontaneously breaking down into tears when in the middle of a morning jog or at the most intense part of an otherwise routine workout. When they were already feeling emotional, vulnerable, and thin skinned, the physical arousal and sense of strain during exercise created an experiential configuration that overdetermined and then potentiated the activation of grief, which was present but otherwise subdominant until arousal was added.

Activating visceral arousal is obviously more of a global process compared with strategically activating specific brain regions. However, the fact that emotional change can be precipitated by an otherwise unrelated increase to someone's basic biological arousal, is also consistent with the observation that mood disorders can be alleviated by applying exogenous stimulation to the brain. To that end, various forms of noninvasive brain stimulation have now been used as neurological treatments for major depression. Interventions like these introduce either an electrical current or magnetic stimulation to correct pathologically low levels of brain activity among depressed patients (Brunoni et al., 2016; Perera et al., 2016).[4] Other applications of transcranial magnetic stimulation suggest that, in theory, one could probably also induce depression by suppressing neural activity. This parallel line of research converges with the notion that thematically unrelated sources of activation are generally assimilated into and bolster one's final overall emotional experience. Bridging these two fields, other research has shown the carryover effect that anger can have on one's default neural functioning (Gilam et al., 2017). When Israeli infantry soldiers participated in an experiment that led them to feel angry over being unfairly treated, the resting state of their brains during the aftermath of that experience revealed an enduring impact on their endogenous neural activity. Critically, the carryover effect of soldiers' lingering anger in that scenario predicted their maladaptive recovery from traumatic stress a year later, after their combat training.

Harnessing Arousal: Building It Up or Explaining It Away

A convergence of factors is needed, but the point of interest for mechanisms of change is that arousal can be channeled into the differentiation of more specific emotional experiences. As very early research on the use of adrenalin already pointed out, "The lack of any object or reason for the emotion usually deprives it of its genuineness" (Cantril & Hunt, 1932, p. 302). This is because genuine emotion is always some response to the environment, whether that psychological environment may be external or internal. One is angry at, afraid of, or sad about something. Emotion takes an object. In the words of American philosopher and pioneer of psychology James Mark Baldwin (1891), "Strong emotions spread themselves out over the whole content of consciousness" (p. 254). The clinical implication is that if one can stoke physiological arousal, it opens a window of opportunity, and given the right circumstances, that flash of arousal could be harnessed to facilitate some more deliberate change in emotion. There are two sides to this, additive and subtractive, and both are relevant to changing emotion.

Building Up the Feeling: An Additive Process

On one hand, physiological arousal can increase affective feeling when it is attributed to stemming from what is perceived as an emotionally evocative situation. This augmentation of emotion occurs by recruiting extraneous arousal into the overall experience, even if it may not otherwise be psychogenetically related (at least not at first). The finding of participants who came to feel either angry or happy in Schacter and Singer's (1962) study are prime examples of this additive process, where arousal plus the appropriate cues can incite and generate an initial trajectory for emotional feeling. Feeling hangry (i.e., hungry + angry) is an everyday example of that process. Experiments on psychological mechanisms suggest people only conceptualize their hunger as emotional when an unpleasant context cues them into negative affect (MacCormack & Lindquist, 2019).

Explaining Away the Feeling: A Subtractive Process

On the other hand, however, when people have a reasonable explanation for what they feel in their body as being unrelated to emotion, it will often explain away the emotional nature of that experience. This is the subtractive process, such that the feelings of physiological arousal which may indeed have been justified as an endogenous part of emotion are now suspended from and no longer support the moment-by-moment formulation of what might have been one's emergent emotional experience. The other participants in Schacter and Singer's study, who had been told to expect some bodily arousal, received a sensible explanation for understanding it, and they were consequently unaffected by the confederate's antics. This example illustrates the subtractive process. In other words, arousal that is incidental and unrelated, per se, can be explained away, which ensures it will not interfere with one's genuine flow of experience (i.e., Schacter and Singer's participants who were in the know). So, a reasonable explanation helps one to bracket out the contribution of arousal.

However, notice that the subtractive process holds, irrespective of whether the feeling of arousal is or is not indeed related to an emerging emotion. That means when arousal is directly and genuinely related to an emerging emotion, that (real) emotional feeling can be diminished or undermined by some ruse of what appears to be a compelling explanation. The proposed explanation, in fact, is a red herring that undermines endogenous emotional feeling. This helps explain why 25% of patients who repeatedly show up in hospital emergency rooms with chest pain as their chief symptom are apparently unaware that they are suffering from panic attacks (Fleet et al., 2003). These individuals misconstrue their sudden psychophysical experience of anxiety as a major adverse cardiac event. This initial physical explanation (i.e., that it's a heart attack) is so compelling that it fully eclipses any consideration that the sensations may be emotional in nature. This is a clinical example of the subtractive process. An example in everyday life might be erroneously disregarding the cautionary uneasiness of one's gut feeling, when in fact it was information described in Damasio's (1999) somatic marker theory. Consider this example: "It feels like I'm nervous about making this business deal, but I'm sure it's just the espresso, I don't usually have that much"—when, actually, there is real cause for concern!

Overdetermining Emotion: The Sum of All Influences

Even more subtle than the clear-cut additive or subtractive processes described here, one can assume that in everyday life there is a veritable scrimmage of this kind of process among a whole host of emergent emotions. After all, a newly emerging emotion is often an (implicitly) reasonable explanation for the arousal initially generated by some other emotional state, activated just moments before. In this way, the ebb and flow of qualitatively different feelings and embodied actions can either borrow activation, merge with, derail, or entirely displace some earlier presenting emotion. In short, arousal through subcortical activation will boost the activation of all applicable emotion schemes. This means one source of arousal can laterally activate other expressions and experiences of emotion, such that the final expression, and experience of emotion itself, is overdetermined (as defined in Chapter 1; J. Pascual-Leone & Johnson, 2021). The spreading of activation is also described in the application of dynamic systems theory to psychotherapy (Gelo & Salvatore, 2016).

Everyday examples of this overdetermination abound, particularly when arousal derails and makes a process unproductive, often resulting in undifferentiated anger or aggression. Imagine a bicycle courier on a tight deadline, exerting themself physically, sweating hard, and enjoying the rush of a fast ride. However, when they are cut off by a careless taxi driver, they abruptly flare up with uncontrollable road rage. The outrage may be justified (or not), but it is fueled by the preexisting physiological arousal that they bring to the moment, exactly as described in studies on the misattribution of arousal (e.g., White & Kight, 1984).

In another example, rocking a baby back and forth to sleep may become dangerously vigorous when a parent, who is also exhausted, inadvertently expresses their frustration through what started as an attempt to soothe the crying baby. It is no coincidence that shaken baby syndrome is a prevalent form of abuse suffered by infants, who first called their parents for physical soothing. Here, the behavioral act of soothing a baby—by rocking back and forth—is physically similar enough that it can become magnified and distorted to subsequently produce an expression of aggression (through increased arousal and an overdetermination of schemes; J. Pascual-Leone & Johnson, 2021). This is a dark but incisive illustration of how dynamic emotional changes occur when underlying emotion (e.g., a parent's frustration) is laterally activated, and then it hijacks the trajectory of some other impetus (e.g., the initial intention to physically soothe). Finally, the confluences that can occur in adults between sexual arousal and physical pain or violence are still other examples of this process (Doidge, 2007).

Adverse life experiences and personality pathologies are likely moderating factors, increasing the likelihood that potential activation of any number of other emotional states is redirected or shunted off to potentiate one specific kind of emotional experience. For example, children who have experienced trauma have an attentional bias and heightened sensitivity to the perception of threat-related stimuli when compared with children who have suffered less adversity (Pollak & Sinha, 2002). Furthermore, traumatized children are more likely to misclassify negative or even neutral emotions as specifically anger (McLaughlin et al., 2020). Similarly, adults suffering borderline personality disorder have more intense baseline experiences of sadness, fear, disgust, and shame compared with healthy controls. However, shame is the only feeling for which these individuals are more emotionally reactive than controls (Di Bartolomeo et al., 2022). The intensity and reactivity together mean that feelings of shame, in particular, become a gateway that catalyzes the emotional volatility associated with borderline personality disorder.

Fortunately, the spread or migration of emotional activation can equally serve the creation of healthy developments. Classic psychoanalytic perspectives often formulated this as a client discovering the underlying meaning of their arousal (Freud & Breuer, 1895). A more constructivist perspective would describe this as the differentiation and creation of newly embodied meaning from an otherwise unformulated experience (A. Pascual-Leone & Greenberg, 2007a; D. B. Stern, 1997). In a healthy shift, what was initially a largely unrelated source of arousal can be laterally recruited to help resolve a more figural and target emotional concern. When the aroused (but relatively undifferentiated) feeling gets applied in this way, it is quickly channeled to a more specific and salient embodiment of personal meaning.

In an ingenious study, researchers yoked two groups of participants together, both of whom had suffered comparable traumas (M. A. Greenberg et al., 1996). While one group was asked to write expressively about their own experience of trauma (i.e., a classic expressive writing task), the other group was asked instead to write about some fictional accounts of trauma that was not their own experience (using content from the first group). Both groups enjoyed similar positive changes that were greater than those of a control, even though the second group had never addressed their own narrative content. As the researchers pointed out, this suggests personal content, per se, may not be as important as suggested by the context-bound theories of cognitive processing or behavioral exposure. An alternative explanation, however, is that the expressive activation of similar enough distress accounts for these health benefits of expressive writing, precisely because arousal spreads to the tacit activation of more personally relevant content, even if that is only implicit.

Individual Differences: Which Cues Are Most Salient to Whom?

Although research on the misattribution of arousal has focused on the salience of social and other external cues influencing this reassignment of arousal, in psychotherapy the internal context of meaning (e.g., the themes one is feeling and thinking about in the moment) will often be the most salient cue in the (re)attribution of arousal. In therapy and in everyday life, most people are not likely to be duped into grossly misunderstanding their genuine experience, although a radical social constructivist perspective would disagree. In her book, psychologist Feldman-Barrett (2017) gives an intriguing personal example of developing flu symptoms and feeling warm while on a date with someone who she was initially not too interested in but then misattributed those sensations as an unexpected romantic attraction to her date. This is the scale of misattribution that Schacter and Singer's (1962) participants experienced, although they were being deceived by design. In everyday life, the emotional awareness someone brings to a task will also be relevant, as one disentangles different sources of information about different kinds of feelings.[5] Nevertheless, beyond the additional clarity that should come from emotional awareness as a synergistic process, there is reason to believe that individual differences in one's cognitive processing style also play an important role here.

Research suggests that whereas some people may be more responsive to having their emotional experience influenced through situational cues (e.g., contextual cues, social pressures, sociocultural scripts), other people are not as responsive and instead are more likely to be influenced by cues observed in their own bodily expression (e.g., the self-perception of one's facial expressions, movement, expressive action; Laird & Berglas, 1975; Laird & Lacasse, 2014). This has implications for the applicability of how one might leverage either arousal or expressive processes to facilitate emotional change. (The impact of dispassionately taking on expressive actions to then assume some congruent emotion is discussed in a later section.) Whatever the case, the process discussed in this section of general arousal being ascribed to some situational context to influence emotional feeling is probably a significant part of the confusing and very slippery nature of working with emotion, both in psychotherapy and everyday life. Even so, treatments can capitalize on the role of more generic arousal to launch clients into the meaningful engagement of more targeted and difficult emotional states.

Harnessing Arousal in Clinical Work

While experimental research offers solid support for this specific way of changing emotion, it is not usually openly recognized in theories of psychotherapy. Nevertheless, this process has often been folded into the rituals, interventions, and target processes used to promote therapeutic change. In more ancient times, psychological treatments primed people with fantastic talks and elaborate staging:

> Shamans and folk healers typically began their healing ceremonies by performing feats of magic to demonstrate their power, heighten expectancies of success, and generate an emotionally charged atmosphere. Once primed, emotional arousal was enhanced by drum beating, chanting, shrieking, and convulsive dancing. (Nichols & Efran, 1985, p. 47)

These ancient practices have been woven into popular culture to heighten arousal and generate an emotional experience, often for entertainment (e.g., in live shows, or just when throwing a great party!). However, the critical issue here is that these strategies were used for the purposes of health care by facilitating some target psychospiritual change. Moreover, the fundamental mechanism remains pertinent to contemporary treatments, especially when interventions put a premium on the client having a certain kind of emotional experience within the session.

Using Psychedelics to Work With Emotion

The ancient tools for stoking both perceptual and emotional arousal sometimes involved administering psychedelic drugs as part of a spiritual healing process, often in the form of a sacrament. That practice has endured to this day: Research on psychedelic drugs in the treatment of mental health problems—including psychological trauma, depression, end-of-life issues, as well as addictions—has recently become the focus of renewed attention (M. W. Johnson et al., 2019). To those that look on psychedelic drug-assisted therapy with apprehension, consider that serving alcohol at a party essentially produces a substance-assisted social encounter. In that familiar setting, the synergy between chemical effects and emotional processes will seem less foreign, although the mechanisms here seem to go beyond lowering someone's inhibition.

After having been abandoned in the 1970s, psychedelic research is still very much in its infancy. Even so, mystical experiences occasioned by psychedelic drug use are associated with improved psychological outcomes in volunteers from both healthy and psychiatric populations. One of the proposed biological mechanisms for this effect is the drugs' broad facilitation of emotional arousal during a state of reduced defensiveness (M. W. Johnson et al., 2019). Particularly related to psychedelic treatments for depression, preliminary evidence suggests these drugs boost endogenous activity in the default network and limbic systems, increasing the likelihood that people enter introspectively emotional states (Kubiru et al., 2022). Thus, the role of psychedelics as an agent probably occurs either synergistically with or in potentiating the basic mechanisms of emotional processes known to psychotherapy research and as described in this book. Nevertheless, drug-induced experiences remain a very blunt instrument, and what happens during the experience or the way arousal is subsequently channeled remains a critical process.[6]

Leveraging Arousal in Psychotherapy Sessions: The Springboard Effect

There is some early research on psychotherapy that specifically explores the role of induced arousal in psychotherapy. For example, when persuasive communications were used in the session, clients remained resistant to changing certain maladaptive attitudes. However, when clients were first pharmacologically induced to experience heightened arousal, they were more likely to make attitudinal changes following the same in-session persuasions (Hoehn-Saric et al., 1972, 1974). Psychotherapy does not usually involve outside stimulation or agents (e.g., drugs, exogenous brain stimulation, confederates). However, it certainly involves natural moments of intense emotion, and these too can act like springboards. One emotion can be used to decisively boost the intensity of an affective experience that immediately follows. Sometimes this leverage of arousal occurs in psychotherapy through dynamic two-step sequences of emotion (see Chapter 13). At other times, it represents a critical window of opportunity. An example with practical implications for psychotherapy comes from an observational study on single session interventions. Although clients often are at a loss for words and have trouble articulating what they most deeply want, a quasi-experimental design suggested the optimal time for therapists to help their clients identify unmet needs is immediately after that client expresses a moderate increase in emotional arousal (Nardone et al., 2022).

Habib Davanloo, a psychiatrist at McGill University, developed intensive short-term psychodynamic therapy (ISTDP), which is known as an intense and emotionally evocative treatment approach (2005). A central effort in the approach is something Davanloo called "unlocking the unconscious." It prescriptively will involve an intense experience of murderous rage[7] that often is first directed at the therapist and then an attachment figure from the past, followed by strong feelings of guilt and grief over attachment injuries and loss (Abbass & Town, 2013). Pressuring and confrontation by a therapist are key and effective interventions for initiating this sequence (Town et al., 2011). The unrelenting persistence that characterizes the intervention style of therapists using this approach can often be an adverse experience and will activate the deeper maladaptive emotion that therapy intends to work through. So, at this juncture, there is an equifinality among the various causal forces precipitating emotional arousal in a general sense. The only critical issue is that therapists continue to focus on attending to a client's internal emotional experience, rather than allowing any deflection to external narratives or acting out behaviorally.

Arguably, if emotion is mobilized, it can be subsequently leveraged, as the arousal will be attributed to the attractor of underlying meaning. My formulation of what happens here is as follows: When this kind of faceoff arouses rageful anger in the client, that reaction also produces lateral activation, catapulting the client into energizing other emotions that are proximally related by theme, such as grief. Particularly, if grief is also the therapist's next prescribed target of intervention, the first activation of emotion precipitates a second and more critical emotional experience (e.g., rage followed by guilt about that rage, which is ultimately followed by grief over the deeper losses that initially triggered one's rage). It is the psychogenic proximity between certain emotion schemes which makes them more easily conflated, switched, or cascaded together like a line of dominos in expressive arousal. The key clinical interest with respect to activating emotion is that rage is more easily and directly engaged by the confrontational strategies used in ISTDP. Then, once murderous rage is freely and fully expressed, it potentiates arousal while clients are also searching for meaning, and entering with this tailwind are the deeply painful feelings of attachment-related grief. If grief is to be explored as a pivot for change, then experiencing rageful anger can serve as the point of entry through a client's defensiveness to the experience of more vulnerable feelings. It is probably not coincidental that clients with somatization turn out to be particularly well treated using ISTDP (e.g., Abbass et al., 2017). Research on other approaches (e.g., Brauninger, 2014) has similarly converged on the idea that working with expressive arousal is an especially helpful process for such clients.

Experimental findings on sequences of emotion within single sessions based on emotion-focused therapy support this interpretation of how arousal may be carried forward from one emotion to the next. Diamond and Rochman (2008) recruited participants who reported feeling angry at someone and asked them to first express their anger toward the imagined person and then, second, to follow with expressions of their sadness. Finger temperature was recorded as a measure of the nervous system's sympathetic activation and showed that arousal during the initial expression of anger carried over to a participant's heightened experience of grief during the second half of the intervention.

Moreover, expressing anger first offered more benefit compared with when the reverse sequence was used.

A follow-up experiment by another group confirmed that the second emotion (in this case grief) seems to be potentiated by arousal from a previous and more easily activated emotion (e.g., when the resentful person was first invited to express their anger; Nardone et al., 2025). However, the later study also clarified that anger is not always the potentiator of sadness. Sometimes it works the other way around because these findings also interacted with a person's presenting disposition—one emotion borrowing arousal from the other depending on the circumstances (Nardone et al., 2025). This means the springboard effect of expressive arousal probably works synergistically with another process I discuss later called a sequential transformation (see Chapters 12–16). Nonetheless, in what is essentially the spreading of neural activation, a given impulse of feelings can be used to boost or energize some subsequent experience, and that is a subtle form of emotional change.

EXPRESSION CAN GENERATE EXPERIENCE: START WITH ACTION AND THEN BRING IT IN

Sometimes expressiveness itself, even if done dispassionately, will stimulate the emergence of emotion. This process starts with commitment to action, rather than starting with genuine feeling, affective impulse, or deeper meaning. At first it may even be prescribed as a hollow or half-hearted action, but the experience of doing it hooks the involvement of some inner workings. When this happens, physical engagement leads to emotional engagement.

Peripheral Theory of Emotion

Emotion is reflected in the expressive actions of a person's face, posture, and voice, and that directionality is the way emotional experience is commonly thought of. Consistent with this, the brain regions involved in decisions about our affective values and needs, also influence our motor control. However, there is good evidence that the reverse is also true. The neurobiological basis of someone's physical movements covertly shapes the subsequent valuation and decisions about their affective preferences and needs (Shadmehr & Ahmed, 2020). What remains unclear are the conditions under which this opposing direction of influence is most impactful (i.e., the timing, to what extent, and under what circumstances).

In working with emotion, the kinesthetic cues aroused in movement and freeing up the voice evoke a host of preverbal associations. In some sense, loosening up physically helps loosen up emotionally and can even prime certain facets of emotional experience. So, at times, expressive action can be deliberately chosen as an intervention, and this serves as an experiment in inciting and generating internal experience. Of course, this potentially bidirectional role of expressiveness presumes that the behavioral expression one chooses is not too incongruent with any existing internal experience. By the same token, the effect can be significant when an outward behavioral expression turns out to be a good match for one's internal affective configuration, which may have been dormant and awaiting possible activation. Under the right circumstances, action leads to feeling and then feeling creates genuine momentum.

The idea that feeling is partly a byproduct of doing is one of the oldest theories of emotion in psychology. William James, a pioneer of psychology as a discipline, essentially theorized that emotional experience is created by the perception of gross and autonomic bodily adjustments. This has sometimes been appropriately referred to as a peripheral theory of emotion, and he sketches examples of this when he says we feel "angry *because* we strike, afraid *because* we tremble" (James, 1890, p. 449, italics in original). Clearly, behavioral expressions (e.g., crying) and facial expressions (e.g., furrowed brow) contribute to the actual experiencing of emotion.

James also believed different emotions were the result of particular and different physiological signatures of the visceral, but that has never held up empirically.[8] Emotion is made up of more than its physiology, although the body is what gives emotion its inertia. In a relevant case example, I provided psychotherapy to a migrant agricultural worker who had been paralyzed from the torso down when his bicycle had been struck from behind by a pickup truck on the highway. He visited me in a motorized wheelchair, and we held sessions in his native Spanish. He came from an emotionally expressive culture, had easy and nondefensive access to his feelings, and was sometimes tearful in our sessions. However, I was struck by how his expressiveness was always fleeting and returned to baseline in an unusually rapid period of time. He described himself as "always a doer and a feeler in life, not the conceptual type, that's not my thing." Yet despite my evocative and emotion-focused interventions, the most productive processes in our work were the highly reflective ones. The most meaningful work was his coming to grips with his change in identity from an able-bodied and highly physical laborer, the provider for his family.

Perhaps this is what working with emotion in therapy is like when the client does not have full access to feedback from their body and its expression of emotion. My speculation is consistent with research findings: "Individuals with [spinal column injuries] experience a blunting of affect, possibly due to attenuated feedback from the autonomic nervous system" (Salter et al., 2013, p. 255). Whatever the case, the original ideas from James about behavioral and facial expressiveness are still relevant today.

The Effect of Peripheral Expressiveness on Emotion

A recent review of research evidence on William James's theory that bodily behavior influences one's emotion concluded that "the basic notion that emotional feelings are [in part] consequences of expressions and autonomic responses has been supported over and over" (Laird & Lacasse, 2014, p. 31). Posed facial expression has also been found to activate internal emotion, which has been dubbed the facial feedback hypothesis. In a now-classic study, participants were asked to rate how amusing cartoons were while either holding a pen between their teeth (i.e., in what resembles a smile) or while pursing their lips onto the end of the pen (i.e. in what resembles pouting frown). While the purpose of the experiment was masked, those who were incidentally using the smiling facial position rated cartoons as funnier than those who inadvertently expressed the pouting frown (Strack et al., 1988; see also Noah et al., 2018).

As a counterpoint, participants who are instructed to refrain from moving their face report less emotional arousal than participants who were free to move their faces (J. I. Davis et al., 2009). When participants were given Botox injections (i.e., botulinum toxin to paralyze muscles of facial expression), it produced a similar muting of emotional feeling when the evocative video clips used as stimuli were mildly positive or negative. However, no muting was found when the stimuli were highly evocative of emotion, indicating that an internal experience that is burgeoning forth will override restrictions on expression that might otherwise constrain emotional experience (J. I. Davis et al., 2010).[9]

A large amount of research has been conducted to date that supports the facial feedback hypothesis. In short, making facial expressions increases emotion, whereas preventing expressions can reduce those feelings. This can have clinical implications. For instance, a meta-analysis suggested Botox may have a large impact in reducing symptoms of depression, although the trials were fraught with bias, and there is reason to be skeptical (Coles et al., 2019). For working with emotion in psychotherapy and everyday life, one of the most direct implementations is to incorporate behavioral changes to one's expression to influence the emotion one feels. In dialectical behavior therapy, for example, clients are instructed on the skill of wearing a very subtle Mona Lisa half-smile to help them begin to negotiate emotional distress (Linehan, 2015). The idea that one can make purposeful choices in expression and that emotional tone might follow is something also suggested by the first epigraph to this chapter.

Going further, posture and expressive actions also modulate emotion. A body of research shows that when people slump in their posture, they start to feel sadder, but when they sit upright, it increases their pride, while leaning back and raising one's hand as if to protect one's face heightens feelings of fear, and standing erect with fists clenched bolsters feelings of anger or disgust (Laird & Lacasse, 2014). In a randomized experiment, participants were assigned to adopt either a slumped or upright posture in advance of a stressful speech task (Nair et al., 2015). Participants who were asked to assume a slumped posture quickly reported less positive affect and that abatement lingered even after participants gave their speech. They also reported highly aroused negative affect that persisted after the speech task. In studies that look beyond self-reports, the effects of physical expression have also been typically found to have behavioral impacts on people's performance. In this study, posture also had a large effect on the content participants generated during their speech: Relative to those holding an upright posture, people in a slumped posture also used more negative emotion words, especially more sadness words, and fewer positive emotion words. The impact of postural effects has also been examined in psychiatric populations with similar results. When depressed participants sat in a slumped position to do a memory task, they recalled more negative words than positive words from a list, while those who sat upright recalled relatively equal numbers of positive and negative words (Michalak et al., 2014).

Considering more dynamic physical expressions, an unobtrusive biofeedback technique can be used to manipulate participants into walking in a manner that was either characteristic of depressed clients or was a particularly happy walking style (Michalak et al., 2015). Participants who were shaped into walking in a happy way recalled a higher proportion of positive self-relevant material, while walking like a person with depression produced a negative memory bias. Other research shows convergent findings for the manipulation of respiratory patterns or vocally expressive sounds, where participants experienced affective shifts that subsequently made emotion congruent with the implemented expressions (Hatfield et al., 2002).

In a study that looked at separate and combined effects of facial expression and bodily posture, arousal for the corresponding emotion (e.g., fear, sadness, anger) was higher when both methods were implemented simultaneously and when they were congruent with the same emotional expression. Mixed emotional expressions were typically less arousing (Flack et al., 1999). This speaks to the additive effect of physical forms of expressions in face, posture, gait, voice, breath, and so on. It also highlights the importance of their overall coherence if one seeks to spark up a specific emotional feeling. When it comes to the role of physical expression in generating an emotional experience, if it looks like a given emotion, walks like that emotion, and sounds like that emotion, then if it is not already, it may very well turn into that emotion.

Fake It Till You Make It: Expression With the Intention to Feel Different

James's peripheral theory of emotion posits that expression evokes feeling, and under certain circumstances, the research supports this. The clinical implication is one can start with action and then somehow bring it in. But how does that internalization happen? Part of the explanation may be that basic directional actions of moving oneself forward can activate the approach motivational system, whereas pulling backward activates withdraw or inhibition by the avoidance system.[10] For example, one study found repeated flexions of the arm, as if to bring things closer, essentially led men (but not women) to report more approach and fun-seeking motivations (Haeffel, 2011). In contrast, quite literally taking a step backward is a physical behavior that seems to have a large effect in enhancing cognitive control and inhibition (Koch et al., 2009). While intriguing, this line of inquiry becomes increasingly meaningful to clinical work when it is situated in an individual's more personal and narrative context. When research participants were encouraged to tightly clench their fists while recounting an angering event, they reported stronger subjective experiences of anger. In contrast, when participants did the same fist clenching while reporting a sad event, they felt less sadness (Berkowitz, 2000).

While some of the experimental findings may seem contrived, there are numerous examples of this being applied in every life. For example, the short battle scream used in martial arts when making an attack (e.g., "Hi-yah!") is a technique called *kiai* in Japanese. Fighters are explicitly taught to use high piercing sounds to startle and strike fear into their adversary. At the same time, low guttural sounds are also used to muster one's courage and sense of strength to deliberately self-induce emotional change. In Korean, this concept is known as *k'ihap*, which literally means "to amplify one's energy." It is essentially a technique for facilitating emotion and one with immediate practical application. For similar reasons related to their impact, treatment interventions from various psychotherapy approaches will directly or indirectly organize a client's physicality or vocalizations to facilitate emotion (e.g., a therapist saying, "Say it louder" or "Try putting your feet down on the floor").

Perhaps unsurprisingly, the observation that emotion can be targeted and evoked through physical movement has been a longstanding technique of contemporary acting.[11] If a scene requires an actor to weep, they might initiate this affective process by performing congruent physical actions, such as taking a deep sigh or holding their head in their hands (S. Moore, 1984). As cited before, the essence of this way of working with emotion has stood up well to the experimental scrutiny of basic research. However, an experiment on the biological correlates of manipulating expressive arousal has further shown that one can raise one's testosterone levels simply by acting aggressively (Van Anders et al., 2015). The study demonstrated that when female trained actors were instructed to act angry following a script that highlighted experiences of competition and wielding power over others, it boosted their testosterone levels as compared with those in a control task. In short, under certain circumstances just behaving differently can modulate hormones related to mood, fostering the generation of a robust change in emotional experience. The implications for intervention in psychotherapy is that expressive enactments can indeed engender real biologically anchored emotional experiences.

When Does Faking It Work, and for Whom?

An elderly client of mine was coping with grief over the loss of her husband. One day between sessions, she abruptly decided she would start to dress up more, wear makeup, and make a conscious effort to smile at others. When I asked about these behavioral changes despite her very deep sadness, she reflected, "Maybe sometimes it doesn't matter how you feel, it just matters how you look and act, and the rest will catch up." This fake-it-till-you-make-it approach worked for my client in getting through her uncomplicated grief, but it will not be so in all cases. The degree to which one can adopt a new emotional experience by way of staging its expression will very much have to do with, firstly, its congruence (or incongruence) with other emotions and the affective predispositions that are in one's field of immediate experience. Secondly, the success of this strategy will be related to individual differences in the internal versus external frame of perceptual reference one typically uses.

Unlike in the research laboratory, psychotherapy is a dynamic context of emotional upheavals and change. Generating emotional experience through outward expression depends on the readiness and personal framework of intentions that a client brings to the task at hand. It may work to the degree that the intended direction is not dramatically incompatible with one's presenting experience. To use a commonly misunderstood example, relying on expressive behavior alone to bolster assertiveness assumes there are no substantial incongruencies with a client's internal affective disposition, which of course there would be, particularly if assertiveness was a treatment goal. So, to facilitate emotion through expressive action, the target emotion will only be achievable if it has some proximity to the presenting set of emotions.

The other side of this is that if the prescribed expression one is experimenting with turns out to be highly compatible with one's dormant internal experience, then the outward physical expression will quickly hook into real emotion, lighting the process aflame. Recall that counter to theories of catharsis, letting loose and venting one's rage does not reduce those feelings but rather such expressiveness further increases one's anger (Bushman, 2002). There is a powerful reciprocal relationship between expression and feeling, each feeding the other so long as there is some suitable level of congruence or compatibility. Generally, expressing emotion that is close enough or within the field of attraction will rapidly recruit one's internal process. In short, if you have it in you, then pretending to feel quickly becomes feeling it. The generation of emotional feeling is a complex, dynamic, and multidetermined process that can sometimes also gather momentum. In everyday experiences, the bidirectionality between emotion and expression can be quite subtle and is ubiquitously present when working with emotion in therapy. This is particularly the case when clients test out and try different words or expressions to symbolize the tendrils of their hereto unformulated experience. The domino effect that can ensue has to do with the way psychological schemes are dynamically and spontaneously applied in interacting with the external and internal environments.

Second, although timing and the presenting landscape of emotion is a critical issue, so too are individual differences in how someone typically construes emotion. Ultimately, this is a well-established aspect of information processing styles. In the perception of oneself in the world, some people primarily rely on an internal frame of reference, while others rely on an external frame of reference (Witkin & Goodenough, 1977). There is some evidence that most of the effect found in studies that manipulate emotion through physical expression is attributable to a subgroup of participants, whereas other participants were largely unaffected. Similarly, the emotional response individuals had in response to holding a certain facial expression was also found to be consistent over time and across kinds of emotional expressions (Laird & Lacasse, 2014). These people, for whom the facial feedback hypothesis did not seem to apply and who were generally unresponsive to manipulations in expressiveness, were also less likely to experience cognitive dissonance when asked to perform behaviors that were at odds with their personal attitudes (Laird & Berglas, 1975). Such observations point to an individual difference, wherein certain people are more responsive to having their internal emotional experience swayed by performing an outward physical action, posture, or facial expression. Meanwhile, those who are less responsive to such cues may well be primarily influenced by situational cues in the external environment when interpreting their feelings (Laird & Berglas, 1975; Laird & Lacasse, 2014). In other words, while those who use an internal frame of reference may be more influenced emotionally by physically enacting certain expressions, others using an external frame of reference may be more influenced by the contextual cues (e.g., as described by Schacter and Singer, 1962). By hook or by crook, these entry points to generating a change in emotion via arousal and expressiveness are each important and unique mechanisms.

In summary, under certain conditions some people can consciously make a choice to change emotion using deliberate expression. Motor expression can be used to intensify congruent emotion or to dampen incongruent emotional experiences. In other words, fake it till you make it probably will not work if one pretends to have a feeling that simply is not there. However, most experiences are complex and layered, so if even a small part of the experience fits with what is being faked, then the bodily performance could energize it and make it more present. These findings are important for facilitating emotion in psychotherapy. They also mean that if people stoically pretend they are not feeling something (e.g., keeping a stiff upper lip), it may suppress or mute their emotional experience (Berkowitz, 2000; Perls, 1969).

EXPRESSIVE AROUSAL INCREASES AWARENESS: TURNING UP THE VOLUME

If the early steps of emotional awareness are about detecting what is there (i.e., get in touch and notice the feeling; Chapters 4–6), then the bigger and louder an experience, the easier it becomes to detect (up to some limit, of course). Furthermore, while an emotional experience can vary in intensity, expressiveness is subject to some personal control. In this way, expressive arousal can be used purposefully as an amplifier to boost the otherwise tacit signal of emotional meaning. Increasing the volume helps an emotion ring out more clearly.

Embodied Meaning

The expression of arousal occurs largely through nonverbal communication, which can be a rich source of information both diagnostically and in the process of therapy. Often, the preverbal meanings conveyed through a gesture or tone of voice are only on the periphery of one's awareness. What remains tacit is difficult to grasp until it is increasingly concretized through expression, first by exaggerating that gesture, and then by translating it into the right words. This means increasing arousal and spontaneous expression can be leveraged to magnify implicit meaning. The initial expression of emotion is often regarded as a form of getting in touch with one's feelings, an emerging awareness as might occur in expressive arts (Gendlin, 1996). The role of spontaneity is key because arousal also drives action, which then not only reveals but also precipitates some unfolding meaning. The first part of this is that the covert meaning needs to be made salient enough for one to hear it. Simply put, it is easier to explore and make sense of emotion when it is blatantly aroused. The second part, which seamlessly follows, is that expressing more also often means feeling more—more intensity but also more range in one's feelings. From an experiential perspective, the goal of evoking and exploring affect is to eventually arrive at the deepest level of core primary emotion.

It is also important to recognize that we are not only living beings, but we are also living doings. The role of the body and action in emotional experience is a primordial one that runs deeper than conceptual or verbal elaborations. From this perspective, action itself is an important key in creating, identifying, and symbolizing meaning (not only expressing it). In Darwin's (1872) classic work entitled *The Expression of the Emotions in Man and Animals*, he observed that readying oneself for some physiological action is the primary function of emotional expression.[12] Thus, the practical meaning (the praxis) is literally embodied in the expression. This also means that although it is usually only the beginning, expressing is acting (Nichols & Efran, 1985).

All of this is about the formulation of meaning that precedes and is not initially available to logical, verbal awareness. For example, the neuroscience of movement and decision making shows that the vigor with which we move our limbs and eyes is linked to both the value we assign to stimuli as well as the ongoing formulation of our goals. This points to a coconstruction in the brain between actions and affective preferences, in which decision making essentially includes a sensorimotor process. This has even led some neuroscientists to suggest that physical vigor might be used as a proxy for measuring someone's implicit affective state (Shadmehr & Ahmed, 2020). As in the second epigraph from Blaise Pascal, "The heart has its reasons that reason itself doesn't know." This observation is particularly incisive given that it comes from a mathematician over 300 years ago. Nevertheless, the philosophical adage anticipates Damasio's (1999) somatic marker theory that bodily reactions reveal aspects of affective experience that are occurring outside one's awareness.

Working With the Body

Wilhelm Reich, a psychoanalyst and former student of Freud, proposed a somatic theory of psychopathology premised on the notion of a body-based life force that he believed in. Furthermore, he argued that people engage in habitual, somatic response patterns in an effort to regulate emotion. These rigid ways of regulating and holding oneself eventually become pathological, something he referred to as *body armor* (Reich, 1973). For example, suppressed anger could manifest as tightness in the chest, so a therapist using this approach would seek to increase awareness of that nonverbal behavior and dissolve body armor by accessing the associated unconscious material. This theory has since informed several contemporary body-based psychotherapies that give close attention to nonverbal behavior. Gestalt therapy is only one example, particularly given that Fritz Perls had completed psychoanalysis with none other than Wilhelm Reich (Sletvold, 2011).

Body psychotherapy encompasses a broad collection of therapeutic techniques in which the body is a central point of focus and a means of expression. It is thought to promote change by increasing motivation, bodily awareness, and self-confidence while also enabling the expression of suppressed emotions (Heller, 2012). Dance and movement therapies similarly put a special emphasis on the gestural, postural, and facial expressions of emotion and the development of individual as well as group dances to express various feelings (among other processes such as empathic mirroring). These expressive approaches to psychotherapy may more easily address physical symptoms than traditional talk therapies. Indeed, randomized clinical trials using such approaches have shown large effects in reducing depression (Punkanen et al., 2014; Pylvänäinen et al., 2015; Röhricht et al., 2013) or the negative symptoms of schizophrenia (Lee et al., 2015; Röhricht & Priebe, 2006) maintained for several months after treatment. Large effects are also reported for reducing anxiety, with emerging evidence in other areas (Payne, 2017).

The potential mechanisms of change identified in the literature on these treatments invariably cite the increase in emotional expression, awareness, and vitalization, or in other words, the cultivation of vigor and zest for life (Schmais, 1985; Chapter 11). The somatic marker hypothesis of emotion (presented earlier in Chapter 5) has been used to explain the possible process of change in dance and movement therapies (Shafir, 2016). If, as the theory postulates, physical feedback from sensory networks informs the neurological representation and conscious experience of emotion (Damasio, 1999; see also Bechara, 2004), then physical movement in these treatment approaches should activate or weaken emotional experience. Furthermore, at the conclusion of both body-based and dance movement therapy sessions, individuals or groups are typically encouraged to verbally discuss the significance of movements that occurred in the session.[13]

In process research, general dance techniques (i.e., choreography) were associated with an increase in the quality of daily life, whereas therapy techniques that specifically facilitated emotional expression, symbolic movement, and synchrony within groups were associated with a decline in somatization (Brauninger, 2014). Furthermore, after 20 biweekly sessions of dance movement therapy for clinical depression, participants improved in their ability to identify emotions and became less alexithymic (Punkanen et al., 2014). This supports the idea that increasing bodily awareness fosters emotional awareness. It also converges with other lines of research showing people's awareness of their own heartbeats had an association with emotional awareness (Critchley et al., 2004; see Chapter 4), and that training can help them increase that interoceptive capacity (Bornemann & Singer, 2017). Together, these results point to the idea that activating one's bodily expression is closely intertwined with emotional awareness.

Increasing Arousal Boosts Emotional Awareness

While expression and enactment are sometimes thought of as end products in the effort to capture or symbolize one's existing experience, they can also serve as means or processes by which one might heighten emerging awareness. In fact, one of the main reasons why arousal is presumed to be useful in experiential approaches to psychotherapy is that it is used as a tool to help facilitate emotional awareness. The assumption here is that by increasing emotional arousal, the embodied message or hereto unspoken meaning becomes more salient and clear. Sometimes a spontaneous emotional expression itself precipitates insight about oneself and one's wishes. Leveraging arousal in this way goes beyond traditional cognitive and behavioral theories, which conceptualized emotional arousal as a symptom to be attenuated (Nardone et al., 2025). Whatever the case, expressive arousal helps boost emotional awareness, magnifying the experience and making it easier to work with, articulate, and make use of. In short, arousal and awareness work synergistically. Given this, it should come as no surprise that entire treatments have been based on precisely this pairing of processes (e.g., consider emotional awareness and expression therapy; Lumley et al., 2011, 2017).

Amplify Emotional Meaning

In working with emotion, it helps to turn up the volume. When clients in emotion-focused therapy described what it was like to do an expressive enactment of their own self-criticism, they highlighted both how emotionally intense the experience was and how clarifying or direct and incisive the process became (Stiegler, Binder, et al., 2018). One client reflected,

> A powerful [mental image I have is from] when I was in the critic-chair. . . . It was very . . . naked. It was like getting a root canal. You get at the very nerve in a way. Like a straw into my soul. (p. 247)

Similarly, another client described the experience of heightened emotional intensity as one that made therapeutic work more relevant or productive. As the client explained, "It became stronger. It became more real. More direct. Like there was no filter. And it threw me off a bit. So, it was like it was more targeted at my emotions. It was very useful" (p. 247).

A study of emotion-focused therapy for depression showed increases in emotional arousal were associated with increased specificity being used in the autobiographical narratives told by clients (e.g., referring to specific events, giving detail in words and imagery; Boritz et al., 2011). Particularly among clients who enjoyed good treatment outcomes, the co-emergence of arousal with increased specificity in the detail of their narratives was observed at all stages of the treatment, and that relationship between these processes was not observed among clients with poorer outcomes. Furthermore, the relationship between these variables taken together was a better predictor of treatment success than either of them alone, suggesting a synergistic process is at work.

Balancing Arousal With Attention to Meaning

The parameters by which increasing arousal helps boost emotional awareness remain unclear, although one can presume they are nonlinear. Excessive arousal can unhinge someone's focus from the specific meanings that first sparked an emotional experience. For example, clinical theory on the nature of anger problems has highlighted how efforts toward articulating some specific meaning can be derailed by too much arousal. In the case of anger, this can be one source of problematic processing: The deterioration of meaning specificity explains an all-too-common rapid regression from assertive anger into general rage, where the individual essentially no longer remembers what they were fighting for (A. Pascual-Leone et al., 2013).

What else are productive clients doing during moments of high arousal? To that end, a study of experiential psychotherapy for depression showed that during the middle phase of treatment, the combination of emotional arousal and meaning making (e.g., recognition, development, differentiation, reevaluation, integration) predicted improvements in depression and other symptoms better than either process variables alone (Missirlian et al., 2005). This suggests that how affect is being processed and the meaning that clients construct from their immediately aroused emotion determines the ultimate experience and points to one reason why aroused emotional experience is helpful. The role of expressive arousal probably occurs most often through moments of spontaneous speech or gestures that capture emotion but also happens through more deliberate enactments that draw implicit meanings into awareness. The following is an excerpt from Fritz Perls (as cited in Marinary, 2013), the founder of Gestalt therapy, working in session as the therapist:

THERAPIST [PERLS]: I have to interrupt you because there is some expression going on now. Let your right hand talk to your left hand.

CLIENT: [*speaking as if she were the voice of her right hand*] I'm rubbing you, squeezing you. It feels good. . . . I like to squeeze you.

THERAPIST: Now, what does your left hand answer?

CLIENT: I'm passive. I like that. It feels good. (18:04)

In this simple example, the principal role of expressive enactment is that it brings to light a spontaneous process, and doing so both orients the client to meaning and then deepens emotional awareness of that implied meaning about a part of herself. Similarly, when the presenting concern is unfinished business or an emotional injury by a significant other, research suggests that increasing expressive arousal in clients predicts the emergence of a fresh and meaningful shift in how one views the other person (L. S. Greenberg & Malcolm, 2002; Lumley et al. 2017; Paivio & Pascual-Leone, 2023). A related process has been observed when working with couples, where a therapist commenting on the somatic cues of one partner (e.g., their facial expression, posture) predicted that person would then have an immediately deeper emotional experience within the context of couples therapy (Kailanko et al., 2022).

As discussed in Chapter 8, based on a study of experiential therapy for depression, Pos and colleagues (2017) estimated that expressive arousal explains 20% of the variation in treatment outcomes. More arousal predicted a better outcome, although clients generally stayed within the low to moderate ranges of arousal. However, they also found that almost all of this benefit in a client's heightened arousal (about 95% of it) was mediated by the degree to which it also related to deeper levels of client experiencing. In fact, the relationship between emotional arousal and deeper experiential awareness was so strong the researchers concluded that expressive arousal might be thought of as a proxy to emotional awareness, the two processes working tightly hand in hand. This means that arousal probably causes better outcomes by influencing (or augmenting, synergizing, activating) the processes of emotional awareness and experiencing. This is strong evidence against simplistic venting or purging hypotheses of how arousal changes people.

Although this mediation is a powerful finding, it applied primarily to the middle phase of therapy. In contrast, early on, during the first four sessions of treatment, there was no meaningful relationship between arousal and emotional awareness (Pos et al., 2017). Then, in the middle phase of treatment, heightened emotional arousal became a critical process in the causal chain, ushering in and vivifying awareness. Finally, in the last four sessions of therapy, the relationship between arousal and emotional awareness became diminished, although not entirely. Increased levels of arousal still helped with emotional awareness later in treatment, but its impact also seemed to diversify in how it facilitated change.

WORKING FROM THE OUTSIDE IN

Engagement, awareness, arousal, and the expression of emotion are processes that are tightly knitted together. Often one process leads to another through successive approximations toward change, and they also interact synergistically. To begin, emotional engagement (Chapter 4) is a prerequisite for most ways of working with emotion (although not all; see down-regulation in Chapter 3). Of course, emotional engagement is not necessarily the same as physical engagement, the latter having been the topic of this chapter. Furthermore, with a decision to orient to and engage emotion comes a new horizon of emotional awareness, and then the experience itself becomes increasingly complex (Chapters 6 and 7).

Arousal and raw action can create momentum, even when the sense of direction (i.e., meaning) itself may be less clear. By the same token, arousal helps with awareness by amplifying any signal in affective meaning that may lie within. When emotion is already clear, the overt expression of arousal creates a full emotional experience. The expression of arousal is about propelling a process forward toward some discovery. Physical and nonverbal expressions (artistic or otherwise) can be used as steppingstones to reach more articulate and differentiated verbal expression. In this way, the means of expression is scaffolded toward further specificity, where one makes meaning on the back of arousal.

In this sense, sometimes getting physical is about starting from the outside (i.e., the body) and then working inward (i.e., to the felt meaning), as the title of this chapter suggests. That process could begin as a superficial gesture without much meaning or even heart. However, through that doing of physical engagement, the body's activation is carried inward and potentiates congruent facets of some internal experience, facilitating a genuine change in feeling. As a counterpoint, one could also start with what one is feeling inside and then work outwardly towards an increasingly differentiated expression. That might reflect a more common understanding of expressing one's feelings but as the next chapter shows, experimenting with self-expression also opens the door to more vivid and imaginal enactments of meaning.

ENDNOTES

1. This epigraph is from *Recollections of President Lincoln and His Administration*, by L. E. Chittenden, 1891, Harper & Brothers. For more information, visit this website (https://quoteinvestigator.com/2020/08/17/face/).
2. There is some evidence that cold water immersion helps mood by vagus nerve stimulation, multiple hormonal responses, and reducing the inflammatory response. There is also some hypothesis that it helps manage stress response through *cross adaptation*, which is essentially a general dampening of the autonomic stress response over time and perhaps would generalize to everyday life (for references, see Burlingham et al., 2022; Shevchuk, 2008). The idea that one can use cold water plunges to train one's nervous system to better cope with psychological stress still lacks solid empirical support. That is why it has not been included in Chapter 3 on reducing emotion or habituation, which is where it would apply. Even so, rather than being a simple translation across domains, it would be more likely that any such process was a complex and layered form of character development, like ideas such as mental toughness (Jones et al., 2007) or distress tolerance (Bernstein et al., 2011; McHugh & Otto, 2012).
3. Strictly speaking, if one was focused on cold water as the intervention, all these other processes would be considered part of a placebo effect. It is unfortunately that in mental health research, referring to placebo effects often overlooks the complex array of collateral benefits that are tied up with a participant's purposeful efforts to focus on self-care.

4. In a related line of research on memory reconsolidation, experiments on mice have shown that the individual hippocampal cells associated with a positive or negative memory can be directly stimulated using a laser, triggering their activation and the associated behavioral response (B. K. Chen et al., 2019; see also Chapter 18, this volume).

5. Recall from Chapter 5 that an individual's ability to differentiate their own heartbeat from rhythms that were either synchronized or unsynchronized is also related to their level of emotional awareness. The misattribution of flu symptoms in this example from Feldman-Barrett (2017) further recalls my client from Chapter 5 who puzzled over his somatic experience, wondering, "Is this heartbreak or heartburn?"

6. In 2010, I attended a symposium at the American Psychological Association convention in San Diego, California, which presented outcomes for the treatment of psychological trauma using psychedelics. In a closing statement, one of the researchers ventured, "We don't think it's the actual drug that is curative, we think it's something that happens while a client takes the drug." I remember thinking: "Well then, welcome to the world of psychotherapy process research! Because we don't think it's the office chairs themselves that are curative; it's something that happens while a client sits in the chair."

7. "Murderous rage" is terminology of ISTDP used to describe a specific client experience in therapy. It should be clear clients are not encouraged to act on such feelings. One can debate whether such intensity is desirable when all factors are considered, but that is a separate issue. The point here is to note a convergence of theory and evidence on a potential mechanism of change.

8. Cannon (1927) demonstrated that visceral and physiological responses did not discriminate between emotions. His experiments also showed that emotional reactions occurred in an unchanged fashion even if large parts of an animal's sympathetic nervous system were removed. At most, attempts to artificially induce emotions by eliciting organic changes led to an experience that human participants described as being reminiscent of emotion, but not emotion per se. Subsequent studies have continued to disprove the idea that emotion is the simple sum of visceral experiences.

9. While it is useful to have an experiment confirming that Botox does not mute strong emotional experiences, anyone who has reacted with a spit take when caught unexpectedly by a funny joke will attest to the same conclusion.

10. While there is still debate in neuroscience, some argue that the overarching motivational systems are essentially housed on different sides of the brain (Davidson, 2000; Davidson & Begley, 2012). For more on this, see Chapter 13 (this volume) for discussion on the sword and shield hypothesis (Brookshire & Casasanto, 2018).

11. This is not just folk psychology. Working with emotion has a very long tradition in theater schools, and techniques in acting have been tested, honed, and passed on—largely through mentorships and quite independently of psychological research. Arguably, the craft of the actor in generating a real emotional experience on stage provides a wealth of practical knowledge on how to change emotion in purposeful ways.

12. Counter to any notion of catharsis, Darwin also believed that the relief associated with expression was largely incidental. And finally, he saw the social communication of emotion as important but believed it to have evolved as a secondary signal.

13. The way reflection and debriefing are done in body-based and movement therapy contrasts with how it is done in traditionally seated approaches to experiential therapy. Treatments that work primarily with movement and the body usually debrief the process retrospectively, at the conclusion of a session. However, in seated experiential psychotherapies, clients are usually encouraged to talk about emotion simultaneously with its emergence as it peaks and decays in the here and now. While one approach allows for freer bodily expression, the other allows for the more explicit moment-by-moment formulation of feeling (i.e., mentalization).

10

Enactments

Working From the Inside Out

Don't tell us, show us!

—JACOB MORENO (ATTRIBUTED)

The literal played . . . as small a part as it perhaps ever played in any, and we wholesomely breathed inconsistencies and ate and drank contradictions. The presence of paradox was so bright.

—HENRY JAMES, *A SMALL BOY AND OTHERS*

The previous chapter explored three distinct ways expressive arousal acts as a mechanism of change: First, increasing affective arousal can provide a general impetus for change; second, expression itself can generate internal experience; and third, arousal can be used to amplify emotional awareness. One way of thinking about the first two of those processes are that they work at generating novel emotional experiences by starting to work from the physicality of expression until it influences experience (e.g., working from the outside in). This, in the sense that externally taking on some expression or choosing to embody some emotional trajectory helps one either access or generate internal emotional experience, is what amounts to using peripheral bodily experience to tacitly shape the emergence of emotion.

However, another way that expressive arousal often creates changes is when clients work from the inside out. That would represent a more bottom-up constructive process, where clients are internally searching for some internal referent and then bring it expressively outward, amplifying it and eventually exploring it through action. (Of course, in practice, all of these processes operate

https://doi.org/10.1037/0000460-011
Principles of Emotion Change: What Works and When in Psychotherapy and Everyday Life, by A. Pascual-Leone
Copyright © 2026 by the American Psychological Association. All rights reserved.

dialectically, creating a synthesis rather than each operating in isolation). However, the current chapter will explore another process of change that is constructively more complex and can also be thought of in broad strokes as working with emotion from the inside out.[1] So, fourth, dramatic enactments have a special role in creating affective momentum and affirming one's commitment to some underlying emotional meaning. Implicitly, enactments involve expressive arousal as well as increased vividness as one activates a complex psychological experience.

ENACTMENT CREATES COMMITMENT TO MEANING: START INSIDE AND THEN BRING IT OUT

Once emotion is brought into awareness, it also needs to be viscerally experienced, and one needs to feel the emotion for processing to be carried forward. *Expressed arousal* means being in contact with an emotion rather than just talking about or reflecting on the experience. Emotional awareness provides an entry point for this, but using arousal in an enactment is the follow through (L. S. Greenberg et al., 2007). *Enactments,* in psychotherapy, are deliberate tasks to externally convey the significance of one's feelings beyond just finding the right words. Compared with isolated acts of emotional expression, enactments usually entail a more complex process, sometimes with several steps, to fully capture an evolving experiential narrative (A. Pascual-Leone & Baher, 2023).

Hypothesized Mechanisms of Enactment

There are several aspects to enactment as a mechanism of emotional change. First, often following the prompt of a therapist, one typically embarks purposefully, actively choosing to enact something. So, a key aspect of expressive enactment is the fact that one deliberately engages in it. Second, enactments are not only the explicit expression of emotional feeling, but they also generate momentum and thereby commitment to the embodied meaning of an emotion. As one commits to the task, like pushing off from dry land, the experience is carried forward into lesser known and less deliberate territory.

Third, it follows that enactments are often some kind of experimental elaboration based on what was hereto only an implied message. This complex form of expressive arousal is a powerful way of owning (or sometimes re-owning) an initial aspect of one's experience, often reifying an otherwise unspoken emotional meaning, and then seeing what comes out of propelling that process forward. In short, therapeutic enactments are about both the experience of agency and a commitment to one's full experience in a process of discovery. The significance of engaging in an enactment is as if to say, "I have some sense of what I feel and what it might mean, and I'm going with it! I'm now leaning into that experience and am dedicated to seeing it through to completion, whatever that might be. Right now, I'm making this happen."

It is important to distinguish that the process of expressive enactment is not about a true reenactment or reproduction of events, nor is its function an exercise in graduated exposure to trauma cues (although that may nonetheless play a minor role as well, one that usually goes unacknowledged in humanistic or psychodynamic accounts). Rather, the primary purpose of an enactment is to create an embodied experience that can be concretely explored in the moment. For example, consider a client who feels ambivalent about accepting an apology from someone who betrayed them. Enactment could be used to explore the possibility of forgiving or of not forgiving. The client might imagine the person and declare, "I accept your apology, and I forgive you." People often have immediate visceral reactions to the experience of making such statements out loud. So, if it feels uncomfortable or untrue, then the client might try going the other way and experiment with saying, "I will never forgive you for what you have done!" Trying on these alternative meanings is done in the same exploratory spirit with which one might try on a shirt at the store just to see how well it fits. Doing this is not a rehearsal for real life but rather is to see if the meaning suits them or if it has potential. In doing so, the client may also find themself discovering and exploring personal obstacles or still other trajectories of meaning.

In group therapy, enactments also often serve as a kind of public ceremony that seeks to externalize and make concrete what has often become an internalized script (Westwood et al., 2010). Furthermore, in some systemic approaches to therapy, and in existential or attachment-based interventions, explicitly focusing on the human encounter can involve performing enactments with the meta-awareness that what is happening in real time is a special kind of existential encounter (A. Pascual-Leone & Greenberg, 2007b). While remaining present in the here and now, clients enact a situation (imagined or real) to explore and perhaps change their mental representation of the event and then to experiment with alternative responses to it (Armstrong et al., 2015; Blatner, 2000; Meisiek, 2004; Minuchin, 2012; Moreno, 1958).

Process analyses have been used to explore the complexity involved in various kinds of enactments to explain how these interventions lead to good outcomes. To discern significant therapeutic events in psychodrama group therapy, cases who resolved their concerns and enjoyed improvements in both interpersonal functioning and sense of self (i.e., good outcomes) were compared with unresolved cases who had poor or relatively unsuccessful outcomes (McVea et al., 2011). Sessions that revealed the resolution process in psychodrama were characterized by a series of within-session steps that highlighted reexperiencing the problem with awareness, activating internal resources, and an emotionally aroused experience of social repair, which was followed by an integration of the experience.

Similarly, chairwork is a method of enactment used in various approaches to individual therapy (A. Pascual-Leone & Baher, 2023), whereas task analysis represents a formal method that aims to anchor process steps in an ordered sequence (Elliott, 2010). Several task analyses have now studied the uses of chairwork interventions in emotion-focused therapy, examining (a) self-critical chairwork, where a client assumes and enacts the opposing positions of their own self-critical process (L. S. Greenberg & Foerster, 1996); (b) empty chairwork, where a client has an imaginal dialogue with a perpetrator from the past (L. S. Greenberg & Malcolm, 2002); and (c) self-interruptive chairwork, where clients explore how they might hold themselves back from feeling or acting (Vrana, 2021). A narrative synthesis of these studies has also abstracted commonalities observed across explanatory models (A. Pascual-Leone & Baher, 2023). While the original studies each examined different clinical problems, the review identified six components that are common across chairwork, and typically they are ordered in time:

1. Activating the problem state

2. Exploring one's inner reaction

3. Enacting the specific core concern

4. Expressing emotion in the service of an unmet need

5. A change in perspective on the original problem

6. Negotiating future engagements (A. Pascual-Leone & Baher, 2023, p. 567)

These common components represent a series of process steps from start to finish. As such, they articulate a general causal model of what happens during emotion-focused therapy chairwork that leads to good outcomes. The findings also converge with what was found to be central in psychodramatic enactments (McVea et al., 2011). Also, they align with several qualitative studies that reported firsthand client accounts of how enactments helped (A. Pascual-Leone & Baher, 2023).

Action Gives Momentum to Feeling: Put Your Muscle Where Your Mouth Is

Emotion is embodied meaning, but meaning may not be fully developed, exercised, or applied to the living of life. An expressive action can be decisively used to energize and introduce meaning in a new way. This often adds momentum to the significance of one's feeling, when previously it may only have been tentative. Enactments can also make the ever-changing psychological processes within a lived moment less abstract and easier to grasp conceptually.

Energizing the Meaning

When aroused enactment is used strategically in clinical work, it acts as a Trojan horse that injects energy through the mobilization of otherwise more dormant meanings and feelings. In practical terms, physically moving from place to place when taking on or changing roles helps to symbolize different perspectives of characters or different facets of a problem. This spatial aid also helps make personal problems less confusing and more concrete (Blatner, 2000; Pos & Greenberg, 2012).[2] So, agreeing to engage in an enactment is one way of getting behind or physically endorsing implicit meaning, making it explicit (i.e., to walk the walk, not just talk the talk). This explicit physical activation then allows for the client to make use of an affective state that was previously only tacit and on the margin of awareness. This concretization is the essence of enactment (e.g., start with what's inside and then bring it out). Concretization requires clients to specify their problems in dramatic form (e.g., a specific scene with specific characters).

The grandfather of therapeutic enactments in psychotherapy was Jacob Moreno, a psychiatrist and contemporary of Freud who was the originator of psychodrama and an early pioneer of group therapy (Moreno, 1958). A common phrase used to prompt clients in psychodrama is "Don't tell us, show us!" (Blatner, 2000). Psychodrama, and drama therapy in general, insists that emotional narratives be evoked, embodied, and enacted. Enactment brings the client out of vague abstractions or generic stories (which may be subtle ways of avoiding experience) and fixes the client in the here and now, re-anchoring the clients in their experiences.[3] This also concretizes and demonstrates the problem for the client and therapist alike, so that new approaches to the problem can be encouraged. Mobilizing the embodied experience is what allows for further developments in that experience.

The individual willingly experiences oneself as an agent in the emotional process rather than feeling overwhelmed or tumbled by a disowned wave of feeling. Enactments of self-interruption are a good case in point: When clients inhibit themselves and hold back in conversation, feeling, or behavior, it is often a rapid internal process that occurs covertly, often mostly outside of awareness. However, instructing clients to explicitly enact the process that is underfoot helps them identify their own agentic process in what may be happening. It also makes the covert process available for the client to experiment with through an exaggeration (Therapist: "So, you stop yourself from speaking up? Like putting on a muzzle. Try doing it now, put your hand over your mouth. What happens inside?").

The simple fact that deliberate expressive arousal moves things along and energizes and mobilizes some direction, creates a vector for change. In short, enactments get the ball rolling, but this also has a lot to do with timing. The lyric poet says just the right thing at the right time and allows us to see the present experience more deeply. In much the same way, a therapist must strike while the iron is hot, proposing dramatic enactments and experiments to create windows of opportunity that open into the client's flow of experience (L. S. Greenberg, 2021; Nardone et al., 2022).

Maintaining the Momentum

Another challenge in working with emotion can be simply keeping enough momentum in the flow of conversation and emotional exploration. Because emotion is so ephemeral, exploration can unfold in staccato spurts, which becomes increasingly challenging if clients are not verbally active enough when conveying an emotional narrative or elaborating on the meanings of a feeling. An experiment on the use of gesture during verbal improvisation (e.g., the act of making something up on the spot) offers some insight into why getting physically active can help with moving the session process along (C. Lewis et al., 2015). When participants were asked to engage in spontaneous speech production that could not be planned in advance, they gestured more than when answering very familiar questions with well-rehearsed responses. Furthermore, the rate of using gesture was related to the quality of participants' creative improvisation. The clinical implication is that using gesture facilitates the spontaneous generation of verbal content, which in psychotherapy promises more exploration of the possible meanings at hand.

Physical engagement can be very helpful for clients who are either stuck or just less talkative in therapy. Convergent with this, it is standard practice in drama therapy of various kinds to always keep the client moving during an enactment. The client rarely sits, but even more so, rather than simply standing during enactments, clients are continually encouraged to keep walking. This practice reduces the client's sense of being on display or performing, and it also maintains the sense that one is still on task, even when one is at a loss for words. During periods of emotional elaboration, clients will be seen slowly strolling alongside their therapist or a fellow group member, circling the inside of the treatment group as they search for meaning (Blatner, 2000; Moreno, 1958; Westwood et al., 2010).

Whereas psychodrama as a specific approach emphasizes pure and uncharted spontaneity, therapeutic enactments of other kinds may rely more on the safety of emotionally exploring a predetermined script that the therapist guides a client through (Balfour et al., 2014). Treatment approaches vary quite a bit in the degree of this therapist directivity, which should also be a function of previously evaluating clients presenting concerns, vulnerabilities, and preparedness for such evocative interventions. In some cases, for example of trauma or of intense self-criticism, a preintervention evaluation of this kind is an important part of good clinical practice (Balfour et al., 2014; Paivio & Pascual-Leone, 2023; Stiegler, Molde, & Schanche, 2018).

Tough People Use Enactments Too!

The notion of enactments is occasionally met with skepticism, perhaps because of its theatrical nature (discussed later in this chapter), as if this way of working were not suitable for serious concerns, or perhaps not for serious people. However, the physicality of enactments offers some unexpected opportunities for working with clients who have hardened characters or who pride themselves on their toughness. One such application for structured enactments is in group therapy with military veterans who have suffered war-related trauma. The treatment is now used across Canada and in Australia, attracting national levels of funding in both countries (Balfour et al., 2014; Westwood et al. 2010). Participants complete three weekend-long sessions about 1 month apart (approximately 80 hours in total).[4] This intervention is used to alleviate posttraumatic stress syndrome through a number of components (e.g., social support, psychoeducation, the development of emotion regulation skills, expediting access to other treatments, goal-setting), but the use of therapeutic enactments is central (D. W. Cox, Buchanan, et al., 2014). These are self-declared people of action. They do not identify themselves as people of words, and much less as people who want to sit in a circle and talk about their feelings. So, acting out their feelings turns out to be an appealing treatment approach.[5]

In this group therapy, a member first narrates their trauma while others enact it, then the member enacts different roles in the trauma, and finally they narrate an idealized version of the traumatic situation while others enact it. In one posttreatment evaluation, male veterans experienced very large effects in the reduction of depression, as well as medium effects in the reduction of anxious arousal related to trauma symptoms (D. W. Cox, Westwood, et al., 2014). Another study of male veterans showed decreases in depression were maintained with a medium effect 3 months after intervention. Although mediation analyses were not done, during posttreatment interviews, over 65% of participants identified therapeutic enactments as a key beneficial aspect of the treatment (Westwood et al., 2010).

While the application of psychodrama as a treatment for war-related trauma may be unanticipated, there is reason to believe similar treatment strategies might be useful for other groups of tough people who are recalcitrant to conventional talk therapy. For example, therapeutic enactments could offer benefits to some professional athletes (e.g., in football, hockey, combat sports; consider Tamminen & Watson, 2022). Another example is in working with incarcerated populations. A treatment study (A. Pascual-Leone et al., 2011) illustrates this by using emotion-focused group therapy within a prison setting to treat men who had history of intimate partner violence. The treatment had the men enact imaginary dialogues with an empty chair to address issues of shame, personal trauma, and the vulnerability that underlie their acts of interpersonal aggression. Following up 8 months after their release from prison, the treatment group's rate of relapse into criminal assault or sexual assault was significantly lower than that of a matched comparison group, with effect sizes of this treatment being comparable to those reported by mainstream forensic psychotherapies. Moreover, the positive direction of this treatment effect was still apparent at 3 years after release.

Making the Process Palpable

Enactments help reify the psychological process. Grappling with the unhealthy processes that produce and maintain one's emotional problems is a slippery and indeterminate task. That is why problem clarification has turned out to be such an important process early in treatment, and it anticipates useful good treatment changes that occur later (e.g., Grosse Holtforth et al., 2006). In short, it's hard for clients (and therapists) to get a sharp focus on the problem, so physically symbolizing a psychological process helps make abstract meanings more concrete and real. Whereas arousal and enactment seem to work synergistically with basic levels of emotional awareness, reifying the process and viscerally experiencing oneself as an agent facilitates a higher level of meta-awareness.[6]

It turns out that this concrete formulation of a problematic process is quite important because negative self-treatment is a much more nebulous and highly idiosyncratic aspect of psychopathology than was previously thought (L. S. Greenberg & Watson, 2006; Watson & Greenberg, 2017; for a research perspective on this puzzle, see A. Pascual-Leone, Herpertz, et al., 2016). For example, in a study of depressive processes, undergraduate students previously identified as either high or low in their vulnerably to depression were asked to engage in an enactment of their self-critical process using a two-chair task during a single session of emotion-focused therapy (Whelton & Greenberg, 2005). Contrary to the widely accepted cognitive theory of depression, this study showed the best predictor of someone's vulnerability to depression was not so much the content of what people said to themselves (e.g., the verbal nature of their self-criticisms), but rather it was manner in how they talked (e.g., the paraverbal cues and emotional tone) when they chastised themselves. Specifically, the harshness and contemptuousness of self-criticisms is what makes it so pernicious, not the critical beliefs per se. Furthermore, whether someone was subsequently able to respond assertively to their own self-critical process (e.g., switch chairs and respond to the critic) with self-affirming anger predicted resilience, even in the face of harsh self-contempt.

However, without first having some minimum level of affective arousal and expression, self-contempt and self-loathing remain largely covert processes; they are not easily measurable, they are not held up as a target for intervention, nor can they even act as the spurs that might otherwise trigger healthy assertive rebuttals (Kramer & Pascual-Leone, 2016; A. Pascual-Leone, Herpertz, et al., 2016). Unlike the palpable mudslinging of verbal content that is so evident in personal criticisms or dysfunctional beliefs, it is much more difficult to capture and pinpoint, for example, the message being implied in a smirk or curl of the lip, tacitly expressing harsh self-contempt or hostility (see Beuchat et al., 2024).

In short, this is where enactment can help by externalizing the psychological process, objectifying it, and making it easier to explicitly engage with. The enactment of interpersonal difficulties helps reveal underlying emotion and communication patterns. Similarly, the enactment of different parts of the self helps offer a higher order perspective on the negative ways one implicitly treats oneself, which are the most common depressogenic and anxiety-provoking processes (L. S. Greenberg & Watson, 2006; Watson & Greenberg, 2017). The enactment of self-criticism (e.g., negative self-talk) or self-interruption (e.g., how one holds oneself back from feeling, from engaging with life) are prime examples of how enactment tasks are used in drama therapies, Gestalt therapy, and emotion-focused therapy. These complex tasks facilitate change through several processes, but one of those is the experience of oneself as an agent, whether that be an agent for better (e.g., feeling how I fight back) or for worse (e.g., realizing how I beat myself up). By incarnating different parts of the pathogenic process in a dramatic enactment, clients become aware of themselves as internally generating or re-activating depressive or anxious states.

Although the deliberate activation and enactment of a deeper pathological process is sometimes a daunting proposition for clients (and some therapists), that experience of ownership and involvement also orients clients to their implicit involvement in negative self-treatment, which can empower them for change. Client subjective experiences of enacting self-criticism in a two-chair task has been explored in a qualitative study of emotion-focused therapy, and findings closely support this formulation. When clients were invited to reflect on their treatment process, they spontaneously reported becoming more aware, during the chair tasks, of their own role in generating depressive symptoms. As one client suggests, this was not about gaining a theoretical or conceptual understanding; rather, it was about experiencing the self as an active agent:

> I can talk, and I can realize a lot of stuff. I can have insight into how I function, but it doesn't . . . it doesn't become real until you actually get in the chair and see what you are doing to yourself. (Stiegler, Binder, et al., 2018, p. 148)

Another client comments on how the process of enactment was a lived experience that brought a new meta-awareness about the significance of what was going on:

> I think the most important part for me was realizing what I was doing inside my head, and how nasty it was. It was a real shocker. I remember not being able to state it at first, when I was acting as my critical voice. I remember not being able to actually say it. And I just started crying, "It is so nasty, I can't do it." (Stiegler, Binder, et al., 2018, p. 149)

Finally, as will be picked up again later in this chapter, another advantage of using physical enactment is that it acts in the service of organizing conceptual content (e.g., a template, a spatial pneumonic) for therapists, who often consolidate case formulations based on how a client process unfolds during a task (R. N. Goldman & Greenberg, 2015; Paivio & Pascual-Leone, 2023).

The Impact of Enactments: How Well Does It Work?
Enactments in various kinds of psychotherapy have been associated with therapeutic changes in outcomes. A meta-analysis of 25 experimental studies comparing psychodrama to controls (Kipper & Ritchie, 2003) demonstrated a large overall treatment effect as reflected in a range of behavioral, attitudinal, and personality measures. This suggests that psychodrama is effective in promoting therapeutic change, holding comparable effects across studies that worked with students as well as the treatment of clinical and other special populations. Moreover, the specific techniques of role reversal (i.e., where a client acts and speaks as some other person in their life) and doubling (i.e., where a client interacts with some other version or part of the self) were found to be the two most effective interventions.

A dramatic embodiment can be thought of as any period of the therapy session in which a client purposely performs a theatrical or bodily focused exercise (e.g., physical enactment of the content of a therapy session) while actively attending to and expressing oneself through the body. In a study that systematically coded demonstration videos of psychodrama, episodes of dramatic embodiment were associated with significantly greater levels of emotional arousal as well as deeper levels of client experiencing (see Chapter 7) as compared with episodes that did not make use of dramatic embodiment (Armstrong et al., 2015, 2016). Interestingly, these are the same two variables that Pos and colleagues (2017) showed to have such a tight mediating relationship, particularly during the middle phase, in the prediction of final symptom outcomes in emotion-focused therapy.

Chairwork interventions were derived from the original notion of enactments in psychodrama in an application to individual therapy (more on this history and development later). Since then, these interventions have come to be incorporated across a wide range of treatment approaches including Gestalt, emotion-focused, and schema therapy, as well as variations of cognitive behavior therapy. A series of meta-analyses involving 28 studies estimated the overall impact of chairwork in individual therapy (A. Pascual-Leone & Baher, 2023). Compared with a therapist using empathic responding alone, chairwork offered a large advantage in deepening client experiencing, which is an intermediate (process) outcome. Moreover, across studies, a single session of chairwork had a noteworthy impact on reducing symptoms pre- to postintervention.

Furthermore, the impact seems to be magnified over an ongoing course of therapy. Five studies explored the unique impact of chairwork when it was included as a component of treatment. They did this by way of dismantling designs, comparisons with treatment as usual, and multiple baseline controls and then reported the long-term changes to a client's target concerns, which ranged across studies on posttraumatic stress disorder, social anxiety, depression, obsessive-compulsive disorder, or both depression and anxiety (A. Pascual-Leone & Baher, 2023). Treatments using chairwork were compared with prolonged exposure, client-centered therapy, and standard cognitive therapy using automatic thought records. The meta-analytic review showed that including chairwork as part of a treatment package produced a small to medium benefit above treatments as usual (i.e., without chairwork).

Interestingly, there is also some reason to believe that treatment orientation may be a moderator. Chairwork in emotion-focused therapy emphasizes an exploration of the emotional impact of a dialogue, irrespective of its veracity (e.g., Therapist: "What does it feel like to be on the receiving end of that criticism?"; see L. S. Greenberg, 2021; L. S. Greenberg & Goldman, 2019). In contrast, the application of chairwork in cognitive behavior therapy is typically in the pursuit of truth and developing more accurate beliefs, as when different perspectives are considered during a judicial trial (e.g., Therapist: "So, how likely is it that the criticism is really true?"; see Pugh, 2022). Preliminary evidence suggests chairwork done in the manner of an emotion-focused approach may offer an advantage, although a direct comparison has not yet been conducted (A. Pascual-Leone & Baher, 2023).

ENACTMENTS RESTRUCTURE A NARRATIVE FROM WITHIN

Enactments can influence narrative changes in several ways. First, these tasks shift the weight given to different aspects of the presenting experience. Second, they elaborate new content through the process of imagination. Third, they can help generate new experiences in the present. I discuss these kinds of restructuring in each of the three following subsections.

Shifting the Balance in What Is Already There

As various parts of an experience get concretized and mobilized, facilitating the enactment of emotion is a way of also shifting the balance among different facets within that emotional experience (i.e., Paivio et al. 2001; A. Pascual-Leone, 2009). Although a story's content about what happened (or is happening) may not change, the experience of oneself and the emotional account within that narrative is malleable. For example, when therapists first used a relational reframe to focus clients on the attachment issues underlying a presenting emotional injury, and then second, encouraged them to enact an imaginary dialogue about it, the ordered pair of interventions intensified clients' attachment-related sadness while decreasing their presenting anger (Narkiss-Guez et al., 2015).

Most people who have suffered some interpersonal grievance or betrayal feel various degrees of both anger and sadness, with some people reporting feeling mostly angry about what happened, whereas others reported feeling mostly sad. Following that observation, an online experiment manipulated the balance of emotion reported by people who had unfinished business with someone in their life by having them respond to a systematic combination of open-ended questions and emotionally evocative prompts (Nardone et al., 2025). Even in the absence of any dialogue or attentive listener, when participants responded online to a series of prescribed steps, it successfully incited and then mobilized feelings that were either compatible with or contrary to a participant's presenting state depending on the condition they were in. In other words, irrespective of whether they initially felt mostly angry or mostly sad, prompts could differentially encourage specific expressions of emotion and modulated the salience of what people felt regarding their concern. Participating in such exercises shifted people's feelings either from anger to sadness or from sadness to anger (Nardone et al., 2025). Furthermore, the notion of memory reconsolidation provides a neurological account of how within-session shifts like this can eventually create enduring change (Lane & Nadel, 2020).

Nevertheless, notice that the change process I am highlighting here remains distinct from simply expanding one's horizon of emotional awareness because, in this scenario, one is already aware of the various (often mixed) feelings. For example, when a client feels both angry and sad about being betrayed, the way a therapist helps explore and elaborate that presenting feeling can potentiate one or the other emotional facets depending on how the therapist's reflection is phrased (e.g., shifting the client's attention from sadness to anger):

THERAPIST: So, I can really hear how hurt you are.

CLIENT: Yeah.

THERAPIST: But I guess there is also this deep sense of injustice? Is that it?

CLIENT: Yes, that's right. I'm. . . . Yeah, I'm also really pissed off about what happened!

So, activating emotion at this moment is an intervention aimed at altering the relative balance or primacy of components (e.g., dominance of anger vs. sadness) within that same experience.

In an example from my clinical practice, a father described to me how he discovered he could turn around his bouts of obsessively ruminating on the tragic death of his youngest child. What he described was the use of action to essentially shift the balance of emotions that were already within the scope of his awareness. He explained,

> Grief is important . . . but whenever I found it going sideways, slipping down the depressive rabbit hole of what happened, the horrible self-doubt, I realized the best thing for me was to stand right up and go straight to wherever my other children were playing, make eye contact, and just be with them.

Here, the physical enactment of getting up and moving to engage the living children that needed him was one behavior that dislodged and offset his elaboration of pathological grief, refocusing his attention on the love he already had.[7] In short, this process is about introducing expressive action within a narrative by way of enactment. Physical enactment may act as an antidote to the cognitive loop of rumination. Taking explicit action (even in one's imagination) changes the experiential story of what happened (i.e., it changes the overall balance of feelings about what happened).

In a research example, 40 highly self-critical students were invited to engage in a single session of chairwork from Gestalt therapy to explore the various feelings and meanings related to their self-criticism (Neff et al., 2007). A 2-week follow-up showed reductions in anxiety, depression, and self-criticism, but those symptom changes still did not fully explain the additional changes participants enjoyed, including increases in positive affect (e.g., self-compassion, self-esteem) and psychological well-being (e.g., sense of belongingness, social connectedness). The authors interpreted the emergence of positive emotional experience as indicating a separate effect of the enactment, one that may serve as a protective factor against self-critical processes.

The Drama of Enactments: Elaborating As-If

Unlike an isolated expressive gesture or a single act, enactments necessarily entail some minimal narrative context. A dramatic enactment is a mental simulation that is situated in some time and place (cf. McLean et al., 2007). That setting might be a richer and more explicit reenactment of the past (e.g., of things that happened but may have been left unsaid or unacknowledged), the new enactment of some alternative reality (e.g., what one wished for, what could have been), or it might even be the present moment (e.g., when orchestrating an encounter between members of a couple or a family). Because enactments begin with some definitive point of departure and then elaborate forward, even when they are more scripted exercises, the creative engagement generates momentum in the process of discovery. Expressive arousal, in some narrative context, is a process that can be used to carry forward an implicit meaning with conviction.[8]

One of the key aspects of enactment is the experiment in real time, where neither client nor the therapist really knows what will happen. This is not a rehearsal or practice for scripted events. The essence of an enactment task is to explore some narrative scene or imagined dialogue as-if, with an eye to what might imminently happen next. Moreno and psychodrama refer to imagining as-if as a central principle in the spontaneity of emotional exploration. However, not coincidentally, acting as-if is also a central premise in the Stanislavski system of method acting, an immersive, imaginative approach into characters and their situations (S. Moore, 1984).[9]

The emergence of experience-based schools of theater is related to the experiential enactment interventions used in modern psychotherapy. In the early 1900s, opera and theater relied on highly stylized stock portrayals (e.g., faking affect) and did not reflect the idiosyncratic or embodied experiences of a given actor. Based in the Moscow Art Theater, Russian actor and director Konstantin Stanislavski introduced a radically new experiential approach in the 1910s and into the 1930s. In short, in this contemporary approach to acting for film or stage, actors are taught to enter the imagined experience (i.e., of the story being told) to internally generate genuine emotional experiences that emerges spontaneously in the lived event of a performance. Rather than just outwardly displaying the trappings of a stock feeling, the thrust of this novel method was to bring a moment-by-moment as-if realism into dramatic enactment.

This is explicitly cited as a source of inspiration for Moreno's development of psychodrama, as he came from Eastern Europe and was a contemporary of Stanislavski. Later, interventions in psychodrama such as doubling and role reversal inspired key interventions of Gestalt therapy in the 1950s and 1960s (Blatner, 2000; Scheiffele, 2008). This is evidenced in striking similarities of the theory and practice specific to enactments, as shared by Moreno's psychodrama and Perls's Gestalt psychotherapy. Although reluctantly, Perls acknowledged the influence psychodrama had on him in developing the hot-seat technique (i.e., one-on-one enactments using chairs; Scheiffele, 2008).[10] Finally, beginning in the 1970s, researchers of what would become emotion-focused therapy systematically studied and refined enactment interventions inherited from Gestalt therapy. The two-chair and self-interruptive tasks (both derived from doubling) and the empty chair task (derived from role reversal) are chief examples of this evolution in enactment techniques as used in emotion-focused therapy, with similar variations in schema therapy and compassion-based therapies, among others (A. Pascual-Leone & Baher, 2023).

In current psychotherapy, tasks of therapeutic enactment essentially ask clients to consider the following questions of themselves: What if I were in this scenario?; What feeling comes up as I imagine it?; What does the feeling make me want to do?; What was there, that perhaps I did not notice at the time, that I did not give a voice to?; and What is it like to elaborate this experience beyond its premise? Enactments of this kind capture an implicit meaning, one that is too ephemeral for words but still needs to be concretized or symbolized, but, most importantly, it needs to be committed to with agency. Notice that the first part of that process is about mediating emotional awareness (as discussed earlier), but the second part is about getting behind that emergent self-awareness. In this sense, therapeutic enactment is about commitment to and indisputable ownership of a certain aspect of personal meaning or truth.[11] For example, when clients find themselves mystified by their own precipitous expressions, it illustrates this point: "I don't know why I did that, it just happened! But now that it's out there, I can see that's how I really feel!" Obviously, this function of expressive arousal is contingent on the degree to which the proposed enactment is congruent with one's covert (but real) experience.

Add Something Different

Beyond the discovery-oriented process, restructuring a narrative through vivid imaginal enactments of some kind also entails a purposeful (goal-directed) corrective emotional experience. Again, distinguishing arousal and expression from the indiscriminate venting or bleeding of emotion is critical because this corrective experience will have to be creatively generated in all its specificity. Here, it is the details that matter. According to psychodynamic theorist Malan (1979), "What went wrong must go right." Sometimes going right is as simple as articulating what was felt but left unsaid, such as assertion of one's value or rights, particularly when those were previously too dangerous to assert. Alternatively, it may be to deeply feel one's grief, particularly when previously there was no time, space, or permission to acknowledge loss. As many authors on expressive arousal have argued, facilitating feelings that are on the perimeter of awareness but have hereto been suppressed allows one to develop a meaningful and coherent narrative (e.g., L. S. Greenberg & Angus, 2007; Janoff-Bulman, 1992; Moreno, 1958). However, the chief impact of enacting as-if is that one does something different.

Using Surplus Reality

The work of Westwood and colleagues (e.g., 2010) with war veterans suffering from posttraumatic stress is a poignant example of getting clients to do something different with respect to what was originally experienced. Enactments of that kind involve not only making the internal experience explicit but also rescripting what happened and often enacting a newly discovered wish. Here, *rescripting* is the purposeful and structured enactment of something different. Through a collaborative development by therapist and client, the client performs a change that deviates from the historical account. This introduces new emotional elements and new narrative turns that are congruent with the lived experience but never actually happened.

Similarly, chairwork in individual therapy could involve imagining what a deceased person would say if they were alive today, imagining a conversation with oneself as a 6-year-old child, or imagining what a better father would say (e.g., Therapist: "Now imagine the dad you deserved but perhaps never had"). These enactments are the exploration of various constellations of genuine experiential meaning, but they are unfettered by the constraints of narrative reality. Moreno (1958) introduced the term *surplus reality* to describe this enactment of fantasy or impossible scenarios. In a video of his work made in Paris, a client of Moreno protests that talking with her mother-in-law was unfeasible because she lived so far away. Moreno grins at this and waves his hand in a playful dismissal. Over a brief exchange, he explains,

> Where is your mother-in-law now? . . . She's in New York?! Ah! Well, let's go to New York and see how she is! Let's project ourselves. Where does she live in New York? . . . Well, let's go up to the 16th floor and see her! . . . Will you go alone? . . . Why don't you join me and face her? [*A moment later*] . . . Well, okay, then let's suppose we are all here in Paris. . . . No, no, we can arrange it very easily. In psychodrama the ocean is nothing! . . . We can always go thousands of miles away from this point. . . . And now, I would like you and your mother-in-law to have an encounter. . . . You have to realize, the encounters you have had with your mother in real life are one thing, but here you can be far more expressive! (Moreno, 1964, 00:56)

When therapists set the scene in this way, they are offering a hypothetical and invite the client to creatively act as-if, and clients are often able to explore those possibilities.

Surplus reality is not only prompted by therapists' intervention; it can also emerge spontaneously from clients. Welling (2012) observed that just before a significant shift in affect and personal meaning, clients sometimes say things like "I know that my father would never say this, but as [I enact] my father, I feel like apologizing" or "I know that my mother in reality is unable to express such affection, but I thought she wanted to say that she loves me" (p. 124). In the end, however it gets precipitated, the client experiences something that did not happen and perhaps would never happen in real life (Welling, 2012).

Some aspect of participating in these quasi-lived encounters with surplus reality is captured by the second epigraph to this chapter. Henry James (brother to early psychology theorist, William James) describes growing up surrounded by similarly playful experiments in meaning on account of his family's casual tolerance for paradox and contradictions. The issue of truth in these fabricated narrative scenes is taken up later, in Chapter 19. However, here it will suffice to state that creative exercises like these offer a process to deliver novel experiences that may hold deep personal significance.

The Purposeful Act

In the context of psychodynamic therapy, Malan (1979) was referring to the enactment of a relational experience and what should (must) unfold purposefully between client and therapist. This kind of process can also be thought of as an expressive enactment in vivo in the sense of embarking on a purposeful and deliberate human encounter (Buber, 1957; May & Yalom, 1989). Like searching for the right words (Chapter 6), such acts are deliberate experiments with interactional meaning, and over time, they offer successive approximations toward a new meaning that holds some truth. Performing an act of this kind, willingly and with a broader meta-awareness of what it might mean, is a common intervention in both existential and attachment-based therapies (A. Pascual-Leone & Greenberg, 2007b).[12]

Admittedly, in this kind of corrective relational experience, the line begins to blur between what is an attachment-related process and what is a dramatic enactment per se. However, the issue becomes clearer using examples from couples therapy. Emotion-focused couples therapy is an empirically supported treatment for resolving relationship distress, and one of its principal interventions is the use of in vivo relational enactments to restructure interactions (Wiebe & Johnson, 2016; also partly anticipated by Minuchin's [2012] approach to family therapy). It is important to note that despite these being exchanges between members of the couple, enactments are neither behavioral role plays nor scripted rehearsals. In this context, enactments consist of emotionally expressive dialogues between partners, as orchestrated by their therapist (Tilley & Palmer, 2013). Research suggests shaping enactments in this way plays a crucial role in resolving interpersonal discord. For example, when therapists use evocative empathy and encourage the blaming party in a couple to reach out to their partner, that enactment between partners leads to softening in an expression of compassion from the blamed partner (Bradley & Furrow, 2004).

Consider the example of "Bill" and "Kate" who I saw for couples therapy. She longs for tenderness and affection and describes him as hard and cold. In this verbatim example from clinical work, the process of arousal, expression, and enactment is facilitated in the service of several different moment-by-moment objectives (marked with an asterisk). In what was one of the few times in their relationship to date, Bill became vulnerable and cried in session. Kate responds by speaking to him and touches his knee only gingerly, but he does not pull away.

THERAPIST TO KATE: And while you say this, I notice that you also rub his knee, but using the back of your hand, right? It's almost like you are saying, "I want to touch you, but I'm not sure you want to be touched." Is that right? [*Expressed arousal is used in the service of orienting to personal meaning and heightening client's awareness of immediate emotion.*]

KATE TO BILL: Yeah. . . . (*she smiles suddenly*)

THERAPIST TO KATE: Maybe you can tell him that? [*explicitly facilitating, giving permission, encouragement*]

KATE TO BILL: (*she now puts the palm of her hand on his knee and gives a squeeze*) I guess what I really want is to hug you.

BILL TO KATE: (*still tearful*) Well, I'd like that too. (*He smiles. They seem to hold their breath. There is a strange pause as each waits to see what will happen next.*)

THERAPIST TO BOTH: Well, uh, now is actually a particularly good time for hugging! [*orchestrating an enactment to embody meaning*] (*The three laugh as the hug happens. Kate now rubs his back with her hands and Bill kisses her shoulder as they hold each other.*)

The therapist's playful tone in orchestrating this simple enactment is both permission giving and supports the embodiment of meaning. I invited the couple to try hugging as an experiment, which is consistent with the Gestalt use of enactments as a method of exploring the possible tacit meanings in one's lived experience. Furthermore, this exploration in action is analogous to what Gendlin emphasized in focusing therapy as an exploration in words and symbolization. Ultimately, the intervention expands awareness about underlying needs through successive approximations or attempts at concretizing some tacit internal process, whether verbal or nonverbal, and in doing so, carries the emotional process vividly forward.

What is happening is more explicit in this approach to couples therapy, because while orchestrating enactments the therapist serves as a sort of third-party facilitator of what unfolds between members of the couple (e.g., recalling Moreno's director approach to group psychodrama). In psychodynamic therapy, many of these same enactment processes occur in a similar fashion, except through interpretations about the immediate relationship. However, because the psychodynamic therapist is at once facilitator and active participant, the process of enactment is both more covert and more conceptual. Safran (2002) discussed the process of attempting to understand a relational enactment as it takes place as involving sharing observations, including countertransference disclosures, asking questions, and speculating aloud.

Disembedding From an Unintended Enactment

Interpreting transference is a more inferential intervention in which the therapist draws attention to aspects of how a client experiences other important relationships that are now being ascribed (often unwittingly) to the therapist. When this interpretation is delivered and explored in real time (i.e., in the here and now), the conversation has a self-conscious and self-referential quality (i.e., "We are now enacting the exact thing that we were just talking about"). Articulating that process is also a special kind of enactment that re-structures the narrative from within. An example of this comes from the first experimental study on transference interpretation, conducted in Norway (Ulberg et al., 2014, p. 263):

PATIENT: When I'm together with somebody, I get this painful feeling that it's my fault when we're silent—that others think I'm a fool because I have nothing to say.

THERAPIST: Mmm.

PATIENT: I take the responsibility for the silence.

THERAPIST: Yes, you do. That's interesting because [in that scenario] it's the two of you, and here we are also just two [people] talking together.

PATIENT: Yes, because . . . I feel uneasy even here with you.

Here, the therapist makes explicit reference to what the client (patient) is doing here and now in session, and then those actions become pregnant with implicit meanings and usher in an implication for what could happen next.

As suggested by Høglend and colleagues (2011), a "focus on transference can enable the patient (and therapist) to distinguish what is real in the therapeutic relationship from what are enactments influenced by earlier experiences" (p. 698). As I have argued, enactments generate momentum in something that was previously only implied, and this allows one to explicate the embodied meaning. When introducing this section, I highlighted that one typically makes a choice to deliberately attempt an enactment, but psychodynamic transference is an exception to that. In the experiential enactments of Gestalt or emotion-focused therapies, for example, the therapist proposes a client agree to embark on an experiment by way of enactment, and that initial choice is what sets the process in motion. In the case of psychodynamic work, however, the client's choice to engage in an enactment only occurs later. In this version, therapist and client are more likely to suddenly find themselves already amid a transference enactment. The successfulness of working with transference is in the degree to which a client grasps this realization of what is currently happening right there and then makes a choice to disembed from the immediacy of that enactment. In some sense, whereas experiential therapies create meaning from the experience of getting into an enactment, transference-based therapy creates meaning by getting out of an unintended enactment.

Whether the spontaneous transference of social expectations between therapist and client or an orchestrated expression of genuine affection between a couple, enactments help objectify the process. In this way, a choice-point opens, a moment of self-awareness, in the immediacy between what went wrong and what might now make it right (Malan, 1979). Moreover, research on psychodynamic therapy showed that the impact of referring to and discussing events in this way had a positive impact up to 3 years after therapy had ended (Høglend et al., 2008). Clients who suffer more severe or chronic interpersonal difficulties (i.e., poor quality object relations) and are struggling in therapy to establish a strong working relationship are the ones who benefit most from transference interpretations. So, explicitly bringing attention to and formulating what is happening here and now, as an enactment that is distinct from the real relationship, is helpful specifically to clients who do not have clear conceptual representations of what healthy relationships look and feel like (Høglend et al., 2011).[13]

VIVID IMAGERY POTENTIATES CHANGE: I CAN SEE IT IN MY MIND'S EYE

Mental imagery can involve multiple sensory modalities including not only visual images but also bodily sensations, feelings, and the imagined experience of complex actions or even events unfolding over time (Holmes & Mathews, 2010). The vividness of imagery is related to the degree of psychological distance[14] one has in relation to some experience, whether that be imagined, recalled, or immediately presenting (Gu & Tse, 2016; Trope & Liberman, 2010). On one hand, the vividness of intrusive imagery is a hallmark of emotional problems, such as posttraumatic stress disorder or obsessive compulsions. On the other hand, research has established that the conspicuous absence of vivid imagery is a core pathological process that maintains generalized anxiety disorder and ruminative forms of depression. In these pervasive problems, excessive verbal-based thinking essentially prevents healthy image-based emotional processing (Borkovec et al., 2004; Fresno et al., 2002). So, the vividness of imagery that people make use of when considering their concerns has an important relationship to psychopathology and harnessing that process in clinical intervention has powerful potential.

Neurological Correlates of Vivid Experience

Neuroimaging has shown such a substantial correlation between activation in the brain's visual cortex and participants' subjective ratings on the vividness of imagery that it has led some researchers to claim that vividness can be measured objectively (Cui et al., 2007). Going further, brain imaging using functional magnetic resonance imaging (fMRI) also shows that when it comes to imagining personal events (whether historically accurate or fictitious), the neural activation supporting emotion occurs first, while brain activation supporting vividness occurs only later. Thus, when bringing autobiographical events to mind, emotional activation and vividness are both part of the subjective experience, but the time course in each of these underlying processes is different (Daselaar et al., 2008). Nevertheless, what follows is a complex and iterative process, where emerging affect and the visual clarity of some storied event gain momentum together, while further brain activation relates these to an autobiographical reflection (St. Jacques, 2012).

In other words, affect acts as the spark, and then vividness provides the fuel to yield a more complete emotional experience. This helps explain why imagery fosters emotional change to a greater extent than verbal–linguistic processing alone (Holmes & Mathews, 2010). It also suggests why adding imagery components (e.g., visualization) to interventions that are otherwise purely cognitive–verbal (e.g., thought challenging) will increase a treatment's efficiency for a range of disorders (Holmes et al., 2007; Hyett et al., 2018).

The Role of Vividness in Emotional Change

The vividness with which one recalls past experiences or emotionally explores some scenario (whether historically based or hypothetical) plays an important role in fomenting emotional arousal. It is also an integral part of successful enactments in psychotherapy. For example, in the treatment of complex trauma, for example, the reported vividness with which clients engage in enactments is as an index of their immediate affective involvement. That vividness was also a robust predictor of symptom change long after the treatment had ended (Paivio et al., 2001).

Facilitating therapeutic enactments is typically discussed in terms of physically staging some inter- or intrapersonal process, but ultimately the heart of this process is in the vividness of an imaginal experience that a client conjures up through creative fantasy.[15] Without vividness, dramatic enactments are no more than a hollow staging where clients acquiescently go through the motions. This suggests that the physicality of a dramatic enactment is not the only way of doing it; instead, it can also be approximated through smaller increments. A host of other creative experiential interventions can be used to create poignancy and heighten emotional arousal, including the use of poetic and metaphorical language, visual art with guided imagery, role play with props, and so on (for a case study of couples therapy, see Hinkle et al., 2015). Furthermore, when therapists intentionally introduced an appropriate metaphor in session, clients found the formulation was easier to remember, and they perceived that session as more helpful (Martin et al., 1992). The point of these strategies (to the degree that clients welcome them) is to create emotional engagement and vivid imagery to activate and then elaborate the implications of what are otherwise only tacit emotional meanings.

Treatment research also suggests evocativeness and vividness can be purposefully used within session to facilitate good moment-by-moment process (Adams, 2010). When clients in therapy for depression described external events using more vivid language, those emotionally evocative events were immediately followed by increases in emotional arousal, a pattern that occurred more often in sessions where there was some productive resolution as compared with less useful sessions. This observation highlights that encouraging the vivid description of events, particularly when they are problematic or puzzling to clients, can heighten arousal and seems to initiate successful emotional processing in treatment (Watson, 1996). Metaphor, generated by either clients or therapists, is another subtle way of evoking vivid mental imagery. According to clients, metaphors emerge from the association of relevant meanings as they try to verbally depict an experience being felt in-session. In this sense, the use of individual metaphors can be thought of as *micro-enactments*, where one creatively portrays some complex affective meaning state. This tool allows clients to clarify their self-concept both in terms of identity and in the relationship patterns they experience in their lives (Angus & Rennie, 1989).

Adding to these qualitative and process accounts, a review of experimental findings in cognitive neuroscience confirms that using mental imagery evokes stronger emotional responses as compared to representations in verbal form. Moreover, the literature suggests several related explanations for why this seems to be the case (Holmes & Mathews, 2010). First, vivid imagery is closely related to sensory perceptual signals, which have a more direct influence on the brain's emotional system and are relatively unmediated by conceptual language. This mechanism is intuited by arts-based and other experiential interventions that put a premium on preverbal experience (recall the phrase, "Don't tell us, show us"). Second, imagery is closely linked to and helps one evoke autobiographical memories about past experiences.[16] Third, there is a fundamental processing overlap between firsthand perceptual processes and working with mental imagery, which can lead one to respond as if being confronted with real-life emotionally arousing cues. This mechanism is what allows therapeutic enactments to restructure a narrative from within its existing meaning context, changes that are then reconsolidated into newly updated memories (Lane & Nadel, 2020).

The creative (re)entry into an imaginary circumstance is a complex psychological process. The intensity of that emotional experience depends on several factors, including the image perspective one chooses to adopt. Experiments suggest using mental imagery from a first-person perspective (e.g., as if one were embedded within the imagined scenario or scene) is more emotionally evocative than imagery from a third-person observer's perspective (e.g., as if one were removed, a fly on the wall, watching oneself as the scene unfolds; see Chapter 22). The clinical implication of this for introducing vivid imagery and using enactments in therapy is that emotional processing (of this particular kind) is optimized when clients assume first-person perspectives by taking on the role, embodying it, and imagining the perceptual field from their personal point of view (Gu & Tse, 2016; Holmes & Mathews, 2010; Libby & Eibach, 2002).[17] Used this way, mental imagery can act as an emotional amplifier and can be harnessed in the therapeutic process (Holmes & Mathews, 2010). Moreover, a body of research on the neuroscience of arousal and memory encoding shows that intense emotional experiences are essentially burned into memory (Lane & Nadel, 2020; Talmi, 2013).

WITH OR WITHOUT THE ACTUAL ENACTMENT: IS THERE A SIMPLER WAY?

It is not uncommon that therapeutic enactment tasks are initially met by clients with some awkwardness, particularly in individual therapy (Stiegler, Binder, et al., 2018). However, the performance-related aspect of such tasks can pose extra difficulty to some clients. Based on clinical observations during supervision, when a therapist first proposes chairwork to their client, the best predictor of whether a client is going to accept and fully engage with that enactment is probably the confidence with which the therapist presents it (L. S. Greenberg, personal communication, October 19, 2006). So, therapists who present the task weakly and with uncertainty are more likely to have their clients decline to participate (e.g., Therapist: "Uh. . . . Do you want to try something? It's a bit weird, um . . . but maybe it will be okay. If you wanted, you could. . . .").

Meanwhile, a therapist who introduces and recommends chairwork with conviction inspires the client's curiosity and confidence (e.g., Therapist: "I know something that would be very helpful here! This is useful for getting to the core of what's going on. Ok, let's try this. . . ."). Of course, there are also important client variables that influence someone's willingness to freely engage in enactment tasks. Conversational analysis has also been used to explore how therapists might best negotiate a client's reluctance to engage in enactment tasks such as chairwork (Muntigl et al., 2020).

Chairwork Compared With Treatment as Usual

The question of whether dramatic enactments are necessary as such is important to discerning the essential change processes underlying these interventions. For group treatments using drama therapy, enactments are so central that removing them would undermine the central axis of intervention as well as the group's relational dynamic in these shared experiences. However, the research question is more easily addressed in the context of individual therapy.

As cited earlier (A. Pascual-Leone & Baher, 2023), a meta-analysis showed at least five dismantling studies have been conducted using randomized clinical trials (readers may also consider Høglend et al., 2008).[18] One of these was a landmark study that compared two arms in the treatment of depression: emotion-focused therapy (using chairwork as usual) versus a version of the treatment without chairwork (i.e., emphasizing empathic exploration of the client's experience; R. N. Goldman et al., 2006). Both versions of treatment were helpful in reducing depression, with or without the use of enactments, although using chairwork gave clients some distinct advantages. When therapists used the enactment intervention, it helped clients get significantly better according to all measures of treatment outcome (e.g., decreasing their depression and interpersonal problems while also increasing self-esteem). Overall, judiciously adding the use of enactment tasks to the treatment of depression seems to increase the size of beneficial effects of experiential psychotherapy from large to very large (R. N. Goldman et al., 2006). Furthermore, following-up clients over the longer term has shown that adding enactment tasks that characterize emotion-focused therapy (beyond an empathic relational treatment) led to a longer maintenance of gains up to 18-months posttreatment. Indeed, according to client self-reports during the year and a half after treatment, having done enactments as part of their therapy led clients to later use more active and effective strategies for coping with their distress (Ellison et al., 2009).

Enactments are densely layered interventions, and using them often turns out to recapitulate some of the prior treatment process as well as provide material to be further elaborated in the sessions that follow. So, showing that an in-session enactment has a specific and local effect (in time) would further strengthen the causal argument that enactment-related processes are mechanisms of change. Using a multiple baseline design, two-chair tasks (in which clients enacted their self-criticism) were only introduced, by prescription, half-way through the course of treatment. This allowed researchers to create two distinct phases of emotion-focused therapy in the treatment of depressive and anxiety symptoms (Stiegler, Molde, & Schanche, 2018). Then, looking for discontinuities in the progress of symptom change allowed researchers to locate more precisely when the benefit of enactments may have been accrued. The treatment phase in which clients enacted two-chair dialogues had a more dramatic impact on reducing symptoms than the earlier phase without dialogues. Interestingly, this study also showed using two-chair dialogues impacted the somatic-affective components of depression more substantially than cognitive components, which converges with other findings on the impact of expression, arousal, and enactments.

Is It Better to Talk to the Real Person?

Sometimes one might dispense with the theatrics and just have a real conversation. Imagining a conversation in an empty-chair task might be useful, for example, if the significant other were deceased. However, if they were available, would it not be better to directly facilitate a real conversation? One clinical trial has considered this very practical question by cleverly comparing attachment-based family therapy with emotion-focused therapy (for individuals) to tease out the relative effects of real or imaginal dialogues on symptom improvement (Diamond et al., 2016). Young adults who were angry at their parents and the avoidance of attachment to them were assigned to one of two conditions. In one treatment arm, the young adults attended individual therapy where they imagined speaking to and enacting their parent (who did not attend; i.e., an empty-chair task). In the other treatment arm, young adults attended sessions of family therapy accompanied by their parent, in which the young adult expressed their emotions and needs directly to their parent in real conversations facilitated by the therapist.

Both conditions showed similar improvements in psychological symptoms, anger resolution, and attachment anxiety. However, the process pathways toward these symptom changes seemed to be different. Empty-chair tasks in individual therapy produced more productive emotional processing than having direct interpersonal dialogues by a large effect. In contrast, only direct interpersonal dialogues in family therapy were associated with decreases in attachment avoidance by a moderate effect. Finally, positive changes in emotional processing (in either treatment) predicted symptom change, whereas reductions in attachment avoidance did not (Diamond et al., 2016). In sum, whether it is better to talk to the real person depends on one's treatment goal. If the client needs some sort of relationship resolution and to stop avoiding a significant other, then it would be better to engage in a real interpersonal dialogue. However, if what the client needs is to work through emotional difficulties to promote symptom change, then it would be better to use imaginary dialogues through chairwork.

Chairwork Without the Chairs?!

Although using chairwork in-session facilitates expressive arousal, heightens vividness, and deepens emotional exploration, it also typically involves quite another kind of process: the multi-step sequential ordering of discrete emotions. As suggested in the introduction to expressive arousal, the process often works synergistically with other forms of emotional processing. Sequential transformation is another type of emotional processing central to emotion-focused therapy, and it often occurs in tandem with expressive arousal (see Chapters 12–16). Furthermore, the chief intervention for facilitating those sequences of emotion is also the use of chairwork or other enactments, the pattern unfolding as clients move through various stages of an enactment toward resolution. So, while dismantling and comparison studies affirm the beneficial impact of using enactments as interventions, they do not disentangle the processes of vividness and expressive arousal (i.e., the intensity of emotional expression) from the concomitant process of sequential transformations (e.g., the discrete ordering of emotional states). Doing so would require an analogue to the usual enactment interventions, one that does not explicitly use chairwork or explicitly orchestrated enactments yet still entails some structure to guide the client(s) through the same passage of emotional sequences. The next two studies I discuss did just that.

A very brief course of emotion-focused couples therapy studied the role of interpersonal enactments by randomizing half the participating couples to receive three sessions in which the couple communicated directly via enactments (i.e., enactment-based sessions), followed by three more sessions in which the couple communicated indirectly via the therapist (i.e., therapist-centered sessions). In short, the flow of interaction was the primary structural distinction between these two modes of intervention. Meanwhile, the other half of the couples in the study received the reverse pattern of therapy (Butler et al., 2011). Couples who started therapy with enactment-based sessions reported greater initial increases in attachment security that those who started their treatment with therapist-centered sessions. Furthermore, those same couples who started with enactments in sessions 1–3 continued to show improvement after switching to therapist-centered work in sessions 4–6. However, starting early in treatment may be an important part of the process, as those who started with therapist-centered work (sessions 1–3) did not enjoy a corresponding increase in attachment security upon switching to enactment work (sessions 4–6). Interestingly, there was also an interaction with gender, where men improved the most when enactment sessions came first, but that order was less important for women. Whatever the case, while introducing enactments on a prescribed treatment schedule can yield insight into this change mechanism, the multiple baseline design also comes with a rigidity that is admittedly Procrustean. As experienced clinicians will confirm, the timing is often critical to the usefulness of activating this process in treatment.

In working with people suffering from trauma, retraumatization and problems related to hyperarousal poses a treatment risk in general, specifically when using evocative interventions such as enactments or vividly reimagining one's trauma. For this reason, another study looked at emotion-focused therapy in a randomized clinical trial to treat adult survivors of child abuse and then examined the benefit of empty-chair enactments in which clients imagined confronting their perpetrators (Paivio et al., 2010). In one version of treatment, the explicit use of an empty-chair task was routinely used (e.g., physical enactment of roles by shifting chairs, imagining and "looking at" the other person, talking to the other in first person as if in dialogue). This was compared with an alternate version of treatment, which involved a non-enactment analogue. As with the study of couples, that comparison task used empathic exploration to implicitly follow similar process steps as the original chair task, all the while keeping therapeutic work in the context of conversations directly between therapist and client (e.g., not introducing any guided imagery tasks or enactment and typically speaking about the perpetrator in third person; see Paivio & Pascual-Leone, 2023).

In this randomized clinical trial of 16–20 sessions, therapists were permitted to use the corresponding version of intervention (i.e., with or without chairs) as needed and whenever it was suitable. Findings showed that both versions of the treatment were highly effective and produced very large treatment gains for working through complex trauma (Paivio et al., 2010). The clinical implication is that if clients are unable or unwilling to participate in enactments where they imagine and confront their perpetrators, therapists can accomplish much of the same kind of emotional processing using an implicitly structured task. Although focusing on the vividness of imaginal experiences is less evocative, it offers an important alternative. Even so, the explicit use of dramatic enactments in chairwork still provided a small meaningful advantage in terms of outcome. So, when possible, best practices in this treatment approach would be to make use of formal enactments (Paivio & Pascual-Leone, 2023).

Therapists who are new to using chairwork interventions in emotion-focused therapy are sometimes relieved by a finding like this, because it suggests that without sacrificing too much, they may not have to move the furniture around after all. However, most therapists quickly discover the technical advantages to using structured physical enactments. It is critical to note that the treatment comparison to doing formal enactments was not as simple as omitting the enactment; rather, it involved a complex and multistep process for therapists except without ever using physical structuring or formally introducing any task as such (Paivio et al., 2010). Even when enactments are only done implicitly, they must entail a vivid and imaginal reentry into the experience with the same attention to emotional detail, evocativeness, and emphasis on expressive arousal. So, the hidden problem or disadvantage for psychotherapists in what at first appears to be an ideal solution is plainly that using enactment procedures implicitly is much harder to do. Moreover, doing it right matters. In one of the few studies on psychotherapists' technical proficiency, the skillfulness with which therapists use specific procedures of a therapeutic enactment is itself a predictor of good outcome (Paivio et al., 2004).

A Conceptual Scaffold for Clients and Their Therapists

Using enactments has advantages for both clients and their therapists. While there are benefits for emotional processing, enactments also have implications for grasping the complexity of case formulation and how it applies moment by moment.

A Framework for Guiding Client Process

For clients, using explicit enactments helps with emotional processing. Beyond symptom management, enactments carry the implicit goal of helping clients realize they may be complicit in a meta-process, for example, of making themselves anxious. This is especially the case when one's emotional awareness of underlying processes is less developed, as in people suffering from generalized anxiety disorder (Watson & Greenberg, 2017). Clients report that the psychogenetic process (e.g., how one actively makes oneself anxious or depressed) becomes blatantly apparent when they participate in an enactment between parts of the self (Stiegler, Binder, et al., 2018). So, first, working this way facilitates a meta-awareness, clarifying the problem.

Second, as we know from the research presented on imaginal vividness, working from a first-person perspective (which is central to enactments) is more evocative, incisive, and emotionally engaging (Holmes & Mathews, 2010). Artificial or orchestrated as they may be, enactments are fast, direct, and straightforward tools for evoking emotion and helping clients creatively engage with experience. Mechanisms of how enactment facilitates feeling have been the focus of this chapter. Third, another issue related to facilitating client process is its impact on the flow of conversation. As reviewed, controlled research shows engaging the body through gesture helps facilitate one's production of verbal content (C. Lewis et al., 2015). For example, this principle is exercised in drama therapies by keeping clients slowly moving around the room (e.g., Therapist: "Let's walk. . . . If your feet keep moving, the words will keep coming.").

Advantages to Case Formulation and Tracking the Process

In addition to how enactments guide and scaffold the processing for clients, these tasks also seem to help therapists with their cognitive load—an advantage that is often overlooked. When therapists try to guide their clients implicitly through the same process steps as a formal enactment—but without the use of chairs—it adds substantially more to their mental burden (e.g., see Paivio et al. 2010, cited earlier). Tracking a client's process through the nonlinear and highly dynamic changes in their meaning and feeling is a lot of information to manage. So, using the physicality of enactments between parts of the self or relational positions serves as a spatial mneomic. The physical structure helps organize clients as much as therapists in their effort to track a complex and rapidly unfolding experience of emotion. Common examples of this are when a therapist observes, "Oh! So that's the critic's voice creeping in again, isn't it? That's from over there. Okay then, switch chairs." Or similarly, when a client reflects, "Yikes! I sounded like my mother just then. And it makes me mad. I want to respond now and tell her to back off!" and then the client spontaneously changes their position. In short, using enactments to explore the development of a complex psychological experience is like using the physical layout of pieces on a chessboard to formally represent a dynamic and metamorphizing set of internal relations among parts of the self or self-objects.[19]

So, when therapists and clients use enactments of internal experience, those enactments also serve an organizing function to reduce complexity and assist in the collaborative formulation of an understanding about how the client dynamically constructed their own sense of self. Formally using physical enactments in this way facilitates key emotional processes, but it is also an important way of managing conceptual complexity. It serves as a physical bookmark to locate one's place in an unfolding conceptual space. This may be particularly useful early on as therapists are collaboratively developing case formulations with their clients (R. N. Goldman & Greenberg, 2015; Paivio & Pascual-Leone, 2023).

Finally, if one understands enactment as an explicit portrayal of intrapersonal or interpersonal issues, it becomes clear this is a conceptual scaffold for understanding otherwise implicit processes. In short, enactments (and conversations about enactment) become tools for exploring immediate processes that cannot be easily discussed retrospectively. Psychodrama slows down and maps out the relational processes using physical space as group members walk around the therapy room. In emotion-focused therapy or schema therapy, clients are encouraged to vividly imagine and dialogue with parts of the self or others who are not present. In a psychodynamic therapy, mapping out the enactment is done conceptually, verbally juxtaposing the transference relationship against the real relationship. A further implication is that even when it is unclear what may be at play, enactments can serve as a canvas to tease out the contrasting voices that contribute to an emotional problem and its possible resolution.

From a symptom-focused perspective, these techniques are sometimes dismissed as fanciful and impractical when working with serious pathology. Admittedly, the novelty of enactments likely does contribute to the salience of these tasks in client accounts. These are highly memorable treatment events. However, while enactments themselves may be imaginary, their effects on process as well as measurable symptom change are very real (Armstrong et al., 2016; A. Pascual-Leone & Baher, 2023). Quantitative research on humanistic and psychodynamic therapies confirms that using and discussing enactments offers a special benefit to clients' symptom change in cases of depression, anxiety, and eating disorders (e.g., L. S. Greenberg & Goldman, 2018) but also with personality disorders, complex histories of relational trauma, somatization, and when clients have trouble feeling understood by their therapist (Abbass et al., 2012; Høglend et al., 2011; Paivio & Pascual-Leone, 2023; Pos & Greenberg, 2012).

Finally, during the COVID-19 pandemic, therapists and clients around the world found themselves assessing the advantages and disadvantages of using enactments as part of their usual practice. This natural experiment unfolded as therapists from a range of treatment perspectives (e.g., compassion-focused, emotion-focused, cognitive behavior, and schema therapies; psychodrama) were forced to move their sessions online. Using enactments via teletherapy clearly has logistical challenges. Nevertheless, a survey of the practice experiences reported by expert therapists concluded that enactments are still acceptable, effective, and valuable, even in the absence of a physically shared space and the constraints of working through a computer screen (Pugh et al., 2021).

WHEN SHOULD ONE DO CHAIRWORK AND HOW MUCH?

Not engaging with these tasks for long enough has already been cited as one reason why enactments may not be productive (Stiegler, Binder, et al., 2018). So, given the demonstrated usefulness of these evocative tasks for processing emotion, another common question from clinicians is how often should therapeutic enactments be used for emotional processing? And when should they be introduced? One of the clinical trials on emotion-focused therapy for depression reported that after session 3, once the relationship had been established, enactment tasks were performed in about 30% of the subsequent sessions (R. N. Goldman et al., 2006). That could be construed as suggesting enactments were used about every third session, although the distribution is unlikely to be even across cases.

In a trial of emotion-focused therapy for complex trauma, treatments were found to use enactments an average of about five times over the course of 16–20 sessions (Paivio et al., 2001). Indeed, the variation across individual treatments was substantial. If one considered the central two thirds of the treatment sample (i.e., excluding extreme cases), using enactments ranged from as little as once or twice in the entire course of treatment to using enactments as often as every second session. The reason why there is so much variability across cases in how often enactments are used is answered by research I discussed in Chapter 4 on emotional engagement. Briefly, when it comes to enactments, the best predictor of treatment gain was not only a client's level of engagement (e.g., vividness of experience, expressive arousal, spontaneous involvement) but rather the interaction between engagement and the frequency with which these enactment tasks were introduced. Thus, a client whose engagement is more superficial but who does the tasks much more frequently could get the same benefit as a client who is highly engaged and does enactment tasks just a few times (Paivio et al., 2001).

Some therapists feel it is more conservative or cautious to leave the unpredictability of enactments for later in therapy. However, it turns out the opposite is true as converging lines of evidence suggest introducing enactments early in treatment is best. Enactments are inherently dramatic, both for their facilitation of expressive arousal given their salience as well as defining an encounter in the here and now. As such, the novelty of explicitly participating in enactments often sets a precedent for the level of engagement and the momentum with which treatment will proceed. So, the first enactment a therapist introduces is critical and it sets the bar for subsequent enactment tasks that may follow. When this is done early in therapy, it also establishes the overall pace and expectancies for treatment progress. This is why, when emotion-focused therapists introduced an enactment in session 4 and clients fully engaged with their trauma (e.g., imagining a confrontation with their perpetrator), that single experience of enactment was still a predictor of good symptom outcomes even 6 months after treatment had ended (Paivio et al., 2001).

The importance of having enactments in the first three sessions is echoed by experimental research already cited on couples therapy (Butler et al., 2011). Another study interviewed couples early in therapy (i.e., during the first four sessions) when they were more distressed and compared with couples who were interviewed later in therapy (i.e., during the last four sessions) when they were presumably less volatile and less distressed. The open-ended interviews used video of the sessions to facilitate discussion about what the couple found useful, and they also indirectly inquired about the use of highly structured versus minimally structured enactments (Andersson et al., 2006). In the first four sessions of therapy, couples reported that they preferred highly structured enactments, which often helps manage a couple's sensitivity and emotional volatility. In contrast, when couples were interviewed during the last four sessions of therapy, they did not indicate any clear preference in how structured a task was, which researchers attributed to their reduced vulnerability. The contrast in preference for enactments seems to reflect the changing needs of couples as they develop emotionally over the course of therapy.

Overall, findings like these suggest that if a treatment is going to make use of therapeutic enactments, it is generally advantageous to introduce that kind of processing experience early in treatment, as soon as the therapeutic alliance will allow for it. Furthermore, enactments can be more or less structured and one strategy for keeping heightened arousal from exceeding the optimal zone of arousal is to provide more structure to clients in doing these tasks. Finally, while enactments facilitate the creation of meaning, they are sometimes also profound proclamations of the self. The next and final chapter on expressive arousal considers how expressiveness helps cultivate an active, free, and joyful self!

ENDNOTES

1. Generating an emotional experience by working "from the inside out" or "from the outside in" are notions used in theater schools and are metaphors that refer to the different techniques (i.e., constructive strategies) an actor might use to generate a desired emotional experience (see S. Moore, 1984). Although these metaphors can be conceptually useful as starting points for clinicians, they should not be taken too

literally or too far. On final analysis, it is certain that all clinical work that uses expressive arousal is probably operating in both directions to varying degrees and at various moments of the process.

2. Pos and Greenberg (2012) point out that despite the potentially evocative nature of these tasks, used another way, enactments can also be helpful in down-regulating people who feel overwhelmed by emotion, such as those suffering from borderline personality processes. Indeed, another facet of enactments is that they offer a concrete and externalized narrative frame, which allows one to organize and grapple with some emotional experiences.

3. Referring to the here and now of an experiential moment has become a familiar turn of phrase in psychotherapy literatures of various stripes. It often goes unrecognized that this was a term originally coined by Moreno in reference to immediacy of psychodramatic enactments.

4. The intensity of this intervention schedule also has some bearing on group cohesion and the induction of members into a creative and dramatic process, particularly when emotional experience and aroused enactments are central process goals within a session.

5. In 2012, I had the pleasure of working with Marvin Westwood, psychologist and originator of this program, at the University of British Colombia. Encouraging the use of mental health care services is a difficult issue in general, and particularly among war veterans. Ingeniously, this treatment program is billed as a training course, and holding it on a university campus also helps destigmatize it. Finally, most men did not volunteer directly for their own treatment; rather, they agreed to participate with the knowledge that they would be helping other veterans, since they already have a sense of what their brothers-in-arms had been through.

6. Here, *meta-awareness* refers to a higher order of awareness, for example, when one considers the interaction between various parts at work during a therapeutic enactment (A. Pascual-Leone & Greenberg, 2007b). The term can also refer to gaining awareness of the scope and limits inherent in one's usual frame of reference, which is more akin to psychodynamic insight or emerging awareness of personal themes. Both are forms of meta-cognitive insight and this is discussed in later chapters, which describe "reflection on emotion" as a unique kind of emotional processing.

7. In Chapters 12 and 13, I discuss the *sequential transformation of emotion*, which is a different kind of emotional processing from expressive arousal. Sequential transformations involve a pair of emotions experienced in a specific order, which then interact. In this case, for example, it might be maladaptive guilt and sadness followed by, and transformed through, primary adaptive love. Importantly, the interaction between successive emotions is not always a direct consequence of altering the relative activations of presenting emotions. However, when it does happen, the overarching change process that results is a synergy between those two kinds of emotional processing. This is a common example of the overdetermination of change, through differing but compatible mechanisms.

8. Although enactments require a setting (i.e., presuming some time, place, etc.), the narrative elaboration can be quite minimal. This process is not the same as "storying" a coherent narrative about the experience of events or one's identity (see Chapters 17, 18, and 21).

9. Method acting was made famous in the Western world by actors like Marlo Brando, Dustin Hoffman, Robert DeNiro, and Meryl Streep, among others.

10. Although Perls first studied with Moreno in New York in the 1950s, it is unclear why recognition of this lineage came only later. I speculate that understating the influences of Moreno and Russian theatre in the 1960s and 1970s may have been related to a political climate during the Cold War, which was when gestalt therapy was being elaborated in the United States. Whatever the case, the influence has since been documented (see Scheiffele, 2008).

11. Similarly, "say yes" is one of the axioms in improv theatre. Rather than resisting or denying the imaginary circumstances presented by fellow performers, the position one takes as a performer in improv theatre is to respond with, "yes, and. . ." Thus, as a rule, an actor accepts the nature of a presenting hypothetical situation (however absurd) and then adds some contribution through creative elaboration. In much the same way, enactments in therapy are about (a) willing and deliberate engagement and (b) the elaboration of meaning.

12. Again, the higher order reflection on this process is itself a different kind of emotional processing, which entails subsequently decentering oneself from the enactment (see Chapters 17, 20, and 23).

13. Notice this is opposite to former conventional assumptions, which took for granted that emotionally mature and interpersonally healthy individuals would derive more benefit from transference interpretation. On the contrary, clients with healthy attachment histories may be disadvantaged by such interpretations, perhaps because these interventions are perceived as unnecessary, overzealous, or pedantic (Høglend et al., 2011).

14. The construct of psychological distance is discussed at length in Chapters 20 and 22.

15. The analogue of vividness during a relational human encounter, as described in the couples therapy example (earlier), is arguably one aspect of therapeutic presence (cf. L. S. Greenberg & Geller, 2012). This also becomes apparent in some examples of transference interpretation, where the real encounter is vividly contrasted with unhealthy enactments (c.f. Høglend et al., 2008).

16. The relationship is one of close association, although the causal directional is complex. While vividness can certainly evoke emotion, neural mechanisms also allow a memory to be enhanced (i.e., becoming more vivid and accurate) when one is emotionally aroused during the consolidation of that memory (Talmi, 2013).

17. This finding on perspective-taking is also relevant to reflecting on emotion, which is a different kind of emotional processing from expressive arousal (see Chapters 17 and 20). So, in contrast, if one is processing objective was to reduce arousal and think about emotion, then taking a third-person observer's perspective would be most helpful.

18. The work of Høglend and colleagues (2008) offers yet another dismantling study, which is relevant here if one considers enactments to include the self-referencing discussions that follow a transference interpretation. Their randomized clinical trial was used to dismantle psychodynamic therapy, showing the long-term benefits in specifically using transference interpretations (cited earlier).

19. By analogy, consider that the game of chess is about the configuration of relations between parts, not the shape or color of tangible pieces. It is even possible to play without a chessboard, using letters and numbers as coordinates (e.g., "knight moves from B1 to C3"). In this sense, displaying pieces on a physical board is no more than an elaborate memory aid for players to consider the moment-by-moment states of a formal system. In psychotherapy, the case formulation a therapist uses to makes sense of a client's emerging process is itself a formidable cognitive task. The "chairs" in chairwork serve as a conceptual aid to therapists. Other than taking notes in session, there are relatively few tools to assist therapists in managing that cognitive load, particularly if they do not want to interrupt the flow of client emotion or the relational connection.

11

The Proclamation of Self

I Felt It, I Said It, I Did It!

The oldest known graffiti at Pompeii also happens to be among the simplest: Gaius was here. Or, more precisely, "Gaius Pumidius Diphilus was here," along with a time stamp, which historians have dated to October 3, 78 B.C. It's a classic. . . . So-and-so was here . . . has been one of the messages humans have scrawled, etched, and eventually Sharpied and spray painted onto public spaces for millennia . . . People want to write on things to be known.

—ADRIENNE LAFRANCE, *POMPEII'S GRAFFITI*
AND THE ANCIENT ORIGINS OF SOCIAL MEDIA[1]

In his book *Feeling and Will* (1891), James Mark Baldwin attempts to describe dimensions of emotion's phenomenology. He suggests that the self is the most fixed point of reference and is therefore the ultimate reality. In this way, acts of expressive arousal often supersede other mental processes, as seen in the way a client might suddenly overcome defensive inhibitions. Furthermore, affirming the self through making the unsayable into something sayable or expressing a declaration of personal experience can, even more than freedom, spark a sense of joy in one's vitality. Put simply, the argument being made here is along the lines of "I feel, therefore I am" (a refurbished alternative to Descartes's much older axiom). Overall, the neurological substrate of expressive arousal in this role will be quite complex, but it may involve von Economo neurons, which are particularly common in the brains of social animals, are fast acting, and they seem to be the spark of agentic initiatives and action (Butti et al., 2013).

https://doi.org/10.1037/0000460-012
Principles of Emotion Change: What Works and When in Psychotherapy and Everyday Life, by
A. Pascual-Leone
Copyright © 2026 by the American Psychological Association. All rights reserved.

This brief chapter highlights one final process by which expressive arousal facilitates change, and that is through its affirmation of the self. Acts of freely expressed arousal stand as a testament of the self. They are embodied experiences of one's identity and its proclamation. Furthermore, when emotional expressions are sufficiently articulated to be goal directed, they are also lived experiences of personal agency (i.e., praxis). The clinical implication on a basic level is that being active helps to counter a sense of helplessness and passivity. It also counters some of the demoralizing feelings that accompany emotional and psychiatric problems (Blatner, 2000). On a higher level of complexity, this also means that expressive arousal can play a key role in healthy declarations of the self and augmenting—or better stated, exercising—one's sense of self.

ACTIVE EXPRESSION AFFIRMS THE SELF

Hopefulness is an important component in healthy expressions of the self. However, even the expression of hope is a process that depends very much on the meaning context in which it occurs. For example, after discovering that emotional expressiveness was a unique longitudinal predictor of health in women coping with breast cancer, researchers went on to speculate on how that specific process might confer its benefit: "Emotional expression may drive effective goal pursuit [but] only for those who have a strong sense of agency and avenues for attaining goals, as supported by the obtained interactions between dispositional hope and expressive coping" (Stanton et al., 2000, p. 880). This role of hopefulness and the implied sense of self as deserving, valuable, and worthy is also inherently captured in expressions of primary adaptive emotion (e.g., assertive anger, adaptive grief, self-compassion), which entail healthy ownership of one's experience and productive action tendencies. In contrast, this is not the case for expressions of maladaptive or secondary symptomatic emotion (e.g., rumination, whining protest, global distress, ambivalent engagement, when the self is experienced as bad or weak; A. Pascual-Leone, 2018).

There is consensus among clinical theorists that a client's relationship to their own burgeoning affect is critical to their sense of self. However, developing criteria to dynamically measure someone's sense of self is a daunting task. Observational tools that do this in psychotherapy research have counted the expression of activated and self-affirming emotion as evidencing a healthy sense of self (e.g., McCullough et al., 2008). These are visceral and palpable experiences of one's own feelings as being a lived affirmation of oneself in the flesh.[2] Research on cognitive, experiential, and self-directed therapies have shown that the arousal and expression of anger (specifically) was related to the development of agency, self-efficacy, and self-assertion (Beutler, Engle, et al., 1991; Van Velsor & Cox, 2001).

A critical finding on this topic comes from the moment-by-moment ratings of client expressive arousal in general during experiential therapy for depression. Increases in the expressive arousal of emotion during the middle phase of therapy predicted subsequent increases in a client's self-esteem at the end of therapy (Missirlian et al., 2005). Furthermore, in the treatment of personality disorders that feature anxiety and worry (Cluster C), if a client experienced more approach-motivated emotions (i.e., activating affects as opposed to inhibiting affects) in a session than was usual for them, it predicted a subsequent increase in the client's sense of self (Berggraf et al., 2014). This held irrespective of whether clients were being treated with short-term dynamic psychotherapy or cognitive therapy, and growth in a client's sense of self over those treatments was linked to good outcomes (Schanche et al., 2011). Process–outcome relationships like these speak to expressions of aroused emotion as helping individuals to affirm their sense of self, which in turn facilitates good treatment outcomes. However, the inception of that self-affirming experience is not obvious and is probably predicated on the earlier groundwork of exploring emotion.

Affirming the Self Is a Later-Phase Process

A previously cited study on the impact of experiential therapy for depression (Pos et al., 2017; see Chapter 9, this volume) also explored the impact of arousal longitudinally over various phases of treatment. As it happens, the explanatory power of a client's expressed arousal remains relatively stable over the course of their treatment. As a predictor, it explained almost 20% of the treatment's outcome in both middle and later phases of treatment. However, the tight relationship between arousal and awareness that was observed in the middle phase of therapy became markedly weaker later in therapy. As treatment progressed, the importance of expressive arousal in relation to awareness dropped by about half the strength in association to what it previously had. As Pos and colleagues (2017) ask, if expressive arousal is no longer about facilitating awareness later in therapy, then what is it doing? Indeed, the weakening of a previously strong mediating relationship with awareness while still maintaining its strength as predictor of treatment outcome suggests that expressive arousal may start to facilitate change in some new way. Again, this highlights how a given process (in this case, expressive arousal) could have various functions across treatment approaches and even across phases within the same treatment.

It seems reasonable to speculate that whereas arousal facilitates awareness in the middle phase of experiential therapy, arousal in the late phase of therapy may be functioning through the more behavioral processes of expression, action, and embodied agency. I suggest that as clients approach the conclusion of their treatment, the mechanism of expressive arousal shifts. It comes to be less in the service of developing awareness and less about discovery, and it instead serves more as an affirmation of the self and more about declaration. Thus, in the latter phase of a successful therapy, clients arguably delight in their newfound freedom of expression, expanding their expressive range both personally and interpersonally.

Another observation by Pos and colleagues (2017) adds to this interpretation of their findings. They found that clients' average level of emotional arousal increased over the course of treatment. We also know that successful clients in that sample were not continually in high states of arousal but rather did this in bursts (Carryer & Greenberg, 2010). Taken together, this means the individual cases would seem to be increasing in their expressive range, most likely expanding incrementally as they repeatedly express emotion through successive waves of self-expression. If this pattern was like the saw-toothed patterns already described in research on emotional meaning making (A. Pascual-Leone, 2009; Stiles et al., 2004), then perhaps increased arousal near the end of therapy can be understood as exercising the self through self-expression.

Owning the Feeling

Enactment is a way of owning some implicit meaning that may have been previously dismissed or denied. The client experiences that they have an active hand in constructing some meaning, as if saying it makes it real and openly doing it makes it one's own. Thus, the story of what happened acts as both a testament of personal truth as well as a template for understanding situations (both past and current) in new ways.[3] Enactments that explore the satisfaction of one's existential needs also contribute a sense of overall cohesiveness within the self (Pearls et al., 1951).

Although the role of expressive arousal as an experience of freedom or openness toward life is something that clinicians and therapists will value, these existential processes are not typically captured by standard measures used in clinical research. Nevertheless, examples of those processes are easily found in everyday life. For instance, one of the ways disclosures and expressive acts (e.g., in speech, writing, behavior) facilitate change is by creating a tangible event, document, memento, and so on, which serves as a historical record of one's experience. As the epigraph to this chapter suggest, when people tag a wall with their name in graffiti, even when there is no interlocutor, the creation of these pure and concrete expressions, involves a proclamation of "I exist, I was here, this is me!" Expressing emotion in this case is itself an experience of freedom and vitality, where an individual deliberately chooses to let the arrow fly.

The pure action that goes with an emotional expression can have similarly palpable implications that affirm the self in a lived choice. It may represent inherently irreversible acts, which one knowingly accepts ownership of. An example is recounted by a man who talked to me about his starting a family later in life, when he had almost given up hope:

> The decision to have kids was an act of well-considered recklessness. I couldn't be sure if it was a good idea, the romantic relationship was so new, and yet it seemed like a gamble that I didn't want to miss out on making! So, that was the moment. I just looked her straight in the eye and said, "Do you want to make a baby?" And then we did.

Here, the expression of emotion essentially consolidates an existential commitment to a chosen life direction.

OVERCOMING DEFENSIVE INHIBITION

The role of using heightened arousal, physical engagement, and emotional expression to help people overcome their social and emotional inhibitions as a curative experience has a long tradition across ages and cultures.[4] In such examples,

> healing rituals and religious rites were preceded by the expectation that catharsis would occur and began with various devices to overcome resistance to emotional release. . . . Ordinary social restraint was further weakened through the use of alcoholic drinks, narcotics, and psychedelic mushrooms. These ritualized ceremonies enable participants to shed traditional inhibitions and depart from social norms which called for emotional restraint. . . . They provided a culturally sanctioned occasion for experiencing and expressing significant but taboo thoughts and feelings. (Nichols & Efran, 1985, p. 47)

Thus, expression of what hereto seemed too intense, terrifying, shameful, or ugly to express, becomes permissible and tolerable for exploration in treatments that value congruent disclosures of emotion. In short, "the unsayable becomes sayable" (L. S. Greenberg, 2010, p. 36).

The Courage to Speak (and Be Witnessed)

First and foremost, emotion has an internal organismic function, which is why experiencing and expressing arousal (e.g., with the right focus and toward the right target) essentially mobilizes the productive procedural value of emotion. However, concomitant with this, emotion also has an external and social function. This other function means that having one's arousal witnessed by someone (e.g., a therapist) can often lend a second layer of significance to one's expressive experience. This is a moment where the processes of expressive arousal and the therapeutic relationship coincide and interact synergistically.

Particularly when a compassionate other is present, the context offers permission to overcome defensive inhibition through expressive arousal, and that can be highly validating. However, the experience of validation only comes to fruition when a client completes the experience, which means following through with an act of observable expressive arousal. A client makes contact with their heart-wrenching grief about intimate losses, and the therapist responds with gentle eye contact and offers compassionate acceptance. Another client clenches their teeth and then lets out a guttural bellow of anger, calling out against injustice while the therapist sits in solidarity, echoing the gravity of what is at hand. Allowing one's expression to be witnessed is an experience unto itself. The feelings in such examples are expressions of a personal reality, but by having them witnessed in the presence of another, they become a shared and validated reality (Geller & Greenberg, 2012). When therapists make empathic conjectures about their client's emotion, it models an exploratory process and implicitly gives permission for clients to feel and express their underlying experiences. It tells the client that the intensity of their experience is permissible in this context and welcome for discussion. This helps clients who are inhibited or ashamed of their experiences. Further, sometimes admitting one's experience to another person also serves as an admission of feeling to oneself.

Maladaptive emotion often requires permission giving to help destigmatize the experience. For example, early in treatment a client tried to apologize to me for her outpour of feeling and what she referred to as "making a weepy scene." However, rather than matching her overly precious treatment of emotion, I responded respectfully although also much more casually: "It's okay, so you feel stuff. [*nodding*] This is the place for it, and I'm okay with that [*smiling*]. Welcome to the Human Race!" Examples of well-chosen moments for permission giving often are in response to client vulnerability (e.g., weakness, shame) or forbidden feelings (e.g., anger). However, the relevance of this process can be true of any newly developed emotional experience, even for the riskiness of expressing positive feelings. Consider, for example, the role of the therapist in our verbatim exchange cited in Chapter 10 from "Bill" and "Kate" in couples therapy.

When Overcoming Inhibition Is Pivotal

In research on expressive writing and other forms of self-disclosure, a commonly explored theory is that confronting previously inhibited emotions is salubrious. While chronically inhibiting emotion has been shown to be harmful, the notion of just confronting inhibitions as a way of overcoming them is simplistic and questionable as a change process (Frattaroli, 2006). As discussed in Chapter 8, emotional expression usually involves much more than just engagement, venting, or catharsis; there is a wide range of other processes that are implicated and yet go undeclared in the notion of inhibition confrontation. Nevertheless, individual differences probably also play an important role. For example, the influence of gender and culture as treatment moderators is thought to stem from prescribed social norms regarding expressivity, with men and members of Asian culture being socialized to inhibit emotion more as compared with women and Caucasians (Lu & Stanton, 2010; Range & Jenkins, 2010). Arguably, the more fundamental issue is that "individuals who are ambivalent about expressing feelings might benefit most from [that process], because the perceived safety of expressing oneself . . . reduce[s] the conflict between the desire to disclose and the failure to do so" (Lu & Stanton, 2010, p. 671).

After receiving successful courses of either emotion-focused therapy or attachment-based family therapy for their unresolved anger toward a parent (i.e., individual vs. family therapy), young adults were asked during a follow-up interview about how they explained their personal change (Steinmann et al., 2017). Clients in both groups attributed their treatment gains to having expressed and explored emotions and specifically how they had been "saying difficult things aloud to their parents that had never been said before" (p. 281). Such moments were pivotal, even when the client was only having an imagined dialogue with their parent (i.e., in individual therapy), although they were even more impactful when the parent was present (i.e., in family therapy; see Diamond et al., 2016, discussed in Chapter 10 of this volume).

Sometimes the power of expression is naming the proverbial elephant in the room because it acknowledges what is being tacitly felt and breaks the ice for a brave new conversation. In line with the previously cited work and following a number of studies on group psychotherapy with patients suffering from metastatic cancer, Spiegel (1993), who collaborated with Yalom in working from an existential therapy approach, offers the following recommendation to individuals confronted with a life-threatening illness: "The best way for you, your family, and your friends to cope with illness is to do the hard emotional work of recognizing and feeling what those losses might mean" (p. 203). In short, overcoming defensive inhibition through the shared acknowledgment and expression of emotion, is an important part of working through with the existential challenges of life (and death).

THE JOY OF SELF-EXPRESSION

Clinical writing has keenly pointed out that clients commonly present with too much emotion of various kinds—too much fear, too much sadness, too much anger—and these are well discussed in the treatment and research literature. However, not enough joy is another common and painful presenting problem. The inability to experience joy or pleasure is sometimes referred to as anhedonia. People suffering this will often report feeling numb or simply less interested in things that they used to enjoy. It is commonly a symptom of depression but also of many other mental health conditions. Even among subclinical populations, joy may emerge spontaneously, but it can be difficult to sustain or to spontaneously generate without the pleasant surprise of an unexpected cue.

The problem of not enough joy is directly relevant to the role of expressive arousal as a change process because sometimes arousal for arousal's sake alone can be pleasurable. A very basic example is sexual arousal that does not necessarily lead to climax. Some clinicians have argued that for established couples, being excessively goal directed during sex has led them to present with the problem of what is essentially an unsatisfying sex life. Often, those couples also reportedly overlook the joy of arousal for arousal's sake (S. Snyder, 2018). Sexual feelings are only one example where just feeling something intense can be a fulfilling experience. Experiencing and expressing arousal can essentially help people feel more alive. There are several ways that arousal and emotional expressiveness help promote joy. One is that under certain circumstances, joy can be an inherent part of self-expression as an experience. Another reason is that when clients are encouraged to play with being expressive and experiment with that spontaneity, it can be fun!

The Pleasure of Functioning

The German word *Funktionslust* refers to the joy of performing well-rehearsed movements or the pleasure one takes in functioning proficiently and having an impact. While there is no English translation, the term was coined by German psychologist Karl Bühler in the 1920s while making observations about the psychology of experience, a precursor to humanistic psychology.[5] Funktionslust is positive emotion that underscores the lived experience of agency and mastery, but apart from any resulting achievement or success, enacting or expressing as an activity becomes a source of pleasure in itself. Daniel N. Stern (2010) described the level at which these singular actions are completed as fundamental forms of vitality. He identified these in a range of expressive instances that reach a satisfying conclusion, such as completing an anticipated sequence of musical notes or the follow-through of some physical action. More complex examples, such as playfulness (e.g., especially as observed in children), artistic expression (e.g., the joy of dancing), or the carefree pleasure of being creative are chief examples of funktionslust as a self-referencing pleasure (Bühler, 1926/1965).

There can be an inherent joy in the arousal of self-expression and relishing that experience as harmonious, beautiful, and most of all, worthy. The joy in action can perpetuate therapeutic change. For example, a person suffering from a terminal brain tumor talked to me of their recent turn toward regular exercise: "I've been cycling a lot, it's not something I've ever done much in my life before . . . but I like to feel that exertion, like I'm actually accomplishing something palpable, I'm pushing forward into the wind."[6] While this example may seem to be about exercise more than emotional expression, the commonality is in experiencing one's body and exertion as existentially meaningful and as a lived and gratifying expression of the self. The idea is echoed in treatment literature that puts a premium on freeing up expressive arousal, such as dance and movement therapies, therapeutic drumming and rhythmic activity, drama therapy, and other approaches that use psychotherapeutic enactments. These approaches to intervention often describe participants feeling an improved sense of vitality and zest for life (e.g., Blatner, 2000; Geller & Greenberg, 2010; Margariti et al., 2012; Perls et al., 1951; Schmais, 1985).

Playing With Ways of Being

In his development of psychodrama as a method of treatment, Moreno (1958) became convinced of the importance of spontaneity as a creative and vitalizing process central to life. Spontaneity is not simple impulsivity; rather, it requires precision to be a fresh and effective response to a presenting challenge. Breaking out of old habits by doing something different yet effective is a positive experience that helps build confidence. There is also strong evidence that one function of positive emotion is helping individuals broaden and build the cognitive, affective, and behavioral repertoires with which they engage the world (Fredrickson, 2001; discussed in Chapters 13 and 18, this volume).

Sometimes healing comes from the sense of empowerment a client feels when discovering their own creative ability. During the treatment session, warm-up exercises in group therapy or the playfulness of a therapist's engagement are critical in generating a collaborative spirit of spontaneity (Blatner, 2000). Generally, improvisation is an important aspect of enactments, and it is an even more critical aspect of playfulness. This observation has significant practical implications.

Humor, Parody, and Having Fun With It

Dance, clowning, mimicry, and playful exaggeration are at the core of many expressive enactments, and there can be as much humor as insight in doing this. For example,

THERAPIST: Ha ha! Yes, I know it's more complicated and there are a lot of sides to this, but if you exaggerate it? Even doing it more, just like you are already doing. . . . Play up this caricature of your father. What is he really saying to you? Be him. What's the impossible message here?

Enactments also offer clients the opportunity to make a caricature or make absurd parodies of their own self-critical voice, which introduces humor, facilitates playing with experience, and puts it in a broader context of meaning. The role of emotional expression in this kind of play comes in knowingly experimenting with ways of being. For example, Client: "I don't really think this (wink, wink!), but I guess a part of me thinks that. . . ." and thus begins a farcical enactment of the self-critic. Perhaps it is not surprising that the epitaph on Moreno's tombstone reads, "The man who brought joy and laughter to psychiatry."[7]

From a psychodynamic perspective on healthy development, Winnicott (1971), much like Moreno, associated playfulness with spontaneity, authenticity, and vitality. Minuchin (2012) had a similarly spirited approach to family therapy. Furthermore, despite their very different treatment frameworks and intervention styles, these authors discussed increasing a client's interest and ability to be playful as one of the goals of psychotherapy.

Another approach to fostering playfulness is to be much more explicit about it. Improvisational theater (improv) training has been introduced as a group treatment for people with anxiety and depression. Studies show promising results. One found medium effects in reducing depression and anxiety symptoms among outpatients after four 2-hour sessions (Krueger et al., 2017), while a larger school-based program for adolescents with social anxiety reported symptom reductions after ten 45-minute classes (Felsman et al., 2019). Both studies lacked comparison groups and had notable dropout rates (20% and 45%, respectively), so further and more rigorous study is needed. Nevertheless, improv training is an innovation that appears to offer an accessible, low-cost, and low-stigma approach to symptom reduction. Also, it is tremendous fun! —although the studies did not measure fun or playfulness.

The Case of the Missing Outcome

Unfortunately, joy, humor, and playfulness are typically overlooked as dependent variables in clinical research and are often missing from the collection of tests and procedures that measure treatment outcome. This may be because research on emotionally expressive, body-oriented, and arts-based interventions, which could make the most use of such outcomes, are often trying to further their recognition as the serious and legitimate treatment options they usually are. So, perhaps this conspicuous omission has been to hedge against the risk of being regarded as trivial or irrelevant to clinical concerns. Even when qualitative inquiries are done into clients' subjective experiences, researchers from most approaches seem to be shying away from asking clients pertinent questions about treatment like, "Did you have fun?" or "How does being playful relate to your change process?" (e.g., consider Stiegler, Binder, et al., 2018; Westwood et al., 2010).

Another reason for these missing outcomes may be a measurement issue. Pivotal moments of spontaneity, playfulness, or the gratifying feeling that may come with self-expression are typically very ephemeral. They are not within the conventional set of issues clients themselves see as pertinent, even in their responses to open-ended inquiries. However, as much as a state of being, an increased tendency toward playfulness can be thought of as a personality trait. Although the effect of personality changes as a result of psychotherapy are typically smaller than symptom changes (e.g., reduced distress), increases in a personality trait such as playfulness arguably represents a very sustainable and powerful effect (Ogles, 2013).

Treatment Research on Playfulness: From Process to Outcomes

In a study of drama therapy, researchers isolated video segments which characterized central intervention principals of drama therapy to study the intensity of emotional arousal in general. To their surprise, the segments that best demonstrated dramatic enactment and dramatic projections also revealed joy and excitement as the most commonly observed emotion. Although the study design does not allow sweeping generalizations, the authors speculated that perhaps enactment-related interventions have a unique way of tapping into positive emotion (Armstrong et al., 2015).

Similarly, when positive emotion is measured as an emerging treatment outcome, its observed effect has occasionally been found to carry forward. A study on the treatment of psychiatric inpatients suffering primarily from obsessive–compulsive disorder, depression, and negative symptoms of psychoticism used a dance and movement therapy called "primitive expression" to focus on facilitating playful action, rhythmic movement, and expressions of vitality. Over 10 sessions, these inpatients reported a significant increase in their happiness. Moreover, there was some evidence of a change to brain activity, where both immediate and cumulative treatment effects were related to increased states of relaxed wakefulness (e.g., relative increases in alpha electroencephalogram activity; Margariti et al., 2012).

A multisite study of psychotherapy outpatient clinics also explored positive changes in playfulness and creativity as possible treatment outcomes. Unexpectedly, these nonsymptomatic traits increased over treatment by a magnitude comparable to that of symptom change (Yonatan-Leus et al., 2020). Treatment in the study was naturalistic and heterogeneous although primarily psychodynamic. This last point is important because it highlights that playfulness is not proprietary to treatments like drama or dance and movement therapies; rather, it can (and should) be fostered in more traditional approaches as well.

However, instructing therapists on how to facilitate playfulness is an elusive training issue. A retrospective study in Israel found therapists who were the most effective in promoting good outcomes in their clients had an aggressive style of humor in the sense of being direct and daring (e.g., teasing, using irreverence, playful confrontation). In contrast, therapists who emphasized their humility and honesty tended to be less effective (Yonatan-Leus et al., 2018). These features are likely to be quite culturally and socially loaded, and yet encouraging enactment, expressive arousal, and carefree experimentation are interventions that universally lend themselves to humor, playfulness, and a certain joy.

THE VARIOUS FUNCTIONS OF EXPRESSIVE AROUSAL

Part III of this book has explored both feeling and expressing more as core principles of emotional change. When emotionally expressive arousal is clear and productive, there are several aspects to the unfolding process: action, choice, commitment, and, of course, deeper feeling. Because this is a complex and dynamic process with various levels of feedback, the development of arousal and expression as a form of emotional process is nonlinear, is overdetermined, and could begin with any one of those points of departure. Expressive action may create some impetus for emotional change, or similarly one may choose to generate an internal experience by starting with a deliberate outward action (e.g., fake it till you make it). When it is present, expressive arousal also serves as an emotional amplifier, facilitating awareness as emotional expressiveness is carried out. Embarking on an expressive enactment is a complex process, but whatever direction it takes, putting it out there is a commitment to meaning and a dedication to the process that will ensue. Overall, expression focuses one's attentional resources, which creates (or allows) some form of momentum, thereby setting a certain trajectory for one's experience. As one engages in a certain kind of expression, one comes to attend more to that same expression, its content, its possible meaning, the feeling, its execution, and so on. There is a spontaneous and emergent development in this way of working with emotion, and in the end, it feels good to express oneself.

ENDNOTES

1. To read the full article by LaFrance, visit this website (https://www.theatlantic.com/technology/archive/2016/03/adrienne-was-here/475719/).
2. Although they may overlap, using expressive arousal in this way is not the same as generating positive self-talk or writing self-affirmations. That aspect of content elaboration is discussed in Chapter 18.

3. Chapter 21 is dedicated to the elaboration of this idea in terms of narrative identity.
4. I am grateful to Dr. Shigeru Iwakabe from Ritsumeikan University for our conversations that have helped me articulate the ideas in this section.
5. Bühler also coined the term "Aha! experience," referring to a sudden realization or insight that comes from bringing together several previously unrelated cognitive–perceptual pieces into an organized whole (e.g., discovering that the sum is more than its parts).
6. The last line on Moreno's tombstone in Vienna, Austria, reads, "Der Mann der Freude und Lachen in de Psychiatrie Bracht" [The man who brought joy and laughter to psychiatry].
7. Although they may overlap, using expressive arousal in this way is not the same as generating positive self-talk or writing self-affirmations. That aspect of content elaboration is discussed in Chapter 18.

IV

ORDER THE SEQUENCE OF EMOTIONS

INTRODUCTION: ORDER THE SEQUENCE OF EMOTIONS

Part IV of this book (Chapters 12–16) discusses how emotion can be transformed through the sequential order in which it is experienced and presents this as a unique form of emotional processing. Though this process has long been implicit in many forms of therapy, it has not been clearly articulated as an overarching process unto itself until the more recent developments in several experiential theories of psychotherapy. What changes when emotions are sequentially transformed is the configuration of schemes that otherwise organize and propel the experience of emotion. This emotional restructuring through a lived experience of ordered emotion states has now been explained on both psychological and neurological levels. Figure IV.1 depicts this process heuristically as a series of emotional states in a cascade of experiences that produce a qualitative change to the presenting state while also expanding one's emotional repertoire.

In this part of the book, Chapter 12 first introduces and describes what the process of a sequential transformation is and when it is either indicated or contraindicated as an intervention goal. The second half of that chapter mounts an argument for how this process is unique among other forms of emotional processing described in the literature and in this book.

In Chapters 13 and 14, I highlight the psychological and neurobiological processes of various pathways of action through which the sequential transformation of emotion leads to positive personal change. The five hypothesized mechanisms of this specific kind of change process are as follows:

- One emotion can serve as the antidote to another, such as how positive or approach emotions have an undoing effect on negative or withdrawal emotions (see Chapter 13).

- Coactivation of emotions creates higher order schemes for meaning and feeling (Chapter 13).

- New emotion developmentally expands one's emotional repertoire (Chapter 14).

- Emotional flexibility creates more dynamic responding (Chapter 14).

- Existential needs drive the direction of transformations (Chapter 14).

My aim is to synthesize theory and research supporting these ideas from various treatment perspectives. However, given the different ways the phenomenon has been conceptualized, the supporting literature comes from disparate traditions and at times may appear disconnected. To address this, in Chapters 15 and 16, I review work by various research groups around the

FIGURE IV.1. Order the Sequence of Emotion: The Principle of Sequential Transformation

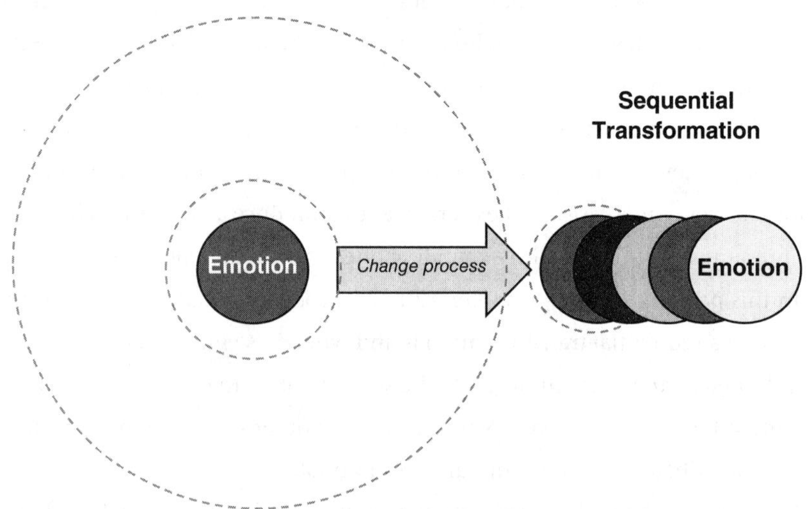

Note. Sequential transformation is a principle that involves using one emotion as the means to change another preceding emotion in what is an emotion transformation. The process is depicted here as beginning with a target feeling, which is then placed in an ordered pattern such that one emotion influences the next to produce a cascade of qualitative changes until the concern is resolved. This is one of five categorically different processes that change emotion.

world that use a range of methods and therapeutic perspectives, and I collectively demonstrate how each of these mechanisms can be observed within a single theoretical model applied across treatment approaches and for a range of disorders.

12

Sequential Transformation

The Pattern in Emotion Makes It Change

And when you're in a Slump,
you're not in for much fun.
Un-slumping yourself is not easily done.

—DR. SEUSS, *OH, THE PLACES YOU'LL GO!*

An emotion cannot be restrained nor removed unless by an opposed and stronger emotion.
—BARUCH SPINOZA, *ETHICS IV*

A sequential transformation of emotion occurs in the transition between two emotions. As one moves from one state to another, the emotions build cumulatively creating the emergence of new meaning. At a more complex level, this occurs through a series of emotions each chained together. It is observable both within a given session and across sessions. An account of this kind of process is illustrated in the case study of "Carla," a 31-year-old single woman, journalist, and writer (first presented more fully in A. Pascual-Leone et al., 2017).[1] Her presenting issues were self-criticism, feeling worthless, and past emotional abuse by her father. She reported feeling like "garbage" and that her father treated her "like he wanted to throw me to the curb with the trash" (A. Pascual-Leone et al., 2017, p. 176). Because her mother was chronically ill, Carla was also left alone for long periods of time when she was growing up, which left her feeling abandoned and neglected.

In session 1, Carla became upset and tearful talking about her father's treatment of her, and she was quickly overwhelmed by distress. When the therapist

https://doi.org/10.1037/0000460-013
Principles of Emotion Change: What Works and When in Psychotherapy and Everyday Life, by A. Pascual-Leone
Copyright © 2026 by the American Psychological Association. All rights reserved.

gently asked what she was feeling, Carla was confused, frustrated, and tearful: "I don't know, I don't know, I don't know!" (A. Pascual-Leone et al., 2017, p. 178). Even so, she had some insight about how she coped with emotion: "I have a tendency to carry stress in my muscles, to not experience emotions, to physically restrain myself, to avoid. I'm a somatizer" (p. 178). Helping Carla attend to, accept, and allow her feeling of undifferentiated distress and repeatedly connecting her to her internal world was an important part of therapy. Treatment focused on her self-criticism and feelings of worthlessness. As Carla remarked, "I've been nominated for a couple of awards for my work, but I never get any satisfaction, I always feel like it was a mistake and that I didn't deserve it" (A. Pascual-Leone et al., 2017, p. 179).

She also had a sense that those feelings originated from her father's pernicious treatment of her. Around session 4, the therapist focused on helping Carla experience the primary maladaptive shame stemming from that abuse. Finding words for her deep sense of inadequacy often sparked a sense of disgust and destructive anger over how her father had treated her (i.e., session 8, Carla: "I'm *really* pissed off!"; A. Pascual-Leone et al., 2017, p. 179). These unhealthy emotions eventually gave way to an intensely assertive anger toward her father, which she symbolized as a primary adaptive and healthy emotion. Over the weeks, revisiting that process multiple times allowed Carla to forgive her father and let go of her hostile and blaming anger.

The next critical turn in therapy was when she started to talk about sadness and actively grieve how she had been treated. As she articulated losses of her upbringing, she also became more able to set boundaries for what she still needed in life and started responding to herself with compassion. In session 10, she creatively imagined her parents reassuringly saying, "I love you. It's going to be alright." Finally, session 11 saw her reach a feeling of acceptance and agency:

> I feel like I can breathe again. . . . I'm gonna try to say goodbye to that part of me, that child that was hurt and was defenseless. I'm not going to ignore her, she'll always be there and if she wants to say something, I'm going to listen. But I'm not that child anymore. I'm an adult now. I have control over my own destiny. . . . Goodbye to being a victim. (A. Pascual-Leone et al., 2017, p. 180)

Although one may consider each passage independently, the deeper process in this clinical account is the progressive building of one emotion out of the other, starting in global distress, then moving to shame, then anger, grief, compassion, and finally, ending with a feeling of personal resolution. The synergy between affective parts represents a unique mechanism.

WHAT IS A SEQUENTIAL TRANSFORMATION? WHEN IS IT IMPORTANT?

Historically, theories of emotional change in psychotherapy have not clearly tracked how people negotiate their way through these twists and turns in an unfolding cascade of emotion. On one hand, ideas of exposure and habituation do not explain the emergence of categorically new experiences. On the other hand, explanations that appeal to a humanist growth tendency beg for some type of elaboration to account for emotional transitions. Furthering our understanding of how individuals shift their experience from inherently maladaptive emotional distress to some more meaningful and adaptive emotional state opens the way to advancement in both clinical theory and methods of intervention (A. Pascual-Leone & Greenberg, 2007a).

Sequential transformation is a form of emotional processing that L. S. Greenberg (2021) has described as "changing emotion with emotion" (p. 1).[2] This means that experiencing a certain and nonarbitrary sequence in emotional states can lead clients to ultimately feel more resolved about their personal difficulties. The principle here is that problematic emotions can be changed through the subsequent experience of other emotions that are either ambivalent or synergistic in nature. Taken further, this kind of emotional processing is the result of certain sequences of feeling that ultimately produce a personal transformation.

Maladaptive emotion is transformed through several moments of change all related to restructuring the experience of an underlying emotion scheme (i.e., a cofunctional network of related sensations, action tendencies, personal cues, embodied meanings, and tacit needs; see Introduction). First, the lived experience of that maladaptive emotion allows one to explore its meaning in depth. Second, the aroused experience allows one to identify and articulate the unmet existential needs that underpin maladaptive emotion. Clarifying what previously was only an implicit need is the pivot point in a sequential transformation (see Chapter 14). Third, and finally, emotion is procedural, so in the moment that one clarifies what is missing in one's life, one simultaneously organizes to address that need met. The feeling of mobilization that comes with orienting toward one's need is an adaptive emotion (see Introduction). In short, transformation occurs through an ordered sequence of states in which maladaptive emotion is resolved. The person was stuck in the same old story and now begins a new trajectory of emotional experience.

Emotional processing of this kind has been a major research focus in the study of emotion-focused therapy, but several other approaches to therapy also often move toward transforming emotion in one way or another (e.g., Davanloo, 2005; Ecker et al., 2024; Fosha, 2021; McCullough et al., 2003; A. Pascual-Leone, Paivio, et al., 2016; see also Chapter 14, this volume). Indeed, after first exploring emotion, the focus in many experiential and emotion-centered treatments shifts to transforming certain emotional experiences by using emergent and alternative emotions to expand a person's affective repertoire. So, although the transformation of emotion technically relies on the coordination of some other processes including awareness, regulation, and reflection, the productive sequences of emotion represent a unique form of change (A. Pascual-Leone, Paivio, et al., 2016). Irrespective of treatment approach, sequences from one emotion to another (i.e., transformations) are proposed in the next three chapters as a potentially universal therapeutic change process that may ultimately reflect pathways of adult emotional development.

When to Focus on Sequential Transformation: What Are the Markers of Dysfunction?

As we have seen in the first part of this book, facilitating awareness helps increase the salience and direction of an existing emotional experience. When that emotion is adaptive, clients should make use of the emotion and express it by following the productive process to completion, whether in action or in meaning. However, when awareness and clear symbolization reveal that an emergent emotion is maladaptive, carrying that experience forward with either meaning or expressive arousal cannot complete or resolve the emotion. Maladaptive emotions (e.g., the feeling of being shamefully unlovable) have no productive action tendency and only entail a destructive meaning, so continued expressive arousal or reviewing the meaning will not create closure. Instead, maladaptive emotions must be transformed. So, if self-soothing and the down-regulation of emotion is like turning down the volume on negative experience, then a sequential transformation is more like changing the channel or moving forward into another experience (see Chapter 2). In short, secondary or symptomatic emotions (e.g., anxiety, feeling helpless, feeling overwhelmed) can sometimes be efficiently worked with by down-regulating or inhibiting those bad feelings enough to move on with one's life (see Chapter 3). However, when the emotional experience is both more primary and inherently maladaptive (e.g., core feelings of being bad, shamefully unworthy, unlovable), then a different kind of processing is needed—one that creates a transformational sequence of emotions.

This means the most common targets for sequential transformation and intervention are primary maladaptive experiences of fear (i.e., I am terrified and will not survive), shame (i.e., I feel fundamentally inadequate and unacceptable), or irreconcilable loneliness (i.e., I'm not just alone, it's a feeling that I'm somehow not part of the human race). In terms of clinical presentation, these states are the core source of dysfunction when clients suffer from negative self-treatment (e.g., harsh self-criticism, self-blame), a lack of integration of the self (e.g., feeling torn, indecisive, disempowered), or feeling haunted by unresolved interpersonal problems. However, the core underlying emotions (i.e., fear, shame, loneliness) are complex and dysfunctional affective meaning states that usually tacitly (and sometimes explicitly) embody a sense of being incompetent, bad, or unlovable. These are embodied preverbal experiences (schemes) that are not easily amenable to logical or rational change.

As the first epigraph to this chapter playfully points out, transforming such maladaptive emotions is one of the more difficult challenges when working with emotion. In an example cited by Paivio and Pascual-Leone (2023), a client who had been raped stated, "I know that he was the adult, and I was just a child, but I still feel like I was responsible" (p. 70). Another client said, "I know in my mind that I'm successful—I have a PhD, for God's sake! But I still always have this sense that there's been some misunderstanding or clerical error" (Paivio & Pascual-Leone, 2023, p. 70). Case examples from other treatment approaches (e.g., Kramer, Pascual-Leone, et al., 2018) similarly highlight how some core maladaptive feelings defy rational thinking, making it difficult to change such emotion through reason. This underscores a need for emotional over cognitive approaches to work through maladaptive feelings.

Provided that clients are willing to tolerate and go through the presenting maladaptive emotion, two key distinctions should be made in the case formulation that might lead to this treatment effort. First, to confirm that the presenting emotion is primary, the therapist should help clients clarify the unmet existential need that underlies a maladaptive emotion. When such needs are not yet apparent, it is often because the presenting emotion has not yet been differentiated and symbolized in enough detail and is too vague to be transformed. If this is the case, therapists should first further facilitate emotional awareness. (Secondary emotion and overly general experiences of distress may anticipate deeper and more problematic maladaptive emotion, but only the latter is a target of change in a true sequential transformation.)

Second, in anticipating how smoothly (or not) the process will unfold, it will be useful for therapists to determine to what degree the emotion is free of a negative self-evaluation. Indeed, maladaptive emotions usually have some implicit injunction that makes it impossible for an individual to have their needs met. So, it is often the case that this contradiction will be an impediment. Still, when therapists sense this conflict is not fully salient, they should guide clients to experience the dialectical tension between having a need versus feeling that one is essentially undeserving, unable, or alone. This tension represents an existential confrontation. That process could be accomplished gradually and recursively through cognitive reframing, narrative reconstruction, and continually integrating the different (often contradicting) facets of meaning into a larger whole. New transformative emotions that would follow in a sequence emerge from that tension. The goal of doing this is to eventually use emotion to help a client find personal direction and agency.

There are also specific moments in session when facilitating a transformational sequence would be bad for treatment, and at those moments, interventions that target changing emotion with emotion are contraindicated. For example, when clients are dysregulated and overwhelmed by a presenting maladaptive emotion, it is not a time to push for deeper meaning exploration (see Chapter 2). This is because sequential transformation requires sustained engagement in the affective process and will unfold through moment-by-moment experience and meaning elaboration, so clients need to be able to sustain that level of activation in a meaningful way.

At other times, clients need to step back and get their bearings regarding a maladaptive emotional experience, such as when they first find the right words to capture the essence of a pathogenic feeling (i.e., "I've carried this sense of dread all my life, and I'm just starting to get a sense of what it's really about").

During a moment of this kind of personal discovery, the instance is best used for reflection on emotion (see Chapter 18) and particularly its historical and personal–social context. Stepping back to get a bird's eye view of one's life is an important level on which to elaborate meaning. However, because that would represent a top-down process, a life narrative perspective is not conducive to simultaneously attending to the bottom-up moment-by-moment process of emotion.

Finally, the last point is not a contraindication so much as a technical caution to therapists. As the next two chapters will demonstrate, there are indeed a series of specific and typical pathways toward emotion resolution. However, the exact process usually cannot be applied formulaically. This is because the process of true sequential transformation is contingent on the personal experiences and internal meanings for each individual. So, just as people cannot be easily instructed to have more emotional awareness, when therapists facilitate a meaningful sequential transformation, it will involve a dialectic of leading and following the client process.

What Kind of Emotions Are Therapeutic?

In the last 20 years, research on discrete emotions in the treatment process has shown that certain kinds of emotion predict good outcome, whereas others do not (A. Pascual-Leone, 2018; see also Chapter 13, this volume). However, since the dawn of client-centered approaches in the 1950s, process-oriented therapists who want to work with emotion have essentially been offered the universal instruction to stay with the feeling and just follow the emotion. For the novice, this is a useful place to start. However, with more experience in working with emotion, therapists learning to do this quickly find themselves asking, "Follow the emotion, okay, fine. . . . But which emotion?"[3] At this point, the distinction between different kinds of emotion becomes paramount. Simply put, not all kinds of emotion are equally productive.

From an evolutionary perspective, the different functional organizations of various emotions capture distinct action tendencies and embodied meanings (Darwin, 1872/1965; Panksepp, 2008; Porges, 2011; Tracy & Matsumoto, 2008; see the Introduction, this volume). In general, or even in a given moment, some emotions are more useful than others for facilitating change. Furthermore, while the discrete nature of emotions (e.g., anger, fear, joy, sadness) represent distinct self-organizations, emotion can also be either productive (e.g., provide healthy directions of insight and action) or unproductive (e.g., be destructive, overwhelming, disorienting). The productivity of aroused emotion, rather than arousal alone, distinguishes good from poor outcome cases (Auszra et al., 2013; L. S. Greenberg et al., 2007). Optimum emotional processing requires the integration of cognition (e.g., reflection on emotion) and affect (e.g., awareness and arousal of emotion).

In sum, the process research discussed here and over the next few chapters shows certain qualitative kinds of emotional experiences are productive (i.e., only certain kinds of anger or sadness seem helpful), whereas other emotional experiences represent stagnation or ongoing expressions of distress (Kennedy-Moore & Watson, 2001). This suggests it may not be so much an issue of which emotions are productive (i.e., Is it productive to express anger? What about sadness?); rather, the critical issue is one of quality (i.e., What does productive vs. unproductive sadness look like?).

In What Order Are Those Emotions Therapeutic?

The idea that feeling specific discrete emotions (e.g., self-compassion) may be uniquely helpful is aligned with the notion that a good psychotherapy session involves some key events or critical ingredients. Even so, an instance of productive emotion is not an isolated moment generated in a vacuum; rather, it emerges as part of a larger sequence of feelings over time. Experiences of productive emotion are like musical notes, where each have their own circumscribed value, but when ordered into a melody, they can also render a higher level of complexity and meaning.

The Sequence Is an Overarching Process

Once productive versus unproductive kinds of emotion can be differentiated (e.g., Auszra et al., 2013), does the order in which they are experienced matter? And if so, which sequential order of emotions is best related to good outcome? In short, the crux of sequential transformation is that the order of operations does matter when facilitating emotional change. As L. S. Greenberg and Paivio (1997) described in their seminal book, clients in therapy often present with secondary emotions, which are symptomatic feelings that avoid (i.e., defend against) the deeper and more fundamental (primary) emotion that underpins their suffering. It follows that searching for the deeper emotional process represents a productive sequence.

Emotionally attuned therapists will be familiar with the instant someone sounds vulnerable as they move into a deeper (more primary) emotional experience, and some research has even used computerized acoustical analysis to pinpoint this particular vocal marker. For example, in a study of women working through their unresolved anger during single sessions of emotion-focused therapy, they were observed to approach and activate primary vulnerable emotions in the context of their unresolved anger (Diamond et al., 2010). As people doing this kind of emotional processing shift between emotions or deepen their experience, it typically creates a special kind of vocal perturbation (e.g., variability or a wobble in loudness, perceived breathiness or hoarseness). This observable marker seems to reflect the internal struggle in transitioning from one emotional self-organization to another (Diamond et al., 2010). What this study offers is a physiological correlate of the struggle that presents when shifting between different states in one's overall emotional repertoire. The vocal perturbations represented a shift out of a dominant emotion (in this case, anger) and into a less dominant but emergent emotion (such as vulnerability) in the form of sadness and fear as the client confronts some challenge.

Accessing primary vulnerable emotions is an initial sequence that is integral to approaching and engaging core emotion. As we will see, L. S. Greenberg and Paivio (1997) also described more complex sequences for working through (primary maladaptive) emotion, which is entrenched and problematic.

The idea that there may be certain multistep sequences to emotional change is not new and has been represented by clinical formulations from several approaches for some time. In early work, a Swiss American psychiatrist named Elisabeth Kübler-Ross proposed a model (1969) commonly known as the five stages of grief. This model advanced that working through personal loss related to death and dying unfold in a process that begins with denial, followed by anger, bargaining, depression, and then finally, acceptance. It offers an intuitive process model that has come to be widely accepted in popular culture for understanding the process of how one copes with (i.e., emotionally processes) the reality of death and dying. Yet empirical support for the validity of that model is questionable, in that research directly examining it has proven to be inconsistent (Bonanno, 2010). Even so, the stages of grief continue to be taught in medical schools to help guide clinicians in understanding and facilitating the grieving process (MacIejewski et al., 2007).

In defense of the model, Kübler-Ross (2005) also qualified it by stating that not all people would experience all emotions or states, that there may also be other emotions, and that the stages could occur in any order. This seems to make the model unfalsifiable, and yet it still captures something compelling about a complex process of emotional change. Other research has suggested that the salience of meaning making about one's personal loss is a much stronger predictor of emotional change than either time since loss or the supposed stages of grief (Holland & Neimeyer, 2010). However, besides the question of whether a process like Kübler-Ross's stages universally exists or not (Bonanno, 2004, 2010; MacIejewski et al., 2007), it exemplifies a unique puzzle in the study of emotion change.

I suggest there are at least three issues that have made the empirical study of such sequential transformations particularly slippery. First, to examine a model of that kind, one needs to make a more refined distinction between the case of a relatively healthy and straightforward grief process versus grief in the context of a complex and traumatic loss. As put forward by L. S. Greenberg and Paivio (1997), accessing deeper emotion will often suffice to work through (so called) normal personal difficulty. More pathological processes present problems of a different sort, which are rooted in the presence of maladaptive emotion, and working through them will usually require a more complex process.

Second, while the notion of sequences may still be meaningful, such models often have a simplistic categorical definition of emotion, lacking rich differentiation among the kinds of emotions that are or are not productive (e.g., What kind of sadness? What kind of anger?). Often, the meaning behind an emotion, its significance, is more important than its affective tone. Having a sophisticated theory of emotion and the varieties of productive versus unproductive emotional engagement is a critical issue. And one needs this before sequences of change can be discussed in an empirically meaningful way.

Lastly, and probably most critically, rather than being linearly ordered into stages of life, emotion is highly dynamic such that newly budding experience is ephemeral and shifts rapidly. Contemporary models of how this process unfolds have been more successful because they are more probabilistic and allow for dynamic moment-by-moment patterns of emotional experience (e.g., A. Pascual-Leone, 2009, 2018). The idea that order matters but that advancement may be erratic (e.g., advancing two steps forward and one step back) makes it a challenge for both conceptual clarity and measurement, but this also seems closer to the subjective phenomenon of someone's unique pattern of change (for case examples, see A. Pascual-Leone et al., 2017).

The idea of curative emotional patterns clearly has its antecedents. Since then, research on emotion-focused therapy has made some key theoretical contributions that advance our understanding of this change process (see L. S. Greenberg & Goldman, 2019). In a renaissance of these ideas, Welling (2012) considered the process from a number of treatment perspectives, including emotion-focused, accelerated experiential dynamic, coherence, and eye movement and desensitization therapies. In this critical analysis, he cogently argued that "transformative emotional sequences" (p. 109) represent a unique kind of emotional change that cannot be explained by single step interventions such as exposure alone. Furthermore, from an integrative perspective of psychotherapy, Welling argued that this is a common principle of change, which is also the position of this book.

Why Might Sequences Matter as Much as Individual Emotions?

Sequential transformation is not simply the process of generating new experiences in therapy because it does this by using facets of another, already present, maladaptive emotion. This is possible because there can be co-activation of adaptive emotion along with and in response to maladaptive emotion (L. S. Greenberg, 2021). One of the explicit principles in humanistic therapy is to empathically respond to distressing, even maladaptive, emotion while continually supporting the tentative emergence of adaptive emotional responses. In this way, bad feeling is not purged or vented as such, nor does it attenuate, but rather another feeling is evoked in parallel and in contrast to the maladaptive feeling (L. S. Greenberg, 2021; A. Pascual-Leone & Greenberg, 2020). For example, a therapist might observe, "So, there is this sense of fear or terror about the horror of what was happening to you, and at the same time . . . I think I hear in your voice, there's also a sense of protest about what happened, the injustice. . . . Is that right?"

As I explained in the Introduction, the term "emotion scheme" is often used to capture the dynamic nature of emotion as a multimodal network of feelings and meanings (i.e., a self-organization). That network could exist in one's repertoire at various levels of activation, ranging from salient and dominant experiences to subdominant and tacit states.[4] Attending to a current maladaptive emotion scheme that is in need of transformation, such as feeling worthless, makes it accessible to new inputs that might change it. Identifying and articulating unfulfilled needs that are embedded in a maladaptive emotion will stimulate and bolster alternative self-organizations.

These alternative self-organizations are tacit emotion schemes, and they begin to organize the individual toward meeting some identified need. It is the synthesis of this new possibility with the old one that leads to lasting change (L. S. Greenberg, 2021; L. S. Greenberg & Watson, 2006; A. Pascual-Leone & Greenberg, 2007a). Experiential approaches typically make use of affect's power to catalyze change, producing a restructuring of core emotion-based schemes. Sequential transformation produces a rearrangement of relations between the different elements of a presenting complex emotional experience, which creates access to alternative responses through a synthesis of old with new schemes. This kind of structural change is represented in the brain at a neuronal level (Lane & Nadel, 2020; Panksepp, 2008), while at a psychological level, it changes how people engage with the world, the self, and others.

One implication of this for practice is that for some clients (as well as for skeptical therapists), this may seem like slipping precipitously down the rabbit hole of emotional experience. Indeed, changing emotion with a sequence of subsequent emotions suggests that when it comes to working through the deeper meaning of one's distress, it gets worse before it gets better. This conclusion about the temporal patterns of distress was supported by early experimental research on coping with induced dysphoria (Hunt, 1998). Those who gave sustained attention to painful feelings in the short term felt better in the long run as compared with other individuals who used problem solving or avoidance as means of coping with a negative mood induction, which tapped into primary maladaptive emotion. These findings led Hunt to title her article as "The Only Way Out Is Through," which as we will see captures the gist of research findings on the sequential nature of emotional processing.[5]

As the main thesis of this chapter presents, awareness and engagement are only the beginning when working through an emotional experience. The pithy implication for practice is that one must arrive at a place before one can work through and leave it (L. S. Greenberg, 2021). This observation also provides the rationale needed for purposefully engaging and exploring one's core maladaptive pain. The intervention goal here is to become aware of maladaptive emotion (awareness and symbolization) and then change it from within by using the emerging thrust of adaptive emotion.

ONE EMOTION COUNTERS ANOTHER: THE SEQUENCE MAKES THE CHANGE

Baruch Spinoza, one of the most important thinkers in Western philosophy, argued in 1677 for the kind of process that underlies a sequential transformation: "An emotion cannot be restrained nor removed unless by an opposed and stronger emotion" (1677/1967, p. 195). Today, the observation that one emotion can serve as a counter or antidote to another and that the sum of some emotional sequence results in more than its components is evidenced by a variegated collection of empirical findings. Some experimental research and behavioral observation have highlighted the interaction of specifically opposing emotional processes (Chapter 13). Meanwhile, psychotherapy process research has often used dynamic moment-by-moment frameworks of analysis to show the special synergy between specific pairs of emotion (Chapter 16).

Counterconditioning and Opposite Action

The notion that one state may be used to change a preexisting but incompatible emotion was already introduced by early research on conditioned emotional responses. Joseph Wolpe, a psychiatrist and pioneer of behavior therapy, referred to this in the title of his book, *Psychotherapy by Reciprocal Inhibition* (1958). Usually, this was inducing a relaxed state in the context of high anxiety—the induction of a subsequent and incompatible emotional experience. Counterconditioning is commonly used today in behavior therapy to reduce such symptoms as phobia, anxiety, and aggression. Common protocols using the intervention include systematic desensitization and aversion therapy (Spiegler, 2015; see also Chapter 3, this volume).

True to a behavioral focus, once symptomatic concerns are directly addressed, these intervention strategies hold that it is unnecessary to further discern or differentially address what may be deeper (primary) emotion. However, the term "inhibition" was probably not the best conceptualization for the range of processes Wolpe had observed. As discussed in Chapters 2 and 3 on downregulation, inhibition may be very appropriate when the presenting concern is secondary (i.e., symptomatic) emotion. In contrast, when the emotion is primary and maladaptive, the transformational sequence of emotion is quite a different process and is the one that seems to be underfoot. Still, Wolpe and the behavioral tradition have not embraced that distinction.

Nevertheless, following this line of behavioral theory, a crucial function of exposure therapy is now seen as the desensitization and eventual extinction of natural (but excessive) action tendencies associated with problematic emotion (i.e., anxiety) and the promotion of action tendencies that are incompatible with the problem emotion. Dialectical behavior therapy (Linehan, 2015) articulated this process in terms of a teachable skill that might be used to deliberately change unwanted emotion, referred to as either "opposite-to-emotion action" or "opposite action." After identifying a presenting emotion and the urges or action tendency associated with it, one then determines what actions might be opposite to the initial urge for action and behaviorally engages in that opposite action. This purely behavioral intervention hinges on the fact that affective experience can follow suit to behavior so that soon after the behavioral change, one begins to feel something more congruent with the new action.[6]

Opposite action represents a key strategy in dialectical behavior therapy, and Linehan has since generalized its use from working with anxiety to working with any number of unwanted feelings (without distinguishing secondary from primary maladaptive emotions). For example, if individuals typically lay in bed when they feel depressed, then to reduce feelings of depressive sadness, they would effortfully exercise the opposite action by getting out of bed, showering, and so on. For shame, rather than following an urge to hide the shameful event from others for fear of rejection, individual would find an appropriate context to disclose to another person and then actually reveal what one felt so ashamed about (Rizvi & Linehan, 2005). There is also some implicit theory about different kinds of emotion in this: Opposite action may be applied to change emotion when the emotion is unjustified—that is, when the emotion is not a realistic response to the immediate situation or when the intensity is too strong. While behavioral theory focuses on the mediating role of action, the actions are not being selected at random. An opposite action is always implicitly tied to an alternative (and incompatible) emotion, such that the first emotion informs and is ultimately linked to the second emotion. This also goes further than the Jamesian peripheral theory of emotion (discussed in Chapter 9) because there are specific couplings of emotion that produce especially transformational sequences.[7]

A few pilot studies have been done that specifically focus on training clients to use opposite action as a skill and were used to help clients work with several emotions including anger, fear, sadness, and shame. The change process facilitated by this specific intervention shows promise, even when it is used as a standalone treatment (Rizvi et al., 2011; Rizvi & Linehan, 2005). Furthermore, the fact that this intervention is premised on behavioral action alone, rather than a search for personal meaning, makes it amenable to formats that are purely procedural such as computerized coaching via a smart phone application (Rizvi et al., 2011; although, for an experiential spin on this, also consider Nardone et al., 2025). Cognitively oriented incarnations of this process are also found, for example, in acceptance and commitment therapy. Techniques for cognitive defusion include modifying the experience of a negative thought by using a silly voice or by cheerfully singing the thought over and over again until the associated emotion changes (S. C. Hayes et al., 2012).

Sequential Transformation Is Different From Exposure

Although the interventions of counterconditioning and opposite action do work, the question is, why?[8] In discussions on how emotion is attenuated through exposure-informed interventions, sustained arousal that results in desensitization is explained in the literature as occurring through specific mechanisms of habituation, inhibition, and the disconfirmation of beliefs (Foa et al., 2006). However, the idea from emotion-focused therapy that the introduction of some new emotion could itself be a process that leverages change diverges from traditional cognitive and behavioral theories, which typically view emotions as symptoms to be reduced or eliminated (Nardone et al., 2025). Though exposure-based habituation or inhibition may be useful for addressing secondary (i.e., symptomatic) emotion, two critiques can be made of how classic behaviorist theory uses this same explanation to rationalize the way deeper primary maladaptive emotions are changed during therapy.

One Experience Unfolds From Another

The first critique is that the symptom-focused perspective of systematic desensitization (e.g., reducing fear in posttraumatic stress disorder) is sometimes too unidimensional and risks overlooking the continuous and highly dynamic flow of emotion. In short, the fact that one may observe less of the problematic emotion (i.e., its habituation or inhibition) is usually not the whole story when it comes to working with core maladaptive emotion. Rather, there are other emerging emotions that go unrecognized (A. Pascual-Leone & Greenberg, 2020). As a point of illustration, a study that assessed the emotional profiles of clients attending a trauma clinic found that less than 50% of cases with posttrauamatic stress disorder presented with anxiety as their principal emotion and a slight majority showed sadness, anger, or disgust as more dominant experiences than anxiety. After examining the relationship between these emotion profiles and outcome in cognitive behavior therapy, the authors questioned the usefulness of exposure-based treatments when anxiety is not actually predominant (M. J. Power & Fyvie, 2013). Furthermore, even when anxiety presents as a dominant emotion, it may not be central but instead be a secondary (symptom) emotion.

Even when an exposure-based approach is well suited, the notion that such interventions are only dampening a single target emotion overlooks what happens in the wake of desensitization. By analogy, this is like bailing buckets of water out from an ocean of affective experiences with the expectation that there should somehow be a hole some kind left in the ocean in the spot where one has just bailed out water. But water, like the flow of emotional experience, continually fills itself in wherever the bailing bucket has been, and there is always some new and changing experience to fill its place (Gendlin, 1996; A. Pascual-Leone & Greenberg, 2020). While this simile should not be taken too far, the essential critique is that while fear may be attenuated in treatments of systematic exposure, what remains is not just an absence of core fear but rather a vibrant range of other emotions that spontaneously emerge (e.g., hurt, shame, resentment, anger, pride). Often each of these other feelings are very much alive, and they collectively represent undeclared aspects of the change process in the behaviorist account of how exposure might facilitate change beyond habituation. Healthy self-organization is born out of a preceding maladaptive state because the adaptive emotion presents a catalyst for working through meaning that to some extent was already embodied in the problem state. A classic exposure-based perspective misrepresents the continuous and multifaceted nature of how one ultimately works through maladaptive emotional experiences (Colwill et al., 2023; A. Pascual-Leone & Greenberg, 2020).

One may wonder how such an oversight has been possible. From a research perspective, the clinical nuance is often overlooked because of how emotion is measured (or not): Measuring a limited range of emotions (i.e., measuring only anxiety) can sometimes create the impression of a unidimensional reduction on the target emotion (i.e., fear), when in reality, so much more is going on for the client. Similarly, oversimplifying the complexity of various feelings and meanings associated with a given emotional experience can also hide the true effects of an intervention from researchers. The heavy reliance on subjective units of distress ratings in clinical work is a good case in point, as this artificially truncates and reduces all complexity to a single scale of distress.

Presuming the objective was to reduce a single dimension of arousal also dismisses out of hand what an emotion might mean for an individual. Consider emotional changes that seem to help people with borderline personality disorder improve their social functioning. Prior research on dialectical behavior therapy had struggled to show the treatment helped people with their anger problems despite other kinds of improvement. This was a conundrum until one study measured several different kinds of anger that were being expressed by clients (Kramer, Pascual-Leone, Berthoud, et al., 2016). Whereas behavioral interventions would typically aim to reduce rageful anger, that turned out not to be the effect of dialectical behavior therapy. Rather, the treatment's effect when improving a client's social role seemed to be mediated by increasing a client's assertive anger. So clients were actually expressing more anger, albeit in a productive way (Kramer, Pascual-Leone, Berthoud, et al., 2016). This nuanced understanding was only possible when researchers moved beyond a single or unitary dimension of distress, or in this case, of anger. Indeed, the mechanism of change turned out to be just the opposite of reducing emotion through habituation.[9]

Dynamic Interaction Between Emotions

Language that describes painful and maladaptive feelings as being replaced, supplanted, or substituted convey that lasting change essentially occurs by suppressing painful emotion and forcefully moving on by persistently attending to other, perhaps more pleasant, experiences. So, a second critique of how theories of habituation or inhibition explain productive changes from maladaptive emotion is that while other undeclared emotions may, in fact, be part of the change process at hand, they also interact (A. Pascual-Leone & Greenberg, 2020). This issue is inherently overlooked by the constructs of desensitization, habituation, or inhibition, which assume a singular kind of emotional change (i.e., reducing arousal; Colwill et al., 2023).

Furthermore, contrary to its name, the idea of counterconditioning (and similarly of using opposite-action; Linehan, 2015) is not always so simple as a forceful replacement or overriding of one feeling with another as behaviorist theory first suggested in the 1950s. Even so, when the role of changing emotion has been observed, researchers from a cognitive behavior perspective have relied on a modified notion of emotion substitution (Riggs et al., 1992). In these past formulations on the mechanisms of helpful (or unhelpful) sequences, the idea that strands of discordant emotion might interact, was yet to be discovered (A. Pascual-Leone & Greenberg, 2020). The focus on purely overt behaviors such as in opposite action or cognitive defusion prevents this deeper theoretical issue from being examined.

When incompatible states are put in sequence, what is the covert change process that unfolds within the individual? As we shall see later in this chapter, the contribution of Fredrickson (2001) on the interaction of positive and negative emotion (i.e., enjoyable vs. unpleasant) is particularly illuminating for understanding this process where she shows that one emotion undoes another emotion and helps usher people into a new and different state of resolution. To state this in terms more compatible with learning theory, which is the foundation of exposure-based interventions, one can think of changing emotion with emotion as involving new experiential learning that transforms the older learning (cf. Craske et al., 2014).

The Whole Is Greater Than the Sum of Parts

In summary, there is an ongoing flux of emotional experiences that are not simply additive or subtractive, and different pieces of experience cannot be arithmetically summed up to represent the totality of a process. Rather, order matters and the placement of a particular kind of emotional experience takes on a qualitative and operationally different meaning depending on when it happened relative to other emotional states. As the saying goes, the whole is greater than the sum of its parts, which in this case includes a consideration of temporal sequences. Indeed, research on this change process suggests a better description is that core painful emotion is not only reduced but rather transformed from within (A. Pascual-Leone & Greenberg, 2020).

Theories of exposure are focused on reducing secondary symptomatic emotions, such as reducing panic or traumatic fear. In contrast, the alternative perspective presented here is that one must first promote the experience and expression of primary maladaptive emotion (e.g., primary shame, attachment anxiety) that are underling a client's presenting distress. Then, rather than trying to habituate or inhibit secondary symptomatic emotion, the deeper feelings must then be transformed with new adaptive emotions. To appreciate this different view of emotional processing, one needs to distinguish primary from secondary emotion and primary adaptive from primary maladaptive emotion (recall from Introduction). Thus, the clinical effort according to emotion-focused theory is to transform painful maladaptive emotion by way of primary adaptive emotion (A. Pascual-Leone & Greenberg, 2020).

MECHANISMS AT WORK: HOW DOES A SEQUENTIAL TRANSFORMATION CREATE CHANGE?

Transformational sequences of emotion represent a complex form of emotional processing that predicts positive treatment outcomes. The mechanisms that explain this process of change can be described as several levels of analysis. First, at the level of moment-by-moment intervention, when opposing emotions are experienced in a sequence, their competitive interaction represents a special kind of change. In some sense, this is the use of one emotion as an antidote to another. Second, the way one overcomes ambivalence between conflicting emotions might be explained not simply as the opposition but rather the synthesis of the two ordered emotions. This results in the creation of new meanings and actions, which can be explained both in psychological and neurological terms.

Third, in a broader scope of analyses, a sequential transformation can be observed not only within a specific moment but also over a longer developmental trajectory (e.g., over multiple weeks). So, while emotional change can occur in two-step sequences (e.g., emotion A → emotion B), multiple sets of those sequences are sometimes chained together to create longer canonical patterns of change (e.g., A → B, B → C, C → D). Rather than being reducible to a single intervention effort, this longer sequence represents an overarching process of change suggested by several treatment theories (Chapters 14 and 15). Fourth, over longer periods of time, changing emotion with emotion expands one's emotional repertoire. So, rather than just providing a new feeling (by substitution), going through sequential transformations of emotion can help people develop other feelings, expanding their emotional range. Finally, the pursuit of unmet existential needs is what drives ongoing sequential transformations, creating an evolving continuity in one's life regarding the negotiation of unmet needs.

ENDNOTES

1. The case of Carla presented in the introduction to this chapter is derived in part from A. Pascual-Leone et al. (2017).
2. L. S. Greenberg coined this turn of phrase to describe a unique process of emotional change, and it is deliberately contrasted with what was a more established view of cognitive therapy where emotion is changed with cognition. However, the issue at hand is both (a) a different kind of emotional processing (i.e., changing emotion with emotion rather than with cognition) but also (b) applying this kind of processing to a more specific emotional target (i.e., transforming primary maladaptive emotion rather than managing secondary symptomatic emotions).
3. L. S. Greenberg has highlighted this as a practical concern for experiential therapists learning to work with emotion. The issue was also recognized by Laura Rice in the practice and training of classical person-centered therapy.
4. I remind readers that an emotion scheme is not the same as a cognitive schema. This points to a critical distinction in schemes as originally defined in Piagetian theory (see J. Pascual-Leone & Johnson, 2021). *Cognitive schema* is a term used in theories of cognitive therapy but focuses (excessively) on the representational nature of information. *Emotion schemes* are closer to the intention of Piagetian theory in that they are procedural as much as they may be representational (see also Introduction).
5. In illustrating the convergence in theoretical perspectives, a central effort in this book, it is worth noting that the conclusion of Hunt's (1998) experiment (i.e., the only way out is through) published in the journal *Behavior Research and Therapy* supports a long-time principle of humanistic–experiential therapies.
6. The observation that emotion can be influenced through physical enactment will also remind readers of Chapters 9 and 10, where I discussed expressive arousal (i.e.,

increasing arousal, enactment, and vividness) as a change process unto itself. While the pathway of change in dialectical behavior therapy's opposite-action is one of action-to-emotion, the relationship between emotion and behavior is bidirectional. Other sections of this book highlight emotion-to-action as a different pathway of change (e.g., Chapter 7).

7. The distinctive nuance in transformation sequences is that they (a) involve the deliberate use of incompatible emotions that are (b) placed within a particular ordered sequence (for experimental evidence, see Chapter 13).

8. The section "Sequential Transformation Is Different from Exposure" is derived in part from A. Pascual-Leone & Greenberg (2020).

9. The finding of Kramer, Pascual-Leone, Berthoud, and colleagues (2016) that increasing some kinds of anger predicted improved outcomes in dialectical behavior therapy runs directly counter to the way both habituation and inhibition are understood to work in behavior therapies. Naturally, critical readers may become suspicious of the method used in an unusual process study such as this. However, a review on the mechanisms of change on all known research conducted on dialectical behavior therapy and cognitive behavior therapy has ranked the cited study as #2 in the world to date in terms of its methodological quality (Rudge et al., 2017). As such, this must be taken quite seriously, and it also points to the need for more research examining the conceptualization of change mechanisms imported from other approaches.

13

Changing Emotion With Emotion

The Process in Action

Darkness cannot drive out darkness; only light can do that. Hate cannot drive out hate; only love can do that.

—MARTIN LUTHER KING JR., *LOVING YOUR ENEMIES*

People experience primary maladaptive emotion as hauntingly familiar (Introduction). The same old feeling looms over one like a foreboding shadow, its sting always as deep and fresh as the last time. Moreover, genuinely habituating to maladaptive emotion—for example, getting used to the shame of feeling deeply inadequate—smacks of clinical depression rather than any curative process. Meanwhile, logical workarounds of reframing to make it seem less true are predicated on one having the cognitive resources to step outside the condemnation of that mental set (i.e., decentering; Chapter 20).

But what if there was an antidote to these entrenched kinds of painful emotion? In this alchemy of emotional change, each maladaptive emotion would have a counter emotion, one which could undo or neutralize the painful experience. By using one emotion as an antidote to another, the new facets of what becomes an inherently mixed experience transforms the painful feeling itself such that it is "digested" (Gendlin, 1964, p. 6), "absorbed" (Rachman, 1980, p. 51), or "metabolized" to a new end. Repeating small doses of this antidote over time comes to change the very nature of what was a familiar but maladaptive emotion. The previous chapter raised key issues for understanding sequential transformation as a unique process. This chapter delves into more detail on the mechanisms of change by first reviewing evidence of the process in action.

https://doi.org/10.1037/0000460-014
Principles of Emotion Change: What Works and When in Psychotherapy and Everyday Life, by A. Pascual-Leone
Copyright © 2026 by the American Psychological Association. All rights reserved.

Then, the chapter goes on to consider neurological underpinnings in how new emotional experience is psychologically constructed.

POSITIVE EMOTION HAS AN UNDOING EFFECT ON NEGATIVE EMOTION

Positive emotion (i.e., enjoyable or approach emotions) have often been poetically lauded as playing a unique role in facilitating personal change. The powerful words of Reverend Martin Luther King Jr. (1977), cited in the epigraph to this chapter, points at the main thrust of sequential transformations. However, the issue here is the functional difference of positive emotion, and psychologist Barbara Fredrickson had made this a focus of experimental research at the University of North Carolina at Chapel Hill.

As Fredrickson (2001) observed, key components of positive emotions are simply incompatible with negative emotion. Although adaptive emotions (e.g., grief, assertion) are not necessarily positive (i.e., enjoyable), the transformation of emotion is based on a similar principle: Activating a new emotion changes the preceding emotion. One understanding of the sequential effect of negative and positive emotions is simply that it is an artifact of one emotion replacing another. To show this was not the case, Fredrickson and colleagues conducted a series of laboratory studies that were critical in demonstrating the unique nature of this kind of sequential emotional processing (Fredrickson et al., 2000; Fredrickson & Levenson, 1998; Tugade & Fredrickson, 2004). They showed that when negative emotion (i.e., anxiety) was followed by positive emotion (i.e., contentment and amusement), it had a special impact on the pre-existing negative experience, something that did not occur with positive emotion alone.

In one study, participants' cardiovascular activity was monitored in an experiment where they watched stressful, funny, or neutral and boring movie clips in various sequences (Fredrickson et al., 2000). Eliciting joy and content (positive emotions about a funny video) in the context of neutral or resting baseline had no significant effect on individuals' cardiovascular activity. However, if those same emotions were elicited when people were already feeling upset (e.g., anxious after watching a stressful video), the positive emotion sped up the rate at which a person recovered from an anxiety-related cardiovascular response. By contrast, having emotionally neutral experiences after anxiety was activated did not help reduce the cardiovascular responses associated with anxiety. Furthermore, experiencing sadness (another negative emotion) after the activation of anxiety further delayed cardiovascular recovery from anxiety. Taken together, the authors observed that the sequential experiencing of negative to positive emotions uniquely accelerated an individual's physiological recovery from negative emotion.

A quite different line of inquiry on children's morality seems to provide convergent evidence. During a controlled social experiment, researchers used thermal infrared imaging to take continuous physiological readings of emotions in sequence (Ioannou et al., 2013). When children were made to feel guilty (by breaking a pre-rigged toy), their facial temperatures dropped. But, when they were subsequently soothed by the experimenter (i.e., being cheerfully told, "The accident is not your fault, it was already broken, and it can be fixed, so let's repair it together"), their autonomic response not only neutralized but overcompensated, leaving children feeling comfortably warmer than when they first begin the experiment.

These kinds of studies describe part of the biology when one emotion counters another. In short, physiological measures indicate that positive emotion seemed to act as an antidote to the distress of negative emotion. Also, as illustrated in the contrasting examples earlier, such sequences are sometimes, but not always, elicited through an interpersonal encounter (see also Porges, 2011). Nevertheless, the question at hand is not what cues positive emotion, but rather why these sequences facilitate change.

Researchers have also compared cardiovascular reactions of individuals who differed in their general levels of psychological resilience (Tugade & Fredrickson, 2004). The title of that study cuts to the core of their findings: "Resilient individuals use positive emotions to bounce back from negative emotional experiences" (p. 320). Indeed, the study demonstrated that people who were able to experience higher levels of happiness and interest in the context of preexisting distress showed a faster recovery from their anxiety-related cardiovascular responses as compared with others who struggled to experience positive emotions in the context of activated anxiety. On a similar note, a cardiac study of emotions suggests at least one biological mechanism by which transformations like these may occur (McCraty et al., 1995). Whereas anger is known to increase arousal of the nervous system, positive emotions, such as experiencing appreciation, seem to introduce variability in one's heart rate (i.e., vagal tone), which de-escalates the experience of anger. Findings like these point to the salubrious effect of sequentially experiencing positive emotions in the aftermath of negative emotion.

It is worth noting that although laboratory research is incisive, most of the research on positive emotion to date remains largely unexamined in psychotherapy (Fitzpatrick & Stalikas, 2008; Stalikas et al., 2015). Even so, the idea that positive emotion is not only a consequence but also a potential generator of therapeutic change is an idea that is garnering renewed attention. For example, sparking positive emotion has been explored as an adjunct strategy for undoing negative emotion when working with individuals who self-harm. A narrative review on this idea concluded that using positive emotion in therapy is a promising intervention for reducing the effects of negative emotion and helping clients recover from the intolerably painful emotions that underpin self-harming behaviors (Morris et al., 2014). The hypothesized mechanism for this effect is that positive emotion momentarily halts and reverses the narrowing of one's thought–action repertoire, which is implicit in the experience of negative emotion. Even so, negative emotions themselves will still eventually need to be addressed more deeply.

Fredrickson's group underscores two issues in sequential forms of emotional processing. First, as Wolpe (1958) already highlighted (Chapter 12), positive emotions and negative emotions are fundamentally incompatible in their action tendencies. More specifically, negative (i.e., unpleasant) emotions narrow an individual's repertoire of responses into a very specific set of behaviors (i.e., deepen and differentiate) to orient them toward attending to some unmet need. In contrast, positive emotions increase an individual's repertoire of responses (i.e., broaden and build) so that one can optimally engage with the given situation. This basic incompatibility in action tendencies is what gives positive emotions the power to undo preexisting negative emotion.

Secondly, Fredrickson and colleagues (2001) observed that this undoing occurs in the specific sequence of negative-to-positive emotional experiences. So the order matters. While positive emotions undid the cardiovascular responses associated with negative emotion, positive emotions had no noteworthy effect when experienced under emotionally neutral circumstances. In other words, positive emotion on its own may indeed feel good, but if it was not in the context of recovery, it did not offer a transformative benefit. These observations highlight that not only do the types of emotions matter but also the sequences in which those emotions are experienced play a critical role in the process of working through distress.

APPROACH VERSUS WITHDRAWAL: OPPOSING SYSTEMS

Clinically, we observe that approach and withdrawal emotions, motivations, and behaviors are generally incompatible with one other. Consider that the action tendency of withdrawal-related feelings, like sadness or shame, is to shrink back with slumped shoulders and a narrowed chest, raise one's inner brow, and perhaps even cover one's face. In contrast, the action tendency of approach-related feelings like anger or pride is to expand one's chest, push the torso out, sometimes even raise the arms up, or hold one's hands in fists. These action tendencies show dramatically opposing forces of self-organization and embodied meaning (Shafir et al., 2015). Furthermore, there is evidence that such action tendencies are biologically innate and not easily attributable to social learning. For example, one study systematically examined the spontaneous nonverbal expressions of pride versus shame among congenitally blind Paralympic athletes when they either won or lost their events (Tracy & Matsumoto, 2008). These observations point to a dialectical process when one emotion is elicited in the context of another contrasting emotion.

Emotional Expression: An Opponent Process System

The inherent polarity between opposing emotions were attributed to evolutionary origins as far back as Charles Darwin's (1872/1965) book *Emotional Expression in Man and Animals*. The causes of specific expressions, according to

Darwin, usually have some basis in a physiological phenomenon, and the conclusion is almost always an explanation as to why the expression of a given emotion must take the form it does. Given certain emotional states, specific complex actions can be behaviorally adaptive for an organism. The functional effects of such an action also begin to generalize and accompany emotional states that are similar or incipient versions of that state. He called this the principal of emotional association, and it creates convergence in certain sets of emotional expressions.[1]

However, Darwin also described a principle of antithesis, which focuses on the expression of emotions in opposition to one another. Thus, another driving force shaping emotional expression is the minimization of misconstrued emotion. When the functional goals of two emotions are opposite to one another, the animal's expressive actions are also opposite in nature. These opposing expressions are designed to be mutually inhibitory rather than excitatory. For instance, the actions that result from, say, humility and affection become very expressive in signaling as clearly as possible the state of nonhostility.

In short, withdrawal emotions (e.g., fear, shame, sadness, grief[2]) and approach emotions (e.g., rage, anger, assertion, pride, compassion) represent processes that are inherently opposing. This is why these two groupings cannot be fully activated at the same time (although they could be sequentially activated).[3] Meanwhile, the overlapping activation of such experiences produces a dialectical state of tension that is highly dynamic. Finally, withdrawal emotions can be transformed through the activation of otherwise incompatible approach emotions, one emotion undoing the other (Fredrickson, 2001).

Neurological Evidence: Competing Systems in the Brain

At the levels of both clinical theory and psychological functioning, it has been useful to set positive or approach experiences in contrast with negative or withdrawal experiences. But whether that functional distinction is lateralized in the brain speaks to a different level of analysis, one that remains hotly debated. Some researchers maintain that activation of areas in the right frontal hemisphere of the brain are associated with negative or withdrawal emotions, whereas activation of the brain's left frontal hemisphere is associated with positive or approach emotions, essentially representing two competing systems (Davidson, 2000; Harmon-Jones et al., 2010). However, a meta-analysis of neuroimaging studies suggests the issue is more nuanced than a simple lateralization of valence where the right brain supports negative emotion while the left brain supports positive emotion (Lindquist et al., 2016).[4]

Still, the more critical dimension for asymmetry in brain activity may be less related to positive versus negative valence (i.e., pleasant vs. unpleasant feelings) and more related to someone's approach- versus withdrawal-related motivations (e.g., motor actions and affective tendencies; Harmon-Jones et al., 2010). This means that emotions with a positive valence (e.g., enthusiasm) as well as some emotions with a negative valiance (e.g., anger), which both represent approach motivations, would be lateralized to the same side of the brain (i.e., left). Following this update (by Harmon-Jones et al., 2010), a still newer formulation of the lateralization idea has been dubbed the sword and shield hypothesis (Brookshire & Casasanto, 2018). It refers to someone wielding a sword in their dominant hand for attack (i.e., one side of the brain generating approach motivations) and holding a shield in their other hand to defend (i.e., the opposite side generating withdraw motivations). Furthermore, this hypothesis posits that when reviews have shown approach motivations were associated with the left hemisphere (e.g., Harmon-Jones et al., 2010), it is not on account of any inherent specialization of the left brain but rather because participants have been mostly right-handed (i.e., their sword hand).

Prior evidence suggests people typically use their dominant hand for approach actions but use their nondominant hand for actions related to withdrawal and avoidance. Observing that the lateralization of emotion depends on handedness, proponents of the sword and shield hypothesis have argued that "affective motivation may re-use neural circuits that evolved for performing approach- and avoidance-related motor actions" (Brookshire & Casasanto, 2018, p. 1). This is congruent with cognitive developmental theory, although a theory of schemes would argue that motor actions and affective motivations are not so distinct but rather are nested processes and perhaps inseparable (J. Pascual-Leone & Johnson, 2021). In any case, an experiment tested this by applying transcranial stimulation to the brains of healthy individuals in the form of a low but direct electrical current. This stimulation boosted frontal lobe activity in either the left or right hemisphere of participants over several days. The result was that stimulation either increased or decreased participants' experience of approach related emotions depending on their handedness (Brookshire & Casasanto, 2018).

Whatever the case, emerging agreement suggests there are discrete neural systems of emotion in the brain that are interconnected and sometimes have similar autonomic features (Kirby & Robinson, 2017; Lindquist et al., 2016; Panksepp, 2008). Lateralization aside, a more complex rendition still suggests discrete systems, providing a neurological explanation for the interactions observed between opposing emotions. This supports sequential transformations as a unique kind of emotional change.

An Emotional Struggle Between Parts

An example helps illustrate the implication for resolving personal difficulties. In a social experiment, healthy participants were first induced to feel sympathy for someone or not (a control) and then were led to believe that the other person either insulted them or not (Harmon-Jones, et al., 2004). During these steps in the experiment, researchers measured electrical activity in different areas of the brain. For those in the control group (i.e., no sympathy induction), being insulted by the other person increased activity in the left frontal areas of their brains as they thrust out and got angry at the personal violation. Simultaneously, however, the same insult also decreased activity that is usually associated with withdrawal emotion (e.g., hurt, shame) on the right side of the brain. The first observation here is that an approach emotion counters a withdrawal emotion.

However, for participants who had first been experimentally facilitated to feel the softer emotions of sympathy and compassion, the effect of subsequently being insulted was preemptively eliminated (Harmon-Jones et al., 2004). So the second observation in this study was that facilitating sympathy reduced the kind of brain activity that is otherwise typical of angering events. Again, these observations reveal that ordered emotions are not simply additive but rather interactive (A. Pascual-Leone & Greenberg, 2020). Furthermore, it is worth noting that experimental research on this process also translates well into clinical practice. Evidence from a clinical trial of individual therapy suggests that facilitating forgiveness is one of the pathways toward resolving longstanding interpersonal injuries (Malcolm et al., 2005).[5] In this way, one emotion shapes the experience of and can serve as an antidote to another emotion.

It is important to highlight that the process being described here is different from exposure to feared cues or attaining insight, and it goes beyond the ideas of catharsis, habituation, or detachment, which describe the attenuation of problematic feelings. Here, feeling is not purged or attenuated but instead transformed through dynamic interaction with more adaptive emotion. This interaction between two emotions is sometimes experienced as ambivalence or struggle between two parts of the self (e.g., puffing out one's chest in anger or pride vs. shrinking back and covering one's face in shame). In short, the process is not as simple as deciding to think more positively (although that may be part of it) but more so has to do with activating an alternative affective mode of representing and responding to the same or similarly eliciting affective cues. When the alternative emotion is activated, it fuses with the initially presenting emotion and this synthesis produces a categorically new experience.

Again, notice that not all approach behaviors are synonymous with positive emotion, and the role of anger, which is associated with approach motivation, is a prime example (Harmon-Jones et al., 2004; Zinner et al., 2007). This opens the possibility that perhaps not only negative-to-positive sequential transformations, like those identified by Fredrickson and colleagues, might be useful. Indeed, it points to the fact that withdrawal in a negative emotion (e.g., sadness) could be followed by some kind of approach in what may nevertheless still be a negative emotional experience (e.g., anger). This represents a productive withdrawal–approach sequence that does not necessarily involve any positive emotion (i.e., pleasant experiences like humor, compassion, or love).

Recent advances in psychotherapy research and theory have revealed that there are indeed productive temporal sequences of several negative (i.e., unpleasant) emotion that facilitate the resolution of distress. Other neurobiological findings suggest that painful emotion such as primary sadness, sometimes associated with activity in the right hemisphere, can attenuate the activation of language-related brain centers in the left hemisphere and impair verbal fluency, causing transient difficulties in speech (Bartolic et al., 1999). This also helps explain the characteristic vocal perturbations one might notice in the speech of people as they transition between emotions and deepen their experience (discussed earlier; Diamond et al., 2010). Changing one emotion by way of another occurs as a client gains new meaning from a freshly emerging emotion and results in newly formed neural connections as well as increased efficiency of neural information transfer (A. Pascual-Leone & Greenberg, 2020).

THE ANTIDOTE TO PAINFUL EMOTION MAY BE ANOTHER EMOTION

Sequential transformation implies that adeptly navigating specific sequences in painful emotion can have a unique benefit. But what counters this or that maladaptive emotion? If Martin Luther King Jr. (1977) is right, love is what transforms hate. But what counters shame? What about anger? What counters fear? Experimental and pseudoexperimental designs have examined this kind of emotional processing and have given evidence that, beyond the role of positive affect (e.g., joy, contentment), a negative emotion can be productively addressed using a different negative (i.e., unpleasant) emotion.

The Sequential Transformation of Shame and Sadness

A host of controlled experiments on undergraduate and community samples using single therapy sessions or structured online interventions have demonstrated that assertive anger can be prompted to function as a healthy and adaptive antidote to maladaptive shame. For example, one study prescreened undergraduate students to identify them as having either higher or lower vulnerability to depression. Participants were then brought in for a single session of emotion-focused therapy, which focused on enacting and addressing participants' self-criticisms (Whelton & Greenberg, 2005). Video of the process showed that people who had already been identified as more vulnerable to depression showed more self-contempt in their enactments. Yet the critical finding was that the harshness of self-contempt, as expressed by a curled lip or a disparaging sneer (i.e., the emotional quality), was a better predictor of vulnerability to depression than the content of criticisms per se (i.e., the cognitive content).

Furthermore, and this is where the issue of counter-emotions becomes critical, those who were more vulnerable to depression were also less resilient in how they responded to their own self-criticism as compared with participants who were known to be less vulnerable to depression. Specifically, less vulnerable individuals were able to muster up assertive anger and pride as an emotional resource to combat (transform) their depressogenic self-contempt and negative cognitions (Whelton & Greenberg, 2005). The fact that neither group was depressed in this study and that a second emotion unfolded (or not) in response to the first suggests this is a special kind of processing that ultimately underpins vulnerability versus resilience. Another experiment on working through painful self-criticism showed similar results by purposefully instructing participants to use assertive anger as a way to reduce their shame, fear, and distress (Kramer & Pascual-Leone, 2016).

An experiment on how to best work through maladaptive shame offered participants a single session of experiential psychotherapy in which people first disclosed their experience of shame over an interpersonal event (Sawashima, 2018). Once shame was activated, the researcher-therapist followed a protocol to subsequently facilitate the experience and expression of emotion using chairwork according to one of three conditions: fostering adaptive anger (i.e., an incongruent emotional state that entailed a search for meaning), fostering adaptive sadness (a congruent state that still involved a search for meaning), or rumination on shame as usual. Activating anger in the context of presenting shame was what best promoted a participant's emotional recovery from shame, providing them with both a sense of direction for resolving distress and greater self-awareness about their personal struggle (Sawashima, 2018).[6]

Finally, outside the context of psychotherapy sessions, a series of experiments with Chinese university students has shown that anger can serve as an antidote to sad (i.e., depressive) rumination. The studies asked participants to recall an unresolved personal concern and then used unrelated social feedback to subsequently induce emotion in several conditions. The experiment demonstrated that when anger was activated as a counter to sad rumination, it was more effective than the induction of either joy or a neutral state. Furthermore, when the induction sequence was repeated on successive days, anger increasingly enhanced the alleviation of depressive rumination (Zhan, Tang, et al., 2017).

These studies illustrate L. S. Greenberg's (2021) idea of changing emotion with emotion, in which primary maladaptive emotions such as shame or self-contempt can be reorganized and changed through the activation of primary adaptive emotions such as assertive anger, which are nonetheless also difficult experiences in and of themselves. The key to this process, as we will see, is that feelings need to be placed in the right sequence.

The Sequential Transformation of Anger

Of course, shame is not the only problematic feeling. Sometimes anger itself is the presenting clinical challenge for someone regarding a longstanding interpersonal grievance or betrayal. A social experiment cited earlier showed that feeling compassion and sympathy toward another can be used preemptively as an inoculation against angering-eliciting events that follow (Harmon-Jones et al., 2004). But what is there to do when anger is already fully present?

In a study at Ben-Gurion University on working through unfinished interpersonal business, Rochman and Diamond (2008) conducted a multistep mood induction task designed to facilitate experiences of anger and sadness in strategically ordered sequences. The sample involved undergraduate students who reported having unresolved (i.e., secondary) anger toward a significant person in their life (e.g., family member, romantic partner, long-term friend). Semistructured mood inductions were administered in the context of a single session of experiential therapy. In the first part of this study, participants were randomly assigned to conditions where they would experience either sadness-before-anger or anger-before-sadness.

Participants in the sadness-before-anger condition were guided to first experience sadness and then to subsequently experience anger while discussing their relationship with the significant other who they imagined to be in the empty chair in front of them. Meanwhile, participants in the counterpart anger-before-sadness condition were guided to experience and express the same emotions but in the reverse order. As a control, additional groups of participants underwent conditions where they were guided to experience either only anger at both stages of the mood induction task or only sadness. Anger and sadness are often both important parts of interpersonal grievances and represent two sides of the same coin when resolving interpersonal injuries with significant others. However, the question was, does the order of emotions matter when working through one's unresolved anger?

By using finger temperature as a measure of physiological arousal, the researchers demonstrated that all participants had some increased activation in their sympathetic nervous systems from baseline to when they experienced a negative emotion (i.e., whether anger or sadness) during the first step of the mood induction. However, only those in the anger-to-sadness condition showed an additional increase in sympathetic arousal during the second part of the task (Rochman & Diamond, 2008). Thus, the experience of sadness triggered even greater arousal when sadness was induced after anger as opposed to any other sequence. The researchers speculated that individuals who present with unresolved anger may somehow better engage with and process their presenting problematic anger when they subsequently access primary adaptive sadness. The sequence offered an advantage over either starting the process with sadness (e.g., a grief-focused approach) or only staying with anger (e.g., a venting or desensitization-and-extinction-oriented approach).

Another study by the same research lab used a standardized single therapy session to help participants work through unresolved anger toward an attachment figure (Narkiss-Guez et al., 2015). Findings over the session show that as participants' experience of attachment-related sadness (i.e., grief over loss) intensified, the intensity of their presenting anger decreased. A graph of these arousal trajectories forms a remarkable mirror image, where the corresponding changes in anger versus sadness seem to offset one another over the course of a session. By the end of the session, angry participants reported feeling significantly more sad than angry while they explored the meaning of their personal difficulty.

Outside the context of psychotherapy, this form of emotional processing has also been examined in experiments focused on reducing aggression. One study manipulated situational factors to mitigate a participants' risk for aggressive behavior. Anger-driven aggressive behavior was diffused by instructing participants to recall a sad personal event, which was more effective at countering aggression than a control task (Lutz & Krahé, 2018). In another study, participants watch brief emotion-inducing film clips. Once activated to feel angry, participants who subsequently watched sad film clips had larger reductions in aggressive behavior than those in conditions who were led to feel either fear or neutral after their anger. Interestingly, inducing fear after anger exacerbated participants' anger (Zhan et al., 2015).

Experimental research of this kind has also considered how acute stress might interfere with emotional processing (Zhan, Wu, et al., 2017). Research suggests people who are more vulnerable to stress, who lack self-control, or who lack other meta-cognitive and attentional resources are more likely to get angry. However, surprisingly little research has examined the dynamic impact of acute stress on cognitive strategies such as reframing when working with emotion. In contrast, when emotion is transformed sequentially, it is driven by a bottom-up processes and may be less easily derailed by the introduction of stressors.

In a remarkable experiment by Zhan, Wu, and colleagues (2017) at Capital Normal University, a large sample of university students in Beijing were first given critical social feedback as part of an anger induction and then randomized to six experimental conditions. Once participants were angry, they were then shown brief film clips to facilitate either (a) the induction of sadness, (b) the cognitive reappraisal of their anger, or (c) a neutral state (control). In a 3 × 2 × 3 design, the three intervention conditions were administered either in the presence or absence of physiological stress by having participants submerge their arm in either ice-cold water or room temperature water.[7] Furthermore, all six experimental conditions were followed over three time points (i.e., baseline, anger activation, intervention). Finally, the reduction of anger was measured using four indices: tracking subjective changes in anger, the observation of aggressive behavior (through a paradigm in which participants chose how much to punish others), and both saliva cortisol and skin conductance (physiological measures of arousal associated with anger).

In the absence of stress, cognitive reappraisal effectively reduced subjective feelings of anger after participants were provoked. However, the benefit of this cognitive strategy disappeared when participants were under acute stress. In contrast, the strategy of using sadness to change anger reduced both aggressive behavior and physiological arousal, regardless of the stress condition.[8] In short, being under stress impaired the efficiency of cognitive reappraisal. This supported the main hypotheses that sadness had an undoing effect, which countered anger, and that this strategy of changing emotion with emotion was more robust under stress than using cognitive reappraisals to change anger (Zhan, Wu, et al., 2017).

The Sequential Transformation of Fear

Research to date on working with fear through a sequential transformation is underdeveloped. That gap is likely on account of the disproportionate attention given to anxiety, which is secondary symptomatic fear and as such can be soothed, managed, or extinguished (see Chapter 3 on down-regulation). Primary maladaptive fear, however, is not so easily resolved by just reducing its intensity. For example, when someone with a history of abuse cannot receive healthy expression of love and instead reacts with traumatic fear, then habituation alone is not sufficient (Paivio & Pascual-Leone, 2023). Rather, internally generating reciprocal feelings of love or compassion toward the other is essential for countering what initially were deep fears of intimacy (L. S. Greenberg & Malcolm, 2002; Wiebe & Johnson, 2016).

The similar behavioral signatures of fear and anger mean that a courageous act of assertion and fighting for oneself can also serve as the antidotes for undoing fear. There are many examples of this in everyday life, and research on behavior therapy for anxiety disorders also offers a host of relevant clinical evidence (see Linehan, 2015; Spiegler, 2015; Wolpe, 1958). Problematic fear can also be transformed through self-compassion (e.g., Schanche et al., 2011). Finally, avoidance and withdrawal due to fear are sometimes overcome through the experience of curiosity, which itself may become a transformative positive experience (Fredrickson, 2001).

Optimal Sequences Depend on Presenting Concerns

An intriguing observation emerges from the aforementioned studies. When participants were struggling with unresolved anger, then facilitating sadness seemed to be an effective intervention that countered the presenting anger (e.g., Lutz & Krahé, 2018; Narkiss-Guez et al., 2015; Rochman & Diamond, 2008; Zhan, Wu, et al., 2017). At the same time, other research that examined participants with depressive symptoms or who were struggling with sadness concluded that facilitating anger was beneficial (e.g., Choi et al., 2015; Sawshima, 2018; Whelton & Greenberg, 2005; Zhan et al., 2015). Though the use of different methods and populations limits direct comparisons, perhaps the optimal sequence for transforming emotion (e.g., anger-before-sadness, sadness-before-anger) depends on one's primary emotional concern.

That hypothesis was tested using an online experiment that recruited undergraduate students distressed about unfinished interpersonal grievances with a significant person in their lives (Nardone et al., 2025). First, two naturally occurring groups were identified: on the one hand, individuals who reported feeling primarily angry about their interpersonal concern, and on the other, individuals who felt primarily sad. Next, participants from each of these two groups were randomly assigned to one of two online conditions that used a series of open-ended questions and prompts for emotion to facilitate the experience and expression of either (a) anger-before-sadness or (b) sadness-before-anger. In sum, the groups of participants differed in whether they felt mostly angry or sad, whereas experimental conditions only differed by the sequence in which participants wrote about their feelings. Finally, in this 2 × 2 × 3 design, participants were also followed over three time points: baseline level of emotion, the first emotion induction, and then the second emotion induction. This timeline allowed researchers to examine the intensity of emotion at each step and then to rule out the individual effect of either anger or sadness in isolation by comparing it to baseline.

The main outcome of interest was whether there were changes to the kind of distress that participants presented with—that is, was anger reduced for the angry group? Did sadness reduce for the sad group? When participants only experienced one emotion it had little to no immediate effect. Furthermore, experiencing both emotions—but in the wrong order—also made little difference in this brief intervention:

> Findings point to the conclusion that the order of emotions matters, but the optimal order seems to depend on one's presenting concern (i.e., presenting anger or sadness). For individuals who were angry about an interpersonal problem, expressing their anger and then their sadness was more productive than if they had expressed the same emotions in reverse order. However, when individuals presented predominantly with sadness over what happened, then exploring and expressing their sadness before moving on to feelings of anger was more productive, as compared to if the same emotions were experienced but reversed. Overall, ending an intervention with the "new" (i.e., opposing) feeling seems to be most helpful. (Nardone et al., 2025, p. 12)

Indeed, prescribing the corresponding optimal sequence reduced the intensity of someone's presenting anger by a medium effect, or if their presenting concern was sadness the right sequence reduced that feeling by a small effect. These interventions typically took participants less than 20 minutes. Finally, the fact that the best sequence of ordered emotions depended on a person's target or presenting emotion also provides a neat explanation for what appeared to be an inconsistency across prior studies.

Together these studies support the idea of starting with the validation of a presenting emotion and then moving to transform the problematic feelings. The fact that certain ordered emotions predict both better processing and outcomes supports the conceptualization of sequential transformation as a unique form of processing in psychotherapy. In this section I have reviewed a body of experimental and pseudoexperimental findings that show the antidote to a painful emotion is sometimes another opposing emotion. Results from a range of research designs support the hypothesis that some specific sequences of emotion will be more productive and therefore more transformative than others. Even so, more research is needed to determine which sequences are best for working through what problems.

EMERGENCE OF NEW EXPERIENCE: PSYCHOGENESIS AND NEUROLOGICAL UNDERPINNINGS

The key points in defining sequential transformations are the notions of a dynamic interaction between emotions and the moment-by-moment unfolding of an increasingly complex experience through a sequence of composite emotions. Furthermore, the precise way one conceptualizes and describes this psychological process has implications for both understanding the mechanism of change and for executing interventions that facilitate it.

Mental Effort, Information Processing, and Cognitive Development

The phenomenology of how clients switch across emotional sequences highlights that clients do not have equally fluid access to all their feelings that bear on a given difficulty. For understanding the landscape of psychological units that psychogenetically come together to produce an emotion transformation, one key question is: Why does an opposite emotion seem to emerge as the antidote and only after some effort? To answer this from an evolutionary perspective, we could refer to the observations already made by Darwin.

However, on the level of mental processing, when a maladaptive emotion is predominant (i.e., a default or attractor state), it is because there is a hegemony of compatible schemes in one's repertoire that overdetermine and potentiate that pathological way of being.[9] This overdetermination is a large part of why maladaptive emotions are so entrenched. If subdominant schemes are not compatible with the presenting maladaptive (default) state, then they are inhibited through the allocation of attentional resources (e.g., unfortunately, I can't see other possibilities because inhibiting them is one of the ways I am able to be so focused on this negative possibility!). Inhibition of this kind is unrelated to defensive (i.e., motivated) suppression in the psychodynamic sense but rather is the same process that produces the perception of a figure against its background. Inhibition of opposing schemes maximizes their contrast and is a function of basic mental processes, which pertain just as much to cognitive as emotional information.

It follows that potentially adaptive emotions are not only in the periphery of awareness (i.e., less clear, less familiar, and less rehearsed) but that they are also actively inhibited by one's mental hardware simply because those alternative schemes are incompatible with the presiding state (J. Pascual-Leone & Johnson, 2021). This means that accessing alternative and healthier emotional self-organizations (e.g., assertion, pride, self-compassion) in the moment-by-moment context of a presenting dominant maladaptive emotion (e.g., shame, inadequacy, terror) requires the client to exercise mental effort and essentially focus their attention. This means that transformation requires clients to endogenously boost the activity of otherwise peripheral schemes that represent alternative and more adaptive emotion states, which initially may feel counterintuitive or far-fetched. Mental effort in the form of actively attending to other emergent states is a well-documented mental operation in cognitive psychology and is viscerally experienced as the emotional effort in working toward change. So, for adaptive but subdominant emotions to get over the threshold and fully enter one's experience, the feelings must be effortfully and deliberately attended to by the client. Phenomenologically, when this is successful, it essentially produces a switch between the figure and background in one's emotional landscape of experience, a reversal in the gestalt. The mental effort one used to do this is an endogenous but limited psychobiological resource (J. Pascual-Leone & Johnson, 2021).

While the client's effort is being applied through focused attention, it can also be supported by the coconstructive efforts of the therapist. For example, a client of mine who was emotionally abandoned by her father after the death of her mother sometimes needed my focus as a sort of attentional scaffolding to guide her toward a fuller evocation of more adaptive facets of her broader experience, which otherwise would have been missed.

CLIENT: After mom died, he just drank alone a lot in the basement, and just sort of became absent. I was really just a little girl. . . . I would make peanut butter sandwiches for dinner, and he would walk through and just pick one up without even looking at me. . . . I wasn't a person, not enough to make it worth living for him. I was a nuisance, really. I just made life worse for him. [*She weeps.*]

THERAPIST: It's like, "I was just part of the burden [*she nods as she wipes her tears*] and the pain I felt didn't matter to him." [*The client takes a deep breath, frowns, and then looks up at the ceiling, shaking her head.*] Hmm, there's something different going on for you inside right now. . . . Stay with that. . . . [*The client sits back, feet together, folding her arms squarely*] Huh, something isn't right? What is it?

CLIENT: You know . . . no, it wasn't right. I was only a kid. I didn't deserve that! [*A long pause, the client slumps forward slightly*] Well, I don't know . . . maybe I did. [*She hangs her head and sinks back into her seat.*]

Here, the client puts words to her usual feelings in the same old story. But when I attend (as therapist) to some other subdominant parts of her experience, then the client shifts and begins to articulate an emerging sense of injustice and assertion. However, as soon as she gets louder, the emotion erodes and she collapses into self-doubt, falling back into her familiar maladaptive state of feeling at fault and shamefully unworthy of love. So, even when the client can identify, attend, and explore new feelings, the new discovery or positive shift is quite ephemeral and fragile (e.g., Client: "I didn't deserve that! Well . . . maybe I did"). Before I could help unpack the client's fleeting moment of assertion, it had already vanished.

Until newer adaptive states become more stable, their construction is always contingent on the contribution of a client's focused mental effort to uphold it. Essentially any distraction, overload, or excessive arousal (a critical concern) topples the fragile moment-by-moment construction of any new and adaptive emotional reorganization (e.g., assertion, self-compassion, healthy grief) only to be replaced once again by the more familiar and maladaptive emotional states (e.g., a collapse into shame and maladaptive guilt; Client: "Maybe I did deserve it"). This is the main reason why emotional change (and sequential transformation in particular) is a dynamic and nonlinear process (Gelo & Salvatore, 2016). That nonlinear process has been documented in process research as a saw-toothed improvement, where clients progress by moving two steps forward and one step back (A. Pascual-Leone, 2009; Stiles et al., 2004). In time, however, with each push of effortful attention, the client generates some microconstruction of an alternative self-state, slightly shifting the loadings in their neural network. The healthier states, although emergent and still weak, become increasingly reliable as part of the emotional repertoire that a client brings to negotiate their difficult life circumstances.

Coactivating Neural Networks of Emotion

The previous explanation has referred to highly dynamic psychological units using the language of schemes. However, schemes (and by extension, emotion schemes) can also be considered in neurological terms.

Neuroplasticity

In the brain, emotion schemes are represented by distributed networks of activation that are cofunctional and coactivated (J. Pascual-Leone & Johnson, 2021). Furthermore, *neuroplasticity* refers to the dynamic property by which the brain can reorganize itself, changing the way different areas become either more or less interconnected (Doidge, 2007). This helps explain how a sequentially ordered transformation happens in the brain. The process of sequential transformation in psychotherapy first requires the client to become aware of and then process maladaptive emotion by accessing and activating another more adaptive emotion. This competition between patterns of neural activation is a condition for plastic change, where new patterns of activation within the brain can effect dramatic change if they consistently capture more useful or productive (albeit new) representations and procedures for how one interacts with the internal or external word (Doidge, 2007; J. Pascual-Leone & Johnson, 2021). Over time, the coactivation of more adaptive emotion along with or in response to the presenting maladaptive emotion helps to gradually transform maladaptive emotion.

Donald Hebb, a neuropsychologist at McGill University and an early pioneer contributing to the idea of neural networks, is known for describing how neurons contribute to the change of psychological experiences. This has often been summarized by the saying that "neurons that fire together wire together"—and then continue to fire together. This means that when synaptic activity is coordinated between neurons, the strength of their connection grows, facilitating future biochemical communication between those same neurons (Löwel & Singer, 1992). In short, the likelihood of a newly emerging pattern can be shaped through its repeated activation. Because competing emotion schemes may be represented by neural networks that partially overlap, when they are coactivated, the result is a cofunctional synthesis. This is how the process can eventually change what was the default pattern of one's brain (Doidge, 2007; Lane & Nadel, 2020). In a therapy session, once a novel feeling is activated, it offers additional emotional resources that are embodied through a different way of perceiving and engaging with the presenting problem (given that different emotions offer different representational and procedural patterns; A. Pascual-Leone & Greenberg, 2020).

In short, as therapists help their clients to activate alternative and more adaptive emotion, it transforms the embodied meaning from within the presenting maladaptive emotion itself. The approach action tendencies and positive self-evaluations that are characteristic of an adaptive emotion such as assertive anger come to be wired together with elements of what was previously only maladaptive emotion. For example, the soliciting cue for painful emotion and the precise nature of one's unmet need are now experienced differently in a newly synthesized emotional experience. Thus, activating a key shift in emotion (e.g., compassion in the face of anger, assertion in the face of shame) begins to undo the psycho-affective motor program at the basic level of emotionally schematic memories that were previously shaping and determining the person's mode of processing (A. Pascual-Leone & Greenberg, 2020). Notice that in this kind of enduring change, the second neural network of emotion does not suppress and no longer competes with what was an earlier network of emotion. Rather, a newly forged network subsumes and encompasses critical aspects of both reactions. In this way, for example, the old triggers for maladaptive shame now also activate the resilience of assertive anger or pride.

Memory Reconsolidation

Memory formation and re-formation is strongly influenced by emotion, which speaks to the larger elaboration of emotional meaning. *Memory reconsolidation* is the neurological process by which activated memories become malleable and possibly modified (Lane & Nadel, 2020). First, an emotional scheme is activated in the treatment session as part of an associated memory. Then, for some period after that experience of emotion, the associated memory is labile and open to influence. This window of time is at least 10 minutes but can last longer (although not more than 6 hours; Lane & Nadel, 2020). If a new and relevant emotional experience subsequently occurs within that time, it gets integrated into the same overall experience, thereby transforming (or augmenting, or even corrupting) the affective memory that had originally been recalled. So, opposing emotions do not have to be experienced simultaneously (and often cannot be), but it is enough for them to be juxtaposed in time (Ekert et al., 2024).

As the window for change passes, the newly rendered memory is reconsolidated, taking the place of the older memory. The next time the emotional memory is cued, it activates this updated (i.e., reconsolidated) memory. Notice that contrary to the popular understanding of memory as a historical record, where one retrieves some experience as such, the way memory functions is that one retrieves the last version of a memory to have been stored (i.e., reconsolidated; Alberini & LeDoux, 2013). In this way, the story of what happened and particularly its emotional tone will often shift and develop over time as someone works through personal difficulties. (For more on the impact of memory reconsolidation on personal narratives, see Chapter 19.)

Finally, while an isolated shift from one emotion to another may be inconsequential on its own, each transformation event is like a single emotional pushup (A. Pascual-Leone, 2009), where strength is built through repetition. Thus, with repeated coactivation of one emotion after another, two neural networks are coactivated and come to be cofunctional (i.e., neurons that fire together wire together), creating novelty through a synthesis of parts (A. Pascual-Leone & Greenberg, 2020). This emergence of new emotion is transient. Neurologically, it is a pulse of activation (e.g., one pushup) that represents a functional pattern, which organizes one to engage the world with a unique set of affective meanings. Every synchronized pulse of that pattern is an instantiation that further stabilizes the new emotion, further establishing it within an individual's emotional repertoire. The resultant solution is a novel synthesis rendering a new emotional experience made of aspects from each of the preceding states. Thus, the client is changed, and old feelings are now experienced differently.

Construction of Higher Order Schemes

In ordered sequence, the two composite emotions are wired together and then contribute to a larger function; this is the transformation itself. But the wiring together of neural networks is contingent on their synthesis producing a cofunctional and adaptive totality. Yet having complex feelings all too often entails inherent internal conflicts in one's experience. That ambivalence is a perennial problem within human experience.

Aspects of anger can be productive (e.g., healthy assertion) just as aspects of sadness may be equally productive (e.g., grieving a loss). One emotion pushes forward, while the other recedes backwards. Yet so often clients in the throes of emotional difficulty find themselves not only feeling but also doing (enacting) opposing emotions at the same time, where the fusion of anger and sadness manifests in session as stagnant complaint or whining (Paivio & Pascual-Leone, 2023). Each emotion, if it emerged on its own, could be a productive experience. Another common example of fused emotion in psychotherapy is the simultaneous experience of rageful anger and feeling guilt (about one's rage), with the two fused together being an essential psychodynamic formulation of neurosis (Davanloo, 2005). In these and other examples, to be productively worked through, the existing aspects of an emotional conflict need to be separated out and disentangled, so to speak, before they can be reintegrated in a more coordinated manner. Because contradiction is inherent to emotion as a dynamic system, fostering a new level of coherence within a client's emotional landscape becomes an overall treatment objective (Ecker et al., 2024; Gelo & Salvatore, 2016).

How can emotions be reconciled when they form a dialectical contradiction to one another? In short, when opposing schemes are coactivated, all compatible elements synthesize to form a new higher level scheme. This is a complex dialectical process, so to use a more concrete illustration, consider the basic mental coordination needed in the task of how toddlers first learn to walk. In that example, a child already has a procedural scheme for standing and another separate scheme for some kind of controlled falling (e.g., they can purposefully flop down in some direction). These schemes are also opposing, in that one cannot both stand up and fall down at the same time. But when these two independent schemes for physical action are rhythmically coordinated (i.e., stand up, fall forward a bit, stand up, fall forward a bit, etc.), the higher order synchronization represents a larger overarching scheme in and of itself. Thus, using existing subschemes, the toddler essentially dynamically synthesizes these into a categorically new and higher order scheme!—walking (L. S. Greenberg & Pascual-Leone, 1995; J. Pascual-Leone & Johnson, 2021).[10] The advantage of this new synthesis is obvious. Then, as the toddler repeatedly makes efforts to coactivate the existing subschemes into a single system, the components become progressively wired together on a neurological level. In the same way, opposing schemes entailing different emotional states (e.g., anger vs. sadness about being neglected) could be synthesized to form new integrations of experience through a dialectical construction (e.g., feeling affirmed in one's value even as one accepts missed opportunities in life).[11]

Changing emotion through this process often is not simply a matter of willpower (i.e., implementing a skill). However, it does require one to attend to both the dominant and subdominant facets of an emotional experience. It further requires one to endure the ensuing contradiction between parts, which must be internally resolved (Ecker et al., 2024). In other words, the truth of both opposing emotions as embodied meanings must be experienced, articulated, and activated as part of a larger dialectical whole. As discussed earlier, when a problematic emotion is engaged through this change process, it interacts with the new shift in focus (e.g., due to internal exploration, external prompts) and develops phenomenologically into a categorically different (i.e., novel and more complex) emotional state. In this way, one emotion develops out of another, and the generation of new meaning comes from the client both feeling differently and also feeling a wider range of emotions in response to the same old cue. However, primary maladaptive emotion is usually very painful to endure, so engaging and articulating that emotion is a productive first step. The emotion will then be part of a sequence of other feelings and meanings, rendering a deeper experience that precipitates change (L. S. Greenberg et al., 2007; A. Pascual-Leone, 2018).

By the end of the next chapter, it will become increasingly clear that the thread allowing one to bridge from presenting maladaptive to emerging adaptive emotional states—and the common ground between these kinds of emotions—turns out to be the pursuit of unmet existential needs.

ENDNOTES

1. Interestingly, Darwin's account of how emotion naturally generalizes anticipated an observation almost 50 years later by John Watson, the father of behaviorism, that emotions can be classically conditioned.

2. Some readers may question why sadness and grief are categorized along with other affective tendencies to withdraw or avoid (e.g., fear, shame) given that the initial tendency is to call out for contact and comfort. However, more specifically, the action tendency of sadness is to call upon others to make an approach. Adaptive sadness is also associated with actions of withdrawing so one might conserve resources and recover. Meanwhile, maladaptive forms of sadness embody a chronic collapse, as in depression. Finally, brain lateralization points to the association of sadness (in general) with withdrawal-related tendencies (e.g., Harmon-Jones et al., 2010).

3. This describes an opponent process, of which there are many examples in psychology and neurology. The perception of color is a classic example, which follows from Hering's observation that there are color combinations we never see such as reddish-green or yellowish-blue. This is because the perception of such colors is controlled by opponent systems. For instance, a red–green receptor in the eye cannot send messages about both colors at the same time. Similarly, opposing emotions are processes governed within the same affective–expressive system, and as such, both sides of that opposition cannot be fully experienced or expressed at the same time.

4. Generally, lesion research continues to show findings that are consistent with lateralization by valence, but most functional imaging research tells a different story and calls into question the grouping of emotion by positive or approach and negative or withdrawal regarding the neural substrates. It may also be confounded by the research practice of recruiting right-handers as an experimental control.

5. Forgiveness was only one pathway for recovery. Other research on resolving trauma at the hand of a callous or unrepentant perpetrator shows that equally good treatment outcomes often do not involve forgiveness (see Paivio & Pascual-Leone, 2023). This fact highlights that when emotion changes emotion, the process cannot be applied pro forma: Both an individual's context and their idiosyncratic framework of meaning are critical in determining the best clinical direction.

6. An important caution is that expressing anger sometimes works (in the short term) irrespective of whether anger is adaptive or not. This is because when anger is secondary (e.g., rageful or defensive), that also produces temporary reprieve and distraction from deeper pain of feeling ashamed (see A. Pascual-Leone et al., 2013). The practical implication is that when anger is used as an adaptive and productive antidote to maladaptive shame, clinicians need to continually help refocus their clients on the unmet existential need they are fighting for to prevent the feeling from deteriorating into secondary rejecting anger that is blaming and destructive in favor of bolstering primary assertive anger about a specific healthy entitlement.

7. The cold pressor test is a standard paradigm used to induce bodily stress, often as a measure of pain tolerance. It activates the sympathetic nervous system and hypothalamic pituitary adrenal axis.

8. While skin conductance, cortisol, and aggression were all reduced in response to the sadness induction, these changes were not mirrored in participant's self-reported anger. In contrast, when cognitive reappraisal was used under the no-stress condition, participants reported their anger was reduced in a way that was consistent with observed physiological changes. This intriguing caveat echoes the research previously described regarding experiential versus cognitive approaches to affect labeling (see Chapter 6) and suggests different interventions are geared toward different targets of change (i.e., reflected by the different measures). I speculate that a purposeful effort to use cognitive reframing (i.e., thinking about emotion in a different way)

facilitates congruence with the subsequent reevaluation of perceived arousal by both explicitly drawing attention to one's arousal and to reduce cognitive dissonance (see Zhan, Wu, et al., 2017; see also Chapter 9 on the attribution of arousal).

9. Recall that, as discussed in the Introduction, emotion schemes are at once representational and procedural.

10. Although dynamic systems theory offers a good descriptive model (i.e., an account of proximal objects) for the emergence of new schemes or ways of being, it does not offer a deeper causal explanation (i.e., of distal objects) for the mechanism of change. In contrast, constructivist theory does.

11. The term "dialectical constructivism" was coined by Juan Pascual-Leone and refers to an epistemological position where representational and procedural meaning is constructed by working through opposing positions, in this case emotionally embodied meanings (J. Pascual-Leone & Johnson, 2021). The initial contradiction between parts of emotion is reconciled through a dialectic, where compatible elements are combined and competing elements cancel one another out. The resulting synthesis is a dialectical construction of new meaning—a trade-off or working compromise— that coordinates the invariants that have been abstracted across various situations. This functional solution overarches the original contradiction yet contains elements of both positions.

14

Adult Emotional Development

Expanding One's Repertoire

But I must finally realize that I am subject to these sudden transformations. The thing is that I rarely think; a crowd of small metamorphoses accumulate in me without my noticing it, and then, one fine day, a veritable revolution takes place.

—JEAN-PAUL SARTRE, *NAUSEA*

The world breaks everyone and afterward many are strong at the broken places.

—ERNEST HEMINGWAY, *A FAREWELL TO ARMS*

For children, the lion's share of emotional development is explained by their very dramatic increases in mental capacity. As their brain grows, they can experience, manage, and coordinate an increasingly complex array of feelings and meanings (J. Pascual-Leone & Johnson, 2021). For example, they gain more emotional awareness and begin to experience mixed emotions (Chapter 6, this volume; Nook et al., 2018). They also benefit from an increased ability to monitor and reflect on their own experience (i.e., meta-cognitive capacity; Chapters 3 and 20). But the biological maturation of the brain is mostly complete around age 16 (J. Pascual-Leone & Johnson, 2021). After that, some adults continue to develop emotionally, whereas others less so. Largely, the ongoing emotional development that occurs during adulthood has to do with increasing one's repertoire of emotional responses and their underlying meanings. Adults who cultivate a wider and more flexible emotional range are better able to navigate personal challenges. This type of personal growth is the result of working through painful emotion (Freud, 1926) by way

https://doi.org/10.1037/0000460-015
Principles of Emotion Change: What Works and When in Psychotherapy and Everyday Life, by
A. Pascual-Leone
Copyright © 2026 by the American Psychological Association. All rights reserved.

of corrective emotional experiences (Alexander & French, 1946). One important way that personal development occurs is through the experience of sequential transformations of emotion occurring repeatedly over time.

Previous chapters in this part of the book (i.e., in Part IV) discussed the mechanisms of change that operate during a sequential transformation, but they have also focused on individual shifts between emotions—a single instance of sequential transformation. The fact that ordered transitions can occur between multiple discrete emotions raises the possibility of a longitudinal impact on emotional development. In this chapter, I consider several theories of psychotherapy that describe longer sequential trajectories unfolding over the course of treatment. The second part of this chapter considers specific mechanisms of change from a developmental perspective.

LONGER CHAINS MAP OUT THE OVERARCHING PROCESS

Maladaptive emotion is transformed by accessing and evoking primary adaptive emotion. In psychotherapy, this process is believed to typically occur later, during the working phase of treatment, after there is sufficient emotional awareness and when clients are able to manage and make use of their arousal. As reviewed in Chapter 13, research has identified key binary combinations of sequential transformation. For example, maladaptive fear about being preyed upon can be transformed through the emergence of assertive anger in which clients actively defend their boundaries and dignity (Paivio & Pascual-Leone, 2023). Similarly, shame that involves feeling bad, damaged, and unlovable can be transformed by accessing the emotions of assertive anger, pride, self-compassion, or love. The kind of maladaptive shame that drives the contempt of harsh self-blame is transformed when one accesses feelings of anger about injustice (Whelton & Greenberg, 2005). Working through anger, however, can be facilitated by subsequently moving to deeper experiences of sadness and grieving (Nardone et al., 2025; Narkiss-Guez et al., 2015; Rochman & Diamond, 2008), or at other times, it can be changed using compassion (Harmon-Jones, et al., 2004).

As one compiles these assorted findings, at least three problems emerge in their clinical application. First, one might be tempted to consider some of these emotions as universal remedies. Indeed, several folk theories and even some clinical approaches have done that. Compassion is an increasingly popular case in point, although love, assertiveness training, and purging one's grief are other single-experience remedies that have also been championed to date as the panacea for all emotional problems. At best, the treatment's practice is more nuanced, while its explanatory theory is a simplification that neglects important nuances (see Chapters 1 and 8). At worst, a one-emotion remedy acts as a one-trick pony, effective but only with a limited and very specific applicability. Whatever the case, the complexity of moment-by-moment emotional life does not lend itself to a single a priori formula for resolving all personal difficulties.[1]

The second puzzle is that despite empirical evidence showing one emotion can change another, the possible permutations among discrete emotions quickly leads one to a motley collection of emotion pairs. The problem state in one pair might even be the antidote in another. Exactly so, as one experiment showed, sadness can sometimes be used to reduce problematic anger, but at other times, anger can be used to reduce problematic sadness (Nardone et al., 2025). In short, a mix and match of these sequences might resemble a children's game of rock-paper-scissors.

Third, a sequential transformation cannot be applied formulaically to individuals because it is contingent on the idiosyncratic meanings and experience of each person. Ultimately, to address any of these three issues, one needs an overarching framework of how transformation occurs. Mapping out the longitudinal process holds the pieces of evidence together. Indeed, the dualistic conceptualization of sequential patterns (e.g., negative–positive, withdrawal–approach, opposite-action-to-emotion) has been further developed, usually implicitly, within various theories of psychotherapy.

CLINICAL THEORIES CHART A COURSE FOR SEQUENTIAL TRANSFORMATION

Many of the sequences I have described suggest the antidote to a specific painful or negative emotional experience may be yet another (still) painful or negative emotion. This may not seem very encouraging at first. Fortunately, Gendlin's (1981) approach to experiential focusing captures the essence of an ongoing sequence when he points out that "nothing that feels bad is ever the last step" (pp. 25–26). Indeed, researchers and theorists in humanistic–experiential as well as experiential–psychodynamic traditions have focused on understanding the process by which emotions successively unfold over the course of therapy. Probably not by chance, something all these treatment approaches have in common is a long history of using video recorded sessions not only in research but also for training and supervision.

Psychodynamic perspectives typically formulate personal difficulties within a relational framework and as a result those conceptualizations of sequential transformation tend to emphasize interpersonal themes. However, changing emotion with emotion is a process that applies similarly to resolving either interpersonal themes or intrapersonal difficulties, like self-criticism. Emotion-focused therapy, for instance, has explicitly used sequential transformations in both problem domains. I now briefly discussed a few salient examples from these orientations—with a focus on how they conceptualize the emotional struggle as well as the temporal patterns of emotion—that are believed to yield clinical change.

Psychodynamic–Experiential Models of Transformational Sequences

From early on, psychodynamic approaches have understood defense mechanisms as ways of coping, that symptoms represent secondary distress or anxiety, and that there is a deeper primary process underling these (Freud, 1926). This has led several theorists (from various treatment orientations) to use the image of pealing back the layers of an onion to capture a longer process of working with emotion,[2] one that requires a sequence where one cannot simply force the engagement of what in fact may be the deeper issue. Although psychodynamic approaches have typically referred to the layering of defenses, those therapies that are also emotion-oriented refer to sequences in an emotional process that are necessary steppingstones before one can precipitate lasting change. (Indeed, this was inspiration for Kübler-Ross's [1969] stages of grief discussed in Chapter 12).

Change Is Unlocked by a Sequential Process

Intensive short-term dynamic psychotherapy (Chapter 8, this volume; Abbass & Town, 2013; Davanloo, 2005) is an approach aimed specifically at encouraging a client's experience of unconscious emotions related to unresolved attachment issues. These emotional injuries are thought to stem from past unhealthy learning experiences with attachment figures (e.g., parents), and they involve painful emotions such as shame and despair. In this empirically supported treatment (for a meta-analysis, see Abbass et al., 2012), the therapist aims to break down defenses by confronting clients, directly challenging them in a process often referred to as a head-on collision. Davanloo saw pressuring and challenging the client as indispensable in helping the client to overcome the affective–cognitive processes that blocked them from experiencing painful but personally relevant emotion.[3] Thus, *unlocking the unconscious* is essentially a metaphor for a key in-session change event in which specific painful emotions about past attachment injuries are activated, allowed, and expressed (Abbass & Town, 2013).

This approach hypothesizes that in order to resolve their presenting distress, clients need to first experience aggressive impulses or murderous rage toward an attachment figure, which is also laden with—and blocked by—guilt. Second, having this highly aroused experience of rage and working through the related guilt also opens the way to feelings of love and closeness toward one's attachment figure. The third and final phase is a deep experience of grief over personal loss and the missed opportunities in interpersonal relatedness. The imperative of activating both rage and grief is based on an understanding that these experiences, in conjunction with working through transference, precipitate a profound sequential transformation. The prescribed shifts in emotion foster a willingness in clients to explore the deeply rooted emotional injuries that underlie their psychological dysfunctions.

Detailed case study research (e.g., Davanloo, 2005; Fleury et al., 2016) and studies on mixed diagnostic samples have demonstrated that when clients go through this emotional process, it has moderate to large effects in predicting better treatment outcomes (e.g., Abbass et al., 2017). A study of intensive short-term dynamic psychotherapy examined countering one emotion with another as a mechanism of change by looking at how exploring otherwise avoided anger related to the sadness of depression (Town et al., 2022). Exploring a client's anger in a given session predicted the reduction of their depression by the next session, 7 days later.

The Internal Conflict: Activating Versus Inhibiting Affects

Leigh McCullough, a clinical professor at Harvard Medical School, reformulated short-term dynamic therapy in behavioral terms, arguing that clients initially express *affect phobia*—unconscious anxiety about experiencing and expressing emotion (McCullough et al., 2003; Osborn et al., 2015). As such, emotional conflicts are chronically avoided, warded off, or minimized by defensive ways of thinking, feeling, or behaving. Averting emotional engagement in these ways is believed to result in a client's presenting clinical symptoms—hence the notion of affect phobia. This model comes from the triangle of conflict, which David Malan (1979) used in the context of short-term dynamic psychotherapy.

On one side of this conflict, the model identifies four main kinds of *activating affects* (i.e., primary adaptive emotions): self-assertion, grief, feelings of closeness or love, and compassion for self. Other activating affects that are less fundamental include sexual desire, interest or enjoyment, and pride or positive feelings toward the self. On the opposing side, the model also identifies four kinds of *inhibitory affects*: shame, guilt, anxiety, and fear or terror. Emotional pain and misery are less fundamental but serve as additional examples. Reliable criteria for identifying and coding these kinds of emotion from video have been well developed (see the *Achievement of Therapeutic Objectives Scale*; McCullough et al., 2008). In short, certain identified emotions are more productive than others. Although inhibitory affects, like defensive anxiety, are not considered maladaptive per se, they become maladaptive when they are overwhelming or when they block the emergence of more adaptive and activating emotion. In contrast to prior renditions of short-term dynamic therapy (e.g., Davanloo, 2005), this model puts less emphasis on the unconscious role of affect, instead highlighting that adaptive emotion can be blocked by maladaptive emotion (e.g., shame or anxiety). When adaptive emotion is blocked, it produces an internal conflict that is inherently painful.[4] It follows that the treatment aims to help people recognize and relinquish their defensiveness and then to deepen a client's awareness as well as experience of emotion. Finally, the aim is for clients to accept and express both emotion and their underlying needs.

The contribution of McCullough and colleagues includes efforts to anchor this understanding of emotional change in a rigorous program of research. A handful of studies, including two randomized clinical trials, have supported this treatment model (Julien & O'Connor, 2017). One of these compared this dynamic approach with cognitive therapy in the treatment of Cluster C personality disorders. The study showed how patterns in emotional activation changed from early to late treatment and that those shifts in emotion predicted good final outcomes (Schanche et al., 2011). The observed shifts in process unfolded as hypothesized through a decrease in inhibitory emotion (i.e., less terror, shame, or guilt) and an increase in activating emotion (i.e., more assertion, grief, or self-compassion). Furthermore, although changing the relative within-session activations of these categories of emotion is a primary treatment goal in the short-term dynamic model, that process is inconsequential from the perspective of cognitive therapy. Nevertheless, the emotional changes and their predictive power on outcome did not differ across the two treatments, suggesting a general treatment process.

Furthermore, case study has observed and described the session-by-session pattern by which fewer inhibitory emotions as well as both more experience and expression of adaptive emotion progressively relate to positive symptom change (Bhatia et al., 2009). Regarding the actual categorization or groupings of emotions per se (McCullough et al., 2008), more empirical validation is needed. Nevertheless, there is remarkable convergence with the specific emotions identified in an independent line of inquiry on emotion-focused therapy (A. Pascual-Leone & Greenberg, 2005; see Chapters 15 and 16, this volume).

Glimmers of Transformation Anticipate Change

Beginning with a similar point of departure, Diana Fosha, a psychologist and clinical theorist in New York, developed accelerated experiential dynamic psychotherapy (Fosha, 2021). Like the aforementioned authors, Fosha proposes that a wide array of emotional and behavioral dysfunctions arise from long-standing unresolved emotional injuries related to early interpersonal attachments. However, a noteworthy difference in approach is that this treatment uses a style that is markedly more akin to humanistic therapies, resolving emotional injuries within the context of a supportive, inquisitive, and healthy attachment interaction between the therapist and the client. For instance, Fosha proposes that the first state of emotional distress sits side by side with *glimmers of transformation*, which are momentary manifestations of strength, resilience, and positive qualities. This essentially recognizes that even when a client presents predominantly with maladaptive emotion, there are often also subdominant affective states in the periphery of experience that might be picked up on (J. Pascual-Leone & Greenberg, 1995). Indeed, therapists using this approach are to find and affirm the glimmers of healthy emotion while also empathizing with the presenting emotional pain.

Next, rather than challenging defenses, the primary emphasis is on the experiential process of unfolding emotion. Clients are first observed to shift from their initial unhealthy emotional presentation (e.g., emotional avoidance, feeling alone in their suffering) to experiencing more clinically relevant emotional distress (i.e., attachment-related emotional injuries such as shame and despair). Once clients engage with the previously avoided or unprocessed emotional injuries, the safe therapeutic environment is thought to encourage the emergence of alternative and more positive emotional experiences such as self-compassion, love, and acceptance. Recalling the work of Fredrickson, this approach also emphasizes the role of positive emotion as a catalyst of change (Stalikas et al., 2015). However, a critical issue here is that the model also goes beyond the idea of emotions in conflict: Fosha (2021) explicitly emphasizes moment-by-moment transformations as temporal patterns of productive emotion.

To map out the longer sequential process, Fosha describes a linear progression across five ordered stages of emotion change, where three states and the transitions among those states are associated with unique emotional experiences. First, clients work through their presenting *defensive state*, where they are avoiding emotional experience or interpersonal relatedness. Second, they transform out of the defensive state, during which clients work with a therapist to cocreate a safe therapeutic environment. Emotions during this transition herald an openness to experiencing and signal a transition of dropping down into (i.e., engaging) emotional distress. Third, clients enter a new state, this time of *core affect*, as they connect with their emotional injuries. At this point, categorical emotions such as grief and anger emerge as they relate to someone's personal difficulty. Clients also start to attend to their feelings of relatedness to their therapist and the pleasure that entails. They enjoy a genuine sense of self and attend to the blossoming of their experience.

Fourth, Fosha (2021) describes the transformation of those core affects as accompanied by profound feelings related to (a) the aftermath of a personal breakthrough (e.g., relief; hope; feeling lighter, stronger, cleaner, new), (b) the experience of mastery (e.g., pride, competence, joy), (c) the pain related to mourning a past self, and (d) emotions related the experience of healing (e.g., gratitude, tenderness, feeling moved about being recognized or affirmed). This transformation usually unfolds in a cascade of feeling and involves what Fosha has dubbed *tremulous affects*, which are feelings associated with the experience of personal change itself (e.g., fear or excitement, positive vulnerability, shock, curiosity). Finally, step five involves settling into a state of resolution. The feelings associated with that are calm and well-being but also ease, flow, and vitality. The final state further involves an attitude of openness, confidence, and wisdom, in the sense that things feel right and true.

This experiential–dynamic perspective on emotional processing offers an important formulation of the series of emotional experiences that unfold over time as individuals work to through their emotional distress. It also suggests that the interpersonal confrontation approach first proposed by Davanloo may not be necessary. The supporting evidence for this theory of change comes largely from clinical case descriptions and rational analyses. However, understanding emotional change as a multistep transformational process also relies on the humanistic–experiential work by Gendlin (e.g., 1964), L. S. Greenberg (e.g., 2021), and others, which represents a parallel development in the psychotherapy literature.

Humanistic–Experiential Models of Transformational Sequences

The development of emotion-focused therapy has been led by psychologist Les Greenberg at York University and, as an integration of client centered and Gestalt therapies, it is deeply rooted in the humanistic–experiential tradition (L. S. Greenberg, 2021; L. S. Greenberg & Goldman, 2019; L. S. Greenberg & Paivio, 1997; L. S. Greenberg & Safran, 1987; Wiebe & Johnson, 2016). As with the previously described theories of change, the aim of emotion-focused therapy is to encourage the experience of emotion within psychotherapy sessions and generate key emotional experiences as the change process itself. In this context, clients must engage, validate, and bypass secondary emotions (e.g., global distress, rage, anxiety), which are reactions to the initial and deeper feelings and thoughts triggered by an immediate situation. Similarly, clients need to move beyond any instrumental emotions, which they may consciously or unconsciously be using to elicit some desired response from another person. This is because the goal in emotion-focused therapy is to help clients access primary adaptive emotions. As first presented in the Introduction, primary adaptive emotions facilitate the resolution of distress because they orient and mobilize an individual to meet their own existential needs.

However, primary emotions, which are the direct emotional reactions to a given situation, can be either adaptive or maladaptive. Primary maladaptive emotions are conditioned emotional responses from past unhealthy learning experiences. While these emotions often entail an existential need (just like adaptive emotions), that need is simultaneously blocked by core negative self-evaluations that are inherent in maladaptive emotion. Thus, primary maladaptive emotions are distressing and cannot promote need fulfillment because of the fundamental incongruence that arises between a negative self-evaluation (e.g., "I am shamefully unlovable and undeserving of love") and a basic existential need (e.g., "But I need to feel loved!"). This impedes an individual's ability to work through emotional distress and resolve personal difficulties. It follows that when primary emotions are maladaptive, they must be transformed through the emergence of an alternative experience of adaptive emotion.

From Symptoms to Deeper Experience: A Two-Step Process

Clients may present with various kinds of emotional troubles. L. S. Greenberg (2021; L. S. Greenberg & Paivio, 1997) explains that when emotional difficulties are not too complex, a two-step sequence is sufficient. In the two-step change sequence, one needs to get to primary emotion to finish or complete the expression of that experience. Although it may seem natural to express adaptive emotions, sometimes such feelings have nonetheless been suppressed, often due to some interfering life circumstance, hardship, or social imperative. Secondary emotions can also serve to inhibit or obscure more primary emotions, a conceptualization which has an affinity to the psychodynamic notions of defensive emotion or of staving off the formulation of painful experience (consider D. B. Stern, 1997; McCullough et al., 2003).

In Step 1 of this two-step sequence, a client's secondary symptomatic emotion is the point of entry for working with emotion, which needs to be engaged and differentiated (i.e., emotional awareness). When one arrives at a deeper (core) and adaptive emotion, that experience has often been interrupted or truncated in some way. As discussed earlier (Chapter 12), the shift to deeper emotion is often heralded by vocal perturbations as clients deepen and differentiate their initial distress to access more primary vulnerable emotion (Diamond et al., 2010). In Step 2, this primary adaptive emotion (e.g., anger at violation, sadness at loss) can now be aroused, expressed, and completed. In short, emotional processing in this two-step sequence is the result of deeper experiencing and then making use of primary adaptive emotion to orient, guide, and inform the resolution of problems through new meaning and action.

In my reading of the literature, when research or clinical work has led authors to conclude that awareness and expression (i.e., the two-step process) is sufficient, that perspective tends to be a product of working largely with nonpsychiatric populations. Effective treatments based on this narrower understanding of what is needed for emotional change, are typically inspired by working with emotional difficulties in populations who are not afflicted with entrenched mental illness. Examples include psychological interventions to counsel clients through personal challenges coping with chronic physical pain, for medical populations that suffer secondary emotional distress, or for caregivers and parents trying to overcome the emotional blocks that make it difficult to continue being supportive. In short, awareness and expression are indeed sometimes enough, particularly when the client has little or no entrenched maladaptive emotion (see Chapters 4 and 8, this volume; Lumley et al., 2011, 2017; see also Foroughe, 2018). But when the client suffers a psychiatric disorder such as chronic depression, debilitating anxiety, eating disorders, or complex trauma, the primary underlying process often turns out to be maladaptive emotion. Maladaptive emotions (e.g., shame or fear related to low self-worth, trauma, child abuse) are typically intractable and they cannot be worked through using only awareness or expressive arousal; thus, they call for a three-step process.

Identifying and Undoing Maladaptive Emotion: A Three-Step Process
In the three-step process, after an initial secondary emotion (i.e., symptomatic or defensive emotion) is engaged and managed in Step 1, exploring deeper emotion leads one to deeply problematic and maladaptive emotions in Step 2. There is no relief that follows the expression of primary maladaptive emotions. Their pervasive, nonrational, and enduring nature means that they can never be seen through to completion, but they can be transformed. This is Step 3 in the sequence, which sees clients coactivate adaptive primary emotions (e.g., positive emotion, healthy entitlement, grief over loss; see Chapter 13). As described by L. S. Greenberg (2021; L. S. Greenberg & Paivio, 1997), the three-step process that creates a sequential transformation typically occurs in the working phase of treatment. This formulation from emotion-focused therapy has now been both operationalized in concrete terms and borne out empirically (see Chapter 15). While the research on sequentially-ordered emotion has been principally conducted on individual therapy, this theory and research is also consistent with what we know about changes in emotion-focused couples therapy (Dailey et al., 2023; Wiebe & Johnson, 2016).

A COMMON PRINCIPLE OF CHANGE?

I have highlighted the sequential process of emotion change according to theories of intensive short-term dynamic psychotherapy (Abbass & Town, 2013; Davanloo, 2005), affect phobia therapy (McCullough et al., 2003), accelerated experiential dynamic therapy (Fosha, 2021), as well as in emotion-focused therapy (L. S Greenberg, 2021). Furthermore, Welling (2012) has already argued this to be a common principle of change regarding several therapies that would also include coherence therapy (Ecker et al., 2024) and eye movement desensitization and reprocessing therapy (R. Shapiro & Brown, 2019). While these treatments have their respective origins across psychodynamic, humanistic, and cognitive approaches, they each use innovations in treatment that are highly experiential in nature, focusing on the moment-by-moment process of when feelings and meanings emerge. For all these treatments, the relative order of emotional events matters.

The overall convergence among these approaches supports a core argument of this book, which is that changing emotion with emotion represents a distinct kind of emotional processing. It is one that may be universal in much the same way as awareness, regulation, or insight. Different lines of empirical evidence support that hypothesis (Chapters 13–16). Later, Chapter 16 reviews research on a specific model inspired by emotion-focused therapy, which has subsequently been studied across treatment approaches. What these lines of work collectively contribute to our understanding of sequential transformations is that this unique kind of change (a) is precipitated by emotions that are in conflict and (b) there is an order to productive emotional processing. Finally, (c) different emotional concerns are resolved through different sequences (e.g., two-step, three-step), and the steps may also unfold nonlinearly.

NEW EMOTIONS EXPAND ONE'S EMOTIONAL REPERTOIRE

One of the most common challenges to changing emotion with emotion is that people have a limited emotional range, which is why they are essentially stuck in some maladaptive feeling; they have nowhere to go if they stay within their usual range of experience. What often makes a sequential transformation so effortful at first is that clients in therapy need to develop their range of emotion before they can use (new) emotion as a catalyst of change. Following this is also the challenge of becoming more fluid or flexible in shifting between emotional states to create a new normal in one's emotional reactivity. Generally, the emotional needs one is addressing come to be the common thread in motivating the cascade of emotion that is characteristic of this kind of emotional processing. This section explores these points.

Expanding One's Range of Feeling

The idea that when people get better, their maladaptive or inhibiting emotion will proportionally decrease as positive emotion increases, is a common misconception. Emotional change turns out to not be a simple exchange in currency or switching out between healthy and unhealthy emotions (Chapter 12). Granted, opposing emotions cannot fully coexist in the same momentary instant, which is why contradicting states within a given situation produce an internal conflict that must be reconciled (Lindquist et al., 2016; Schmukle et al., 2002; Wundt, 1897/1998). In contrast, however, a trait-like disposition toward experiencing emotions with opposing action tendencies is not a source of immediate internal conflict. Opposing feelings can easily coexist as possible alternatives in the same emotional repertoire or even in the same field of experience (e.g., like a marbled pattern of mixed emotion).

Having a range or mix of emotions is healthy. A longitudinal study of everyday life recorded the interplay between positive and negative emotion over 10 years and found that those who experienced mixed emotion subsequently had less decline in their physical health over time (Hershfield et al., 2013). It also showed that when people increased the occurrence of mixed emotions in their repertoire of experience, this developmental change over the lifespan also attenuated age-related decline. Further relating this process to personal change, on the level of narrative themes, having mixed emotion in one's narrative themes prospectively predicted good psychotherapy outcomes (Adler & Hershfield, 2012). All told, adding new and more adaptive emotional experiences to one's repertoire does not necessarily replace prior maladaptive emotional experiences. Rather, it expands one's range to include possibilities that reach beyond the same old maladaptive feelings.

A common expression in clinical writing about working with emotion is that clients just need to "access" some emotion. This image is a vestige of an outdated (modernist) understanding of how knowledge is generated. Typically, new and transformative emotions have been neither repressed nor latent, and they are not there to be accessed. Instead, they usually do not exist yet for that individual—as least not as a stable part of their repertoire. Such states are largely unformulated and must be effortfully constructed into emergence. One does not access some new part of an emotional repertoire; one must build it.

Each emotion is essentially a distinct affective-meaning tool for interpreting and negotiating the reality of one's (internal and external) environment. In this way, each emotion represents a different set of meanings, appraisals, and action tendencies that can and will be applied at different moments when making sense of a given personal problem. For example, a person might feel angry after a betrayal, which orients them to the violation that took place and organizes them to fight or assert. But if that were the only thing they felt, it would be a shallow and limited experience of what has occurred because betrayals also imply some loss of trust, and that needs to be recognized. One could also have a sense of shame about what happened, which is an experiential exploration of the social implications. Thus, having a range of distinct emotions about a given problem means one makes use of a more variegated set of tools for interpreting and engaging with the problem. In the example, experiencing shame, anger, and sadness each in turn would reflect a rich engagement of what it means to have been betrayed.

If we imagine discrete emotions as keys on a piano, then it is as if people struggling to function emotionally are playing on a very limited section of what could be their keyboard. For a client who is chronically ashamed (or chronically angry or sad), their keyboard is shorter in length and they are often pounding away on a single key, playing a one-note tune.[5] Then, when clients build out their emotional repertoire to include new ways of emotionally responding, they progressively add new keys to their piano until they are eventually able to play (i.e., experience) using a full human range. In short, people who change through the sequential transformation of emotion essentially create new ways of feeling for themselves. They become more resilient even within the inevitable experiences of pain. This is adult emotional development in action.

Why might experiencing a greater range of emotions eventually ameliorate symptoms regardless of which emotions were added into the mix? The value of emotional flexibility is analogous to the notion of cognitive flexibility or creative problem solving: Not all creative solutions are good solutions, but they do contribute to an ongoing process. Similarly, some of the various feelings one has regarding a personal difficulty may not be immediately helpful (e.g., maladaptive emotion), but increasing one's emotional range and flexibility allows one to engage old problems in new ways. Having more emotional flexibility means having access to and using a plurality of action tendencies, associated needs, and appraisals of the self. This opens one to the possibility of newly embodied meaning as well as the subsequent differentiation, interaction, and integration of previously contrasting states of emotion.

In the process of working through his own grief, Johann Wolfgang von Goethe, one of the great German romantic poets, describes what it means to fluidly access a broad emotional repertoire: "Everything the gods, the infinite ones, / give to their favorites, they give whole, / All our joys, the unending ones, / All our sorrows, the unending ones, all of them, whole" (1777/2015, p. 35).[6] The full range of emotional experience is an important part of healthy functioning. Expanding one's emotional range and becoming more flexible in how it is applied depends on the degree to which one can ride through various sequential transformations.

Emotional Flexibility Creates Dynamic Responding

A range of states are required for working through emotional difficulties. The process over a longer chain of sequential transformations changes the emotional repertoire with which a person typically engages their difficulties. Consequentially, it also changes the range of emotional experiences that a client has easily available (or not) to subsequently navigate and work through personal difficulties. Notice that the existence of a target emotion is not one of binary presence or absence, and even among those within one's emotional repertoire, not all states can be activated with the same aptitude. Rather, there is a continuum of construction: On one end, emotional experiences are subdominant and need to be brought into the client's awareness, whereas at the other end of the continuum, a client may have only rudimentary ingredients (i.e., cognitive or affective facets) from which to build the lived emotional experience into their repertoire. Even so, psychological flexibility becomes the hinge point to transforming emotion with emotion. Clients presenting for treatment usually (a) have restricted emotional ranges and (b) are not as flexible in activating the emotions that are relevant to their concern.

Moreover, rigidity is particularly characteristic of mental health problems. Some clients fall into a familiar pattern of despair, whereas others become enraged at the slightest provocation, and identifying this inflexibility in a client's mode of responding highlights the shortfalls in their emotional range. Similarly, making use of healthy assertion or being able to grieve without becoming overwhelmed and losing the relevant personal meaning of that feeling are as much dynamically emerging states as they are achievements in an adult's socioemotional development. This understanding of personal development through the mechanism of increasing one's emotional range in general is in line with Fredrickson's broaden and build theory as it applies to psychotherapy, in which the function of positive emotion is seen as opening new perspectives and new ways of engaging old problems (Fitzpatrick & Stalikas, 2008; Stalikas et al., 2018).

Tipping the Balance of Activation

To fully appreciate transformation as a kind of emotional processing, it is useful to consider the true final product of change. Because older (maladaptive) versus newer (more adaptive) emotions are nested networks, when sequential transformations happen, the new feeling does not entirely replace the old feeling. With practice over time, a newly forged healthy emotional experience (i.e., a dialectical synthesis) becomes an increasingly stable and more salient part of how one experiences the world. Fragments of maladaptive emotion are neutralized in some sense, but those pieces are not literally erased from the psyche. Rather, sequential transformations create change by first expanding one's emotional repertoire and then tipping the balance of habitual activations. This formulation of the change process is consistent with the neuroscience of memory reconsolidation and neuroplasticity at large (Doidge, 2007; Ecker et al., 2024; Lane & Nadel, 2020; J. Pascual-Leone & Johnson, 2021).

Although I have described sequential transformations as changing a presenting emotion with some newly emergent emotion, the new experience is an overarching healthier construction that subsumes elements of the maladaptive emotion. For example, what were cues for a maladaptive emotion now become the cues for a more adaptive and balanced experience. These maladaptive configurations still have some potential to be activated as an isolated subset within the network, particularly when the new connections are not yet strong. So, another issue to consider is how the balance of relative activations is tipped such that the integrity of an overarching and more adaptive emotional state becomes an increasingly stable part of one's repertoire. In dynamic systems theory, this is referred to as the functional reorganization or new normal, which follows some period of destabilization (Gelo & Salvatore, 2016). When that happens, the differential activation of these new healthier ways of being compete with and preferentially displace the prior automatization of a maladaptive emotion.

The completion of primary and adaptive emotional experiences is intrinsically reinforcing because it entails successfully addressing one's unmet needs. In short, even if the adaptive feelings themselves are painful, it feels good to make progress in an emotionally healthy way. Interestingly, in operational terms, this can look very similar to what behavior theory has described as the differential reinforcement of incompatible behaviors (Spiegler, 2015). Whatever the case, the propensity of presenting maladaptive emotions is drowned out by the self-reinforcing nature of healthier, adaptive emotional experiences.

To measure character change that results from emotion processing (i.e., adult emotional development), one can observe small changes in how a client emotionally responds to their core concerns (e.g., the client's response to their own self-criticism or to cues for their past trauma). Effects of psychological treatments are found not only on the level of symptoms but also in the manner with which a client addresses their core concern and how it changes over time. As detailed later in Chapter 16, a handful of longitudinal studies on psychotherapy process have shown that when treatment is successful, clients exhibit a widening in the emotional range that they have to draw upon when contending with personal problem. Furthermore, *emotional flexibility*—the ability to shift between different states in one's repertoire—also increases from pretherapy to posttherapy. The research suggests both a client's expanding emotional repertoire as well as the ability to easily move between emotions within that repertoire are positive predictors of treatment outcome (A. Pascual-Leone, 2018; empirical research on emotional flexibility is reviewed in Chapter 16, this volume).

Existential Needs Drive Sequences in Emotion

Changing emotion with emotion is a form of emotional processing that rests on the deeper meaning of existential needs, which themselves are the *raison d'être* of emotional experience. *Positive emotions* are essentially the experience of having one's needs met, whereas *negative emotions* embody the painful experience of one's unmet needs (see Introduction). When confronted with a maladaptive emotion, knowing what one needs is the common thread in a sequence that bridges to adaptive emotion and brings about a sequential transformation. First, secondary symptomatic distress is an emotional experience that orients one toward a problem (i.e., something is "not right," which then focuses one's attention on deeper issues). Then, as the therapist helps a client differentiate the meaning of some presenting primary maladaptive emotion, one of the elements in that emotion will be a fundamental and unmet need or wish (e.g., Therapist: "What is the worst part about all this? What's at stake here for you? What would the feeling need for it to be better?").

The Sense of What Is Wrong Guides the Search

Articulating and symbolizing a painful emotion clarifies the core issue, but in doing so, one also discovers what one really needs.[7] This creates a miniature paradigm shift in the trajectory of one's moment-by-moment psychological experience. As soon as a person gains clarity in what their underlying and unmet needs are (e.g., exactly what is missing from my life, what must be defended), one spontaneously reorganizes and orients toward that need. In the words of Gendlin (1981),

> The change process we have discovered is natural to the body, and it feels that way in the body. The bad feeling is the body knowing and pushing toward what good would be. Every bad feeling is potential energy toward a more right way of being if you give it space to move toward its rightness. . . . It knows the direction. It knows this just as surely as you know which way to move a crooked picture. If the crookedness is pronounced enough . . . for you to notice it at all, there is absolutely no chance that you will move the picture in the wrong direction and make it still more crooked while mistaking that for straight. *The sense of what is wrong carries with it, inseparably, a sense of the direction toward what is right.* (p. 76, italics added)

In other words, the healthy need is implicit within a primary maladaptive state, and it is also what precipitates the generation of adaptive emotion that is required.

Furthermore, recall that emotions are experiential assessments of one's position with respect to a given need, and they are at once both representational and procedural. In a simplified example, as soon as one notices that one is hungry (i.e., symbolizing a current internal state of need), one's mind simultaneously turns toward satiating the hunger (e.g., asking oneself, "What is there around here to eat?"). In the creation of meaning, these are not two separate psychological steps; they are one and the same.[8] Similarly, when recognizing the pain of maladaptive emotion is about some unmet need, one simultaneously organizes to address and ultimately pursue that need. This pursuit, in turn, precipitates a new and emerging emotional experience, which is the second emotion in a transformational sequence: a healthy and adaptive emotion.

For illustration, one might imagine how a client who suffered longstanding abuse during childhood might work through sequences of emotions in a way that highlights the underlying need as a common thread:

> I feel tense, anxious, and hopeless all at the same time. . . . Something isn't right [*secondary emotion*]. Deeper down, there is this haunting feeling, like I'm just so shamefully unworthy of other people's love and attention [*primary maladaptive shame*]. I don't deserve it [*negative self-evaluation*] . . . and yet I just have this longing. . . . I need that affection and love so much! [*existential need*] And when I get a tiny bit of what I need, it just feels right . . . so . . . maybe I do deserve it . . . yeah! [*primary and adaptive assertive anger*] And yet . . . I guess that also means I've just missed out all these years. That's sad. I might have deserved it, but I've also been unlucky. It's been a tremendous loss, a missed opportunity. It wasn't my fault; I just didn't get what I needed [*adaptive grief*].

In this dramatized example, a client goes through a three-step sequence of emotional change (i.e., secondary, primary maladaptive, and then primary adaptive emotion) as described by L. S. Greenberg and Paivio (1997). Each emotional step captures the ongoing assessment of an existential need (e.g., the need must be attended to, the need is caught in painful conflict, the need is being asserted, the need is being grieved). Following this sequential transformation, one can also imagine the experience of positive emotion when the client's need is finally met. That would be the culmination of an emotional cascade as described by Fosha (2021). For example, a client might say, "A relationship like this is what was missing. . . . When I look into those attentive and caring eyes, I feel warm and calm. I'm happy to be part of this!" Though the order of emotions is important within that unfolding experience, the pursuit of a core unmet need or wish is the thread that strings together a longer chain of emotion.[9]

Support for this process formulation comes from the thematic nature of progressive wishes (healthy core needs) described in the case formulations of brief psychodynamic therapy (e.g., Luborsky et al., 1992, 1994) or the unmet needs discussed in emotion-focused therapy (e.g., R. N. Goldman & Greenberg, 2015; A. Pascual-Leone & Kramer, 2017). Another line of evidence speaks to the etiology of psychopathology. For example, whether women perceived their needs as being met or thwarted, it mediated the relationship between their difficult life circumstances such as family conflict, and features of psychopathology (i.e., borderline personality disorder; Kalpakci et al., 2014). Similarly, when people reported unfulfilled needs for autonomy, competence, and relatedness, it mediated the relationship between their dysregulated emotion and features of psychopathology (van der Kaap-Deeder et al., 2021).

The Pivot Point Is the Specificity of an Unmet Need

Being able to identify and articulate one's needs in the first place plays a critical role in whether one can work through adversity. So, articulating unmet needs is not only a component of sequential transformations, it is also a critical point of passage. This has been shown when working with both self-criticism and interpersonal issues. In a study of undergraduates using chairwork to grapple with their self-criticism, being able to verbalize their unmet needs preceded the decline of hostile self-criticism (Sicoli & Hallberg, 1998). Similarly, in a study of emotion-focused therapy for longstanding relationship difficulties (i.e., unfinished business), the client's ability to verbally assert their existential needs within a session was a better predictor of treatment outcome than having an insight about the other person or gaining some new perspective (McMain et al., 1996).

While verbalizing one's needs is important, the issue goes beyond self-expression or making a disclosure. Additional research highlighted that the degree of specificity one uses to articulate one's existential needs is critical when facilitating change. In a single-session intervention for people with lingering anger about an unresolved event, expressing unmet needs facilitated healthy anger over destructive anger. The findings confirmed that knowing what one is fighting for (i.e., articulating the specific need) is critical for working productively with anger in cognitive as much as experiential interventions (Strating & Pascual-Leone, 2025). In treating complicated grief with emotion-focused therapy, the more specific a client was in describing their unmet need, the more it advanced chairwork and the more it reduced clinical symptoms (Gamoneda et al., 2023). So, rather than just admitting, "I needed their appreciation," better outcomes followed more specificity, as in, "I needed their encouraging comments, their desire to be with me, I needed them to say, 'you are worth my time, and I enjoy time with you.'"

Of course, identifying and symbolizing what one needs (a critical part of emotional awareness; see Chapter 7) is more easily said than done. As we have seen, increased arousal anticipates the identification and expression of unmet needs (Nardone et al., 2022). This means moment-by-moment elevations in a client's emotional arousal (e.g., the person becomes tearful, raises their voice in anger, or suddenly feels deeply moved) seem to generate windows of opportunity to best explore and articulate their deeply felt unmet needs. Having clarity in emotional awareness also interacts with the nature of one's ongoing psychopathology. For example, among those suffering from harsh self-criticism, people who also reported having anger problems were found to have significantly more trouble expressing their needs even when prompted as compared with those without anger problems (Kramer & Pascual-Leone, 2016).

THE CRUCIBLE OF CHANGE

A *crucible* is a container in which substances are melted down and then blended. For example, although it was pivotal for human civilization, bronze is not a naturally occurring substance. Before one can create bronze, copper and tin, each a naturally occurring metal, must be extracted from the earth. They are then put into a crucible, melted down together, and blended at a very high temperature to create bronze. This alloy is easier to work into shapes as compared to tin, and it is much stronger than copper. The combination of both metals under special circumstances rendered something entirely novel and heralded a new era in the advancement of civilization. Similarly, painful emotions can be brought together in the same envelope of mental and bodily experience, and when mutually activated under the right circumstances, it precipitates their dialectical synthesis to render a qualitatively new way of experiencing what previously were unresolved wounds. When clients do this, it expands their emotional repertoire, which represents a paradigm shift in how they can then work with emotion.

The crucible here can be understood in two ways. First, a therapeutic relationship helps facilitate and shape burgeoning emotional experiences. (As discussed in Chapter 1, the interpersonal relationship is an alternative lens for understanding change.) When a therapist facilitates sequential transformations, it demands empathic attunement to their client's needs while also closely tracking shifts in the client's emotional state. Because emotion is only partly within one's awareness, a therapist plays a key role in guiding the client's attention to other (subdominant) facets of experience that otherwise might not be attended to (L. S. Greenberg, 2021; A. Pascual-Leone & Greenberg, 2007b).[10]

The second way one can understand the metaphor of a crucible is as the envelope of time during which change occurs. The modification of emotional memories occurs through a neurological process referred to as memory reconsolidation (see Chapters 13 and 19), which involves merging discrete affective experiences that occur within a similar window of time (i.e., about 10 minutes; Lane & Nadel, 2020). So, while opposing emotions are not usually experienced simultaneously, their juxtaposition occurs within a shared time frame (Ecker et al., 2024). For example, what Fosha (2021) has called glimmers of transformation—the brief but observable expressions of healthy client emotion—are often ephemeral moments revealing a collection of other feelings in the background that hereto are being eclipsed by a client's presenting maladaptive emotion (L. S. Greenberg, 2021; A. Pascual-Leone, 2009). The therapist then brings attention to these other emergent (and healthier) self-organizations, supporting their fuller activation so they can be formulated coherently as an alternative (i.e., competing) emotional state. The synthesis of different states is reconsolidated after one has toggled between them enough to explore their points of compatibility (see Chapter 13, this volume; Ecker et al., 2024; Lane & Nadel, 2020).

Sequential transformations in psychotherapy involve shifts that are often clearly demarcated during chairwork, for example, as clients enact different positions. The same process also occurs in treatments that do not use chairwork interventions, where changing one emotion with another occurs through subtle and repeated shifts between emotions. Irrespective of methods, the continuous contrasting of self-organizations over time is a process that transforms emotion. While this chapter has discussed sequential transformations in the context of adult emotional development, the next chapter illustrates that longitudinal process though case examples.

ENDNOTES

1. Many popular prescriptions for a single emotion are usually naive (e.g., just cry yourself dry, just vent your anger, just be more positive no matter what). However, when prescriptions for a single emotion draw on broader spiritual traditions, they often reference something more complex such as attitudes or philosophies of life rather than singular states of emotion. This is because, in spiritual traditions, the explanatory theory of change is considered less important than having faith in the approach.

2. Psychodynamic authors typically prefer the term "affect" to highlight the deeper roots of a preconscious experience, although in this book I use the word "emotion" to refer to varying degrees of affective awareness. Here, the discrete emotional experiences must come to fruition within conscious awareness to build and complete a transformational sequence.

3. The use of interpersonal pressure and confrontation as an intervention strategy is also tied to using the transference relationship as a lever for mobilizing emotion (also known as "tilting the transference"; Abbass & Town, 2013). Interestingly, Perls and

colleagues' (1951) early approaches to Gestalt therapy also was somewhat confrontational in style. However, since then, humanistic approaches to treatment have found alternative methods, that are both highly experiential and very effective, in activating and accessing the deeper feelings and meanings that underlie presenting concerns.

4. In a conversation I had with Leigh McCullough, she zeroed in on the distinction made in emotion-focused therapy between rage (as a secondary and usually unproductive emotion) versus assertive anger (as a primary adaptive and productive emotion). McCullough highlighted that this operationalization (later published in A. Pascual-Leone & Greenberg, 2007a) articulated her own understanding of anger and how that differed as compared with the original ideas of Davanloo (L. McCullough, personal communication, June 23, 2005).

5. At the broader epistemological level of narrative, Angus and colleagues (2017) referred to this as the same old story (see Chapter 17).

6. The poem appears in a letter from Goethe to Auguste zu Stolberg and was translated here by Dr. M. Wolfram.

7. Notice that the experience of discovering the meaning behind a feeling or bringing it into awareness are useful metaphors in therapy. However, they should not be taken literally. As suggested, both in this chapter and earlier chapters on awareness (i.e., Chapters 6 and 7), the true process is one of newly constructing meaning rather than discovering something that was latent.

8. Modern neurocognitive theory suggests all psychological schemes are simultaneously both representational and procedural (J. Pascual-Leone & Johnson, 2021). Tolman and Brunswik (1935) had pointed out that as one elaborates the mental representation of a chair (i.e., What is a chair?), one comes to realize the most essential quality of a chair is the property of its sit-on-ableness (i.e., the fact that it can be sat on and used as a chair). In practice, this means that as one perceives a chair in the room, just by recognizing it as such, one has already evaluated it suitability for sitting on. This confluence of representation and procedure is epitomized with the experience of needs as embodied in emotion.

9. As an interesting point of contrast, the emphasis in cognitive therapy on correcting core dysfunctional beliefs does not explicitly acknowledge the role of needs or wishes as a driving force for healthy change. Maladaptive emotions certainly entail core dysfunctional beliefs about oneself or one's experience, which is an important obstacle to grapple with. However, the same maladaptive emotion also entails some unmet need, and carrying forward that unmet need is what guides the direction in a sequence of emotional transformation.

10. In Chapter 1, I highlighted that working with emotion can be considered through either the individual lens (i.e., the mechanisms of internal processing) or through a relational lens (i.e., the dyadic experience and internalized objects that shape emotion).

15

The Sequential Model

The Only Way Out Is Through

There is a crack in everything . . . that's how the light gets in.

—LEONARD COHEN, *ANTHEM*

Prior chapters in this part of the book explored the notion of using one emotion to synergistically undo or transform another subsequent emotion. This chapter focuses on a specific model of longer sequential chains that map out an overarching process. As discussed, various converging theories in experiential, psychodynamic, or hybrid treatment approaches elaborate this kind of sequential or stepwise manner of working with emotion. However, there are still very few programs of research that empirically examine those overarching models of change.[1,2]

Measuring emotional shifts has been a major methodological challenge for researchers of all treatment approaches. Perhaps for this reason, when A. Pascual-Leone and Greenberg (2007a) developed a jargon-free observational tool for tracking emotion and a transtheoretical model of how emotion changes emotion, it spurred several systematic programs of research. Their model is rooted in theory from emotion-focused therapy (L. S. Greenberg, 2021; L. S. Greenberg & Paivio, 1997), but it is also a frontier of inquiry for psychotherapy in general. From a clinician's perspective, this transtheoretical model aims to address the question, "What kinds of discrete emotional experiences are most relevant to good process?" First, I present a case illustration, and then I describe the specific emotions and sequences that clients seem to have in common during this kind of sequential transformation. Later, Chapter 16 will review empirical research testing this model of emotional processing as a predictor of treatment outcome.

https://doi.org/10.1037/0000460-016
Principles of Emotion Change: What Works and When in Psychotherapy and Everyday Life, by
A. Pascual-Leone
Copyright © 2026 by the American Psychological Association. All rights reserved.

OBSERVABLE MOMENTS IN CHANGE

Many therapists will intuitively recognize the way emotion unfolds in a complex developmental process toward resolution over the course of an entire treatment. However, whereas some therapists are intent on tracking longer chains of sequential transformation, to others, the progression may seem less obvious. One of the main complexities in perceiving this as a key form of emotional processing has to do with the fact that it represents a qualitative continuum in which each emotional state is manifestly different but is also located on an ordinal dimension of resolution. To illustrate this process over therapy, this chapter will first present a narrative account of a single treatment case and then explicate each step in emotion as it contributes to the larger change.

A Case Example: Moving One Step at a Time

A narrative account of how a client changed over the course of therapy helps illustrate the sequential processes of emotion.[3] This case, which was part of a randomized clinical trial of emotion-focused therapy, has also been studied in a paper that coded emotion from video recordings of treatment to map the client's moment-by-moment emotional progress over time (first presented more fully in A. Pascual-Leone et al., 2017).

"Jeff" was a 50-year-old engineer who was married and had a 11-year-old son. He presented as depressed with features of social anxiety and reported drinking alcohol to soothe himself when he had feelings of shame and inadequacy. He often had difficulty knowing what he was feeling or expressing. His wife and son had complained about his anger because he would easily become irritable and could get angry with them. Indeed, he reported feeling that he had a short fuse and that he was easily angered when he felt others were putting him down, such as snapping at others if he began feeling worthless or ashamed. What brought Jeff to treatment was an awareness that he had feelings of unresolved anger and hurt toward his deceased father who had been both physically abusive and highly critical (A. Pascual-Leone et al., 2017).

Although productive emotional experiences are useful, they turn out not to occur as isolated change events and instead unfold following a predictable sequential pattern. The observation of this overall change process is reflected in the narrative account of Jeff's treatment. When Jeff began therapy, he was easily overwhelmed by his feelings, and in session 2, he graphically described the self-interruption of his own internal process: "I can only get so far. I'm afraid to let myself go there, and my body stops. It's like a blind is drawn down and says, 'That's enough of that!'" (A. Pascual-Leone et al., 2017, p. 180). The therapist helped Jeff work through this emotional block using chairwork and empathic responding to his vulnerability, a step that gave Jeff access to underlying emotion.

Initially, Jeff would become overwhelmed by feelings of worthlessness and shame and would break down in uncontrollable sobbing and global distress.

The therapist introduced a self-soothing exercise in session 3 (i.e., "Imagine a safe place"), which they returned to throughout treatment as needed. With each session, he became more emotionally regulated when processing his childhood trauma. In session 5, Jeff articulated his chronic feelings of inadequacy, saying, "I have to monitor everything I say, because people will just disregard me as a nutcase" (A. Pascual-Leone et al., 2017, p. 181).

Soon after this progress in emotional awareness, Jeff's work in therapy moved to focus first on the unresolved feelings of rage and the rejecting (blaming) anger he felt over his father's physical abuse of him as a child (sessions 3 and 7: "He's repulsive"; "I just want to get rid of him" (A. Pascual-Leone et al., 2017, p. 181). Thus, the next major task in therapy was for Jeff to develop his ability to tolerate and soothe his own distress without resorting to rageful anger, which was often a secondary emotion. Initially, he was unable to do this, but by session 7, he had sufficiently developed that capacity, which helped him feel more entitled to his unmet needs for love and feeling safe. In session 7, Jeff poignantly reflected, "I'm missing . . . the love that only a parent could give a child" (A. Pascual-Leone et al., 2017, p. 181).

After that, when Jeff's underlying vulnerability was more tolerable to him, the treatment focus stepped up again to address his extreme feelings of worthlessness and his feeling unlovable—the primary maladaptive shame that connected to his childhood abuse. To that end, therapy helped Jeff access, experience, and articulate these intense feelings, but now with more purpose. Interventions such as chairwork dialogues in which he imagined confronting his father as well as recalling and exploring related episodic memories were key processes that could now take clinical work to a higher level. Later, his core painful feeling of shame was transformed into a more primary and adaptive anger toward his father. This was then followed by primary adaptive grief for the years he had lost in a dysfunctional relationship with his dad, as well as a different kind of grief for the little boy who never had a safe place to grow up.

As treatment concluded, Jeff came to experience assertive anger toward his father, and by session 11, he had articulated and experienced the important unmet need to be loveable and feel loved by his father. He expressed very clearly what he had so desperately needed as a little boy, as well as a sense of healthy entitlement: "I deserved to feel safe and loved" (A. Pascual-Leone et al., 2017, p. 182). In session 12, during chairwork, Jeff imagined how his now deceased father might have expressed deeper sentiments of love for him (Jeff) and repentance for having been so abusive. Speaking from the perspective of his father, he spontaneously confessed, "It really wasn't about you. . . . I wish I had been a better father. . . . You are my son, and I love you. . . . Really, we both missed out in the end" (A. Pascual-Leone et al., 2017, p. 182). This imaginal exercise and enactment of a caring father by the client himself was the experience and expression of a primary and adaptive state of self-compassion. Jeff subsequently found himself forgiving his father and experienced a dramatic change in his own perspective. He accepted the abuse as part of his past and engaged life with a new sense of personal agency. According to symptom evaluations of depression, self-esteem, and recovery from trauma, the 14-session treatment ended in a good outcome with large effects that were maintained 18 months later (A. Pascual-Leone et al., 2017).

Mapping Out the Sequences of Emotional Change

At York University and University of Windsor, A. Pascual-Leone and Greenberg (2007a) developed a process model of key client states and the productive transitions between them, which captures emotional changes like the ones described previously in the case of Jeff. Taking prior theoretical work (by L. S. Greenberg & Paivio, 1997) as its point of departure, Pascual-Leone and Greenberg asked, what are the psychological steps by which clients work through their distress? By coding emotion from session videos of emotion-focused therapy for depression and interpersonal trauma, they produced an empirical model describing a multistep sequential pattern of how emotions unfold and showed it predicted positive outcomes. This helped to establish certain emotional events as particularly helpful change processes. In the 20 years that followed, subsequent evidence for this model has been garnered from dozens of studies conducted in a range of both treatment approaches and disorders. While the case of Jeff gives a narrative account of how one client processed emotion in the context of working through his difficulties, the remainder of this section will describe each of the steps in that process of change as presented in A. Pascual-Leone and Kramer (2019).

EARLY EXPRESSIONS OF DISTRESS

Emotion states in the model (i.e., global distress, shame or fear, and rejecting anger—the top half of Figure 15.1) are all early expressions of distress rather than expressions of working through distress (as first formulated by Kennedy-Moore & Watson, 2001). However, the additional notion that these are early expressions conveys that they are prerequisite steps to change and an unavoidable part of initial engagement, arousal, and orientation toward personal difficulty. Some research points to getting stuck in these emotions as indicative of a poor prognosis. Still, as we will see (in Chapter 16), these states are also part of the therapeutic process, whether one is observing either an unproductive session or the early sequences of what will subsequently unfold to be a productive session.

Global Distress

According to the model, the sequence for emotional processing in a productive session begins with (Phase 1, Figure 15.1) "global distress," a term coined by A. Pascual-Leone and Greenberg (2007a) to refer to undifferentiated negative feelings (a type of secondary emotion, e.g., helplessness, symptomatic anxiety). Individuals in global distress are often highly aroused but unable to clearly articulate the cause of their distress, and they lack a sense of direction for

FIGURE 15.1. The Sequential Model of Emotional Processing

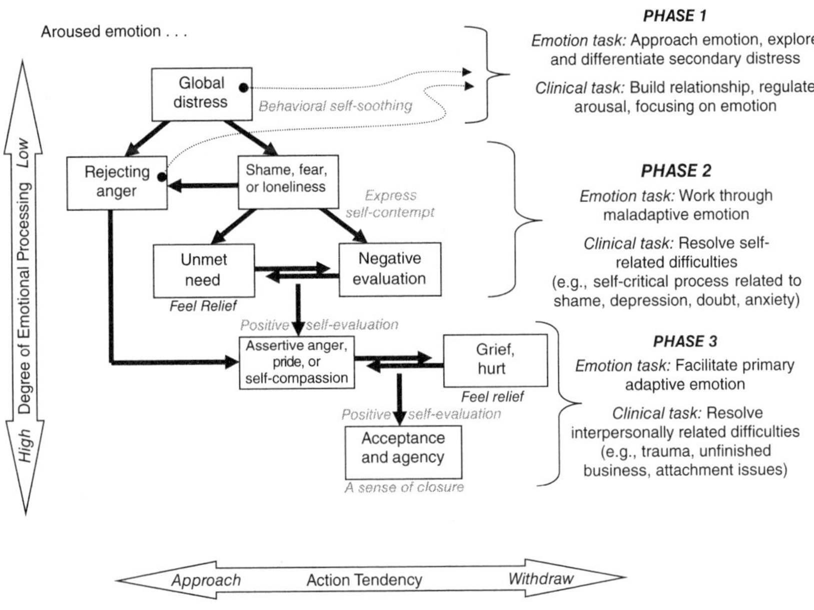

Note. Adapted from "Emotional Processing in Experiential Therapy: Why 'The Only Way Out Is Through,'" by A. Pascual-Leone and L. S. Greenberg, 2007, *Journal of Consulting and Clinical Psychology, 75*(6), p. 877 (https://doi.org/10.1037/0022-006X.75.6.875). Copyright 2007 by the American Psychological Association.

understanding and resolving their personal difficulties. Individuals overwhelmed or stuck in distress must first manage and differentiate their feelings before progressing through the model. Session 2 from therapy with "Erin" is one example of this.

CLIENT: I always feel like crying. And that comes in my upper throat and my eyes. I don't . . . ah. . . .

THERAPIST: Can you tell her that? Can you say, "Mom, I just look at you and I feel like I want to cry"?

CLIENT: I guess. [*Speaking to an imaginary image of mother*] Um, Mom . . . I just have to imagine you in that chair and I feel like crying. [*Sobs*]

THERAPIST: Yeah, "I feel so sad," . . . It's okay. It's all right. "There's just so much sadness I feel."

CLIENT: There's a lot.

THERAPIST: Can you tell her what you're sad about? Are there any words that come with the sadness? Or is it just there?

CLIENT: Hmm . . . that's a tough one! [*client has arousal but little meaning elaboration*]

THERAPIST: Yeah, "I just feel sad."

CLIENT: Yeah, I just feel sad.

THERAPIST: Kind of wordless sadness.

CLIENT: Kind of hopeless.

In another example, "Monica" is obviously upset in session 7 and falls apart quickly with a protesting tone in her voice. In the video she is teary-eyed and seems confused.

THERAPIST: How are you feeling today?

CLIENT: I feel terrible today. [*There is a crack in her voice.*]

THERAPIST: Are you?

CLIENT: Yeah, I'm a mess!

THERAPIST: Tell me what's going on.

CLIENT: [*Shrugs hopelessly*] I burst into tears 10 times. I don't know, I just [*teary and high-pitched voice*]. . . I feel depressed. I have no energy. [*sniffle*] I'm finding it really difficult to just get on with normal things. I feel really . . . I feel tired. I'm just not my, not myself at all.

THERAPIST: So, what's going on for you?

CLIENT: I'm not sure. Normal irritating things happen and . . . I feel all alone and stuff like that.

A critical point in understanding this model is appreciating that moving from global distress to primary maladaptive emotion (i.e., shame, fear, or loneliness) is not yet a sequential transformation, strictly speaking. The kind of emotional processing that moves a client from the secondary symptomatic emotions of global distress (or defensive and rejecting anger) to experiencing their underlying primary maladaptive emotion is increased emotional awareness (see Chapters 4–7). However, this differentiation (through increased emotional awareness) is often a prerequisite for fully engaging the maladaptive emotion that will then be targeted by a sequential transformation. The result is a three-step process, where the last leg changes emotion with emotion.

Shame, Fear, and Sometimes Loneliness

As the exploratory process moves forward, the initial distress is ultimately differentiated into core maladaptive emotions (Figure 15.1, Phase 2), essentially in the forms of maladaptive shame or maladaptive fear. These experiences are of enduring and familiar types of pain (such as that same old feeling, a dreaded state, or chronic vulnerability). Unlike global distress, these are highly personal and idiosyncratic states always anchored in some specific autobiographical context, and people often experience these maladaptive emotions as a hauntingly familiar pain (i.e., the same old story; see Angus et al., 2017). Individuals in states of maladaptive shame or fear have an all-too-poignant awareness of what they see as the cause of their distress, which is often expressed along themes of feeling incompetent, inadequate, or lonely.

Of course, adaptive versions of fear and shame also exist (e.g., adaptive fear organizes one to escape, adaptive shame hides impropriety to protect one's social standing; see Introduction). But this grouping refers to instances of maladaptive emotion, and loneliness offers a useful point of illustration (Timulak & Pascual-Leone, 2015).[4] When loneliness is due to external barriers (e.g., physical isolation), it is an adaptive emotion that prompts action to address an unmet interpersonal need. However, loneliness is maladaptive when the obstacles to interpersonal closeness are inherent to the self (e.g., Client: "I have nothing to offer; I am unlovable; I am too vulnerable for love; I am inhuman and cannot give or receive love"). In sum, pathological aspects of sadness and loneliness are always tinged with maladaptive shame, where a person's inability to connect with others is the fundamental (and internal) obstacle, more than any life circumstances.[5] Similarly, maladaptive forms of guilt (e.g., survivor guilt) are often fundamentally based in fear. While all these states are distinctive experiences, they entail a functional withdrawal and collapse of the self, which is enough to group them together as maladaptive emotions.

An example of maladaptive shame comes from session 5 in the treatment of Jeff (introduced at the beginning of this chapter). The therapist has introduced a chairwork dialogue, and the client now speaks critically to himself in second person. Jeff talks slowly with his head in his hands.

CLIENT: Umm . . . I can't give an example. Everything you say is just a bit off, you know. . . . Off from how other people see things . . . or talk about things [*There is a crack in his voice, and he breaks down sobbing heavily. He rubs his eyes and covers his face.*]

THERAPIST: It's just really. . . . It hurt to say that. . . . What's the sadness? Can you say the words?

CLIENT: [*He sniffles. There is a long pause.*]

THERAPIST: It's just a feeling of inadequacy that gets pulled . . . or . . . ?

CLIENT: Well, I have to monitor everything I say, even while I'm saying it because I'm. . . . I know or feel that everything I say is just a little bit off, it just doesn't. . . . You know, people will just do a double take when I speak or disregard me as a nutcase. (A. Pascual-Leone et al., 2017, p. 181)

Rejecting (Blaming) Anger

The model (Figure 15.1, Phases 1 & 2) also shows how global distress is sometimes elaborated along an alternative path to rejecting, blaming, and destructive anger. This emotional state has also been discussed in other literature as rage or defensive anger to denote a psychodynamic defense against deeper and more vulnerable, painful emotions. Whatever the case, rejecting anger pushes away and essentially is less differentiated in meaning than more productive forms of anger (see "Healthy Assertive Anger" section later in this chapter). As such, rejecting anger simply creates distance from the source of emotional pain. This is secondary emotion but with a potentially complex relationship to primary assertive anger, in that meaning elaboration could yield more assertive anger.

In distinguishing this reaction from a more productive form of anger, it helps to consider what the individual is really fighting for. Often, individuals in a state of rejecting anger (e.g., rage, disgust, hate) are mobilized and have a sharp sense of what they do not want (rejecting, blaming, or pushing away from), but it remains much less clear what they are positively pursuing. It is as if they say, "I don't know what I want, but it's not that!" By comparison, people in assertive anger might say, "I know what I'm fighting for, and I'm fighting for my rights!" Thus, in a statement of rejecting anger, Jeff said of his father (session 3), "He's repulsive, I'd like to punch him out," and on a different occasion, "I'm disgusted, I want to get rid of him" (session 7; A. Pascual-Leone et al., 2017, p. 181). What makes this emotion sometimes initially adaptive (in a rudimentary way) is the agentic rejection of some noxious experience as opposed to shrinking away or closing down, which would be more characteristic of maladaptive shame and fear.[6]

Thus, rejecting anger can be a step in the right direction toward adaptive self-organization and self-protection, but in isolation, it remains generic and unanchored in one's personal and idiosyncratic information. For example, one client referring to a significant other said, "I hate him for what he did to me" without describing what exactly it was that the perpetrator did or how the client experienced it ("Sally," session 9). The object of anger is again unclear when another client declared, "I'm really pissed off!" without elaborating further ("Carla," session 9; A. Pascual-Leone et al., 2017, p. 179). In both examples, the therapist understands the gist of the emotion and there is a clear action tendency of distancing, but one gets no sense of what it is like to be that client in that difficult circumstance. In contrast, assertive anger emerges later (Phase 3) when personal needs have been differentiated and identified and are engaged. Nonetheless, the complex relationship among types of anger is that the defensive momentum of rejecting anger can act as impetus for more productive and articulate experiences of assertion (for more on problem anger, see A. Pascual-Leone et al., 2013).

NEGATIVE SELF-EVALUATIONS AND EXISTENTIAL NEEDS

In a critical step (middle of Figure 15.1), maladaptive emotion in the form of shame or fear necessarily entails both an unmet existential need (e.g., for attachment, esteem) and a fundamentally negative self-evaluation (i.e., an affectively driven core dysfunctional belief about the self). These two aspects of experience are in direct conflict and create a seemingly impossible situation (Ecker et al., 2024; A. Pascual-Leone & Greenberg, 2007a). This poses a dialectical contradiction between internal components and is the point where a client's self-critical process (e.g., related to shame, depression, self-doubt, anxiety) is worked through. The impasse is essentially the reason why people get stuck in maladaptive emotion.

An unmet existential need is at the core of all primary emotions (including maladaptive emotions), but they need to be identified and clearly articulated. Examples of specific existential needs could be interpersonal (e.g., need for love, companionship, understanding, affirmation), related to personal agency (e.g., mastery, competence, dignity, freedom, joy), or about basic survival (e.g., security, inviolacy; Bakan, 1966; A. Pascual-Leone & Greenberg, 2005).[7] Similarly, while unhealthy or hostile ways of treating oneself (negative self-treatment) are characteristic behaviors associated uniquely with maladaptive emotion, the central issue is the experience of oneself as inherently negative. Examples of negative self-evaluations include but go beyond a cognitive belief; they entail a lived experience of oneself as fundamentally bad or weak (e.g., unlovable, inadequate, flawed; L. S. Greenberg & Watson, 2006; Watson & Greenberg, 2017).

It is also worth mentioning that although prior clinical theory pointed at the fundamental difference between descriptions of primary emotion that are adaptive or maladaptive, it lacked operational criteria to distinguish them (e.g., L. S. Greenberg, 2021; L. S. Greenberg & Paivio, 1997). The current model, however, offers insight into the deeper nature of adaptive versus maladaptive emotional states. Whereas all adaptive emotions entail some core (unmet) need, maladaptive emotions are conceptually distinguished by the fact that they entail not only an unmet need but also a core negative self-evaluation—the two held in tandem. These components are yoked together because of unhealthy learned experiences, and the subsequent tension between them defines the very nature of primary maladaptive emotion.

Returning to the model (middle of Figure 15.1), individuals who proceed beyond maladaptive fear, shame, or rejecting anger do so through a dynamic and dialectical synthesis of their negative evaluation toward themselves with an identified existential need, both of which were elaborated from exploring the maladaptive experience. The new meaning construction is ephemeral at first, encapsulated in a novel moment of positive self-evaluation or affirmation (i.e., "I do need love, I just never got it, so maybe that wasn't actually my fault?"). Thus, expression of unmet existential needs (i.e., a wish for attachment, personal agency, survival) is the gateway to deeper and more adaptive emotional experiencing that will follow.

In short, identifying and symbolizing a core unmet need and resolving the ensuing contradiction often ushers in a categorically new experience, which represents the latter part of the model (Phase 3, Figure 15.1). These new emotional experiences lead the client to a sense of self as deserving and mobilizes them to directly address unmet needs. This step is an advanced affective meaning process and takes the form of key emotions that are both primary and adaptive. On the one hand, those emotions are often either assertive anger, where one fights for one's needs (i.e., "I deserved the love that any child deserved, and I still deserve that!"), or self-compassion and soothing, where one offers tenderness and caring for oneself (i.e., "When I think of how good it felt that one time I was acknowledged, I savor it and realize how right it feels"). Meanwhile, on the other hand, the client confronts grief over a loss (e.g., "It wasn't my fault, but I still really missed out. It shouldn't have been that way, but it was, and I'm mourning that loss"). Though they are different lived experiences, assertive anger and self-compassion serve the same function in this approach-related process in that individuals in either state embody a new positive self-evaluation and address their existential need with agency.

SPECIFIC ADAPTIVE EMOTIONS

While early expressions of distress may be thought of as including both secondary emotion as well as primary maladaptive emotion, identifying unmet needs often leads to the emergence of a different set of primary adaptive emotional states. Healthy assertive anger, self-compassion, and adaptive sadness such as grief and hurt are uniquely positive predictors of good outcomes. Finally, acceptance and agency are part of a meaning state that signals the resolution of personal difficulties and a new personal development.

Healthy Assertive Anger

Assertive anger essentially has enough differentiation to embody a positive self-evaluation and expresses the clear assertion of that evaluation or of some personal need. This means that assertive anger is not just about pushing something noxious away. More than that, it is about setting boundaries and engaging in a fight for one's rights or needs. Some statements that represent assertive anger could be, "I won't accept this, I have value! I have been mistreated" or "I am different from you. I exist, and I deserve this." Expressions of this state are both very specific and clearly adaptive. They are also anchored in concrete autobiographical events. In a case example, a client in emotion-focused therapy with borderline personality disorder engaged in a chairwork dialogue with her mother, with whom she had a repeated sense of being dismissed and ignored (Kramer & Pascual-Leone, 2012). The client, speaking from the role of herself as a 6-year-old child, asserted against her imagined mother, saying, "It is my right to play here. This is my space, and I have the right to play here, and right now I need you to see and respect that."

Self-Compassion

This state can appear in several forms including explicit self-soothing, attributed self-nurturing (i.e., a client role plays a significant other or talks gently to themself), or acknowledging and reflecting on existing resources (e.g., social support, past personal successes). Examples include when Carla (introduced at the beginning of Chapter 12) spoke to herself reassuringly from the role of her parents, saying, "I love you. It's going to be alright" (session 10; A. Pascual-Leone et al., 2017, p. 180) or when another client spoke to herself and considered her loved ones: "You deserve to be treated well. You have your husband who loves you, and you have your sister." ("Monica," session 7). Without a doubt, expressions of this are both clearly adaptive and very specific because the need it serves is addressed in unique detail.

Adaptive Grief and Hurt

The counterpoint to assertive anger or self-compassion is the experience of primary adaptive grief or hurt, in which the individual recognizes loss or woundedness yet can express this pain without collapsing back into their negative self-evaluation, resignation, or hopeless despair, which is characteristic of earlier states. Although the role of healthy grief will seem intuitive to some clinicians, others may question how withdrawing in sadness might be adaptive. Unfortunately, the most common answer given to this question is that adaptive grief helps you get over it. This, of course, is a tautology and offers little insight to those who hope to better understand the curative role of (certain kinds of) sadness.

Although grief and hurt do not defend or pursue the fulfillment of unmet needs (i.e., in contrast to assertive anger), these feelings of adaptive sadness do involve orienting individuals to a closer appraisal of their critical needs. Individuals in a state of grief or hurt take stock of the full scope of their emotional pain, which arises from the lost or missed opportunities to fulfill their needs. For example, in the middle phase of her treatment, a client of mine reflected on how her family's frequent relocations had shaped her, concluding:

> We moved around so much, I missed out on having friends or peers when I was growing up. . . . The way we lived, everything was so tentative. . . . In retrospect, I was lonely a lot, but I didn't really know why. I was never connected to a peer group and that's sad. . . . It's been a personal loss.

So, while a state of grief or hurt inherently involves a withdrawal, its adaptive role rests in the reality check of recognizing what had been lost so that one can accept the damage done. Doing so allows one to carry forward with a clearer sense of exactly what needs must still be met in other ways. That next step will often involve reaching out to others or pursuing alternative opportunities, which is one reason why grief is often intertwined with either assertion or self-compassion.

Assertion, compassion, and grief are the emotions through which fear and shame are undone and longstanding interpersonal difficulties (e.g., complex trauma, unfinished business, attachment issues) are resolved. The following is a powerful example of grief and hurt taken from a session of Jeff's therapy (session 7). The client's voice is very soft, and at this point he has been crying. He holds a tissue and sniffles:

CLIENT: You know, in many ways I never had a family. If it weren't for, you know, extended family, it wouldn't have been much.

THERAPIST: Yeah, mm-hmm, you're missing that in your life.

CLIENT: Well, I'm missing that particular type of love. I guess [*His voice breaks; he covers his face and begins to sob with heavy tears*] . . . the love that only a parent could give a child.

THERAPIST: So, there's nothing that can replace that, there's nothing that can substitute that.

CLIENT: [*A deep sigh as he gathers himself*] Well, not from my experience. You know, I had aunts and uncles and that, who I know loved me, but it was never the same. (A. Pascual-Leone et al., 2017, p. 181)

The expression of grief and hurt in this context marks a second moment of dialectical tension wherein adaptive forms of anger and sadness act as opposite sides of the same coin. On one side, individuals push forward in the present, asserting their value and needs through a healthy sense of entitlement. On the other side, they retreat to mourn the loss of attachment experiences or other missed opportunities from the past. As before, individuals often transition between these opposing experiences and, when they are adequately explored, aspects of both contribute to an emerging sense of resolution. Just as clients in assertive anger or self-compassion may shift into grief and hurt, they may just as easily shift back again. A client commenting on their own process illustrated this idea: "This is where I start to get angry. I feel the anger in the place where the sadness was" (Monica, session 6). Thus, clients move from one of these two model components to the other, switching the gestalt between figure and background.

Acceptance and Agency: Moving Toward Resolution

Completing the nonlinear sequence described previously leads clients to resolution in the form of acceptance and agency. In the change process described earlier, although expression is necessary, venting is not sufficient because the most central part is explicitly symbolizing the embodied meaning of a lived emotional experience. Given that the articulation of meaning is particularly characteristic of later emotion states in the model (i.e., assertive anger, self-compassion, grief, or hurt), they have been collectively referred to in some studies as either "advanced meaning-making states" or simply "primary adaptive emotions." Taken as a whole, the model's nonlinear and multistep pattern of emotion has been identified as a form of sequential transformation, leading clients toward the resolution of personal difficulties in the form of letting go and acceptance.

Readers may recall from Chapter 12 the following example of acceptance and agency, which was from the 10th session of therapy with Carla. Her emotional tone is very soft with a bittersweet air of reflection. One has the sense that she experiences this as positive and with a sense of relief, although there is a sadness that goes with it, as if she is accepting reality but with an eye to some brighter future horizon.

CLIENT: It feels like. . . . It feels like I can breathe again. It feels like that ball inside my chest has loosened.

THERAPIST: Okay, so take a deep breath and see if you can breathe into that ball in your chest. Just notice if anything comes up that you want to say. See if there is anything you want to say goodbye to, that will never be again.

CLIENT: I guess I'm gonna try to say goodbye to that part of me, that child who was hurt and was defenseless. I'm not going to ignore her, she'll always be there and if she wants to say something, I'm gonna listen. But I'm not that child anymore.

THERAPIST: Right, right.

CLIENT: I'm an adult now. I have control over my own destiny. . . .

THERAPIST: It's like, "Goodbye to being defensive, goodbye to that."

CLIENT: Yeah, yeah, correct. Goodbye to that. Goodbye to being a victim. (A. Pascual-Leone et al., 2017, p. 180)

EVIDENCE EXISTS ACROSS TREATMENTS AND DISORDERS

Because lasting emotional change is a developmental process, some productive sequences of emotion may represent common processes inherent to clients as opposed to resulting from an artifact of therapist-led interventions. Thus, although the sequential model was originally developed based on cases in emotion-focused therapy, even clients in quite different treatment approaches (e.g., behavior therapy, psychiatric management) have since been found to change in ways consistent with the model. Indeed, over the past decade the model has garnered empirical support by predicting patterns of process and outcome among a range of very different treatment approaches, including emotion-focused therapy, clarification-oriented therapy, attachment-based family therapy, short-term dynamic therapy, dialectical behavior therapy, the motive-oriented therapeutic relationship, and a manualized general psychiatric treatment.

Furthermore, the model has also been examined in relation to eight notably different clinical problems: major depression, suicidality in adolescents, complex trauma, generalized anxiety, social anxiety, adjustment disorder, and several different personality disorders (for references by disorder or treatment, see

A. Pascual-Leone, 2018). To date, the body of work represents findings based on observations of over 460 clinical cases with various disorders examined in a total of 35 studies on psychotherapy process and outcome, in addition to experimental studies on more than another 470 subclinical cases. Groundbreaking research suggests distinct neurophysiological characteristics underlie some of these emotional states, providing a new line of evidence to support their clinical distinction and underscoring the need for further research (Schmutz, et al., 2025). In short, the proposed model of emotional processing is an emerging area of robust inquiry, which has garnered evidence supporting sequential transformations as a fundamental change process of human emotion. The next chapter explores that supporting body of empirical research.

ENDNOTES

1. This chapter is adapted from "How Clients 'Change Emotion With Emotion': Sequences in Emotional Processing and Their Clinical Implications," by A. Pascual-Leone and U. Kramer, in L. S. Greenberg and R. N. Goldman (Eds.), *Clinical Handbook of Emotion-Focused Therapy* (pp. 147–170), 2018, American Psychological Association (https://www.apa.org/pubs/books/4317501). Copyright 2018 by the American Psychological Association.
2. This is a modern smoothing from a line in the poem by Robert Frost (1915), "A Servant of Servants."
3. This section is based on data from A. Pascual-Leone et al. (2017).
4. I am grateful to Ladislav Timulak at Trinity College for highlighting loneliness as a core clinical concern. The research is clear that chronic loneliness of any kind is quite unhealthy. It predicts and maintains psychopathology, making it an important target for clinical intervention with clients. In several countries it is even a target at the level of national policy (N. Goldman et al., 2024). For example, Ministers of Loneliness have been appointed in the United Kingdom (in 2018) and Japan (in 2021). Still, the seriousness of loneliness as a health concern does not necessarily mean it is always a fundamentally maladaptive emotion. For example, consider that isolation among the elderly or loss of a close companion can lead to feelings of loneliness, but much like adaptive grief, it orients one adaptively to the existential needs at hand.
5. For clinicians who overlook the distinction between adaptive and maladaptive loneliness, what gets described as "loneliness" will typically be a medley of both adaptive loneliness (or grief) and maladaptive shame.
6. Although destructive anger and disgust are distinct feelings with unique action tendencies, they also have some similarity in the way they organize a person. In the sequential model, states of destructive anger, rage, and disgust are grouped together because of their shared role in actively rejecting and pushing away from an unwanted experience (A. Pascual-Leone & Greenberg, 2005, 2007a). Whether finer distinctions in problem anger are useful at this stage depends on one's clinical purpose and is also a question for future research.
7. It is worth noting that not all existential needs are interpersonal in nature. Nevertheless, some attachment-oriented perspectives have overreached by presuming all human needs or wishes are ultimately about human-relatedness. A more defensible position, however, is that attachment processes can help resolve both kinds of needs (i.e., the principal of equifinality).

16

Tracking Sequences

The Roller Coaster to Resolution

If time were like a passage of music, you could keep going back to it until you got it right.
—JOYCE JOHNSON, *MINOR CHARACTERS: A BEAT MEMOIR*

Chapter 15 used the case example of "Jeff" to illustrate a specific clinical model described by A. Pascual-Leone and Greenberg (2007a) on how sequential transformations unfold over the course of therapy. Within that specific framework, this chapter reviews the research supporting sequential transformation as a mechanism of emotional change that may apply across treatment approaches. If working through emotion sometimes feels like a roller coaster, the research suggests this is a roller coaster with a purpose, one that eventually leads to resolving personal problems.[1]

In this chapter, I first address the question of whether specific emotional states are discriminating predictors of both good sessions and good treatment outcomes. Second, I review findings on the dynamic unfolding of successful emotional processing. If key emotions do emerge from an ordered sequence, then the patterns of emotion themselves should be predictive of good outcomes. The third section in this chapter explores studies on emotional flexibility that track clients as they increasingly shift between emotion states over the course of treatment. The recursive nature of those patterns points to how a client progressively develops their capacity for working with emotion. Although the lion's share of this chapter is focused on client process, the fourth and final section considers the role of therapists in facilitating a client's progress when changing emotion with emotion.

---

https://doi.org/10.1037/0000460-017
Principles of Emotion Change: What Works and When in Psychotherapy and Everyday Life, by A. Pascual-Leone
Copyright © 2026 by the American Psychological Association. All rights reserved.

SPECIFIC EMOTIONS ANTICIPATE OUTCOME

Therapists working in session with client emotion will often have a keen sense of whether that session is going well. Sometimes this has to do with the emergence of new emotional content or with a novel shift to some healthier, more adaptive emotion. But while an attentive therapist may sense the productive nature of these in-session shifts, they are often ephemeral, and it is not always clear exactly what the moment-by-moment shift was. Skeptics might also question whether small shifts such as this truly predict any real measurable gain. However, when data is collected using minute-by-minute observations of video, it supports a therapist's hunch about what indeed was a productive emotional shift. Clients feeling certain emotions is related to outcome both in the short term (i.e., productive sessions) and the long term (i.e., final treatment outcomes measured by symptom change). A comprehensive series of meta-analyses that used stringent design criteria to evaluate all possible mechanisms of emotion change in individual therapy found the activation of key emotional states (schemes; e.g., as measured using A. Pascual-Leone & Greenberg, 2005) had a medium effect in the prediction of symptom outcomes (Sønderland et al., 2023). For therapists, taking note of these key emotions represents a thin slice of observation that has practical implications for how to work in session.

Emotions Predict Good Session Outcomes

Antonio Pascual-Leone and Greenberg (2007a) present two studies that each examined in-session examples of global distress in experiential psychotherapy in the treatment of longstanding interpersonal difficulties and depression. When confronted with distress about personal problems, individuals who process their emotion through a sequential transformation (a) engage in emotional exploration, (b) explore both the initial presenting distress and then specific types of adaptive emotion (i.e., assertive anger, grief, self-compassion), and (c) generate those emotions from the exploration of personal distress rather than by circumventing the initial bad feelings. Furthermore, (d) the clear articulation of an unmet existential need offers a gateway for the emergence of adaptive and productive emotional experience and is itself a significant predictor of good outcome events. Finally, the research implies that (e) processing according to the sequential model will predict more lasting, positive changes than haphazard or unordered explorations of emotion. These findings had small to medium effects in predicting good within-session events, and they also laid the groundwork for further research on this model of sequential transformation.

A subsequent study examined sudden treatment gains, a larger unit of change. Researchers recruited a subsample of therapist–client dyads from clinical trials on emotion-focused therapy for depression (Singh et al., 2021). By examining the session-by-session changes in depression, 64% of the clients in the treatment sample were identified as having experienced a large and abrupt drop in symptoms, something known in psychotherapy research as a sudden gain. Moreover, the study also localized when those gains occurred, showing that most of that sudden positive change (i.e., 75% of it) took place during the 50-minute session immediately preceding the recorded gain (as opposed to over the week between sessions). This suggests there is something that happens during a key session to facilitate the treatment change (rather than, for example, practicing skills or exposure exercises between sessions).

A second part of the study (Singh et al., 2021) went on to show that sudden gains in emotion-focused therapy are also related to a pattern of processes that were consistent with those described by A. Pascual-Leone and Greenberg (2007a). Comparing a client's video from other sessions with the one that immediately preceded a sudden gain, (a) therapists focused more on their client's unmet needs, and (b) clients experienced a large increase in primary adaptive emotions (e.g., assertion, grief, self-compassion). In contrast, the sudden gains were not related to other kinds of emotional activations such as secondary or maladaptive emotions (e.g., moments of distress, shame, fear, undifferentiated anger). This suggests exposure to emotion or raw arousal were not the critical issues discriminating between these productive and unproductive sessions, but rather it was the specific kinds of emotion being experienced.

In emotion-focused therapy for couples, the softening of a partner who has a pattern of blaming as well as the reengagement of a partner who was previously withdrawn are both critical events that help a couple restructure their relationship. A study of these processes coded the moment-by-moment emotions of individual members during their couples session (Myung et al., 2022). Findings suggested that as one member of the couple advanced through key states, it was followed by positive emotional responding from the other partner, in what seems to be a collaborative co-development through some parts of the model (Myung et al., 2022).

Considering various clinical contexts, certain identifiable emotions predict short-term treatment outcomes whereas others do not. This highlights productive emotional states as playing a critical role when working with emotion. For therapists, it points to the importance of identifying and making meaning out of those key emotional experiences when they arise.

Emotions Predict Final Symptom Change

Although discrete emotional states and their transformations predict short-term outcomes, a more ultimate question for health care and well-being is whether such experiences predict final treatment success. There are now about a dozen major studies that have demonstrated the reach of this prediction to final treatment outcomes in psychodynamic, humanistic, and behavioral traditions.

Psychodynamic Therapy for Adjustment Disorder: Key Emotions

The first study to successfully relate sequences of emotion to symptom change examined emotional processing among clients in short-term psychodynamic psychotherapy for adjustment disorder (Kramer et al., 2015). The aim was to replicate findings of A. Pascual-Leone and Greenberg (2007a) but also to make a large-scale prediction about final treatment outcome. Results showed that for people suffering from adjustment disorder and depressed mood, experiencing adaptive grief for as little as one minute in session had a very large effect in discriminating between successful versus unsuccessful treatment outcomes. This single observation of primary adaptive grief predicted 19% of the change in depressive symptoms at the end of treatment. The study also partially confirmed the sequential order in which key emotions emerged (reviewed in a later section). Although this was a seminal contribution, it remains the only study of psychodynamic therapy to examine the model of A. Pascual-Leone and Greenberg (2007a). Even so, its findings align with theory and research on dynamic-experiential therapies that consider discrete emotion processes (see Chapter 14, this volume; e.g., Abbass et al., 2017; McCullough et al., 2008; Town et al., 2022).

Emotion-Focused Therapy for Complex Trauma: Key Emotions

One study has related key emotions to final symptom change among clients in emotion-focused therapy for complex interpersonal trauma to address past childhood maltreatment (i.e., sexual, physical, and emotional abuse; Khayyat-Abuaita et al., 2019). This study compared the earliest sessions (1–3) with the latest treatment sessions (15–17), in which clients gave narrative accounts about their experience of abuse. The authors grouped emotions of early expressions of distress (top of Figure 15.1: global distress, rejecting anger, shame or fear, negative self-evaluation) and contrasted them with more advanced primary adaptive processes (bottom of Figure 15.1: existential need, assertive anger, self-compassion, grief or hurt, acceptance and agency). The contrast revealed a strong effect indicating that if clients entered the advanced states, it more than doubled their odds of ending treatment with a good final symptom outcome.

Humanistic Psychotherapy for Personality Disorders: Key Emotions

Several studies have looked at personality disorders and the role of specific emotional experiences. One of these examined client emotion in clarification-oriented psychotherapy (a person-centered treatment for personality disorders) and examined process in the treatment of various personality disorders (i.e., mostly narcissistic and histrionic but also cases of obsessive–compulsive and borderline personality disorder; Kramer, Pascual-Leone, Rohde, et al., 2016). Good outcome cases had experienced more self-compassion and expressed more rejecting anger as compared with poorer outcomes, with medium to large effect sizes. Among good outcomes, the total frequency of all primary adaptive emotions in the model (i.e., assertive anger, grief or hurt, and self-compassion) predicted 18% of the symptom reduction in depression by the end of treatment.

A follow-up study used a subsample to focus on the role of emotion in the treatment of narcissistic personality disorder (Kramer, Pascual-Leone, et al., 2018). Clients with narcissism showed a small decrease in their shame during the working phase of a long-term treatment (i.e., after session 20). The healthy shift in emotion explained 9% of improvement in depressive symptoms posttherapy for this difficult-to-treat subsample. It also pointed to the working phase as an optimal time to focus on maladaptive emotion when treating narcissism.

Dialectical Behavior Therapy for Borderline Personality Disorder: Key Emotions

Findings related to dialectical behavior therapy for borderline personality disorder suggest observations of emotion in the first few weeks of treatment can already anticipate the positive and negative outcomes that will occur up to a year of treatment later (Cristoffanini et al., 2023). When the prevalence of global distress was observed to increase over the course of dialectical behavior therapy, it was a prognostic indicator that anticipated poor outcomes after 12 months of treatment (Nardone et al., 2024). In contrast, when clients expressed self-compassion during the working phase, it explained 19% to 34% of symptom changes by the end of treatment.

As we have seen (in Chapter 3 on down-regulation), research on skills training in dialectical behavior therapy shows that it helps people down-regulate overwhelming emotion, but demonstrating the impact of dialectical behavior therapy on anger problems has remained elusive. However, a randomized clinical trial of dialectical behavior therapy for borderline personality disorder successfully explored this issue using A. Pascual-Leone and Greenberg's (2007a) distinction between different kinds of anger (Kramer, Pascual-Leone, Berthoud, et al., 2016). Kramer and colleagues compared dialectical behavior therapy skills training with treatment as usual. Contrary to expectation, results showed that rejecting anger remained unchanged over the course of treatment for both groups. However, they also observed that increases in assertive anger had a large effect, and these predicted 15% of the positive change in clients' interpersonal problems. This supports the prediction that early expressions of distress occur across both good and poor outcomes but that the more advanced, primary adaptive emotions (bottom of Figure 15.1) are what distinguish between outcome groups. Moreover, increasing a client's assertive anger mediated the benefits that dialectical behavior therapy skills training had in improving that client's social functioning at work, school, or home. The implication is that when therapists are successful in helping clients manage distress over troubled relationships, 23% of that effect is explained by a therapist fostering assertive anger.

Experiential Therapy for Depression: Key Emotions

A series of studies have examined specific emotional states during experiential therapy (i.e., emotion-focused therapy and client-centered therapy) for major depression by using data from the York I and York II depression studies (R. N. Goldman et al., 2006; L. S. Greenberg & Watson, 1998). Herrmann and colleagues (2016) coded cases from these treatment studies using criteria for emotion categories (i.e., secondary emotion, primary adaptive, or primary maladaptive emotion), which are different from the measure associated with the sequential model (i.e., A. Pascual-Leone & Greenberg, 2005). Even so, the study produced very consistent results. When clients in the working phase of treatment experienced fewer secondary emotions (e.g., distress, rejecting anger) and more primary adaptive emotion (e.g., assertion, grief, self-compassion), it predicted good treatment outcomes. Similarly, moderate levels of maladaptive emotion (e.g., shame, fear, guilt) during the middle of therapy were also related to good outcomes. In fact, the presence of primary adaptive emotion alone explained 66% of change in clients' depressive symptoms (Herrmann et al., 2016).

Key emotions are also supported as predictors across subsets of these clients. In cases of self-critical depression, the presence of primary adaptive emotions in a target session was related to good (over poor) treatment outcomes (Choi et al., 2016). For another subset of clients suffering from depression, arrested anger that remains unexperienced or unexpressed is sometimes the core clinical problem. A study that modeled how this emotional block is worked through identified the expression of assertive anger, the expression of an underlying need, and then the experience and expression of grief as several of the ordered processing steps that facilitated good outcomes in emotion-focused therapy (Tarba, 2015). Moreover, a client's expression of assertive anger stood out as unique and independent predictor of symptom change, explaining 42% of the reduction in depressive symptoms and 32% of general severity.

To date, the longest term outcome prediction is a study again based on the York I and York II depression studies. In it, researchers examined segments of sessions from the working phase of 55 clients and then used the narrow windows of observed emotion to predict symptom levels at an 18-month treatment follow-up (Piccirilli & Pos, 2023). The within-session observation of assertive anger and of grief or hurt were specific client states that predicted good treatment outcomes would be sustained at the long-term follow-up.

Summing Up: Discrete Emotions Predict Symptom Change
Studies like these underline that clinicians should gently reach past clients' presenting distress to purposefully differentiate and foster more productive emotional experiences. In summary, at diverse range of studies examining humanistic, psychodynamic, and behavioral therapies have used the model to explain symptom improvements related to psychotherapy. In each approach, primary adaptive emotion(s) predicted decreased symptoms and better overall treatment success, and these process-to-outcome predictions represented relatively large effect sizes. Although broad generalizations remain premature, the observation is provocative. The fact that discrete emotions are rated based on narrow windows of observation and nevertheless can be used to predict client symptom levels has palpable implications for what therapists should focus on during treatment.

PATTERNS OF UNFOLDING EMOTION ANTICIPATE OUTCOME

The studies reviewed in the previous section demonstrate how individual key emotions identified in the sequential model are predictive of both short- and long-term treatment gains. Another important kind of research that contributes evidence for a mechanism of change is research on how these emotions unfold sequentially over time (Elliott, 2010). The hypothesis that emotional processes occur through predictable sequences of emotion has been tested using several methods. Chapter 13 already reviewed experiments helpful in isolating ordered pairs of emotion. Adding now to those findings, the study of psychotherapy offers moment-by-moment analyses of spontaneous and naturally occurring temporal patterns.

What a therapist witnesses while sitting across from a client who is struggling to work through and process emotion is an individual pattern of change. However, the question here is whether those patterns of change are singular and idiosyncratic, or whether they might represent a common pattern of change that generalizes across groups of clients. Moreover, examining individual trajectories of change helps develop a richer explanatory model of how this process occurs. Some of the studies already cited are revisited next because they also conducted additional process-to-process analyses (i.e., sequences).

When Processing Is Good, Emotions Emerge in a Predictable Order

Antonio Pascual-Leone and Greenberg (2007a) hypothesized that when clients were emotionally distressed, before experiencing the primary adaptive emotions that predicted good outcomes, there were intermediate emotions that would need to emerge first (see Figure 15.1). Specifically, when the emotions followed in a sequential order, it was characteristic of a productive sequence. When clients became distressed, that initial and very global feeling was followed by rejecting anger, shame, or fear. Those emotions were then followed by negative self-evaluations and expressions of unmet needs. The final step in this chain of ordered emotions was assertive anger, grief or hurt, or self-compassion. Moreover, they further hypothesized that the temporally ordered pattern of emotions was itself a predictor of the good outcomes that followed. Indeed, when emotions in Figure 15.1 were observed, they emerged in the predicted sequence more often than chance, and such occurrence significantly anticipated good outcomes.

Early Shifts in Treatments for Personality Disorders: Change Sequences

A treatment study gave clients with borderline personality disorder 10 introductory sessions using either a behavioral approach to psychotherapy that focused on client motives or general psychiatric practice (i.e., case management; Berthoud et al., 2017). During the intake session, almost 75% of these clients predominantly expressed global distress. Nine sessions later, most clients who had expressed global distress had subsequently shifted from that state into either shame and fear or to rejecting anger, and the patterned sequence was irrespective of treatment (Willimann et al., 2016). While differentiating distress into specific emotions is predicted by the model, it also matches the initial treatment goals when working with borderline personality disorder. However, the fact that these early sequences in emotion were observed even among clients being helped in general psychiatric management (not psychotherapy per se) suggests a broader principle of emotional change may be at work.

Psychodynamic Therapy for Adjustment Disorder: Change Sequences

Other researchers argued that the session outcome effects found by A. Pascual-Leone and Greenberg (2007a) would be even stronger when emotion sequences were examined by final outcomes, and they looked at this in their study of short-term dynamic psychotherapy (Kramer et al., 2015). Working backward, they found that global distress was significantly more likely to immediately precede shame and fear, and this occurred more often in cases that later ended in good (vs. poor) treatment outcomes. There was also some evidence to suggest fear, shame, or rejecting anger directly preceded all primary adaptive emotions, a sequence that was also more characteristic of good outcomes as compared with poor treatment outcomes.

Emotion-Focused Therapy for Complex Trauma: Change Sequences

The study that examined stories of trauma told by clients in the early versus late sessions of emotion-focused therapy for complex trauma (Khayyat-Abuaita et al., 2019) also analyzed the sequential order of emotions as they occurred within those narratives. This work suggests how sequences develop over the course of treatment. Analyses showed that early in treatment, clients had more moment-by-moment transitions from global distress to either shame and fear or to rejecting anger than one would expect by chance. The effect size of this relationship was very large, and the sequences continued to be observed at the end of treatment.

Early narratives also demonstrated transitions from shame and fear or from rejecting anger to expressions of either negative evaluation or existential need, which again had very large effects. Although primary adaptive emotions were present in final narratives, they were not found to emerge in the predicted order. Authors conjectured that by the very end of treatment, clients may have developed more direct access to adaptive emotion. In short, once clients reached the end of their treatment, the issues related to abuse may have been largely resolved, and so narratives about trauma that have been processed may no longer show the pathways of change through which client have navigated (Khayyat-Abuaita et al., 2019).

Experiential Therapy for Depression: Change Sequences

Emotion sequences have been studied within and across the early, middle, and late phases of an experiential treatment for self-critical depression (Choi et al., 2016). Analyses compared the hypothesized pattern against all other possible nonlinear sequences and confirmed several nonrandom emotion-to-emotion sequences predicted by the model. Those observed multistep sequences also predicted good symptom outcomes. For instance, global distress was followed by the recurrent experiences of shame or fear, which then led to the expression of an existential need. Another key sequence was a recurrent shuttling between the articulation of an unmet need and the experience of grief. Finally, grief and the expression of a need led clients to subsequent experiences of assertive anger. These transitions between states are predicted by the connecting arrows in Figure 15.1.

In contrast, the same study also identified sequences that were characteristic of poor treatment outcomes (Choi et al., 2016). As expected, these all involved being stuck at the top of Figure 15.1 among the early expressions of distress. Finally, cases with poor outcomes suffered miniature regressions according to the hypothesized model. For example, clients in a state of negative self-evaluation would collapse into the less differentiated states of shame and fear or global distress. When these collapses occurred repeatedly, they predicted a client's poor symptom outcome at the end of treatment.

After highlighting the role of primary adaptive emotions, the study by Herrmann and colleagues (2016; cited earlier) also tested for sequences. They found that while the engagement of secondary emotion was related to outcome, primary adaptive emotions mediated that effect. So, engagement with emotions like symptomatic distress was useful to the degree that it offered clients an entry point to then explore their deeper primary adaptive emotions. Furthermore, the frequency with which a client transitioned within a session from primary maladaptive emotion to primary adaptive emotion was another positive predictor of outcome (Herrmann et al., 2016). These findings suggest that it may be useful to engage various kinds of emotion (e.g., secondary symptomatic emotion or maladaptive emotion) but only when doing so facilitates the subsequent experience of primary adaptive emotion.

This final finding by Herrmann and colleagues (2016)—about a directional transition from maladaptive to adaptive emotion—was replicated by a different research team using data from a separate treatment study and using a different measure. That study examined emotion-focused therapy as a treatment for self-criticism by focusing on sessions of chairwork (Delatraba et al., 2025). It showed that when clients shifted from maladaptive shame or fear into adaptive states of assertive anger, grief, or self-compassion (middle and bottom of Figure 15.1), that sequential transformation explained 40% of a client's change in depressive symptoms by the conclusion of treatment. Such sequences were observed as moments within a given session, yet their impact endured even beyond the end of treatment, explaining over 20% of changes to a client's self-hate at a 3-month follow-up (Delatraba et al., 2025).

Thinly sliced observations like these have even predicted symptoms 18 months after the treatment of depression using emotion-focused therapy (Piccirilli & Pos, 2023). Analyses considered all possible combinations between states and identified sequences that occurred more often than chance in a good outcome as contrasted with poorer outcomes. One good outcome sequence was when clients felt maladaptive shame or fear and it was immediately followed by their exploration of an unmet need (see the middle of Figure 15.1).

Another sequence was the exploration of unmet needs followed by the client's experience of adaptive grief or hurt, or vice versa, where grief was followed by the deeper exploration of unmet needs—a complementary process (see the bottom of Figure 15.1). These productive sequences were also in the context of findings mentioned earlier in the chapter, where both assertive anger and grief were each key emotions individually predictive of good outcome (Piccirilli & Pos, 2023). Again, these transitions between states support specific links found in Figure 15.1. Furthermore, the study showed that when clients got stuck in a loop of expressing rejecting anger, it predicted a poor prognosis at follow-up (Piccirilli & Pos, 2023).

Attachment-Based Family Therapy and Couples Therapy: Change Sequences

The studies described previously consider productive patterns of emotion in various approaches for treating individuals. However, patterns have also been examined in the treatment of couples and families. Suicidal adolescents in attachment-based family therapy have also been studied in terms of the conditional probability of emotion-to-emotion pathways (Lifshitz et al., 2021). Here, too, the sequences predicted by the model occurred more often than chance. For a good outcome, a client in global distress was more likely than chance to subsequently shift into maladaptive shame. Similarly, a client experiencing rejecting anger was more likely than chance to move forward in the model to assertive anger and then from assertive anger to adaptive grief. Each of these pathways are predicted by the model (Figure 15.1). However, when adolescents were not benefiting from treatment, they showed correspondingly higher rates of global distress within their sessions.

A study of emotion-focused couples therapy examined how a previously blaming partner comes to soften and how a formerly withdrawing partner comes to reengage, each representing significantly positive change events (Myung et al., 2022). Rejecting anger was observed as a characteristic state for partners who tended to blame. However, a series of case examples that plotted productive change events over time showed that secondary anger was often followed by deeper experiences of maladaptive fear or shame before the individual softened their critical tone. In the case of a withdrawer's reengagement, primary maladaptive shame was initially the dominant state. However, moment-by-moment plots from case examples of good outcome suggest that shame was followed by adaptive grief or hurt. Furthermore, conditional probabilities showed grief or hurt in a withdrawing partner was likely to be followed by acceptance and agency before the individual would begin to share with their partner (Myung et al., 2022).

Summing Up: Patterns That Predict Symptom Change

In summary, process-to-process studies have tested the individual trajectories of personal change as people in distress move from one emotion to the next. Several studies have shown the ordered sequences themselves relate to good clinical outcomes at either the session or treatment level. Overall, these clinical studies, in addition to experimental designs cited in Chapter 13, corroborate various aspects of the predicted patterns of emotion, with supporting evidence from experiential, psychodynamic, and systemic approaches to treatment, among others. Each of these showed change to various symptom concerns. For instance, the first sequential step in the model also seems to have some support from the process observed in treatments for borderline personality disorder. Across all treatment studies, the most robust outcome prediction is that patterns in emotion are followed by a reduction in the symptoms of depression.

This convergence, despite a range in the strategies for analysis, suggests several steps in the sequential model can act as strong predictors. The detailed findings of studies in this section and those that follow collectively support the emotion-to-emotion temporal relationship of the model. However, no single study has been large enough to simultaneously verify every individual link. Finally, it remains to be seen whether the treatment of different disorders will emphasize alternative sequences.

Small Patterns in a Session Echo Larger Patterns Across Treatments

Evidence supporting the hypothesis that passages of productive emotion may emerge in a specific sequence is an intriguing new contribution. Still, a mechanism of change must also explain how moment-by-moment observations of emotion build over time to culminate in what presumably precipitates larger units of symptom change. Although studying that issue is methodologically arduous, it has been done in several ways. First, individual sessions have been examined for micropatterns. Second, intensive case studies have tracked every moment of aroused emotion over entire courses of therapy. Third, group design studies have also allowed researchers to compare patterns in emotion across early versus late phases of therapy.

Patterns of Emotion Build During a Single Session

When therapists know what kinds of emotion to look for, they can track their client's process as it unfolds during a session. Individual sessions reveal a dynamic transformation. But attending to these emotion shifts is with the assumption that a productive experience somehow builds over time until it culminates in what presumably is the tipping point in a dynamic system. So these moment-by-moment shifts should gradually accumulate, contributing to some larger units of psychological change.

Work on this problem was first explored at the University of Windsor, where research showed how nonlinear patterns of moment-by-moment change relate to the unfolding of good outcomes in emotion-focused therapy for depression and complex trauma (A. Pascual-Leone, 2009). Looking at regression slopes of emotional progress during selected sessions for 34 cases, findings showed that when clients worked through their emotional distress, therapeutic changes appeared to advance steadily in an overall linear fashion. However, if a single qualitative shift in emotional state is what we call a sequential transformation, the study also found clients increased their ability to dynamically shift from one set of feelings and meanings and one self-organizing framework of action to another—something one can describe as improved *emotional flexibility.*

Finally, when tracking emotion in a session, many therapists notice their clients occasionally suffer brief moments of emotional collapse. For example, clients may make initial advances into primary adaptive emotion but then, after some effort, regress back into earlier expressions of distress. A. Pascual-Leone (2009) showed that the duration of a client's momentary collapse (i.e., setbacks) became significantly shorter over the course of a good therapeutic event, reducing in length by about one third from the first episode of collapse to the last (see Figure 16.1). The saw-toothed pattern shows clients advance two steps forward and one step back. This reflects how clients build emotional resilience.

The ups and downs in productive sessions can be likened to emotional push-ups, whereby clients develop and strengthen a broader repertoire of adaptive feelings. A characteristic example of this is when a client experiences primary grief but then loses their place—they feel overwhelmed or get distracted from the main concern—and collapse back into secondary emotions of distress, only to eventually find their focus again as they work toward rearticulating the deeper meaning of their loss. While recovering from these momentary collapses is part of the overall pattern in healthy change, research cited earlier on unproductive emotional patterns confirms that getting stuck in a collapse of this kind is a harbinger of poor treatment outcome (Choi et al., 2016; Piccirilli & Pos, 2023).

FIGURE 16.1. Two Steps Forward, One Step Back: The Saw-Toothed Pattern of Emotional Progress

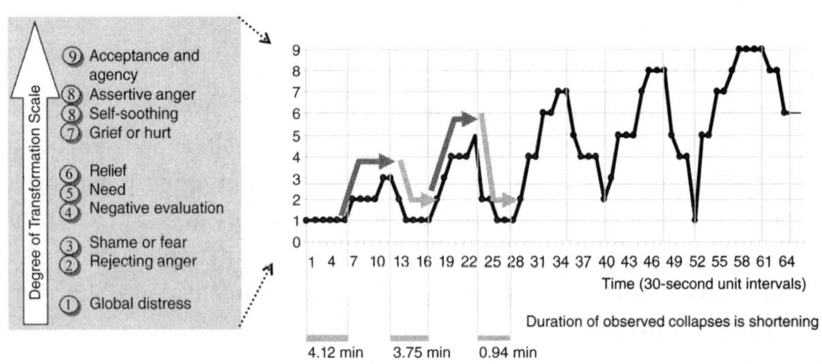

Note. This plot shows the pattern of emotional improvements and collapses (setbacks) for a typical good outcome. At the bottom, one sees the changing duration of momentary emotional collapse (setbacks) in a good outcome case. Adapted from "Dynamic Emotional Processing in Experiential Therapy: Two Steps Forward, One Step Back," by A. Pascual-Leone, 2009, *Journal of Consulting and Clinical Psychology, 77*(1), p. 120 (https://doi.org/10.1037/a0014488). Copyright 2009 by the American Psychological Association.

Case Studies Detail the Patterns of Emotion Over Treatment

While the microanalysis of change events helps us track the nuts and bolts of this kind of emotional change, one also needs to consider the longitudinal context. Case studies can do this by following emotional change over longer time frames, and a number of these have been conducted by a research group at Trinity College.[2] Their research offers detailed descriptions of the various ways in which the sequential model applies to the unfolding narrative of emotion within individual cases.

"Jan" was a very successful outcome case in a treatment study of emotion-focused therapy for depression (McNally et al., 2014). A narrative account elaborates how the client progressed over 16 sessions of therapy to a complete recovery, which was maintained at 18 months posttreatment. The process played out over early, middle, and late treatment sessions in a manner that could be mapped out on the model in Figure 15.1. Early sessions (1–5) were mainly nonproductive, having more arousal and more global distress. Working phase sessions (6–11) showed increased activity across all types of emotion, and although the total amount of global distress was reduced, it was still the most prevalent emotion, followed by shame and fear and then assertive anger. Both this and the later phase showed increases in emotional flexibility, although occasional collapses into global distress were still observed. Sessions at the end of treatment (12–16) revealed dramatic reductions in both global distress as well as shame and fear, which by then had become more prevalent. Adaptive emotions were also increasingly apparent such as assertive anger, self-compassion, and for the first time, grief and hurt.

A similar analysis was conducted of "Lisa," treated over 15 sessions of emotion-focused therapy for depression and ending in a recovery maintained 18 months later (Dillon et al., 2016). Analyses examined the relative frequency of different kinds of emotion from the model. The frequency and duration of global distress and rejecting anger (combined) decreased from the early half (sessions 1–7) to the latter half (sessions 8–15) of therapy. Shame and fear remained constant, whereas adaptive emotions (i.e., assertive anger, self-compassion, grief or hurt, and agency) increased, becoming the most prevalent group of emotion in the second half of treatment. Qualitative observations showed that Lisa had greater differentiation and more emotional flexibility over the course of her treatment. Researchers concluded that the case study supported an ordered sequence of emotions, and they highlighted that progress was nonlinear.

Using a more quantitative approach, researchers at University of Windsor conducted two separate intensive case studies on successful treatments using emotion-focused therapy for relational trauma ("Carla" and "Jeff"; A. Pascual-Leone et al., 2017).[3] The researchers coded every emotional event in the entire course of each treatment and then looked for statistical patterns both within sessions as well as across the entire treatment. In the case of Carla, progress within each session showed moment-by-moment gains replicating prior research that demonstrated the patterns are important for productive sessions and predictive of good treatment outcomes. However, considering the entire course of treatment revealed that Carla also cycled through the model multiple times rather than only in a single key session. Researchers described this as a pattern of practice-makes-perfect, referring not only to the successful within-session processing but also to its repeated rehearsal or consolidation (A. Pascual-Leone et al., 2017). Even so, that recapitulative process did not carry across sessions in the sense that Carla started most sessions in a state of global distress (i.e., at the beginning of the process model). Thus, on its own, each session appeared markedly productive, although the study did not observe those gains as impacting subsequent events from one session to the next. Still, Carla's pattern of change was consistent with the understanding of emotional change as something that needs to be activated and reactivated before it becomes effortless and a stable new way of feeling (i.e., the emotional push-ups described earlier).

The case of Jeff was already described at the beginning of the previous chapter, but the systematic observation of his sessions was also subjected to a detailed analysis (A. Pascual-Leone et al., 2017). The observed pattern was similar to that of a prior case study (McNally et al., 2014). Jeff's emotional processing showed a gradual advancement, moving through the emotional processing model across successive sessions. Statistical modeling showed that each session began and ended with progressively less global distress and increasingly more primary and productive emotion. Thus, the level of sequential transformation for each session improved with each session, a moving average, advancing one step at a time. In this way, the process added up in a stepwise manner, augmenting across multiple treatment sessions. The narrative account of Jeff's change over time (see Chapter 15) provides insight into the different steps he went through, overcoming one emotional challenge at a time as he moved through the series of sessions and toward a successful treatment outcome. Identifying patterns like this of longer term change helps clarify for therapists the various ways a treatment may be on track.

Group Designs Confirm Patterns of Emotion Over Treatment

Several studies have used group designs to examine how emotions fluctuate and interact moment by moment and how that process unfolds longitudinally. Perhaps not surprisingly, many of the observed patterns based on group averages turn out to be strikingly congruent with the individual trajectories described in single case studies. However, although not possible using single case designs, group designs show these dynamic patterns of emotional change are generalizable as characteristic of good (over poor) treatment outcomes.

One study looked at the clinical trial (cited earlier) comparing a behaviorally informed psychotherapy with general psychiatric management as brief treatments (i.e., 10 sessions) for borderline personality disorder (Berthoud et al., 2017). It examined the longitudinal changes in emotion for a group of 50 clients, but treatments did not differ in the observed emotional changes. For all clients who expressed global distress during the intake, the frequency of that expression of distress decreased dramatically by session 9. However, in parallel to that distress, clients enjoyed moderate increases in self-compassion and assertive anger.

Two studies have tracked the longitudinal pattern of change among groups of clients in emotion-focused therapy. One of these looked at the treatment for a group of nine clients suffering from social anxiety disorder and coded their emotion over the course of emotion-focused therapy. It concluded that as successful treatment progressed, there was a trade-off accumulating between different kinds of states: Maladaptive shame was essentially being resolved by increasing the primary adaptive emotions of assertive anger or grief (Haberman et al., 2019). The other study looked at a group of 38 clients in emotion-focused therapy for complex trauma and also demonstrated a progressive shifting in emotion over 16–20 sessions (Khayyat-Abuaita et al., 2019). Researchers measured the amount and type of emotion that was felt when clients told stories about a trauma event, comparing how it was told and experienced during an early treatment session with how it was told during a late session. From the beginning to end of therapy, the amount of primary adaptive emotion clients experienced increased from a total of 8 seconds per session (at the beginning of therapy) to a total of 4 minutes per session (at the end of therapy). The findings of these two studies describe shifts in emotion that clinicians might palpably observe as they conduct treatment. For therapists, this means if a client makes specific identified transitions (e.g., from shame or fear to assertive anger) and is shifting in the relative preponderance of key emotions, it suggests therapy is on track.

EMOTIONAL FLEXIBILITY AND RECURSIVE PATTERNS

Evidence shows the emergence of new emotions appearing in a client's repertoire and that these unfold in ordered patterns as observed at various levels of temporal analysis. This *emotional restructuring* suggests two ideas for understanding adult emotional development. First, while increasing the emotional range available to clients is promising, making use of that will also require clients to become more flexible. Although a common supposition in clinical theory, the idea that clients in successful therapy become more emotionally flexible is a testable hypothesis. Second, findings similar patterns at different levels of analysis represent a complex overall pattern of change that is self-similar across different scales, like a fractal. I explore each of these ideas next.

Clients Gain Flexibility as an Outcome of Treatment

Figure 16.1 illustrated clients increasing in their emotional flexibility during a productive single-session event in emotion-focused therapy (i.e., A. Pascual-Leone, 2009). Increases to someone's *emotional flexibility*—that is, the degree to which they move between and explore a range of different emotional states—

has also been examined over entire courses of treatment and used as a predictor of symptom change. The following three studies examine this in various treatments for borderline personality disorder.

The study that examined client emotion in two brief treatments for borderline personality disorder also considered the variability or range of fluctuation in client's emotional states (Berthoud et al., 2017). While both treatments produced comparable treatment gains, clients at the end of 10 sessions in the behaviorally informed psychotherapy demonstrated a significantly larger increase in their emotional flexibility when working with their personal difficulties as compared with those in psychiatric management. This finding was replicated in another study that looked at emotion over 12 months of dialectical behavior therapy for clients suffering borderline personality disorder (Nardone et al., 2024). The degree to which clients increased their emotional flexibility (i.e., variation between states) from early therapy (e.g., 5 sessions) to the working phase (e.g., session 12) explained 14% of a client's reduction in depression at the conclusion of treatment 8–10 months later.

Preliminary research using functional magnetic resonance imaging (fMRI) of the brain has shown differences in the way people with borderline personality disorder respond to self-criticism before and after receiving general psychiatric management for 10 sessions over 3 months (Kramer, Kolly, et al., 2018). Self-criticism during a standardized task elicited the same amount of shame and fear whether it was presented before or after 3 months of treatment. However, video observation of how clients responded to this standardized task revealed medium increases in their emotional flexibility as well as a corresponding change in brain activation and decreased reactivity at the end of therapy (Kramer et al., 2018). Emotional flexibility is a promising variable for clinical inquiry, and this pilot study underscores the potential value of a multimethod approach.

The fact that the three studies I discussed show the importance of increasing emotional flexibility for successful treatments of personality disorders underscores characterological rigidity as part of that presenting concern. The role of emotional flexibility in other issues of clinical focus needs more research. That said, findings on emotional processing across treatment point to very similar patterns previously observed within single session events during the treatment of depression or trauma (i.e., Pascual-Leone, 2009).

Fractals as a Structure for Understanding Change

Prior subsections have discussed patterns both at the moment-by-moment level within a session as well as broader scoped patterns over the course of an entire treatment. Meanwhile, case studies highlighted patterns both in terms of moment-by-moment micro shifts and the larger macro-scale changes of adult emotional development. Interestingly, the evidence suggests that how these changes unfold across an entire treatment is often similar to the moment-by-moment processes within a given session, although at a larger temporal scale.

Taken together, these parallel observations at different scales recall a recursion, in which a given process depends on the repetition of a simpler version of itself. This seems to represent a fractal or complex pattern of change that is self-similar across different scales.

Classic examples of recursion include the Fibonacci sequence in mathematics, and a popular visual recursion might be the image of a person holding a portrait of themselves, in which they are holding a smaller version of that same portrait, and so on. Recursive fractals can also be used to represent patterns in time, and this may serve as a structure for understanding changes in a dynamic system of emotional processing. The idea resembles a notion that people go through a "spiral of growth," which is a loose metaphor used in some clinical theories and popular formulations of personal development, therapeutic change, and even spirituality. However, the research reported here is the first time such an idea has been empirically documented and rigorously tested.

For therapists, these ideas have some important clinical implications. It suggests the model (Figure 15.1) could be used to understand how their clients are progressing (or should be progressing), both at the session level and over the entire course of treatment. To use this insight, it means staying in the moment while also being mindful of the sequences that are anticipated by a sequential model. Doing so can help a clinician map out a client's treatment and inform one's choice of interventions (Pascual-Leone & Kramer, 2017; Timulak & Pascual-Leone, 2015). For case conceptualizations, this offers an empirically informed context for interpreting divergences from what may be a client's optimal treatment process.

WHAT TO DO WHEN: THERAPISTS FACILITATING CHANGE

Since key emotions and their patterns predict a client's treatment outcome, researchers have now begun to work backward and explore what therapists might be doing to promote those target client processes. Of course, the first step for working with emotion is usually to establish the safety of a therapeutic relationship, but the kind of relationship one develops informs the kind of tasks that will follow (e.g., Fisher et al., 2016; Harrington et al., 2021; Town et al., 2022). However, going beyond good relationship conditions (Flückiger et al., 2020), there is a paucity of research on the specific therapist actions that facilitate a sequential transformation.

One study sought to anticipate what made for a productive session in emotion-focused therapy for depression and relational trauma by looking at the specific type of therapist intervention that might have facilitated a client's deeper emotional experiencing (A. Pascual-Leone et al., 2025). The study concluded that therapists who focused their responses on a client's emotion and unmet needs had more productive sessions. In contrast, therapists who did more uninterrupted listening and also made general reflections about the content a client was discussing had less productive sessions. Another study showed therapist interventions in attachment-based family therapy significantly affected the emotional processing of adolescents who had presented with depression and suicidality (Tsvieli et al., 2020). Effective interventions included using relational reframes and then focusing on primary adaptive emotions. In contrast, interpretations, reassurances, and excessive focus on secondary anger often hindered progress.

When clients engage their distress, the next transition in the model (Figure 15.1) is that clients should explore the experience of maladaptive emotion. In a study that looked at a humanistic treatment for personality disorders (i.e., clarification-oriented therapy), when clients were struggling with their feelings of maladaptive shame or fear, it seemed to be especially useful if therapists responded in a way that guided the client's process. In fact, the therapist's empathic understanding and also their process directivity had meaningful effects in predicting that a client would subsequently share and explore their harsh negative self-evaluations later in the same session (Kramer et al., 2016). As discussed in Chapter 15, a negative self-evaluation always has some tension with respect to unmet existential needs, even when clients cannot readily identify what they need. So another step in the model is that clients should articulate their unmet needs. Minute-by-minute process research using a quasi-experimental design suggested that when a client's emotional arousal increases to a moderate level, it marks an optimal opportunity for therapists to then prompt clients to identify and explore their unmet needs (Nardone et al., 2022).

One of the last steps in the sequential model (Figure 15.1) indicates that clients should move to the experience of primary adaptive emotions. The positive relationship between a therapist's effort to deepen the session process and then their client successfully creating new meaning in the moment was explained by the degree to which clients experienced states of assertive anger, grief or hurt, or self-compassion (A. Pascual-Leone et al., 2025). Taking this further, other research shows the association between a therapist's focus and their client generating new emotional meaning is also echoed more distally at the level of symptom outcome. For emotion-focused therapists treating depressive self-criticism, using interventions that elaborated on client emotion predicted symptom change by the end of treatment (Delatraba et al., 2025; also cited earlier with respect to key emotion states). Moreover, the impact of those interventions was mediated by the degree to which clients subsequently shifted within the same session, moving from maladaptive emotion (e.g., shame, fear) to adaptive emotion (e.g., assertive anger, grief, self-compassion). In fact, the specific kind of emotion a client experienced and the sequence in which client's experienced that emotion, together, explained up to 43% of the effect that a therapist's intervention had on the final outcome of treatment (Delatraba et al., 2025).

These studies demonstrate the role therapists play in facilitating key emotions and their sequences in a change process that leads to final treatment outcomes. To these studies on therapist intervention, one can also add a dozen clinical experiments that show target emotions can be facilitated by design so as to prompt sequential transformations (reviewed in Chapter 13). However, a major implication for working with emotion is that even though one may readily believe in the value of allowing the expression of feelings, not all emotions are equally useful. Furthermore, there is an optimal sequence by which such experiences should unfold. Therapists (and clients) need to discriminate between different kinds of feelings before making the most favorable intervention (see Introduction).

Taken together, research suggests different kinds of interventions could be useful depending on a client's place in the model. The practice implication may be an ordered set of priorities for therapists when trying to facilitate a sequential transformation. For instance,

1. When clients begin to express distress, therapists should use empathic exploration and focus their client's attention on the deeper significance of a presenting feeling.

2. Then, if clients touch upon maladaptive emotion, therapists should express empathic understanding and purposefully guide or direct clients to explore the underlying significance of those emotions.

3. Should clients show some observable increases in their expressed arousal, therapists might take that as a marker to prompt the client in identifying and articulating their unmet needs.

4. Finally, when clients are elaborating on unmet needs and exploring the complexity of an emotional experience, therapists should look to facilitate shifts from maladaptive emotion to the emergent aspects of adaptive emotion.

Based on the available research, these tentatively represent concrete therapist operations that correspond to facilitating clients through the model in Figure 15.1. Even so, the study on what therapist interventions help in this kind of change process is very preliminary.

CONCLUSIONS ABOUT CHANGING EMOTION WITH EMOTION

The idea of changing emotion with emotion speaks to processes that are temporally ordered. Internal meaning states that are temporally ordered and precede symptom change are probable mechanisms of change. The research has shown both proximal and distal effects of this process. Although emotions are sequenced within a productive session event, one should not expect the end of that event to show measurable symptom change, though it may show positive effects. However, these same sequences aggregate over time and do anticipate symptom change.

Causal mechanisms are only conclusively demonstrated to the extent that they offer both a compelling explanation for change and sufficient supporting evidence. The first three chapters in Part IV of this book detailed the convergence of ideas from various perspectives about how this unique kind of emotional change happens and provided explanations for their psychological and neurological underpinnings, supported by evidence using experimental research. The last two chapters presented a specific account of how emotional sequences unfold and reviewed a body of evidence from psychotherapy research. Finally, an important issue in building the case for causality is that emotional states and their order are qualitatively different from symptom relief or character changes, which are the common outcome goals of treatment. As such, the shifts in emotion cannot be mistaken for mini outcomes in any conventional sense. In sum, transformative emotional sequences (emotion changing emotion) seems to be a unique form of emotional processing and is promising as a mechanism of change in psychotherapy.

ENDNOTES

1. The case of Jeff was presented in detail at the beginning of Chapter 12, and a detailed account of therapy with Jeff was presented at the beginning of Chapter 15.
2. Led by L. Timulak, this line of research has produced a series of detailed case illustrations of emotional processing and that work has helped with clinically useful refinements to the categories in the A. Pascual-Leone and Greenberg model.
3. The case of "Carla" was presented in detail at the beginning of Chapter 12, while a detailed account of therapy with "Jeff" was presented at the beginning of Chapter 15.

V

PUT THE FEELING IN CONTEXT

INTRODUCTION: PUT THE FEELING IN CONTEXT

Reflecting on emotion is about creating context. In this sense, a story is the narrative background to a feeling. Although an emotion is a densely packaged unit of information, it only occurs in relation to some context. That context may be primarily external (e.g., a heated argument with a neighbor) or primarily internal (e.g., quietly remembering the loss one suffered after a personal sacrifice), but it is often both. However, this context for one's emotion is ultimately not so much about factual circumstances as it is about the associated meanings and framework of understanding. The details one elaborates help explicate the many interrelated conditions that surround the feeling one is having. Those details coalesce around an emerging affective experience and create an interpretive lens for negotiating the experience of emotion. As tendrils of associated meanings each apply their contribution, the feeling shapes into a more complete and meaningful experience. The context of meaning, whether as a passing association or as a narrated story, serves as an implicit framework. This is a dynamic process that creates the background, couching emotion.

Figure V.1 depicts this process using a variation of a classic optical illusion. The presenting emotion is represented by the gray circle surrounded by a white background (at left). The change process does not involve any direct manipulation of the gray circle, which appear again (at right) surrounded by a dark background. Although the shade of the gray circle remains unchanged, it appears either darker or lighter depending on its background. By analogy, emotion is figural, but it looks and feels different depending on the background narrative context.

This is also the moment to acknowledge that terms like "theory of mind," "mentalizing," and "metacognition" are used in clinical theory and research to describe a person's general capacity to think about their own mental processes as well as those of others.[1] The commonality among such cognitive acts is their reflexive quality (Semerari et al., 2007). In many ways, they represent alternative formulations for understanding the totality of emotional processing, except with a heavy emphasis on higher order reflection. Although I do not work within those very broad conceptual frameworks, what I do explore in this final part of the book are specific processes that are pertinent and well represented to those conceptualizations.

Part V of this book (Chapters 17–23) discusses reflection on emotion, a complex and increasingly abstract group of processes for working with emotion. This final part of the book explores mechanisms that are related to the act of storytelling. By way of introduction, the first chapter (Chapter 17) presents the construct as well as clinical markers for when to reflect on emotion and its narrative context. Then, the chapters that follow present evidence supporting four separate pathways of action through which reflecting on emotion and the

FIGURE V.1. Put the Feeling in a New Context: The Principle of Narrative Reflection

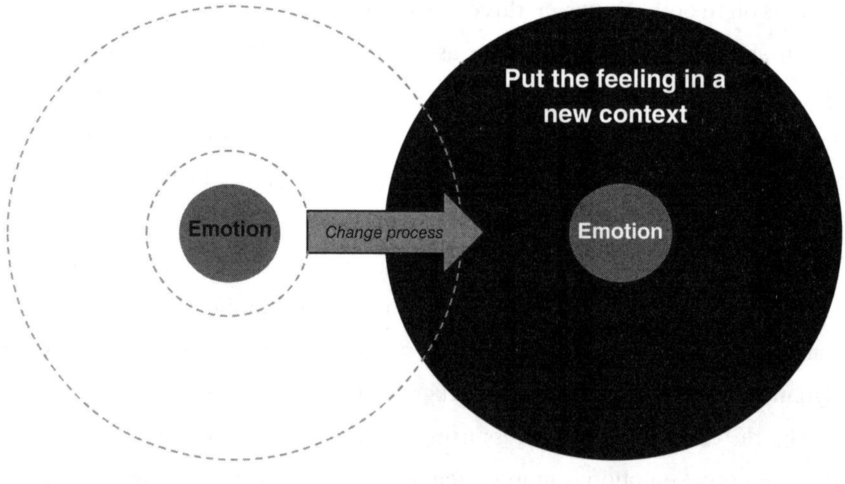

Note. Narrative reflection is a principle that involves elaborating contextual details, reframing an existing experience, or developing a personal story around the experience. Leveraging these changes is illustrated here using a visual illusion. As one shifts from white to black backgrounds on either side of the image, it makes the gray circle in the middle (i.e., emotion) appear to be either lighter or darker in shade—although both are actually exactly the same shade. Similarly, changing the interpretive context alone can change a target emotional experience. This is one of five categorically different processes for working with emotion.

narrative context leads to positive change. I also give some explanation of how these changes happen at the more basic level of autobiographical memory (see Chapters 19 and 22). However, my focus is primarily on the applied level of clinical and personal change (Chapters 18, 20, 21, and 23). The four mechanisms to be discussed are italicized and are described as follows:

- *Psychological elaboration* gives one more to feel about (i.e., increased specificity, positive meaning making, and emotion-narrative elaboration; see Chapter 18). Furthermore, one also has ongoing assessments about the value or significance of the stories being elaborated, which represents another order of meaning elaboration that is also subject to change (Chapter 19).

- *Decentering* from one's frame of reference gives new perspective and existential insights (see Chapter 20).

- The *story itself is an agent of change* (see Chapter 21), which gets construed from multiple perspectives (Chapter 22).

- Existential insights and having purpose also highlight the role of *making choices* as the author of one's own story. Reinventing the self opens new avenues for feeling and motivation (see Chapter 23).

Elaboration, decentering, the story as a blueprint for change, and existential choice are four mechanisms of emotional change that are not exclusive. They are nested and they overlap, wherein epistemologically simpler forms of narrative change discussed in earlier chapters (e.g., psychological elaboration) are also implicit within the more complex examples that follow (e.g., existential insights, reinventing the self). Furthermore, the stories and narrative reflections people make will play different roles at different times in the journey of change.

ENDNOTE

1. *Theory of mind* is a concept taken from cognitive-developmental psychology to refer to insights about mental functioning. *Mentalization,* in psychoanalytic theory, is about formulating and understanding the internal states that underlie a person's overt behavior and the implications that this has for social attachments. Finally, *metacognition* is a concept from cognitive psychology to refer to knowledge about and control of one's own cognition. Moreover, while clinical authors have preferences for these terms largely based on the source of their inspiration, the terms can often be used interchangeably. Thinking about one's own psychological experiences entails an extensive range of semi-independent faculties that have already been described across several chapters in this book.

17

Using Context and Narrative

The Big Picture

And I want you to choose some time in the past when you were a very, very little girl. And my voice will go with you. And my voice will change into that of your parents, your neighbors, your friends, your schoolmates, your playmates, your teachers. And I want you to find yourself sitting in the school room, a little girl feeling happy about something, something that happened a long time ago, that you forgot a long time ago.

—MILTON H. ERICKSON, *MY VOICE WILL GO WITH YOU*

A talking cure unfolds somewhere in the verbal exchange between client and psychotherapist. When we tell other people about what is important to us, what is most difficult, and why, we do it in terms of stories. Freud and colleagues found it was easier to work with defenses against anxiety than to work directly with the material that was making a client anxious. In keeping with this, the narrative and any insight into a client's emotional difficulty is often not being talked about directly; rather, it is being activated by using reflection on how one negotiates painful emotion (Messer & McWilliams, 2006).

WHAT IS REFLECTING ON EMOTION? WHEN IS IT IMPORTANT?

Reflecting on emotion involves an elaboration of the experience as a whole and its significance, which typically includes a great deal of information about its context. Narrative accounts and situational appraisals like these are typically couched in terms of stories about what happened there and then (and this

https://doi.org/10.1037/0000460-018
Principles of Emotion Change: What Works and When in Psychotherapy and Everyday Life, by A. Pascual-Leone
Copyright © 2026 by the American Psychological Association. All rights reserved.

contrasts with when a feeling is viscerally experienced here and now). More-over, even though stories often change, they serve as a sort of ongoing reposi-tory for information so it can be remembered, organized, and shared.

Stories Become the Medium of Change

Narrative becomes the medium through which psychotherapy happens.[1] Every treatment session, a client discloses an average of four to six separate personal stories, an observation that has been replicated across brief dynamic, client-centered, and emotion-focused therapies (Angus et al., 2004; Luborsky et al., 1992). Telling the story often entails a narrative about the plot and characters of what happened and is typically intertwined with a corresponding commen-tary about one's emotional experience during those events. This psychological elaboration extends beyond retrospective accounts when it also takes on a reflexive process, focusing on implications for the present self (Angus, 2012). Finally, the open-ended nature of a narrative as a medium for exploration often reveals whether the author has reached any conclusions about what happened or not, setting a trajectory or implicit agenda for working with emotion.

Going further, sharing a story forms the basis of a connection with one's therapist. Considering the other person as a listener (whether real or imagined) helps one maintain the coherence with which one thinks of one's experience. When clients disclose vivid, specific, and emotionally rich stories, then thera-pists also have the content they need to identify themes about the personal conflicts in their clients' lives (Luborsky et al., 1994). Both stories from the past as well as the lived story of what is happening right now are windows through which a therapist develops an empathic understanding and offers a corrective emotional experience.

Frameworks Help Contain and Interpret Emotion

Many of the processes I have discussed so far in this book (e.g., emotional engagement, emerging awareness, increasing arousal, sequences in discrete emotions) start out as pre-verbal processes. Higher cognition and language subsequently take those processes to another level of sophistication, allowing one to make models of one's own internal experience. Creating stories involves constructing cognitive and verbal frameworks of conceptual under-standing, and these serve as a new symbolic meaning structure for further working with emotion. The result is that cognitive–linguistic processes play an important role in alleviating one's emotional distress, which begins with the early acquisition of language in toddlers and then becomes increasingly sophisticated into adulthood (J. Pascual-Leone & Johnson, 2021). Thinking about one's distress in rational–conceptual terms is not a panacea, but it does allow one to mentally negotiate emotion in at least two ways: It helps with (a) containing emerging affect and (b) interpreting emotional situations. Basic examples of doing this are labeling emotion, compartmentalizing separate aspects of an experience, and being able to reflect more objectively about those experiences.

Cognitive–linguistic strategies are used to contain emerging affect and thereby change emotion when they facilitate the degree to which one can cope with escalating emotion. The way cognitive–linguistic strategies can help one cope with emotional distress goes beyond simply labeling the feeling (recall Chapter 5). Language, gestures, and enactments are symbolic structures that can potentially overwrite what one feels in the moment with functional alternatives. Here, reflecting on emotion is what allows one to compartmentalize it. Often with mental rehearsal (i.e., through self-talk, gestures, or narratives), the use of goal setting or personal imperatives offers a cognitive strategy to focus one's attention away from distress. This creates a psychological distance from the urgency of upsetting emotion and essentially allows one to focus on concrete problem solving.

New cognitive strategies for emotional engagement also allow one to change the way situations are interpreted in the first place, like adding more capacity or capabilities to an existing system. The result of this purposeful approach is that it leads to new constellations of emotional experience. Stepping back to consider the upshot, silver lining, or opportunities that are part of an apparent tragedy is a basic example of this. In this sense, new conceptual formulations can help one internally change the meaning of an emerging or anticipated emotion, thereby changing the emotion by changing its contextual meaning. Sometimes this will involve reframing an experience with new information; at other times, it comes in the form of an insight that helps one better grasp the nature of one's difficulties (Beck, 2020; Messer & McWilliams, 2006; A. Pascual-Leone & Greenberg, 2007b). In short, when cognition is effortfully applied top down, it allows one to reconfigure the experienced reality in a way that makes unmet needs less distressing and oppressive. Initially, that reprieve frees up mental space while one problem solves to address part of the underlying issue in a practical manner. Later, the same top-down cognitive work may also become less effortful as one begins to automatically apply the new framework of understanding to associated experiences of emotion in the future.

When to Focus on Increasing Reflection: What Are the Markers of Dysfunction?

Target emotions and certain clinical scenarios may each signal that further elaborating and reflecting on the story about a given emotional experience could be particularly useful.

Emotion-Based Markers for Reflecting on Emotion

Emotions of any kind benefit from being reflected upon since the process gives a broader understanding of one's experience and often yields self-understanding across similar kinds of situations. However, reflection has a different purpose or objective depending on the kind of emotion, as described in the Introduction.

Secondary emotion. Secondary emotions often reflect characteristic personal patterns of responding to the core pain that lays underneath. When people come to appreciate the nature of their defensiveness, they are more able to manage their symptoms and then selectively choose when and how to grapple with the deeper concerns. Freud (1910) highlighted how hysterical symptoms are well treated through insight. People generally seek help based on a story about how they understand their presenting problems. Insight into the fact that one has a problem is a major prognostic indicator for the anticipated outcome of psychotherapy (Messer & McWilliams, 2006). Although this may be most notable for personality disorders, it is essentially true for all mental health problems. For instance, when a client has symptoms of obsessive–compulsive disorder, the degree to which the individual acknowledges that their obsessions are irrational is a critical issue.

Another issue is that having a coherent narrative about one's symptom distress helps insulate against dysregulation. A contributing factor to panic disorder, for example, is that people feel bewildered by their panic attacks in that the attacks seem to occur out of nowhere (discussed in Chapter 9). A personal narrative that explains what precipitates distress is inherently regulating. As a case in point, a client in my practice reported a great sense of relief when she received a diagnosis for borderline personality disorder because, as she said, "it helps explain so much." Thus, if people are mystified by their symptoms, it is important to help them very early in treatment by reflecting on the broader context and create a narrative account of their personal emotional problem.

Primary maladaptive emotion. Whenever a difficult emotion entails some chronic or ongoing pattern, exploring the contextual meaning is helpful. Primary maladaptive emotion is a central example of this. The same old story or that familiar bad feeling often benefits from being contextualized within one's life story. Doing this helps one understand the origins and clarify the parameters of one's emotional concern. However, there are limits to what narrative reflection can do in terms of changing maladaptive emotion. First, working with maladaptive emotion in this way will come with the critical challenge of contextualizing it in a new way—not by simply rehearsing the same old feeling within the same old framework. And second, even when there is new information to be incorporated into maladaptive emotion, conceptually reflecting on the feeling is not always enough to facilitate change. All too often, knowing about why one feels the way one does or understanding that it doesn't make sense or that the feeling is not adaptive does not necessarily mean one can just choose to feel differently.

Practicing mind over mood or thinking on the bright side are more likely to work for secondary symptomatic emotions (e.g., anxiety, global distress, rage) than for existential concerns of primary emotion (see also Chapter 20). This is because primary maladaptive emotions (e.g., maladaptive shame, terror, crippling self-contempt) are more entrenched and often are the source of dysfunctional beliefs rather than the product of them. When cognitive behavior treatments effectively work with these deeper primary maladaptive emotions, cognitive interventions are often what provides the client with a rationale for behavioral engagement. Then, behavioral components are more likely to provide some new or corrective experience (see Chapter 20 on the roles of reframing).

Primary adaptive emotion. Primary adaptive emotions (e.g., adaptive grief, assertive anger, love) often reflect unnegotiable existential realities such as a personal loss or impinging violation. So, once again, adding context may temper the feeling but cannot resolve it (e.g., "Yes, other people have suffered much worse, but my hunger for love is still a painful hunger for love!"). More generally, reflection, insight, and narrative typically work synergistically with other processes discussed in this book to precipitate lasting change. After primary adaptive emotions are mobilized, symbolized, and expressed, the way they are followed through becomes more meaningful if they are also anchored within a personal narrative (i.e., by reflecting on the emotion). Narratives about the role of adaptive emotion—why and where it came from—often become the story of change. Some psychotherapy researchers have described these as innovative moments, and they can be reliably identified through a narrative analysis (see Gonçalves et al., 2011, 2017).

Instrumental emotion. Reflecting on emotion is uniquely important for working with instrumental emotion, which is emotion generated, in part, to bring about personal gains (see Introduction). When people routinely use certain emotions as a form of social influence, down-regulating the arousal of that feeling will be immediately helpful. Still, instrumental emotion is a felt experience, and it is not an entirely artificial (i.e., fake) expression.[2] So ultimately, unhealthy patterns of social manipulation must be reflected on from the vantage point of a broader perspective. Problematic anger, hate, and aggression are examples in which the instrumental nature of a person's outburst is often not entirely within their awareness, despite it being immediately rewarding in some way (even if only in the very short term; A. Pascual-Leone et al., 2013; Peters et al., 2018). Sadness, fear, and shame, among other emotions, can all be used instrumentally in this way.

Changing instrumental emotion requires a broader perspective, one that allows the individual to look beyond the most immediate outcome of events. In some cases, reflecting on one's emotion as well as its context can be achieved by adopting the perspective of an outside observer to fully grasp the socioemotional process that one is enacting. Appreciating the greater social context of how one may be using emotion as an interpersonal tool begs for some reflection. When the target concern is an instrumental emotion, reflection is often a prerequisite for behavioral change.

Unhealthy strategies for emotion regulation. Finally, in a similar vein, sometimes there are behavioral contingencies that lead to the development of unhealthy emotion regulation strategies. These are essentially habits, which are problematic unto themselves (irrespective of underlying emotion). They are dysfunctional in the person's life, but how they operate remains outside of a client's awareness. Just as the reward mechanisms associated with instrumental anger can insidiously develop it into a habitual reaction for coping with life's challenges, other kinds of unhealthy behaviors may similarly serve tacit emotion regulatory functions (A. Pascual-Leone et al., 2013; Peters et al., 2018). Clinically significant examples of this include self-injurious behaviors (Nock & Prinstein, 2004) and problematic sexual behaviors (e.g., sex addiction, chronic pornography use, and even some sexual offences; Gunst et al., 2017). Finally, procrastination is a ubiquitous example of unhealthy short-term emotion regulation in which the individual prioritizes repairing emotional distress over the well-being of their future self (Sirois & Pychyl, 2013).

When people start using such behaviors to distract themselves, down-regulate their own emerging feelings of distress and numbness, or simply relieve boredom, the relationship between those burgeoning feeling and habitual behaviors are often implicit. Furthermore, although outside of awareness, this type of reward mechanism may cross-sensitize other addictive tendencies in a similar way (Peters et al., 2018). Intervention requires reflection on emotion, and bringing the string of behavioral connections into consciousness occurs through a narrative framework (e.g., a behavioral chain analysis; Linehan, 2015). Furthermore, grappling with short- and long-term consequences to muster the motivation for change also occurs within the context of one's life story (Miller & Rollnick, 2013). In short, reflecting on the role of these behaviors in regulating emotion is key in opening possible choice points. After being more aware of the function of such habits, the individual can purposefully choose to make healthier choices (see Chapters 20 and 23).

Clinical Markers for Reflecting on Emotion

While a range of emotions could be productively worked with using reflection on emotion, there are moments during psychotherapy when the clinical presentation of a client might indicate this kind of emotional processing is uniquely advantageous. When the central source of dysfunction is a client feeling too entangled in an emotional experience, reflecting on emotion can help create an appropriate working distance. In cognitive behavior therapies, this may be as simple as getting pen and paper to write down an agenda or a list of concerns that need to be addressed. In psychodynamic and narrative therapies of various approaches, this is typically achieved by encouraging the client to take a bird's eye view on how they arrived at the current place of difficulty. Humanistic therapies sometimes do this by using a person-centered approach to the unfolding story but also do so less explicitly through enactments or chairwork, which can help implicitly to map out the problematic process in vivo (discussed in Chapter 10). Notice that feeling entangled or confused by the parts of an experience are not simply issues of feeling overwhelmed by intense arousal, although that too will be helped by taking some psychological distance. In such cases, mindfulness exercises to clear a space or self-soothing (Chapters 2 and 3) may be prerequisites to more deeply reflecting on emotional experience as such.

Whatever the case, an assessment that should be made relatively early in clinical case formulation is whether a client's narratives seem coherent, which is often self-apparent to listeners.[3] Clients are usually somewhat disturbed by an experience that does not make sense and the shortcomings in the internal coherence of their self-understanding, which should also serve as a marker for reflecting on emotion. For example, a client may feel fundamentally undeserving of companionship even though the need for it feels so natural, healthy, and deeply rooted. In this case, narrative reflection will help a client put disparate facets of their experience together into a personal narrative, which may then be reframed, reconstructed, and better integrated into a larger whole.

Similarly, narrative reflection is indicated when a client feels there are a lack of meaningful choice points in life (e.g., after a loss, trauma) or when one has a weakened sense of sociohistorical identity or trajectory (e.g., "Who am I? Where am I headed?"). At moments like these, reflection on one's life story will also need to be counterbalanced by occasionally attending to emergent awareness (e.g., "But is this what I really want? Let me check"). Finally, memories are narrative reconstructions that are periodically reappraised for their meaning and personal relevance (see Chapter 19). For that reason, when clients spontaneously introduce autobiographical memories in session, that too is usually a good time to reflect on the meaning of any associated emotion. Many of the clinical and emotion-based markers for reflecting on emotion occur throughout therapy. However, when a course of psychotherapy approaches its conclusion, that is again an important time to ensure the story of what happened and what changed is amply and coherently narrated to help maintain treatment gains (Adler et al., 2007).

FEELING IN CONTEXT

Changing the context surrounding an emotion provides a new interpretive lens for the experience and thereby changes the feeling itself. This proposition is the central thesis for Part V of this book.

What Is the Context?

Emotional experience holds meaning within a given context. But what is the context? And just how much gets included in the big picture? Recall from the Introduction that an emotion (scheme) involves the appraisal of one's well-being (i.e., vital truth) in contrast with the world as it is (i.e., reality truth). As such, the situation or context becomes an integral facet of any given emotional experience, so awareness includes exploring the circumstances related to one's feeling (Chapter 4).

However, although the first-person experience of emotion occurs inside and right now, the contextual meaning that surrounds that feeling could be construed from several vantage points. For instance, as a person attends to and begins to interpret an experience, the relevant context could be circumscribed to the immediately presenting situation, which includes only the most local events (e.g., "My boss is asking me to do more work than I can handle"). Alternatively, one could look to make sense of the same emotion based on a broader narrative context, exploring its meaning in terms of one's personal social history. In that case, the context would span across a range of discrete situations (e.g., "People have always tried to take advantage of me, and my boss's request is another instance of that"). Broader still, context could be framed in terms of personal values and existential choices (e.g., "This work-related problem is a hiccup in terms of what I value in life and my chosen purpose"). Thus, a context can be construed at different levels, and it may come as no surprise that these levels each relate to distinct treatment perspectives. Furthermore, whatever the level of analysis, a context of meaning can always be elaborated, reconsidered, or modified to some degree.

Changing the Context of Meaning Changes the Feeling

Conceptually reflecting on emotion or elaborating a narrative framework clearly represents a higher order of meaning making than negotiating any single instance of feeling, so how do these larger mechanisms facilitate a given instant of emotional change? Processes like emotional awareness change emotion by focusing directly on it, elaborating the details to create further and further differentiations to generate new meaning from within the emotion (see Chapters 5 and 6). However, reflection on emotion offers a different strategy for changing the target feeling. It does this by elaborating the context, circumstances, and frame of reference through which one interprets a given feeling of emotion. In short, to use the language of Gestalt psychology, awareness creates change through an elaboration of emotion as a figure in the foreground of experience, whereas reflection on emotion creates change by elaborating the background and rendering new meaning by virtue of a new context.

This is the reason why reflecting on emotion, offering new interpretations, and creating links in psychotherapy have been historically regarded as more experientially distant ways of working with emotion (A. Pascual-Leone & Greenberg, 2007b). However, contemporary psychodynamic approaches have shown that treatment can purposefully shift between vivid experiencing and taking a reflective distance (e.g., Abbass & Town, 2013; Fosha, 2021; McCullough et al., 2003). Other examples of reflecting on emotion are cognitive reframing or elaborating the broader context of some target emotion, which helps interpret that experience and incorporate it into a more general framework of meaning (e.g., Beck, 2020). This is talking about the feeling and its interpretive context rather than being immersed or deeply embedded within an experiential moment. As one reflects on emotion, the granular aspects of immediate emotional experience and moment-by-moment processing are bridged to the broader psychological realities of identity, sense of self, and sense of purpose.

In short, reflecting on emotion is a categorically different strategy for producing emotional change. Ways of reworking the context of meaning include narrative work, rational or evidenced-based cognitive work, and psychodynamic as well as existential insights, among others. Despite their different scopes of analysis, I take the integrative perspective that these are all strategies for working with the interpretive context as a method of working with emotion to produce change.

The Self as a Framework of Meaning

Although stories are a natural framework for working with emotion and support the conceptual elaboration of those feelings, they also underpin a much higher order construct: one's self-concept. This self-referencing offers a complex source of interpretive context and is supported by a unique neurological substate.

Experience Is Nested Within the Self

Aspects of the experiential self are a primitive form of self-awareness that humans share with other animals. At the same time, the conceptual self is a level of self-understanding that is unique to humans (Damasio, 1999; Gallagher, 2000). Other animals do not have ongoing narratives about their experience; they just have experience.

The construction of this conceptual self comes from making meaning in the form of an overarching framework about a self—one that extends from the past to the present and projects into the future. That formulation of a temporally coherent self is then linked to ongoing themes, goals, abstracted beliefs, and theories about oneself and one's world circumstances (Conway, 2005). What one thinks about oneself is a critical source of context for emergent feeling and informs one's interpretation of that emotion. In his reflections on the role of personhood in agency and communion, David Bakan (2001) asserted, "The person develops over a lifetime [but] . . . the essential identity of the person does not change. . . . All development takes place within the constraint of that identity" (p. 145).

People bring enduring aspects of their sense of self (e.g., "I'm the kind of person who . . .") to the interpretation of their lived experiences. This interpretive framework has implications for both presenting emotion and for the construction of subsequent stories that refer to those emotions (McLean et al., 2007). A body of research has examined how the self is constructed through this act of storytelling. To conceptually model this process, some authors have observed that a person's experience has a somewhat circular (or better said, dialectical) relationship with how a specific story gets formulated (L. S. Greenberg, 2021; McLean et al., 2007). Furthermore, the recursive and dialectical process between emotion and stories about emotional experience is always nested within one's sense of self, explicated by an overarching life narrative (see "Narrative Identity" in Chapter 21, this volume; McLean et al., 2007).

Neurological Correlates of Referencing the Self

Self-reference is a defining feature of autobiographical memories (as well as imaginal enactments), and this sets them apart from the recollection of other events or pieces of information (Conway, 2005). The information one recalls (or not) also has direct implications for one's perception of self. Moreover, remembering stories from one's personal past and imagining the future represent similar tasks of dynamic construction, and they rely on similar patterns of neural activation. In fact, autobiographical recollection, prospection about the self, and thinking about one's own mental states (i.e., theory of mind) are all mental acts that share extensive functional overlap in the brain (Spreng et al., 2008).

There are several facets of neurological processing that come together to produce the emotional experience of self. First, self-referential process in these various forms is brought about by parts of the medial prefrontal cortex (Northoff et al., 2006; St. Jacques, 2012). That region of the brain maintains emotional information as the focus of one's attention and mediates decision making. Second, overall self-awareness and the higher order reflection on one's own mental states is supported by other brain areas (i.e., insula and temporoparietal junction), which integrate information from the external environment with visceral information from inside the body (Craig, 2009; Spreng et al., 2008). Finally, emotion gets translated into goal-directed behavior through still other parts of the brain, creating the experience of oneself as both author and actor (i.e., anterior cingulate cortex and dorsolateral prefrontal cortex; J. Pascual-Leone & Johnson, 2021; St. Jacques, 2012).

The Story of Emotion

Stories are malleable; they change over time. Even so, they continue to serve as reference points that anchor the recollection of emotion (and identity). So, while the story one recalls is silently shifting, so do the emotions one experiences with respect to that story. As suggested in Chapter 10, this means that historical truth may not always map so well onto the story as one remembers it. Fortunately, the malleability of stories is no obstacle when working through personal difficulties.

What Is Subject to Change?

A concern commonly raised by clients is that it's impossible to change what happened in the past, so it seems useless to tell the story, let alone go over that story again and again. Although some clinicians have interpreted statements like this as a client's resistance to treatment, at face value it stands as a reasonable question. The rationale for doing narrative work may simply not be clear to the client, and therapists do need to provide an adequate explanation for reengaging an old painful story. Admittedly, clients who need validation regarding something they are struggling with from their past will often balk at the notion that history is somewhat subjective (although it is).[4] However, the true issue is not about what happened but rather what one remembers and how one feels about it. It is less confrontational to suggest to clients that the content of their memories can be elaborated and may even evolve over time as one gains new perspectives on the past (see Conway, 2005; A. E. Wilson & Ross, 2003).

Furthermore, one's experience of emotion is not synonymous with one's narrative account, although they do intersect in several ways (Angus et al., 2015; Gonçalves et al., 2011). So, the feeling one remembers having had in the past is often not the same as the feeling one has as one remembers in the present. This should offer some consolation to apprehensive clients. Moreover, the feelings one has regarding a narrative, or even what one recalls, will change. The emotions associated with what one remembers may come to have more depth, less intensity, and a change in their significance, or they can develop new facets. Finally, the context within which one tells one's story (e.g., being in a safe haven, having an attentive listener) can influence both what and the degree to which one remembers in a narrated event (Angus & Greenberg, 2011; Pasupathi & Hoyt, 2010). I return to this topic later in Chapter 19.

Neurological Correlates of Emotional Memories

After memories are constructed, they can be enhanced before they are eventually (re)consolidated in long term memory. In short, if the event is emotionally arousing or important, hormones related to bodily stress activate the amygdala to modulate a memory during its' consolidation (Talmi, 2013). This enhancement helps explain why emotional memories are typically more vivid and accurate than the recollection of neutral events (Talmi, 2013). Finally, when remembering painful events evokes emotion (which may or may not be the same as feelings in the memory), affect-regulatory systems of the brain are also recruited (i.e., amygdala, insula, subgenual cingulate cortex, and orbital prefrontal cortex). Furthermore, remembering what happened is increasingly understood as subject to transformation over the course of one's life (Alberini & Ledoux, 2013). Thus, the reactivation of a memory within an emotional context such as psychotherapy further modulates both the emotion and the content of a narrative. As introduced in Chapter 13, this is called memory reconsolidation, and it is a neurological mechanism by which memories themselves evolve over time (Lane & Nadel, 2020). I fully explore the implication of these issues for narrative work later in Chapters 19 and 22.

Implications for the Story of "What Really Happened"

As both psychological and neurological evidence has borne out, change is inherent to the remembering process because remembering is always a reconstruction. The popular understanding of memories as inert recordings from the past, stored in the brain's archives, is incorrect. There is no original memory to be recalled. What one remembers is a reconstruction of the last recollection, which makes reminiscence a more fluidly evolving process (Alberini & Ledoux, 2013; Lane & Nadel, 2020). So, the answer to the skeptical client's question turns out to be quite complex, although the conclusion is simple. One cannot change the historical past, but one can significantly alter (a) what one remembers, (b) what else gets bundled into that memory, (c) how much faith one puts in what happened (or not), as well as (d) the way one feels about it, and ultimately (e) what one takes as the personal significance or meaning of the story.

THE RELATIONSHIP BETWEEN AWARENESS AND REFLECTION ON EMOTION

As discussed early in this book (Chapters 4–7), emotional awareness and symbolizing the emergent experience is one of the key processes that engender making meaning.[5] However, quite different forms of meaning making occur when telling stories, creating narratives, and reflecting on personal themes (Chapters 17–22). These two processes for the creation of new meaning operate at fundamentally different epistemological levels.

While emotional awareness creates new meaning from the concrete and perceptual sensations of experience, reflecting on emotion generates new meaning by elaborating the context which surrounds a feeling. The mechanisms of these two approaches are different, they have distinct neural underpinnings, and the meaning structures they generate are not the same. However, as both mentalization-based as well as metacognitive therapies have observed, distinct kinds of processing will functionally blend into one another, often creating what appears to be a seamless continuum (e.g., Dimaggio et al., 2020; Fonagy et al., 2002; Semerari et al., 2007). And yet, the interventions that facilitate one or another form of meaning making will not be interchangeable. This makes it even more critical to understand the unique constructive process that underpins the different ways we make meaning out of our emotional experiences.

Meaning Can Be Made Either Top Down or Bottom Up

In Chapter 7, I discussed the client experience scale (Klien et al., 1986) and highlighted that both labeling one's emotions and complex symbolization of experiential meaning are captured by the lower half of that scale (i.e., levels 1–4 out of 7). These are graded aspects of unfolding emotional awareness. Moving up on the client experiencing scale (i.e., levels 5–7), sees people start to do something qualitatively different: clients begin to puzzle and reflect on the nature of their own experience, even as it is underfoot. They contemplate hypotheses about how disparate parts of their emerging experience might fit together and they tacitly generate working models (i.e., applied theories) to explain those feelings. As experts of the experiencing scale have observed, this discontinuity represents a fault line between two fundamentally different kinds of processing (A. Pascual-Leone & Yeryomenko, 2016; Pos et al., 2017; Watson & Bedard, 2006). In Chapter 7, I discussed differentiation and integration as the two prongs of meaning development, and while expanding awareness is about emotional differentiation, reflecting on one's experience fosters the integration of emotion into a broader framework.

The Operations for Awareness and Reflection

Antonio Pascual-Leone and Greenberg (2007b) highlighted that meaning making in psychotherapy can be generated either top down or bottom up. Figure 17.1 represents the epistemological differences entailed in emotional awareness, which typically occurs bottom up, as contrasted with reflecting on emotion, which typically occurs top down. At the right of this diagram, *meaning making* is a general term (much like insight, self-knowledge, mentalization, or learning) that refers to phenomena varying on two dimensions. One dimension is the level of abstraction, which ranges from low abstraction (i.e., concrete experiential content) to high abstraction (i.e., relational linking across elements). The other dimension is the type of processing, which ranges from perceptual–emotional processing (i.e., sensory and affective experiences) to conceptual–rational processing (i.e., reflecting, contemplating, and formulating).

Is it abstract or concrete? *Abstraction* is when one internalizes concrete invariances across situations that may span over space and time. The higher the level of abstraction one makes, the broader the scope of the induction set and the larger the set of elements being abstracted from. Low levels of abstraction bear directly on concrete experiential content (e.g., what one is engaged with here and now). In contrast, high levels of abstraction no longer bear just on single direct concrete experience but also capture the relationship between experiential

FIGURE 17.1. The Relationship Between Awareness and Reflection on Emotion

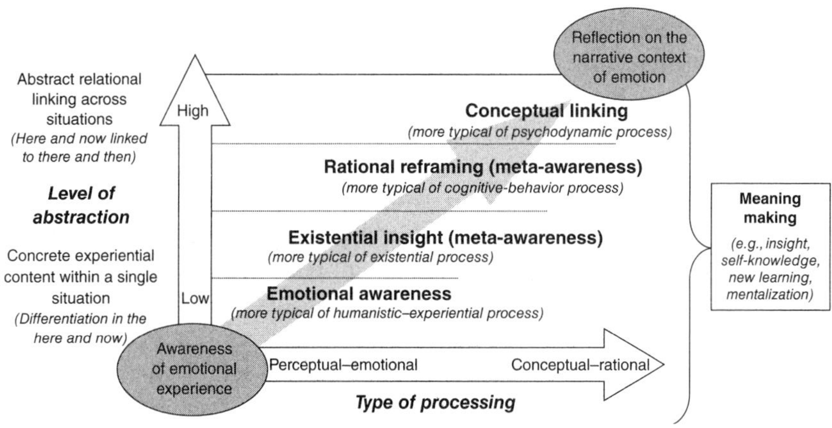

Note. Adapted from "Insight and Awareness in Experiential Therapy," by A. Pascual-Leone and L. S. Greenberg, in L. G. Castonguay and C. E. Hill (Eds.), *Insight in Psychotherapy* (p. 37), 2007b, American Psychological Association (https://doi.org/10.1037/11532-002). Copyright 2007 by the American Psychological Association.

elements. A relationship is abstract because it only becomes apparent across different types of situations (A. Pascual-Leone & Greenberg, 2007b; J. Pascual-Leone & Johnson, 2021). While concrete situations only reveal a single (and possibly isolated) cooccurrence between elements, that relationship may turn out to be invariant across a range of quite different situations. The process of making this kind of observation is called an abstraction. Notice that when one observes invariances like this, patterns or themes across different kinds of situations are no less concrete or reliable in terms of their reality, even though they still cannot be observed directly within any one situation. Abstraction also allows one to traverse psychological distance, in that it allows one to contemplate and make decisions about events that are not part of the here and now (Liberman & Trope, 2014).

Is it perceptual–emotional or conceptual–rational? In Figure 17.1, the *type of processing* refers to the relative weight of affective as opposed to cognitive processes that are entailed in the construction of new meaning. An experience can be processed either by living through the immediacy of one's perceptions and emotions or by thinking about it from a conceptual and rational position (L. S. Greenberg, 2021). Even so—and this is a critical point for clinical work—the kind of personal meaning that each process yields will not necessarily be the same. The two dimensions (i.e., degree of abstraction and type of processing) are conceptually distinct. That is to say, the level of abstraction that characterizes the nature of one's mental construal is not reducible to hot and affective or cool and rational types of processing, even though in practice there is sometimes a strong convergence between these dimensions (Fujita & Carnevale, 2012). More importantly, aspects of each dimension contribute to the therapeutic approach clinicians use when working with emotion and they manifest four commonly observable kinds of meaning making (i.e., emotional awareness, existential insight, rational reframing, and conceptual linking; middle section of Figure 17.1).

Strategies for processing information. The various kinds of meaning making identified here are tacitly constructed using different information processing strategies: bottom up (i.e., starting with low abstraction) versus top down (i.e., starting from high abstraction). These are different implicit approaches to making sense of one's experience, and they are reflected in the two dimensions described. In the bottom-up strategy for meaning making, one begins by blindly exploring the concrete experiences of reality, including one's viscerally felt internal experience. Only after our sensory organs have made direct contact with that reality do we begin to create emerging representations of that reality (Gendlin, 1996; Gilead et al., 2020). In other words, meaning making begins by exploring individual and idiosyncratic details, such as one's moment-by-moment feelings, and then these are gradually combined to create increasingly larger units of general meaning (A. Pascual-Leone & Greenberg, 2007b).

In contrast, a top-down approach to meaning making begins with intuiting some overall conceptual formulation. In this kind of mental work, one's brain activates relevant mental representations of the world before one engages directly with reality (in this case, emotional experience). For example, one formulates a hypothesis that identifies some general theme, which might apply across situations. Then, from the overall top-down formulation one follows with the gradual elaboration of details, which are explored through that interpretive lens (Gilead et al., 2020; A. Pascual-Leone & Greenberg, 2007b).

As reviewed in Chapter 4, neurofunctional imaging has shown the brain areas that help one extract the main gist of a complex scene (e.g., What is the basic scene? What is the plot and who are the characters?). Moreover, the brain areas that support such abstraction are different from areas which capture the details (e.g., What was the expression on their face? What did the place smell like?; Adolphs, Tranel, & Buchanan, 2005; Pessoa, 2013). Despite the appearance of seamless continuity, top-down processes of conceptualizing and understanding one's emotion are not reducible to the bottom-up processes of emotional awareness. On the contrary, bottom-up emotional awareness and top-down reflection on emotion each rely on distinct psychogenetic operations. Neurological evidence supports the idea that these two kinds of meaning making are prewired in the brain as qualitatively different ways of working with emotion (Gilead et al., 2020). Furthermore, examining this idea in psychotherapy intervention shows that experiential strategies work bottom up, whereas cognitive strategies work top down, and that neural imaging confirms these strategies make use of different brain regions (Wang et al., 2022).

How Treatments Approach Meaning

The way different types of meaning making are constructed and function in relation to one another is represented in Figure 17.1. New emotional awareness, such as an emerging experiencing that one feels angry at one's parent, is a mainstay of experiential schools of psychotherapy. Awareness is constructed bottom up. It is rooted in the concrete perceptual and emotional content of immediate experience (i.e., in differentiating the here and now) rather than in abstract conceptual formulations. However, the counterpoint to that process is conceptual linking: for instance, creating connections among a current relationship, a past relationship, and the relationship one has with one's therapist. Meaning making of that kind is typified by psychodynamic schools, and such thematic connections are formulated at a high level of abstraction. This is because they integrate information through relational links that are made top down across several different types of situations from here and now to there and then. Psychodynamic forms of conceptual linking are typically more experience distant, although links could also be constructed close to experience.

In the middle area of this continuum we find meta-awareness, bridging top-down and bottom-up constructions, which is a conceptual awareness about the general character of one's various concrete experiential awarenesses (see Figure 17.1). Depending on the perceptual–emotional or conceptual–rational nature of this kind of meaning making, meta-awareness could be more rational, as in identifying a core belief or considering the evidence for an automatic thought, which are more representative of the cognitive behavioral schools. Alternatively, meta-awareness could be more experiential, such as noticing in a viscerally felt manner that "I am seeing the world as a rejecting place," a kind of meaning making that is more representative of the experiential–existential schools. In this way, the dimensions of abstraction and type of processing act together to define the treatment approach with which one becomes aware of and the lens through which one reflects on experience and its broader associative context (A. Pascual-Leone & Greenberg, 2007b).

The bottom-up and top-down methods for creating knowledge also often represent *inductive* and *deductive reasoning* (respectively). Furthermore, *abductive reasoning* involves inferring explanations that might bridge or coordinate those distinct kinds of meanings. Whatever the case, bottom-up and top-down processes can and should be combined. Ultimately, the process of making meaning in everyday life (and in any treatment approach) always involves a synergy between different mental operations in what has been called a dialectical construction (see L. S. Greenberg & Pascual-Leone, 1995; J. Pascual-Leone & Johnson, 2021). In practice, when people are working with emotion, the processes of awareness and reflection represent two contrasting poles on a structural (i.e., qualitative) continuum. *Experience-near meaning making* is perceptual, emotional, and captures experiential content (i.e., synthesized at a low level of abstraction). In contrast, *experience-distant meaning making* is conceptual, rational, and reflects relational connections (i.e., synthesized at a high level of abstraction).

Neurological Correlates: Where in the Brain Is the Story?

Because of its broad temporal scope and the role that narrative reflection plays in coordinating or bringing together a wide range of elements, it comes as no surprise that the neurological correlates of this kind of emotional processing recruit many areas of the brain. Moreover, this integrative process often occurs through continually shifting back and forth between levels of analysis clearly establishing the dynamics of what is happening as people process emotion. This coordinated meta-process holds together several aspects of emotional processing at large, and neurologically, it represents a formidable task.

How people conjure up autobiographical content is an illustrative case in point, revealing a complex retrieval process that depends on integrating both top-down and bottom-up meaning systems. A body of evidence suggests that search and retrieval of autobiographical memory is cued in the right lateral prefrontal cortex and by self-referential processes (medial prefrontal cortex). These are in addition to posterior areas of the brain (hippocampus, retrospenial cortex) that are required in activating a specific memory trace. Then, a subsequent stage entails the retrieval of contextual details, activating parts of the visual and parietal cortices. As one imagines the events in one's mind's eye, key areas (e.g., precuneus) lend support to episodic memory and any mental imagery related to the self. Frontal regions of the brain related to executive functioning (e.g., left lateral prefrontal cortex) become involved in assembling and reconciling these various sources of information into a working model of the autobiographical event (St. Jacques, 2012).

Meaning making through the process of this autobiographical construction involves the search and mental elaboration of a given memory, and these represent two different phases of the retrieval process. Moreover, search and elaboration each rely on functionally separate components in the brain, which come online at different moments in time. On one hand, top-down mental attention guides the search and construction of the memory, which is mediated by the dorsal parietal cortex. This top-down process is how the brain places a remembered event within some specific time and place and then supports that memory with semantic information about oneself and one's circumstances. Then, as one begins to conjure up an autobiographical event, a bottom-up process comes increasingly into play, retrieving details that populate the memory in mind. This bottom-up process is mediated by the ventral parietal cortex (see Cabeza, 2008).[6] The point of interest here for emotional processing is to observe that even when it comes to autobiographical memory, top-down and bottom-up constructions of meaning recruit distinct areas of the brain. This further supports the identification of awareness and reflection as distinct clinical processes by which one works with emotion.

In psychotherapy, we sometimes invite clients to directly recall an event (e.g., Therapist: "Can you remember the time when . . . ?") and in doing so set up a task for the client to deliberately search and recall the details of an event. This also represents a key metacognitive process when people voluntarily take time to think about what happened. As such, these primarily represent a top-down form of processing (which has also been the focus of most research on memory). However, when working with emotion in psychotherapy, memories often occur involuntarily. On one hand, several pathologies including anxiety, depression, and trauma are associated with involuntary and intrusive remembering. But on the other hand, an inspired episodic memory that unexpectedly pops out of nowhere during a key session is typically of special interest to the treatment process. In psychoanalysis, for example, this event is reflected in sudden recollections that may result during free association. Meanwhile, in emotion-focused therapy, a client focused on describing the painful emotion related to unresolved interpersonal difficulties (i.e., unfinished business) will sometimes suddenly present an episodic memory that is richly illustrative.[7]

Voluntarily retrieving memories requires more deliberate mental control than having involuntary memories. Consistent with the distinction among brain areas that support search or elaboration, voluntarily recalling memories requires more activity in dorsal frontal regions (Hall et al., 2014). Moreover, when there is no intention to retrieve but involuntary memories come to mind, that bottom-up process is accompanied by activity in the ventral parietal cortex. This pattern of activation can happen when a cue unexpectedly elicits a memory or when a memory can no longer be actively suppressed (Benoit et al.,

2014; Hall et al., 2014). Again, we see the neural correlates of working with memory are somewhat different depending on the kind of emotional processing one might be engaged in. A memory of the past serves as a descriptive framework for understanding what happened. That dialectical relationship between different kinds of meaning is even more apparent when one considers new frameworks of understanding.

Creating New Structures of Meaning

When meaning making happens within a session, the nature of that phenomenon can vary on a qualitative continuum, ranging from experience near (awareness of emotion, i.e., feeling the emotion from within) to experience distant (reflection on emotion, i.e., contemplating the feeling from the outside, looking in [Figure 17.1]. A key difference among these types of meaning is the degree to which a client's personal meaning is abstracted from their lived experience. Although these representational substrates are qualitatively distinct, they are hierarchically ordered in relation to one another in what amounts to an ordered series of epistemological levels.[8]

Epistemological Theory Is Lacking in Clinical Work

The idea that qualitative levels of meaning are also hierarchically ordered coheres with neuroscientific models but has still not been fully recognized in mainstream cognitive science, which arguably has hindered the development of that field (Gilead et al., 2020; J. Pascual-Leone & Johnson, 2021). Clinical theory, however, lags still further behind in embracing the implications of this epistemological understanding. Most theories of psychotherapy have been formulated in response to one another, which swings the pendulum, rather than looking for complementarity or integration between approaches.

The emotion revolution in contemporary psychotherapy has been much needed. It has created enthusiasm for working with emotion through bottom-up processes, which is a welcome correction of what historically was an overemphasis of top-down rational (i.e., positivist) knowledge. However, now some clinicians go so far as to regard top-down processing (i.e., productively thinking about emotion) as somehow shallower than bottom-up processing (i.e., deeply feeling an emotion), and that is a mistake. Evoking productive emotion in a client arguably requires more technical artistry of therapists than manualizes interventions for rationally examining client concerns. However, reflecting on emotion remains an essential and unique process.

Self-Knowledge Involves Both Content and Structure

Top-down processing is indispensable for learning how to function in the world and for significant sociopersonal development. The structures that people create (e.g., frames of understanding, belief systems, stories of what happened or could happen) are populated with the bottom-up details of experiential content. But structure itself cannot be achieved by purely working bottom up from the visceral feelings of emotion.

From cognitive–developmental psychology (e.g., J. Pascual-Leone & Johnson, 2021), content learning can be understood as having or acquiring pieces of information like owning individual books or papers. This content may be associative or experiential, but it always pertains to a specific and local context. In contrast, keeping with the same metaphor, structural learning would be, for example, the creation of a bookshelf or organizing framework that allows one to sort and locate the specific contents. Critically, the system by which one organizes informational content is at a different epistemological level than the content itself. So here, a bookshelf is an interpretive context for housing content. Organizational structures help one interpret their content, but they also represent a higher order of meaning, an invariant that is abstracted and holds true across various content situations. In another example, in language acquisition, adding new words to one's vocabulary are instances of content learning, whereas mastering new grammatical rules is structural learning (J. Pascual-Leone & Johnson, 2021).

Reflecting on emotion creates new frameworks of meaning, which then serve both to contain burgeoning arousal and to interpret the significance of those feelings. Moreover, people have (and use) their preconceived ideas about who they are, why they are that way, and what they can expect of the world and others. This is the level of analysis used in psychodynamic interpretations of emotion. Not coincidentally, the elements of a core conflictual relationship theme represent preconceived ideas of this kind, structures through which one interprets the world (Luborsky et al., 1994). Bottom-up awareness provides content learning about the self (e.g., What is happening right now? Do I like it?), whereas reflection on emotion supports structural learning about the self (e.g., Who am I? Who do I want to be?).

Structural learning has the potential to reconfigure one's cognitive–perceptual frame (i.e., one's meta-awareness, the awareness of one's awarenesses). This is because top-down processes begin with an already existing coherent framework of meaning (e.g., a psychodynamic interpretation about overarching motives, a plausible relationship theme, or identifying one's possible role in a narrative). Such top-down frames of understanding are taken first as hypotheses and then explored in terms of how that top-down understanding may indeed apply across a range of specific and concrete situations. This often occurs by taking some psychological distance to reflect on a personal theme. For example, in a study that asked clients to comment on video recordings of their own sessions, one client recalled,

> [The therapist] said, "Your parents don't trust you," and that sounds right. As we talked about my parents not trusting me, I realized that I was getting [my mistrust of myself] from them. It isn't fair that they put that pressure on me; it hasn't served me well. I want to fix the situation. (Watson & Rennie, 1994, p. 504)

In this example, the client contemplates a formulation offered by their therapist and then adopts that new meaning (top down) after observing how well it fits.

The elaboration of a proposed theme in terms of concrete instantiations is itself part of generating new self-knowledge and informs (i.e., provides a meaning-structure for) subsequent experiences of emotion. Obviously, sometimes preconceived ideas are wrong, especially when they are derived from misleading situations, such as when someone is abused by a primary caregiver, a person who is expected to be trustworthy and loving. Those instances are precisely where one most needs the innovation of bottom-up reexperiencing.[9] However, top-down knowledge remains important because it explains how social and personal historical experiences provide us with a set of default expectations and a framework of assumptions (for better or for worse). In short, top-down processing is what effectively allows us to appreciate the frame of reference itself, which ultimately couches the individual experiential elements of what one feels.

OBSTACLES: WHEN NARRATIVE REFLECTION IS PROBLEMATIC

Although working with narrative and reflecting on emotion can be a productive process for working with a range of emotions as well as clinical markers, there are also occasions when focusing on this level of process is contraindicated. Clinical theory and practice as well as some experimental research have led authors to conclude that when using narrative to work with emotion, there may be a wrong way to tell one's story (e.g., Angus et al., 2017; Pasupathi et al., 2017). Unhelpful or potentially harmful ways of engaging in narrative reflection are linked to certain aspects of emotional expressivity. When the narrative process itself is inherently problematic, clients find themselves rehearsing versions of a broken story that cannot be resolved.[10] Continuing to elaborate unhealthy or dysfunctional narratives captures one's cognitive resources and, at best, reiterating such narratives is unproductive. At worst, this kind of engagement can further entrench pathological cognitive–affective styles, and it can rehearse maladaptive perceptions of oneself, the world, or others (Beck, 2020).

There are several different forms of problematic narrative. Psychologist Lynne Angus has led researchers at York University in studying the observable characteristics of storytelling (i.e., narrative styles) that signal features of emotional processing in a psychotherapy session (Angus et al., 2017). Problem markers reflect a storytelling process that is believed to contribute to the maintenance of pathology and core conflictual issues. These kinds of stories are characterized by either under-regulated or over-regulated emotional states, maladaptive self-narratives that are rigidly entrenched, and stories that are so vague they offer limited opportunity for new meaning making.

The narrative emotion process coding system identifies four separate problem markers: (a) unstoried emotion, (b) the superficial story, (c) an empty story, and (d) the same old story (Angus et al., 2015, 2017). Markers are coded based on verbal content, structure, and plot, as well as emotional arousal, expression, and the degree to which narratives are emotionally integrated. Each marker essentially signals the need for a kind of emotional elaboration through story, although each also signals the need for a unique treatment direction.[11] Arguably, these markers offer a process-diagnostic framework for noticing what is conspicuously missing or what seems to be a functional obstacle to emotional processing (Aleixo et al., 2021). Furthermore, this narrative lens is something that is immediately available to clinicians from the conversation in-session as they try to piece together a case formulation.

The Narrative Calls for More Elaboration

Sometimes elaborating and giving more detail is precisely the kind of processing that will be most helpful. In these cases, the most common prescription is deceptively simple: Just elaborate! But what parts need elaboration? The advice turns out not to be as straightforward as it seems. What needs to be elaborated the most is an important consideration for case formulation and intervention.

Unstoried Emotion: The Narrative Needs More Plot

It is hard to think straight when one is very upset. So, although bursts of high arousal are useful in specific contexts (e.g., see Chapter 8), when it comes to reflection of emotion, high arousal risks throwing people off task. *Unstoried emotion* is a narrative process, which involves a person expressing undifferentiated emotion without acknowledging the experience itself. Typically, although the person has some emotional response (e.g., crying, raised voice), they do not refer to their own emotion in their narrative account, so the affective experience remains disconnected, disruptive, and unintegrated with the storyline (Angus et al., 2015).

When emotion lacks sufficient narrative, sometimes it is because that emotion is underregulated (e.g., overwhelming, dysregulated, dissociative). In this case, that lack of connection from the story is itself a marker for down-regulating arousal before one can productively engage in narrative work as a reflective process (see Chapter 3). At other times, unstoried emotion appears when feeling is overregulated and is being too tightly controlled. Speakers may hold their breath, pause, and use silence, all while trying to disengage or avoid the undeclared affective experience (e.g., tears roll down the client's poker face, and seemingly unaware, they continue to tell the story). In short, unstoried emotion reveals raw emotional feeling but without enough context or narrative framework for it to makes sense on its own. This happens for some adults, but it is also characteristic of children who have a feeling but struggle to report a coherent story of what transpired. An unanchored stream of feelings signals the need to flesh out a story about the relevant sequence of events, drawing some causal connections and essentially locating the feeling(s) within some sociohistorical context (Chapters 18 and 20).

Superficial Story: The Narrative Needs More Personal Details

The *superficial story* describes an overly general style that is vague, with sweeping statements and often lacking narrative coherence. If the speaker refers to personal perspectives or feelings, they tend to be poorly integrated. Sometimes the story is intellectualized or uses hypothetical scenarios (Angus et al., 2015). Emotional arousal may be high or low, but it is typically depersonalized, which can seem confusing or choppy to the listener. Linguistic markers include using unclear referents (e.g., "It's so hard") and clients speaking of their distress in third person (e.g., "When things like that happen, one feels . . . "; A. Pascual-Leone & Greenberg, 2005, 2007a). In short, when people tell superficial stories, internal experience is either missing or it lacks depth, and the narrative endeavor has no spirit of personal exploration or discovery (Angus et al., 2015).

Telling superficial stories is characteristic of people who have highly overgeneralized memories, which is a trait-like cognitive style (see Chapter 18). These narratives lack both experiential and conceptual detail (Hamlat & Alloy 2018). The vagueness of a client's in-session accounts makes psychological elaboration a Sisyphean task. In some cases, memory gaps can be the result of traumatic fear, which interfered with the person's capacity to process information. In turn, this compromises their ability to make sense of an experience, leading to a fragmented coherence in their narrative. The gaps are often a source of further uncertainty and anxiety for clients. But by using multiple frames of reference and different scopes of analysis (e.g., switching between the big picture and the recollection of a given moment), one can help clients piece together a meaningful rendition of the past (Paivio & Pascual-Leone, 2023).

The Narrative Calls for a Different Kind of Processing

As discussed, unstoried emotion and superficial stories both indicate problematic narratives that call to be repaired through either more reflection on emotion or further elaboration of the plot. However, at other times, detailing more of the story as such will not help. The kinds of narratives discussed next highlight a need for stories to be repaired through another kind of emotional processing—not just elaborating the story itself. In some cases, continued narrative rehearsal may even be harmful, prolonging or exacerbating one's emotional troubles.

Empty Story: The Need for Emotional Awareness, Not More Story

Empty story is a narrative that describes an event in terms of plot and characters but is nonetheless devoid of reference to internal experiences, emotional arousal, or a search for personal meaning. These stories focus on behaviors and the details of external events from a detached and relatively uninvolved perspective (Angus et al., 2015). In short, the empty story has no heart, meaning it is all plot and characters (i.e., context) but with no details about the lived experience. These stories may seem dull or boring, redacted of their emotional life and motivational drives.

An empty story could result from either alexithymia or a subtle kind of self-censorship that may or may not be within awareness (e.g., an unformulated experience; D. B. Stern, 1997; Chapter 4, this volume). Passing over or sequestering painful feelings and memories makes it difficult to reflect on emotional experience. So, rehashing an empty story is contraindicated. Rather than attempting to foster the client's reflection on the events of a story, therapists will find it more productive to facilitate the elaboration of immediate emotional awareness or perhaps the awareness of a self-interruption. This could be, for example, focusing a client on the first-person feeling of what happened rather than the narrative's plot and characters (e.g., Therapist: "Okay, and while that was going on, what was it like to be you, as a kid, growing up with those sorts of things happening in the house?"). Similarly, another point of entry when working with an empty story will be to use present-centeredness (e.g., Therapist: "And what's it like to just think about this right now? What's happening in your body as we talk about this?"). After deepening emotional awareness, therapists can circle back with clients and connect it to the broader narrative construction (see Chapters 5 and 7).

Same Old Story: The Need for New Emotions, Not More Story

At other times the most central feature of a narrative is a pervasive sense of being stuck. The *same old story* refers to these narratives, in which the speaker seems entrenched in a dysfunctional framework of understanding. The linguistic indicators of this problematic narrative include absolutes such as "always," "never," "no matter what," and "here we go again" (Angus et al., 2015). Stuck in a familiar bad feeling, the client collapses or withdraws into the story, where one emotion of distress often interrupts another. Sometimes this is a collapse into global and undifferentiated distress, a habitual resignation into secondary emotion (A. Pascual-Leone, 2018). At other times, the narrative entails someone repeatedly playing out their specific primary maladaptive emotion (e.g., shame, terror, guilt, loneliness) in a core conflictual relationship theme (Luborsky et al., 1994). In either case, these stories entail a low sense of personal agency, and the specific story may be held up emblematically as one's tragically overarching life theme.

Relatedly, reflecting on emotion also seems to be contraindicated when people are already excessively self-focused, as in cases of ruminative depression or defensive intellectualization. Evidence suggests that for people who tend to be excessively self-focused, worry and brooding on the "Why?" could be harmful, exacerbating their symptoms (Finnbogadottir & Berntsen, 2014; Giovanetti et al., 2019). When people are stuck in these kinds of unhealthy narratives, the process of change will need to entail new emotional awareness and the transformational sequences of emotion (see Chapter 15). If people get stuck in a familiar and unhealthy narrative, the solution is to imbue new feelings into that old story.

The Narrative Calls for a Unified Story

Finally, stories can also be fragmented such that multiple islands of meaning remain disparate at the expense of a single, integrated (macro)narrative.

Dissociative identity disorder represents a distinct challenge in which episodes of dissociation are objectified in a fragmented personal narrative. I suggest that this condition entails not only difficulties in emotion dysregulation but that it can also be understood as a disorder of narrative processing. Here, the client uses the notion of multiple identities as a framework for understanding their own dissociative experiences. However, a fragmented narrative, where each facet of identity is narrated in isolation, poses an inherent obstacle to having a functionally integrated and healthy sense of self. Therapists should avoid being complicit in reifying and further segregating different identities through their separate narrative elaborations.

THE WAY STORIES ARE TOLD REVEALS SYMPTOMATOLOGY

There are unhealthy ways of formulating one's personal stories, and if one uses those narratives, they play a role in maintaining psychopathology (e.g., Adler et al., 2013; Angus, 2012; Angus & Greenberg, 2011; Conway, 2005; Hamlat & Alloy, 2018). The relationship between storytelling and symptomatology was illustrated in a study where undergraduate students were invited to write in first person about a distressing personal difficulty they had. The written narratives, which read like a journal or diary entry, were coded for narrative-emotion processes (A. Pascual-Leone et al., 2023). Findings showed that independent from any personal content being disclosed, the way participants wrote their story (as observed by the presence of certain narrative markers) predicted their level of symptom distress over the previous 1–2 weeks. Superficial stories (i.e., overgeneral, abstract, and speaking of hypotheticals) and the same old story (i.e., feeling stuck in a rigid and familiar theme) were narrative features that signaled these participants from the general population were also suffering clinical symptoms, as compared with when their written accounts did not contain such features. The narrative-based observations had a medium to large effect in the prediction of health and could even indicate whether individuals were approaching or above clinical cutoffs typically used in the assessment of depression, trauma, or anxiety (A. Pascual-Leone et al., 2023). Concretely, this means one could anticipate people's undisclosed symptomatology based simply on the way their stories were being told. The finding brings a new meaning to the otherwise old refrain, "I know what you're feeling."

Consistent with research on overly general autobiographical memories (see Chapter 18), abstract and superficial stories are a prominent problem marker within narrative accounts from clinical samples across various kinds of psychological diagnosis (e.g., depression, generalized anxiety, complex trauma; Aleixo et al., 2021). Moreover, a treatment approach seems to have little influence on the characteristic presence of this marker, suggesting it is inherent to client processing and not an artifact of intervention. In a study that compared clients with depression across emotion-focused, client-centered, and cognitive therapies, a superficial story was the most common problem narrative marker irrespective of treatment approach (Boritz et al., 2014). Furthermore, whether clients suffered from either depression or complex trauma, the prevalence of superficial stories was lower at the end of treatment for the clients who recovered but not for those who remained unchanged (Bortiz et al., 2014; Bryntwick, 2016).

Some intriguing evidence suggests certain narrative markers may also be especially characteristic of specific disorders. For clients with general anxiety disorder, the superficial story seemed to be their default approach to narrative, telling overly general and abstract stories (Khattra, et al., 2020). This is consistent with the surface level processing and emotional avoidance that underpins chronic worry (Borkovec et al., 2004; Chapter 4, this volume). In contrast, the same old story, typified by hopelessness and polarized language (e.g., Client: "This always happens to me!"), underscores the hallmark stuckness of depression (Angus et al., 2017; Angus & Greenberg, 2011). The extent to which depressed clients generated that type of narrative diminished over the course of successful treatment and distinguished between those who would recover and those who would not (Boritz et al., 2014). Finally, unstoried emotion was observed more often among people with complex trauma when compared with those with depression or generalized anxiety (Angus et al., 2017). Exploratory research suggests unstoried emotion markers may be lower by the end of treatment for clients who have recovered from trauma (Carpenter et al., 2016). Dysregulated emotion coupled with the fragmentary and unspoken nature of trauma memories also points to unstoried emotion (Paivio & Pascual-Leone, 2023). Of course, anxiety, depression, and trauma overlap in both symptom presentations and their causal factors, suggesting that narratives are more related to specific patterns of emotional dysfunction rather than diagnostic categories per se.

There are clinical implications for working with process observations like this. The narrative codes make discriminating reference to expression, awareness, regulation, and the specificity of meaning, which map onto the different kinds of emotional processing discussed in this book. The problem narratives are red flags that signal to therapists what kind of psychological elaboration is most called for.

MECHANISMS AT WORK: HOW DOES REFLECTING ON EMOTION CREATE CHANGE?

This chapter has introduced key conceptual issues related to narrative reflection as a form of emotional processing, of which the current chapter explained some of the epistemological issues and neurological correlates of making meaning from autobiographical reflections. In the remaining chapters, I explain the various mechanisms that may be implicated when narrative reflection is used to work with emotion. Such change processes include the specificity and positive nature of a narrative's content, as well as the construction of narrative as a framework of understanding (both in Chapter 18); the issue of how we relate to our memories (Chapter 19); as well as reframing and developing a meta-perspective (Chapter 20). Then, the remaining chapters discuss mechanisms that represent increasingly abstract and latent meanings within a story. These are processes such as narratives about one's identity (Chapter 21), the interplay between different vantage points in the construal of meaning (Chapter 22), and finally, reinventing the self (Chapter 23).

ENDNOTES

1. It is understood there are several aspects of therapeutic change associated with narrative. The interpersonal experience of disclosure is an obvious example. However, as stated in Chapter 1, this book focuses specifically on the intrapsychic process directly related to working with emotion.

2. Recall from the Introduction that it is critical to appreciate that individuals who express instrumental emotion are still having genuine emotional experiences. They are not clandestinely pretending, and they typically balk at the suggestion that they are playing games or manipulating others. The reality is more complex: All emotional experiences are subject to some degree of behavioral contingency. However, when instrumental emotions become problematic, it is because the social and behavioral contingencies of emotional expression have gone unchecked: The individual's emotional range has also become increasingly narrow and too focused on its possible social impact.

3. There are radically different positions on how direct a therapist should be in addressing narrative incongruencies (e.g., Abbass & Town, 2013; cf. Angus & Greenberg, 2011). The risks in being too direct involve precipitating clients to impose premature closure or pseudoclosure, where they satisfy some superficial coherence while obfuscating the deeper psychological problem at hand (e.g., see Conway & Pleydell-Pearce, 2000; Swann et al., 1987).

4. This observation is especially germane to someone's entrenched account of their personal history, but it extends to the discipline of history as a whole. For a classic introduction to this issue, see Carr's (1961) *What Is History?*

5. Parts of this section are adapted from "Insight and Awareness in Experiential Therapy," by A. Pascual-Leone and L. S. Greenberg, in L. G. Castonguay and C. E. Hill (Eds.), *Insight in Psychotherapy* (pp. 31–56), 2007b, American Psychological Association. Copyright 2007 by the American Psychological Association.

6. Using a first-person perspective versus a third-person perspective also seems to differentially recruit ventral medial versus dorsal medial parts of the prefrontal cortex (St. Jacques et al., 2011), something that is discussed in Chapter 22.

7. For a neurophysiological account of what happens when people are involuntarily cued to remember their "unfinished business," see Rohde and colleagues (2018).

8. Formulations of emotional change that rely on singular constructs, linear scales, or degrees of some general capacity have difficulty assimilating this qualitative distinction between subprocesses. Therefore, a criticism of general-capacity formulations (e.g., mentalization) is that they become excessively broad, even amorphous.

9. As discussed in Chapter 7, the bottom-up process of emergent awareness can also generate structure, although they do it through a different mechanism: As one generates new contents from experience, which continue to be at odds with an existing framework of understanding, the system of meaning can reach a tipping point and potentiate a top-down structural reorganization. This is essentially what Piaget and Gibson referred to as "accommodation." In other words, the contents of new moment-by-moment awareness are continually assimilated into one's experience of self,

world, and other until it becomes untenable. The failure of assimilation leads to accommodation (a structural reorganization) in order to maintain stability (i.e., Piaget's equilibrium) across a range of disparate experiential fragments (J. Pascual-Leone & Johnson, 2021).

10. This is to say that the broken story cannot be resolved in its presenting form. The issue here is on a deleterious process being the obstacle to change. By contrast, even when it is very painful, the content of a narrative is not as much an impediment to emotional change as the ways in which people are formulating (or not) their story of what happened.

11. Chapter 18 discusses "transition" and "change" markers, which highlight narrative as a mechanism of change.

18

Psychological Elaboration

Telling More of the Story

"Would you tell me, please, which way I ought to go from here?"
"That depends a good deal on where you want to get to," said the Cat.
"I don't much care where—" said Alice.
"Then it doesn't matter which way you go," said the Cat.
"—so long as I get SOMEWHERE," Alice added as an explanation.
"Oh, you're sure to do that," said the Cat, "if you only walk long enough."

—LEWIS CARROLL, *THE ADVENTURES OF ALICE IN WONDERLAND*

The easiest aspect of working with emotion is simply to elaborate on the psychological dimensions of a narrative, purposefully detailing the feelings, motives, and thoughts that pertain to what happened or could happen. As a mechanism, psychological elaboration is deceivingly simple. The content of memories and stories can be continually elaborated, and as one makes new associations to the events being described, the narrative account becomes richer and evolves. At its most rudimentary level, this is an issue of time on task, where exploratory processing is a predictor of growth, if only because ongoing elaboration presupposes a certain number of attempts at meaning making (Huang et al., 2020; McLean et al., 2020). This is probably one of the basic reasons why clients improve in psychotherapy irrespective of a therapist's orientation or even the quality of psychotherapy they receive. Psychological elaboration is functional engagement, and time on task is a prerequisite common factor.

https://doi.org/10.1037/0000460-019
Principles of Emotion Change: What Works and When in Psychotherapy and Everyday Life, by A. Pascual-Leone
Copyright © 2026 by the American Psychological Association. All rights reserved.

Despite being so open ended, even the hackneyed prescription to "just elaborate" can often result in a minimum of meandering progress. So long as the process remains in motion, people are likely to eventually touch upon critical new developments. Then, as an elaboration comes to feel personal, poignant, and inherently meaningful, emotion orients the individual and begins to pull toward deeper and more focused exploration. The fact that the cognitive load required for psychological elaboration can range from rudimentary to highly complex may explain why this kind of processing is a significant predictor of positive outcomes across the lifespan, with research support for the impact of this process among children, adolescents, adults, and older adults (e.g., Pasupathi et al., 2017; Wainryb et al., 2018; Woods et al., 2018). Probably because of this, when children and adolescents were compared on the quality and internal complexity of their narratives, it showed that similar benefits can be garnered through different pathways that are cognitively scalable (Wainryb et al., 2018).

However, the reason why psychological elaboration can be more impactful than it might at first seem is because it eventually entails a tipping point. Although the initial process is only to generate more content further downstream, that quantitative change will often also precipitate profound qualitative (i.e., structural) changes. As details are elaborated, they are also being simultaneously reorganized, integrated, and reintegrated. Again, differentiation and integration are the two prongs of development, a dialectic that gives rise to structural change.[1] In short, with the elaboration of enough narrative context, the emotion comes to mean something more, or it may even come to mean something entirely new. Emotion and narrative can intersect in several ways (e.g., as the actor who felt, the observer who empathized, the evocativeness of words, the feeling implied, the poignancy of being witnessed). Generally, the more one reflects on experience, the more content one accrues to then potentially have feelings about. At the same time, each emotion is increasingly ascribed personal meaning.

There are at least three specific ways in which psychological elaboration holds promise as a direct approach to emotional change. First, it helps to increase the degree of specificity in the stories one tells. Second, deliberately exploring the positive meaning within a given event is a valuable process. Third, elaborating the narrative in relation to emotional experience or vice versa ensures that emotion is appropriately contextualized and, conversely, that a narrative account has emotional depth. These three points are the topics explored in this chapter. I also note that psychological elaboration is the foundation of more complex, multistep mechanisms, but those are discussed in later chapters (i.e., Chapters 20 and 21).

MEMORY SPECIFICITY AND ELABORATING THE DETAILS

A narrative is a framework of understanding, but one also needs to adequately make use of that framework. It needs to be populated with the details that give narrative richness. A bookshelf that remains barren has little practical use. Similarly, narratives that lack the specificity of psychological elaboration are not optimal mechanisms of emotional processing.

Overgeneralized Memory Is a Transdiagnostic Phenomenon

Sometimes people remember events using broad strokes, recalling and offering up generalities. For example, a person might recall, "I don't feel good in those situations. So, I usually just get something to eat. It is weird." These are categorical representations. Even if they are used emblematically, they refer generically to a host of similar events collated across time. However, on other occasions, people give discrete and specific memories. These are rich with detail and capture what happened at a unique time and place. For instance, the same (overgeneralized) memory given previously could be rendered with much more specificity: "I felt broken. I sat there in the diner holding my ham and Swiss, avoiding eye contact but also feeling grateful, hoping the server wouldn't see I was using her napkin to wipe away my tears."

Memories are stored (i.e., generated) in a hierarchical fashion, and the search process (i.e., the dynamic construction) occurs through a top-down approach.[2] This begins with broad abstract life themes, narrows down through periods of time in one's life to general repeated events, and finally ends with reconstructing specific episodes with detailed sensory information (Conway & Pleydell-Pearce, 2000). However, when that memory process (i.e., the search) operates laterally, what one subsequently retrieves is circumscribed to abstract and general memories, leaving the individual's story with a lack of specificity. The process of elaboration is truncated, and the individual is left with an overgeneral memory, the specifics of which simply are not (re)constructed (Williams et al., 2007). This memory bias is closely related to rumination. Having that trait-like cognitive style poses a barrier to exploring episodic memories, such that people either cannot (or will not allow themselves to) elaborate their experience in detail. For some people, their memories are so vague and elusive they may appear to have amnesia for highly salient or traumatic personal events.[3] Unsurprisingly, this also makes it difficult to productively work with emotion.

Overgeneralized memory represents a transdiagnostic phenomenon. Studies have linked higher rates of overgeneral memories to depression, trauma, anxiety, eating disorders, bipolar disorder, dissociative identity disorder, and schizophrenia (Hamlat & Alloy, 2018).[4] Furthermore, producing a preponderance of overgeneral memories predicts the onset and course of major depression. Similarly, when people have suffered trauma, a high level of overgeneralized memories is related to both avoidance and maladaptive coping. It is common among those diagnosed with posttraumatic stress disorder, and even when initial severity is accounted for, having overgeneral memories predicts the course of posttraumatic stress symptoms. This link to psychopathology holds across the lifespan, as observed in children, adolescents, and adults (Callahan et al., 2019).

Interventions Promote Improved Memory Specificity

Some clients grew up or live in a social milieu without the benefit of a listener persistently inquiring about the narrative details of their memories.[5] However, brief therapy interventions can increase the levels of specificity people elaborate during retrieval. Reminiscence therapy, life review therapy, and memory specificity training are approaches developed to facilitate this kind of process, primarily as treatments of depression or trauma.

Reminiscence and Life Review

Reminiscence therapy is one of the most common treatment interventions for people suffering dementia, and it involves using tangible prompts such as photographs or music to evoke memories and stimulate the discussion of past experiences. A Cochrane review's meta-analysis of 22 studies concluded that four to six sessions of this treatment had a wide range of small positive effects on people suffering from dementia (Woods et al., 2018). A broader meta-analysis on 128 studies showed that reminiscence-based interventions had a moderate effect on improving wellness. However, among those presenting with either major depression or chronic physical disease, reminiscence had a large effect in relieving symptoms of depression (Pinquart & Forstmeier, 2012).

Symptom changes were largest when reminiscence interventions were part of *life review therapy*, which is a protocol of systematic prompts to elicit memories from specific periods of a client's life. The aim is to increase the specificity in someone's autobiographical memories, focusing especially on the generation of positive (i.e., happy) memories (Webster et al., 2010). Four weeks of life review therapy has been repeatedly shown to reduce depression in older adults. Another large clinical trial showed that a combination of life review and narrative therapies reduced depression relative to treatment as usual, and those benefits were maintained 9 months later (Korte et al., 2012).

Importantly, these protocols have been used primarily with older adults and typically emphasizes the recollection of happy memories. But an unexplored application of reminiscence or life review therapy could be in working with distressed couples. It is common to ask couples how they first met. When this happens during treatment it typically leads to the reminiscence of better times. Some couples have the practice of frequently strolling down memory lane together, basking in a shared memory of special moments. That simple process likely tightens their connection and heightens shared joy. Still, reminiscence needs to be rigorously studied in couples, ideally using experimental manipulations.

Memory Specificity

Memory specificity may be an important mechanism of change in reminiscence and life review therapy (Hamlat & Alloy, 2018). When life review therapy was compared with supportive therapy, the two produced similar symptom reductions over four weeks. However, compared with those in supportive therapy (controls), clients in life review therapy generated more specific memories as well as more positive memories (Serrano Selva et al., 2012). Observations like these have led researchers to try training people in generating more specific memories as a treatment for emotional disorders (Barry et al., 2021).

Memory specificity training is often delivered as a circumscribed group therapy, conducted over five to eight weekly sessions of about 60 minutes (Barry et al., 2021; Raes et al., 2009). It teaches clients about the perils of overgeneral memories and uses skills training for the retrieval of specific narrative content. When memories are overgeneral (e.g., Client: "On Tuesdays, my partner and I go on dates"), therapists solicit more detail to enrich the target story (e.g., recalling a specific date at a given restaurant). That could involve focusing on the sensory–perceptual and contextual details that make the memory unique (e.g., recalling the taste of the food, the decor, the conversation, the smell of one's partner; Barry et al., 2021). Individuals are typically assigned homework on the recollection of specific memories (Callahan et al., 2019). The training can also be used as an adjunct to traditional interventions or delivered online by artificial intelligence (Barry et al., 2021).

The training has been studied with clinical samples suffering major depression, posttraumatic stress disorder, bipolar disorder, and schizophrenia. It has also been delivered to adolescents, adults, and older adults across a diverse range of cultural settings (Barry et al., 2021). A meta-analysis of 13 studies showed training in memory specificity has a very large effect in improving the richness of someone's autobiographical memories (i.e., the target process) as compared with control conditions (Barry et al., 2019). The training also predicted a small- to medium-sized advantage over other treatments in the post-treatment reduction of depression and other symptoms. The comparative effects, however, are short-lived since any difference relative to other treatments is lost by follow up (Barry et al., 2019).

Nevertheless, the uniqueness of this particular training may be less important than the process it targets. Increasing memory specificity still explains part of symptom change. Among adolescent Afghani refugees, for example, increases in autobiographical specificity was a process that mediated the effect training had on reducing depression (Neshat-Doostet al., 2013). Furthermore, while generating more positive memories anticipated better outcomes in life review therapy, again, the number of specific memories someone recalled mediated the alleviation of symptoms (Webster et al., 2010). Finally, when memory specificity training was directly compared with an established therapy for posttraumatic stress disorder (i.e., cognitive processing therapy), both treatments were associated with increased memory specificity as well as clinical improvements, although participants in the training accomplished the same gains in half as many sessions (Maxwell et al., 2016). The fact that memory specificity increases in treatments not explicitly designed to do so highlights that other treatments may also leverage this process.

Implicit Interventions That Increase Specificity

Adopting the intervention goal of increasing autobiographical specificity could be easily integrated into most treatment approaches (Barry et al., 2021; Callahan et al., 2019). Arguably, such training to increase autobiographical specificity already occurs covertly during experiential treatments, particularly if they put a premium on a discovery-oriented process (see Chapter 4). Experiential treatments aim to deepen a client's moment-by-moment experiencing, which is contingent on elaborating idiosyncratic details and leads to increased memory specificity. Indeed, over the course of client-centered or emotion-focused therapies alike, the autobiographical specificity of clients' narrative became more detailed, and they generated proportionally more single-event memories over 15–20 treatment sessions (Boritz at al., 2008). From a different approach, exposure-based treatments for trauma ask clients to repeatedly tell a target narrative about a traumatic event, giving special attention to elaborating details in hotspots of the story that evoked distress. Increasing narrative specificity is probably an additional mechanism in such treatments, even if it goes undeclared in the treatment's theory (Hamlat & Alloy, 2018).

Qualitative reports from participants in memory specificity training suggest limitations to a skills-based approach when working with autobiographical specificity and emotion. Older participants in one study commented that exercises to recall memories based on generic cue words of negative, positive, or neutral memories overlooked a rich opportunity for exploring more personally meaningful memories (Leahy et al., 2017). Arguably, specificity skills training targets a different objective than making meaning during the recollection of significant events. The contrast highlights how increasing specificity can be functionally disentangled from the elaboration of personal meaning, even if the two processes are somewhat nested (Chapter 17). Whatever the case, although overgeneral memory is a trait-like style, increasing narrative specificity can be deliberately practiced and improved upon.

Mechanisms of Change Through Increased Specificity

Several complementary pathways have been proposed to explain increasing specificity as a mechanism of emotional change (Dalgleish et al., 2007). First, elaborating the details brings effortful engagement with one's narrative. Second, the forward momentum of exploratory work helps displace ruminative thinking. Third, increased specificity gives a finer resolution to the concerns at hand, which supports better problem solving.

Increased Engagement and Reduced Functional Avoidance

People can avoid emotional experiences simply by not being very specific about painful memories and events. This is what D. B. Stern (1997) described as unformulated experience (see Chapter 4, this volume), and it can serve as a passive strategy to evade emotional distress, which would otherwise spark the recollection of aversive experiences.[6] On one hand, a purposeful exploration demands mental effort, whereas nonengagement is just less work. On the other hand, actively constraining one's elaboration to the level of generalized memories truncates the retrieval (i.e., formulation) at an intermediate stage. Thus, recollection remains vague, which down-regulates any preliminary distress evoked by the unwelcome recall of upsetting experiences. Furthermore, if the functional avoidance is effective, it reinforces a retrieval style biased toward overgeneralizations (Hamlat & Alloy, 2018).

In contrast, interventions that increase an individual's specific autobiographical memories prevent one from circumventing difficult emotions associated with past negative events. From the perspective of behavioral exposure, only when individuals reexpose themselves to negative details of an autobiographical memory can they habituate to those feelings (Barry et al., 2019; Raes et al., 2009). An experiential perspective sees the elaboration of details as rendering a richer integration between emotion and its narrative context (Angus, 2012; Angus & Greenberg, 2011). So, when interventions focus clients on narrative specificity, they foster emotional engagement while also using those evocative memories as important sources of information.

Disrupting Rumination

Increasing the specificity of a narrative facilitates emotional change by interrupting chronic rumination typically associated with overgeneral memories. People can get stuck in a rut, where cognitive resources get captured at a shallow level of general memory, spurring on ruminative thinking (Williams et al., 2007). When this happens, the individual focuses on memory at the categorical level and then loops it through generic but all too familiar scripts. These are often well rehearsed and are gratifying in an unhealthy way (e.g., Peters et al., 2018; Watkins & Baracaia, 2001). The more one broods at this generic level of engagement, the more one strengthens memory connections at that superficial level.

Among those with major depression, the degree of specificity in autobiographical memories mediated the relationship between their rumination and how effective their social problem solving was (Raes et al., 2005). Experiments show a brief distraction task interfered with the ruminative thinking of depressed people, which subsequently increased their retrieval of specific autobiographical memories (Watkins & Teasdale, 2001). Training in memory specificity showed only limited evidence for its impact on rumination (Barry et al., 2019). However, life review therapy and expressive writing are other methods that facilitate more specific memories, and in both, decreased rumination mediated the impact of treatments on reducing depressive symptoms (Lamers et al., 2015). In sum, although rumination maintains overgeneral memories, systematically adding more detail may dislodge old thinking patterns, such that cognitive resources are freed up and reallocated to an exploratory effort.

Improving Problem Solving

Improving problem solving may be another way in which recollection of specific autobiographical memories could reduce depressive symptoms (Raes et al., 2005; Westerhof et al., 2010). The meta-analysis on memory specificity training showed strong evidence for the treatment's direct effect on improving problem solving (Barry et al., 2019). There are at least three ways this process may operate as a mechanism of change. The first reason has to do with clarifying the problem at hand. Lingering issues from the past (e.g., unfinished business with a person in one's life) are easier to grapple with when one has specific details to contemplate as opposed to getting mired in rumination or the generalities of discontent. Then, having more details about one's personal difficulties sets a stage to better inform a solution.

The second link between memory specificity and problem solving rests on the fact that narratives about how one solved problems in the past serves as a critical database for problem solving in the present. Recalling past events where one strived to attain personal goals can help avoid repeating errors of the past and identify problem-solving strategies that were previously successful (Hamlat & Alloy, 2018). Again, the psychological and neurological processes of remembering the past are closely related to how we generate simulations of the future, which narrows the demarcation between reviewing past solutions and working on current problems. When life review therapy focused on recalling instrumental details about how one successfully coped with an event and identifying which strategies were most suitable, then the treatment reduced depressive symptoms as compared to an active control (L. Watt & Cappeliez, 2000). Furthermore, this large effect was maintained 3 months later. Such instrumental reminiscence probably also fosters feelings of mastery and competence.

A third way in how reviewing the details of a memory helps with problem solving may be related to its impact on executive capacity and control. The retrieval of specific memories demands that one effortfully apply metacognitive resources: One searches for information while being mindful of the question or objective at hand and continually monitoring one's performance in the generation of a coherent and relevant narrative (Conway & Pleydell-Pearce, 2000; Dimaggio et al., 2020; Hamlat & Alloy, 2018). Studies suggest overgeneral memories are caused by an individual's shortcoming in executive control (Dalgleish et al., 2007). Certain cognitive–emotional vulnerabilities, such as depression, make it difficult for people to inhibit extraneous information, which then makes it challenging to retrieve details and creates a bias toward overgeneral memories. This causal chain, with poor inhibitory control as a driving factor, has explained low autobiographical specificity in the memories of depressed children, adults with eating disorders who have depressed mood, and older people showing the cognitive effects of aging (Dalgleish et al., 2007; Piolino et al., 2010; Raes et al., 2010).

There may be multiple levels of directional influence because other research suggests autobiographical specificity can also impact executive functioning. Greater specificity seems to counter the hampering effects that depressive rumination has on problem solving (Raes et al., 2005). At the same time, memory specificity was a predictor of how well someone would acquire new problem-solving skills as well as the degree to which a psychoeducational intervention would decrease symptoms of depression and anxiety (Van Daele et al., 2013). Even a very brief instruction to enhance the recall of episodic details from one's past can immediately improve one's ability to solve presenting problems (Madore & Schacter, 2014).

Clinical Implications and Individual Differences

The retrieval of sufficiently detailed memories from one's life is a probable mechanism of change, and an intervention strategy for working with emotion. Working with the specificity of narrated memories is also an easier and less stressful entry point to working with emotion than, for example, exposure-based approaches (Callahan et al., 2019). Across cultures and populations, the average woman typically has autobiographical memories that are a bit more specific, more accurate, longer, and more emotionally detailed than those of the average man. The role of overgeneral memory in depression also seems to be more important for women than men. Brain imaging suggests the reason for these differences may be that men and women use different cognitive strategies during the moment of recall (Beike & Wirth-Beaumont, 2005; Ros et al., 2014; Young et al., 2017). Following this, increasing the specificity of memories might have more potency as a mechanism of emotional change for women than for men, but this hypothesis needs testing. It also remains unclear whether such neurobiological differences are related to genetic sex differences or to the impact of gender role socialization.

POSITIVE MEANING MAKING: STOPPING TO SMELL THE ROSES

The idea of stopping to smell the roses suggests the benefit of taking time to acknowledge the positive values and meaning in life. The point is that along the path of negotiating adversity, there are also positive and enjoyable experiences that could be included if one takes the time to notice and to incorporate them into the context of one's experience. Although positive psychology covers a delightfully sprawling assortment of constructs, its basic notion is that elaborating positive aspects of one's experience is a psychological process with reaching implications for health and happiness and predicting positive outcomes across the lifespan (C. R. Snyder et al., 2021). A meta-analysis shows the effects multicomponent positive psychology interventions have on well-being to be noteworthy: small for the general population or those suffering from mental illness and medium for those suffering physical illness (van Agteren et al., 2021).

Balancing Negativity With Positivity

Striving to strike an appropriate balance in affective valence is not simply a Pollyannish wish for rose-colored glasses. In fact, the odds are stacked against us. Our biological inheritance has endowed us with a predisposition to attend to and identify the negative aspects of our emotional experiences more than the positive ones. Attending more to the negative aspects of life has helped promote our survival, which is a deeper evolutionary goal than being happy

(Panksepp, 2008; Pessoa, 2014; Porges, 2011). That imbalance in emphasis is also reflected, for example, in the broader functional vocabulary we have for negative experiences over positive ones (Schrauf & Sanchez, 2004; as discussed in the Introduction). The implication of all this in everyday life is that if one is looking for something to be upset about, one will easily find it! It also means that offsetting this natural inclination will demand making purposeful (and effortful) choices to also attend to the positive.

For some people, this dispositional bias is more severe than for others. Furthermore, certain mental health and emotional difficulties entail a problematic skew toward negativity and pessimism. For example, identifying and reflecting on positive events is particularly critical for people with depression because they tend to selectively experience positive events as both overly general and more psychologically distant. Similarly, criminal offenders recalled positive memories with less specificity than a control group, but the difference did not hold for negative memories (Neves & Pinho, 2016). Moreover, such processing biases seem to differentiate by disorder. For example, unlike those with depression, people with symptoms of posttraumatic stress disorder are not psychologically distant from positive events; rather, they often report feeling too psychologically near the negative events (Janssen et al., 2015).

A bias against articulating and exploring positive emotion likely has a complex relationship with other information processing variables. Those variables could include everything from someone's task-orientation to the intensity of their somatic experiences. For instance, people living with spinal cord injuries also experience less positive emotion as compared to healthy controls, but they showed no difference in levels of negative emotion, despite their suffering more depression (Salter et al., 2013). Perhaps relatedly, people suffering spinal cord injuries also receive less feedback from their body's autonomic nervous system. If that explained the observed imbalance in the valence of their emotional experiences, it would suggest positive versus negative experiences are constructed through somewhat different processes. but still suggests a unique kind of shortfall.

People's attention to positive versus negative aspects of life can be out of balance, but it might also shift over time. This would help explain the benefits of reminiscence and life review therapy for older adults with depression. As a client of mine in his late 70s put it, "Getting old sucks—everything on this carcass is falling apart. So, you know, it's good to have the stories to look back on." For this client, reliving past adventures served as an emotional counterweight to his present pains of aging.

What Is the Right Balance?

One approach to emotional complexity is reducing it to either positive affect and positivity (e.g., feeling grateful, being proud, expressing appreciation or kindness), or negative affect and negativity (e.g., sadness, irritability, feeling contempt, expressing criticism or dislike). This kind of contrast has led some researchers to ask what the right balance between positive and negative emotion is if someone is to thrive and flourish in their growth and well-being. The issue has been studied in individuals, marriages, and even small groups such as business teams (Frederickson & Losada, 2005). Consistently, an overall ratio of about three positive emotional experiences to one negative experience marks a boundary line. All things being equal, this means that three genuinely positive interactions are needed to neutralize one negative interaction for the individual or system to be made whole again. A larger proportion of positive experiences signals resilience and generative flourishing, with research suggesting optimal levels are four or five positives to one negative experience. In contrast, if the positivity ratio sinks below three, it signals languishing and deleterious effects, which is what we see in clinical samples or when people start looking for treatment. Moreover, this ratio (3:1) is supported across various measures of emotional valence, time scales, and levels of analysis (Frederickson & Losada, 2005).

Unsurprisingly, emotional accounts that are excessively positive and optimistic from the beginning are not associated with high levels of well-being. For example, narrative research shows that when people's stories fail to explore the negative experiences they suffered, it often precludes the possibility of getting closure or personal growth (Lilgendahl & McAdams, 2011; Pasupathi et al., 2017). Similarly, when dynamic systems modeling is used to push the upper limit into being overly positive, the boundary line first shows signs of disintegration at 11 or 12 positive emotional experiences for a single negative one (Frederickson & Losada, 2005). Thus, getting the right balance assumes some appropriate level of negativity, and in personal change, this will be a process that dynamically unfolds over time. For instance, expressive writing has been more helpful when a participant's writing over time increases in its use of both positive emotion language and reflective language (e.g., Pennebaker & Chung, 2011).

Correcting Imbalances

From a mental health perspective, the problem is essentially that bad mood is stronger than good, so more instances of positive emotion are needed to offset negative emotional experience. Psychotropic drugs (e.g., Prozac, Xanax) represent a pharmacological approach to correcting some chemical imbalance, although they are relatively blunt instruments. Experiments with mice show that shifting the emotional balance can be done on a more targeted neurocellular level by identifying and then manipulating certain kinds of memories. Specific memory cells in the hippocampi of mice have been directly stimulated using a laser to dial up either negative or positive memories (B. K. Chen et al., 2019).[7] The objective of that kind of memory reconsolidation research is essentially to use positive memories as a means for overwriting the bad ones.

In humans, a more suitable solution for correcting imbalances in positivity and negativity is to foster narrative-based changes in clinical work and everyday life. For example, correcting the negative bias in someone's thinking is a primary focus of cognitive therapy (see Chapter 20). Storytelling can also be used prescriptively for the psychological elaboration of positive meaning as a change process. This approach is personally active (as opposed to being the passive recipient of chemical or energy stimulations). And such repeated experiences of narrating positive emotions can also stimulate enduring neurological changes. Affective neuroscience suggests this line of intervention is helpful for addressing emotional dysfunction as well as some deficits observed in psychopathology such as depression, anxiety, and perhaps schizophrenia (Garland et al., 2010). As one looks to correct imbalances related to a shortfall in positivity, useful processes include expressing gratitude, optimism, self-affirmation, and looking for the silver lining.

Expressing Gratitude and Optimism

Writing a gratefulness journal or letters of gratitude are ways of elaborating the narrative of one's experiences in a prescribed direction. Positive psychology highlights the value of these experiences, wherein even single interventions of this kind can have a small meaningful effect on emotion and well-being (C. R. Snyder et al., 2021; van Agteren et al., 2021). A critical point for understanding this process is that expressing gratitude or optimism do not inherently reinterpret one's experiences rather they simply bring attention to and narrate the positive aspects that one might otherwise have taken for granted. So this is not so much about reframing as it is about further elaborating positive experiences. At first, people typically have some trouble with these prescribed exercises. There is a mental search for what one might be most grateful for. This is because the positive aspects of one's life are often background to negative concerns that are more salient and pressing, irrespective of how important (or not) they are. So, the crux of this kind of emotional elaboration is precisely to articulate positive aspects and bring them to the foreground.

An 8-month-long experiment in which participants practiced the expression of gratitude and optimism concluded that these processes work best at boosting people's well-being when they are engaged as a deliberate practice and with enthusiasm (Lyubomirsky et al., 2011). The study also confirmed a common suspicion about the effects related to positive psychology interventions, which is that someone's self-selection to even participate in such exercises play a role in their effectiveness. Other practices such as keeping a humor diary for just a week (e.g., recalling three funny things that happened each day) have shown similar results in decreasing depressive symptoms and increasing happiness over the following 3–6 months (Wellenzohn et al., 2018). Psychosocial interventions for boosting positive emotion are more than a placebo, although they are more effective when people subscribe and dedicate themselves to such practices. Further, some evidence suggests that although looking for humor in events of life seems to work for everyone, the process may be moderated by personality, where people who are extroverts enjoy larger effects compared to introverts (Wellenzohn et al., 2018).

Gratitude is a central element in most 12-step programs for addiction recovery (e.g., Alcoholics Anonymous). At least one study has confirmed that people who were more grateful engaged in more 12-step practices, made more promises, enjoyed more posttraumatic growth, and had more social support. Their rates of gratefulness also predicted lower health symptoms and stress (Labelle & Edelstien, 2018). Again, self-selection for such programs likely plays a role. Although attachment style may be another moderator, people who were avoidant of interpersonal attachment showed more gratefulness and enjoyed better outcomes after the 12-step program.

Consistent with Frederickson's (2001) broaden-and-build theory of positive emotion (see Chapter 12), the experience of positive emotion broadens one's cognitive and behavioral repertoire, resulting in healthy exploration, psychological elaboration, and openness to experience. Interventions such as writing gratitude letters or writing a diary over 2 weeks suggest that gratitude and humility are mutually reinforcing emotions and jointly create an upward spiral that leads to positive emotion and subjective well-being (Kruse et al., 2014). Some forms of gratitude and acceptance of life as it is are formulated from a more spiritual approach, entailing a grateful surrender to some benevolent higher power.

In early work on the psychology of religion, psychologist David Bakan (1966) posed the following question: Is prayer useful even if it turns out no one is listening? Otherwise said, could it be valuable to take some time every day to reflect on and summarize what is of most value in one's life and articulate one's aspirations and longings (irrespective of one's spiritual beliefs)? Clearly the answer is yes, and it highlights the role of positive emotions such as gratitude, optimism, and humility. It points to the impact positive emotions have on an individual's internal process as distinct from the additional interpersonal or social function they may have. Irrespective of an ontological reality or personal beliefs, positive affect shifts the baseline focus of one's emotional life.

Self-Affirmation

Self-affirmations are statements intended to positively reflect one's own personal traits, self-concepts, or values. This concretizes what is commonly referred to as positive self-talk. Admittedly, even the most well-intentioned affirmation is ripe for parody. And yet, the potential in affirming a belief is that it serves as a top-down frame of engagement (e.g., saying, "Remember who you are! You can do this!"). Affirmation is a rationally derived effort to reach across, or realign, an otherwise misleading emotional situation (e.g., when things are not as they should be or, not as one wants them to be). This affirmation against more skeptical interpretations of reality is the very reason for its appeal, although it will only be successful when the discrepancy between the hoped-for narrative and manifest reality is not too large (Brooks, 2014).

Self-affirmation theory argues that people can use statements of positive self-evaluation to support the integrity of their self-concept and to buffer against negative feelings when that self-concept is being threatened (Cohen & Sherman, 2014). Interventions that make use of self-affirmation usually involve writing exercises in which participants are asked to reflect on and elaborate core personal values to give them a more expansive view on themselves and their resources. Furthermore, while self-affirmations can be stated from a first-person perspective, other research suggests that self-talk may be most effective when the individual adopts an observer's perspective (e.g., someone speaking to themselves, saying: "You can do this!"; see Chapter 22).

Given the right moment, this reflective process can tip a positive feedback loop into motion, between how one understands oneself and the broader context of social meaning. The timing of self-affirmations is a critical issue, but they have been shown to improve educational and relationship outcomes as well as self-care and health (for a review, see Cohen & Sherman, 2014). For example, randomized trials of a psychosocial intervention that had young adolescents periodically do self-affirmation exercises throughout a school year showed that it improved their grades for the 3 years following the intervention relative to a control condition. Critically, the intervention was most impactful in supporting the achievement of Black and Latinx students who came from economically disadvantaged families as compared with White students at the same school (in the United States; Sherman et al., 2013). Other research supports the hypothesized mechanism of this process that explicitly affirming one's strengths and values helps shield one against stereotypes and threats to identity, which reduces defensiveness and prompts an internal readiness to respond adaptively.

Another study found that when breast cancer patients used self-affirmations during expressive writing, it was accompanied by the alleviation of physical symptoms 3 months later, and the effect of this was not better explained by the construction of genuinely new meaning (Creswell et al., 2007). The interpretation of such a finding is that "people benefited from the expressive writing not so much because it led them to reappraise their cancer but because it helped them to reappraise themselves" (Cohen & Sherman, 2014, p. 350). In short, self-affirmation can mobilize someone to draw on the larger context of personal meaning to marshal resources and bring their best when confronting an imminent challenge. However, having the choice to make self-affirmations or not is an important moderating factor, and so when these tasks are externally imposed, it may undermine their usefulness (Silverman et al., 2013).

Looking for the Silver Lining

Looking for the silver lining refers to an elaboration of meaning in which a person places some difficult experience under a more positive light, but that process can be executed via at least two different pathways.

Reframing Versus Positive Elaboration

On one hand, making positive meaning can be a straightforward elaboration of positive experiences (e.g., Therapist: "Was there anything positive that also may have happened?"). Even when positive aspects of life are obvious, they are not always fully explored in psychotherapy for their latent meaning nor sufficiently celebrated. In training, sometimes junior therapists are stumped by how to work with emotion when what the client feels is neither painful nor negative. As one trainee said to me, "The client says they feel good. So, I guess there isn't any real processing to do, right?" On the contrary! Compared with the distress of treatment concerns, the fact that expressions of positive emotion are less common in psychotherapy makes experiencing them even more precious and worthy of elaboration. These are golden opportunities to deepen client experiencing by savoring, enjoying, and then extending personal meaning within a narrative context. Treatment manuals often overlook instructing this as a purposeful task or objective. Accelerated experiential dynamic psychotherapy is one of several exceptions: It explicitly encourages therapists to elaborate their clients' positive experiences of attachment, accomplishment, or the joyful sense of having changed in treatment (Fosha, 2021). But notice that attending to and expanding on positive elements that are already there is not a reconstrual of events. Rather, it is an intentional elaboration of the existing experience (i.e., symbolizing the latent experience of some silver lining).

On the other hand, when positive meaning is not self-apparent (or may not yet exist), a different kind of process can be used. That would be a sort of damage control, and it requires creatively finding ways to reinterpret or reframe what initially seemed to be a negative experience or misfortune (e.g., when life gives you lemons, make lemonade). Thus, one can differentiate between two types of *cognitive reappraisal*: cognitive reframing and positive reappraisal or—better—positive elaboration (Nowlan et al., 2016).[8] *Reframing* is a purposeful and rationally based reinterpretation of events (see Chapter 20), whereas *positive elaboration* refers to revisiting a default appraisal with a renewed agenda that aims to seek out and elaborate positive content.

Different Targets, Different Operations

Although they are often conflated, two facets distinguish reframing from positive elaboration. First, the targets of interventions are different. Reframing usually applies to negative thoughts held by an individual that might not be true, such that unrealistically negative interpretations of events are replaced with more balanced and realistic interpretations (Beck, 2020). In contrast, positive elaboration is applied to negative interpretations that are (unfortunately) realistic. Admittedly, looking for the positive is premised on a tacit assumption that even negative events are inherently mixed, and there may be a silver lining or an upside that is also worth exploring.

Second, the mental operations are different in each of these strategies for recontextualizing negative emotion. Reframing evaluates the entire event from a different point of view to alter its overarching meaning (e.g., Brooks, 2014). As such, the mental process involves more than elaboration; it requires that one momentarily dis-embed and consider not just the content of the view but also the frame of one's perspective. In contrast, positive elaboration acknowledges the negativity of the event but focuses on the positive, incorporating that new information to alter the initial appraisal. Thus, a positive elaboration is a matter of extending one's initial appraisal, a decision to include more by deliberately looking on the bright side. In short, the aim of cognitive reframing is to reinterpret unrealistic appraisals into more realistic ones, while positive elaboration aims to incorporate some kind of positive content into an otherwise realistic appraisal of negative circumstances.

Practice Implications

Clarifying the difference between reframing and positive elaboration is more than a trivial academic detail. It likely has palpable implications for who benefits most from which process. Reframing is more cognitively demanding, as the individual tries to interrupt and then decenter from the ongoing flow of their mental process (see Chapter 20). In contrast, following a prompt for positive elaboration exerts less mental demand. This difference in the necessary mental resources and attentional effort means that positive elaboration probably is more effective than reframing when working with children and people with developmental delays, when the client is struggling to concentrate, or simply when a client is functioning less well than usual, such as during states of extreme stress. Meanwhile, reframing will be more critical for working through misleading situations and when things are not as they may at first have seemed (such as abuse by a caregiver).

Interventions that focus on the positive aspects of a situation essentially facilitate positive emotion. When life review therapy focused exclusively on the recall of positive autobiographical memories, it decreased people's level of obsessive reminiscence but did not increase the resolution or acceptance of past negative experiences (Preschl et al., 2012). Even so, looking for the silver lining is a valuable elaboration that changes how one feels by adding depth and positive range to one's emotional experience (e.g., Nowlan et al., 2016). Life review therapy assumes that beyond increasing the specificity of memories, the positive content is critical. When working with older adults, some have argued that the "more positive the content of the reminiscence, the greater the therapeutic benefit" (Parker, 1995, p. 523). This positive alternative perspective is a psychological elaboration that gets the ball rolling, increasing its impact over time in a positive loop as already described with self-affirmations (Cohen & Sherman, 2014).

Experience as a Gift: Not Resolved, but Rosy Nonetheless!

Focusing on the positive aspects of a narrative does not cancel out the reality of negative aspects within a personal narrative. However, it does increase positive emotion and provides an overarching attitude. Considering the positives that should be enjoyed in one's life despite whatever negatives one has endured becomes a thematic intention. For some, the existential position may be that experience itself is inherently valuable, even if it is mixed, and living that experience is a gift not to be taken for granted.

Qualitative feedback from participants in a study that compared memory specificity training (which explores positive, negative, and neutral memories) with life review therapy (which focused on positive memories in particular) revealed that the latter may be better suited for older people. Participants commented that the opportunity to reminisce on positive events from the past was not only enjoyable, but it seemed to frame their life story in ways that led to gratefulness and satisfaction (Leahy et al., 2017). Speaking of the process, one client stated,

> I feel that focusing on so many memories which have been temporarily forgotten has helped me to appreciate that my life has been filled with happy experiences. Looking back has made me feel amazingly lucky and grateful for all the positive influences in my life. This gives me a feeling of peace and satisfaction. (p. 173)

Here, the recollection of positive events serves as a framework of interpretation for the rest of life. The top-down process also fosters an attitude with which one contemplates life, influencing what aspects of experience one attends to most. Another client in this study remarked,

> It has helped me to bring many happy memories to the forefront. Any unhappy memories I was able to cope with and realize how lucky I was to be able to overcome them and how much stronger it has made me. I hope it will help me and others for the future. (p. 173)

The older adult population in this study also leveraged a psychological distance from the various challenges of earlier life. This is a critical aspect by which positive meaning making may function differently depending on one's stage of life and relative to the issue at hand. As a client observed, "I recalled incidents that at the time I didn't think [of] as happy, but now, many years later, I have realized they were" (Leahy et al., 2017, p. 173). This is how a straight elaboration of enough narrative context (i.e., without effortfully transforming, reframing, or reinterpreting) can lead emotional content to mean something else from what it did at the time it occurred.

In the various ways discussed in this section, psychological elaboration can be done with a deliberate intention to look for beauty, count your lucky stars, find the humor, express gratitude, and appreciate the wonder of life. This intentionally positive elaboration contributes to change.

TELLING THE STORY OF EMOTION

Psychotherapy research has also explored the specific features of how clients tell stories. The reason for tracking narrative changes moment by moment is that identifying microprocesses in how a story is formulated could help clinicians identify adaptive and maladaptive ways of working with emotion. Studying the intertwined relationship between narrative and emotional experience has led to the development of several coding systems. The narrative emotion process coding system (Angus et al., 2017; introduced in Chapter 17, this volume) and the innovative moments coding system (Gonçalves et al., 2011) are two conceptually distinct methods of tracking how narratives change in a range of psychotherapies for diverse clinical concerns. These methods have independently identified emerging patterns in how clients (re)formulate their narratives during psychotherapy and how those patterns relate to recovery (Angus et al., 2017).

At the end of Chapter 17, I described a handful of narrative formulations that are problematic (Angus et al., 2015). Examples included the superficial story (i.e., an overly general account lacking emotional detail) and its counterpoint, unstoried emotion (i.e., a story with intense emotional content but lacking in concrete narrative signposts). Both these kinds of stories lack detail. The first does not have enough emotion, and the latter does not have enough in terms of plot and characters. When first introducing narrative processes, it was sufficient to highlight these as obstacles for working with emotion. But I now explore the issue further in a discussion of change. What happens if one systematically adds detail to enrich narratives that previously were lacking?

Narrative Process Goes Beyond the Elaboration of Content

Psychological elaboration and adding narrative context represent a quantitative change. When stories are further elaborated, there are simply more details and more nuance, so the change underfoot is easily formulated as more specificity. However, there is more to this than meets the eye. Adding richness also creates downstream effects, where a tipping point in increased specificity eventually renders the emergence of a different narrative. What began as a quantitative elaboration of content eventually yields a qualitative change in process. Clients not only feel more, but they also come to feel differently. This narrative change has an affinity to how expanding one's emotional awareness also leads to emotional change (Chapter 7). Similarly, the elaboration of narrative leads not only to the conscious revealing of more story but the construction (i.e., invention or creation) of a new and hereto unexplored story.

Narrative Markers Are Associated With Recovery

Emotional trouble, whether transient or chronic, has characteristic narrative signatures that reveal themselves both in content as well as in the process of their construal (e.g., unstoried emotion, superficial story, empty story, same old story; as described in Chapter 17). Changing those problem narratives, however, requires a working through. In narrative terms, this denouement is when a chain of events comes to some climax and the strands of plot are then brought to some conclusion. In the context of psychotherapy, Angus and colleagues (2017) conceptualize these later passages as transition markers, which eventually reach their conclusion in the form of change markers.

Stories of Transition

The evolving narrative clients use to formulate their stories of personal difficulty can change in at least two ways. First, the prevalence with which problem markers are observed diminishes over the course of a successful treatment, a macro-change most evident among those with the strongest treatment outcomes. This general trend applies regardless of clinical presentation, diagnosis, or treatment modality. In other words, as people become psychologically healthier, they decrease the frequency with which they relay their experience using unstoried emotion, superficial stories, or empty stories, and they are less likely to recapitulate an experience using the same old story (Aleixo et al., 2021; Boritz et al., 2017).

Second, while depression, generalized anxiety, and complex trauma may manifest through different features of narrative construction, evidence also points to an equifinality in the narrative processes that mark one's path toward recovery. Although presenting problems may be associated with varying kinds of stories, there seems to be a convergence toward healthy change such that good treatment outcomes make use of increasingly similar narrative processes. Thus, narrative problem markers are offset or replaced by an increasing count of contrasting narratives, which are qualitatively different.

Angus and colleagues (2015, 2017) identified four transition markers that capture narratives whereby clients begin to explore and destabilize what was previously a dominant and problematic self-narrative. They are

- *inchoate story* (i.e., focusing inward and a search for new symbols or words, where the speaker actively gropes toward a new development in feeling or thinking),

- *experiential story* (i.e., engaging, enacting, or reexperiencing an autobiographical memory),

- *reflective story* (i.e., explaining a general pattern or developing an insight about one's beliefs, feelings, and intentions), and

- *competing plot lines* (i.e., when a minority voice or alternative perspective is elaborated in opposition to what was a dominant problematic narrative).

Each of these transition markers challenge the continuity of what was a speaker's initial (problematic) approach to interpreting their emotional experience. Transition markers have been observed to emerge more often in the middle or late phases of successful psychotherapy. The pattern has been observed in the treatments of depression (e.g., cognitive, emotion-focused, and client-centered therapies), generalized anxiety disorder (e.g., motivational interviewing plus cognitive behavior therapy), and complex trauma (e.g., emotion-focused therapy; Aleixo et al., 2021).

Stories of Change

Narrative formulations invariably demand some form of conclusion. In line with equifinality, only two markers have been suggested to capture productive end states in the narrative change process. The *discovery story* and the *unexpected outcome* are characterized by their respective articulations of an adaptive and novel rendition of one's personal story (Angus, et al., 2015). The markers entail both emotional and behavioral change in how one is responding to an experience. In a discovery story, the emphasis is on articulating some novel understanding. It occurs more often, for example, in the resolution of depression as compared with clients who were in the same treatment but remained unchanged (Boritz et al., 2014). In contrast, the unexpected outcome story entails a sense of surprise, pride, or relief. The marker occurs more often, for example, among clients who have recovered from generalized anxiety than those who are unchanged (Khattra et al., 2020).

Change markers represent accounts of personal transformation. They have also been thought of as innovative moments, which identify a narrative's tipping point toward positive personal change (Gonçalves et al., 2011). A chief example is *reconceptualization*, an innovative moment that challenges some problematic narrative that was previously dominant. This moment in a story affords the meta-perspective of both the process of change as well as the lived experience of that change (Gonçalves et al., 2017). Reconceptualization is the precise moment of innovation that gives new meaning to reflection, protest, or action. The event also resonates as a visceral experience, and this internal validation signals that change is taking place. Such narrative markers appear more often in the conclusion of successful treatments of depression, generalized anxiety disorder, and complex trauma (Aleixo et al., 2021).

Narrative Flexibility and Specific Patterns of Change

Problem markers are followed by transition markers and in turn by change markers. These are the kinds of narratives most characteristic of the beginning, middle, and end of an evolving story. There may also be canonical pathways of narrative formulation that more efficiently usher clients from problem markers through to transition markers (Aleixo et al., 2021; Macaulay & Angus, 2019). One way of understanding this is that transition markers serve as the narrative antidote to problem markers or perhaps that they simply provide an account that described the process of change. Early in treatment, the status quo of problematic narratives represents a force that must not only be confronted but also needs to be countered by a new manner of narrative formulation. This observation helps us understand narrative construction as a dynamic system, particularly when it comes to consolidating healthy and lasting change over successive versions of a story (A. Pascual-Leone, Yeryomenko, et al., 2016; Stiles et al., 2004). For example, as a person becomes more aware of how a past trauma has adversely impacted them, the individual may begin to protest that same old story of being stuck, and an elaboration of this protest marks the emergence of a competing plotline—a transition heralding their readiness for change (Macaulay & Angus, 2019).

Other examples of narrative change emerge bottom up are empty and superficial stories that are often abstract and externally focused may be followed by experiential stories, which explore autobiographical specificity from a first-person perspective. Or, in examples of change that are actuated top down, unstoried emotion may transition through inchoate and reflective stories, where the individual searches for meaning and then formulates a way of understanding their preverbal experience (Khattra et al., 2020; Macaulay & Angus, 2019; see also Chapter 17, this volume). These clinical observations are provocative but need to be scrutinized using larger contrasting samples, and they may also be influenced by the treatment approach being used (as suggested by Figure 17.1).

The junction between stories is a growth point, where meaning emerges and where a new set of feelings are often experienced.[9] From a bird's eye view, the overall narrative appears to advance through a smooth progression, but from the surface of lived experience, the dialectical construction of junctions is a much more punctuated, stumbling, and recursive process. The *return to problem* marker describes a phenomenon in which a person oscillates between the dominant narrative and an emerging voice of challenge but then returns to the dominant framework by default. Returning to a problem is a marker that typically appears in the early and middle stages of a client's treatment (Ribeiro et al., 2014). This is what narrative continuity looks like when the author is ambivalent.

Shifting between narrative markers is a dynamic process over the course of one or more sessions, and most clinicians will be intimately familiar with that unfolding of a story during the therapeutic hour. *Narrative flexibility* refers to an individual's ability to engage and symbolize their experience using a range of frameworks for storying a given set of events. Ultimately, consolidating a story requires "one's ability to integrate narrations of what happened, with emotional processing of how it felt, in order to determine what it means . . . or more specifically, one's ability to shift between these modes" (Boritz et al., 2017, p. 667). This flexibility is more prominent in the sessions of clients who eventually recover during therapy as compared with those who do not make meaningful treatment gains.

Irrespective of whether examining emotion-focused, client-centered, or cognitive therapies, the probability of narrative shifting increased over the course of therapy for those who eventually recover from depression, whereas it decreased for clients who would remain depressed. In fact, the duration of time a client spent elaborating narrowly within any single kind of narrative was inversely associated with good outcome. In short, clients who recovered from depression shifted more often during their treatment sessions, but they also tended to do so in a positive direction, such as advancing from problem narratives to transition narratives or from transition narratives to change narratives. In contrast, stagnation in treatment and the lack of meaningful change was associated with shifting upstream or, in other words, the return to a problem (Boritz et al., 2017; Ribeiro et al., 2014). From a narrative perspective, getting stuck in a single mode of storytelling may be tantamount to getting stuck in depression.

Stiles and colleagues (2004) have conducted a host of theory-building case studies on how clients slowly assimilate the problematic experiences they are working on in psychotherapy. Researchers have tracked a client's different internal voices (e.g., perspectives, plot lines, parts of the self) both moment by moment and session by session (Honos-Webb et al., 2003). At first, clients may avoid or ward off a key aspect of their experience. Then it emerges as part of a vague awareness, followed by a sharper problem statement. This clarification results from the confrontation between conflicting plotlines. Irrespective of clinical concern, treatment, or research method, findings consistently show the encounter between these internal voices is a critical process of change. The struggle between voices leads to new emotion as well as new insight, followed by resourcefulness and, finally, an integrative mastery (Brinegar et al., 2006; Stiles et al., 2004). However, like all dialogical processes, the patterns are nonlinear. This toggling between narrative perspectives is something that will be picked up later (in Chapter 22) as a basic narrative mechanism of how emotion changes.

Is the Story a Description or an Agent of Change?

From an assessment perspective, resolution and closure are outcomes that are substantively distinct from symptom change, but they still represent a narrative appraisal of someone's health care status (Boucher et al., 2024). Even so, the stories we tell about our emotional problems are essentially working models that we invent to represent interrelations among meanings that unfold over time (i.e., the structural order of a process). Those narrative models can be either rich descriptions about what is happening, or they may be causal mechanisms that directly facilitate the change. Problematic narratives signal psychological trouble, but they also maintain it; both are true. Even markers of transition or change can similarly serve as either descriptive or causal accounts. These two functions are intertwined through varying temporal moments in the process.

Notice there is an epistemological parallel in the way finding the right words at the micro level (see Chapter 6) and formulating one's story at the macro level each contributes to shaping emotional experience. The blurring between *narrative process* (i.e., the creative act of storing as a mechanism of change) and *narrative outcome* (i.e., the story as a descriptive retrospective account) may seem like an artifact and the result of poor theory or of methodological shortcomings, but it is not. Narrative change is inherently iterative, something that is obviated in the meta-processes of narrative identity and life stories (see Chapter 21). Sometimes the function of narrative is primarily descriptive as the retrospective documentation of what happened (i.e., an outcome of change). At other times, a comparable narrative will function as a vehicle for catalyzing change through the act of storying it (i.e., a mediating process of change).

This dual relationship that narrative has with change is why, in depressed people, therapeutic change is evidenced both in the fact that clients who are improving become less likely to narrate their experience in an overgeneralized manner and also in the fact that the life stories they tell will evolve, with the individual perceiving their life through a new lens (Boritz et al., 2014, 2017).

So although treatment success could be the result of processes unrelated to narrative, those positive changes will nonetheless be reflected in a narrative description of personal change. For example, when a client suffering borderline personality disorder mastered certain skills for emotion regulation, it was captured by her new sense of identity. As the client reflected, "I'm different now. I can have intense emotions without falling apart or getting overwhelmed and acting impulsively" (T. Boritz, personal communication, March 14, 2019).[10] This description then becomes a new point of departure and a revised platform for narrative processes to interpret future experiences. The description of change becomes a framework for change.

The issue has also been discussed at the macro level of life stories and narrative identity and has led to similar conclusions from research on autobiographical stories (see Chapter 21). A case in point comes from an extensive study on the stories of ex-convicts, which is particularly illustrative given the binary nature of reoffending (Maruna, 2001). The stories of ex-convicts were described as reflecting either generative scripts or condemnation scripts. At the same time, individuals were either actively involved in criminal behavior or desisting from drug use and crime. The implicit drive for coherence between one's identity and one's story appears to be central to what may be a complex and circular process. The study concluded that for these individuals, success in their criminal reform depended to some degree on the way their personal narratives were constructed and how such narratives were used (Maruna, 2001).

The different levels at which narrative process is discussed and to what end (e.g., modeling to describe what happened vs. modeling to make it happen) need to be better clarified. Research still needs to identify moderating factors that determine what way narrative modeling will be used (i.e., descriptively or causally). Moderators of when narrative may become a more causal factor in shaping emotional change include when someone is within a critical period of their life (e.g., during early adulthood, in palliative care), being triggered by certain events to reformulate one's narrative framework (e.g., after discovering a betrayal), critical moments where one affirms one's identity (e.g., explaining an act of personal courage), and the role of social accountability (e.g., when one fulfills expectations set out by one's previously declared narrative). Studying precisely when moderators like these might switch the narrative processes into playing a causal (rather than just descriptive) role in personal change provides critical directions for future research.

Open-Ended Story: The Promise of a Dot-Dot-Dot

A man who returned to university later in life to complete his undergraduate degree visited my office hours to discuss his career direction with me as a professor. Although he was doing well in my course, he referred to himself as an academic failure because of how and when he had first dropped out of school so many years ago. I noticed the narrative he told was truncated and did not yet integrate the full meaning of his having now returned to school.

Elaborating one's story around some target emotion is about extending the meaning that surrounds (and informs) that feeling. This chapter has explored several specific strategies for elaborating meaning, but the most basic way of generating meaning is simply to keep on elaborating. As the epigraph to this chapter points out, you are bound to get somewhere if you go on long enough. The more time one spends earnestly exploring a story, its contradictions, and its possible interpretations, the more likely one is to stumble upon something helpful, useful, healthier. In its simplest form, this is just an issue of time on task. Keeping the story open allows one to incorporate more content into one's formulation of events.

A client of mine who suffered from depression strongly identified with the story of herself as a failed musician. However, when this failure was further contextualized by a broader and more inclusive perspective on her own life, then her narrative was extended to include several vindicating anecdotes. Neither of us had anticipated how a more complete life narrative would come to include such heartfelt stories about her having closely mentored several talented young artists. Those stories had previously been sequestered from the client's sense of self such that her "lived story" of the past had not been fully reflected in the "told story" of her life. After formulating a richer story, her feelings about herself changed, and she began making new life goals.

Even when there is no counterfactual evidence, there is tremendous power in the simple affirmation that one's story is not yet finished. Canadian speaker Neil Pasricha (2019) has referred to this as adding an ellipsis at the end of personal strife, such that adding a dot-dot-dot to the end of a narrative or adding "yet" to the end of a sentence (or doing both) essentially keeps one inherently open to further change—for example, "I don't know how to waltz . . . yet!" (p. 17). As discussed in Chapter 4, emotional engagement is what keeps one in touch with immediate feelings. Similarly, an ellipsis is a narrative device for keeping one's story open and amenable to future reworkings. Remaining engaged and curious in the narrative unfolding of lived events essentially keeps the story open beyond the next page.

As this chapter shows, psychological elaboration creates not only more contextual meaning, but it also affords qualitative changes because of its ongoing development. The continued unfolding follows from a bidirectional interchange between the storyteller and the experience of that story. In the end, a critical feature of this change mechanism is that the process of psychological elaboration is not teleological or driven by a predefined outcome objective. Rather, the process is deeply exploratory, continually unfolding from the horizon of where one last left off.

ENDNOTES

1. This key idea was first introduced in Chapter 7 at the micro level of symbolizing emotion that is in awareness. But the same observation holds true here at the macro level when emotion is interpreted through stories (see also Chapter 17).

2. The language of "storing" and "searching" for memories, as if they were concrete entities with some location, must not to be taken literally. "Searching one's memory" is a metaphor, referring more properly to the dynamic construction of an event in one's mind. And rather than any literal "recall," that construction is shaped by a multitude of contextual factors (see Chapter 19).

3. There are several likely mechanisms that produce this retrieval bias, including functional limits in terms of metacognitive control, entrenched personal styles of rumination or avoidance, and even defensiveness (Dimaggio et al., 2020; D. B. Stern, 1997; Williams et al., 2007).

4. Deficits in either immediate emotional awareness (reviewed in Chapter 6) or overgeneralized narratives (this chapter) are each pervasively related to psychopathology. The gender differences observed across these epistemological levels are also congruent, such that men have higher base rates than women in both alexithymia and overgeneralized memories. This further supports a parallel between these two kinds of processing. Nevertheless, the connection between alexithymia and overgeneral memories has not been systematically examined.

5. In some family cultures, emotions are considered uninteresting or an undesirable focus of conversation (see "Shallow Levels of Affective Processing" in Chapter 4 and "The Development of Narrative" in Chapter 21). This also applies more generally to the need for narrative specificity.

6. This is not the same as psychodynamic repression. *Repression* is when a person has some specific knowledge or thoughts that they actively try to block or even lie to themselves about because the details are too psychologically painful to revisit. Thus, repression is a motivated forgetfulness where on some level the person knows what they are avoiding, masking, or denying. In contrast, *unformulated experience* represents an earlier step upstream from repression where the person has not had the painful thought as such. The person does not even really know what they are avoiding, only that they are delaying engagement with certain kinds of content. The experience may be unformulated because an individual has not had sufficient opportunity or time on task, or perhaps they have a vague sense of foreboding and avoid even the preliminary trappings of what such a thought might entail, or both. Whatever the case, unformulated experience essentially means one has not yet even gone there (see also Chapter 4).

7. Transcranial magnetic stimulation is another neurological treatment that can and has been used in humans to alleviate depression (Perera et al., 2016), although that treatment does not intervene at a level of specificity regarding the valence of individual memories.

8. The terms cognitive restructuring, cognitive reappraisal, and cognitive reframing are all used somewhat interchangeably in the literature. The term *cognitive restructuring* had appeal in clinical psychology probably because it appears to mechanize the notion of psychological change. But much like the term *emotional processing*, that term is only a label for a puzzle, not an explanation of change (see Chapter 1). One would be hard pressed to identify any personal change that does not involve some level of cognitive change. So there is some artifice in the use of this language. I avoid the term "cognitive restructuring" in this book, which is also somewhat esoteric outside clinical circles. Instead, I favor more concretely descriptive terms such as (cognitive) "reframing" and "positive elaboration" (i.e., positive reappraisal).

9. This idea of sequences in the type of narratives someone uses is reminiscent of the sequences in emotion discussed as a different process in Chapter 15 and 16. However, emotional sequences refers to the order of felt experiences themselves, while narrative sequences refer to shifting across different interpretive frameworks and their corresponding sets of contextual information.

10. I am grateful to Dr. Lynne Angus and Dr. Tali Boritz (both at York University) for their insightful exchanges with me, clarifying how narratives serve this multifunctional role.

19

We Have Relationship With Our Memories

Revising the Metadata

When it comes to influencing autobiographical memory, the cue is everything.

—ALAN SCOBORIA[1]

Truthiness. . . . We're not talking about truth, we're talking about something that seems like truth—the truth we want to exist.

—STEPHEN COLBERT

Stories serve up an easily available frame of reference for remembering and sewing together so many pieces (e.g., insights, new feelings, novel perspectives) that pertain to a complex and nonlinear web of personal change. Research on memory retention shows that constructing stories out of a set of words can help one remember six to seven times more words than if one used rote memory and rehearsal. That stories are more memorable than isolated facts is not too surprising, but there are few interventions with effects of such magnitude, increasing retention from 13% without narrative to 93% with the use of narrative (Bower & Clark, 1969). In much the same way, the rehearsal of stories helps us retain what happened to us. But our personal stories are more than a memory aid; in fact, they are carefully curated selections of events. We also have relationships with those memories; we relate to them in various ways and have feelings about the recalled events. Sometimes the stories we remember feel close at hand or deeply definitive of who we are. At other times, they feel unfinished or are quickly dismissed.

https://doi.org/10.1037/0000460-020
Principles of Emotion Change: What Works and When in Psychotherapy and Everyday Life, by A. Pascual-Leone
Copyright © 2026 by the American Psychological Association. All rights reserved.

STORIES ARE BOTH MEMORABLE AND POINTS OF REFERENCE

Even before considering its impact on working with emotion, narrative serves as a mediator for memory, and that potentiates personal change in a monumental way. Relating this to clinical work, for some people and in some families, certain stories about what happened in the past are never externally shared or even internally rehearsed. In some cases, what happened is never even formulated in terms of a coherent story with a beginning, middle, and end. Whether positive or negative, what happened is harder to remember (and to work with) without having a specific narrative as some point of reference or to act as a container to collect the pieces of an experience.

Furthermore, although other forms of emotional processing (e.g., awareness, insights, changes in arousal, sequences of feeling) have critical impacts at the moment-by-moment level, part of carrying those changes forward is that the emotional processing event in which one started to feel differently can also be explicitly recalled as the story of change (Chapter 18). This thematic organization helps guide the reconstructive process of recall. It also sets a tentative trajectory or agenda for the continuation of that construction because one typically picks up the story wherever one last left off. When emotional processing events are packaged into a story, they can be revisited, extending the impact of what may have happened at a single moment in time. Then the process of revisiting, rehashing, and fleshing out experiences in therapy allows the client to set the stage for future sessions and helps them gain a greater grasp of their feelings and unmet needs (Gonçalves et al., 2017). Psychological elaboration was the topic of Chapter 18, but once a memory or story becomes a point of reference, there is yet another layer of significance that comes into play. That is the focus of this chapter.

We have a relationship with our memories, particularly the emotional ones, as well as the narratives we then construct to recall and tell those stories. Those ways in which we relate to our autobiographical narratives, at their most basic, are appraisals of the event. This *metadata*[2] corresponding to one's memories evaluates and weighs the contents of autobiographical narratives. For memories, that second layer of meaning represents an ongoing implicit set of judgments about what we seem to recall in relation to our sense of self and its significance in our life. In short, we cherish certain memories and earmark others as being somehow definitive of who we are, while still other memories are dismissed as trivial derailments from what is perceived as the overarching narrative (e.g., the true story of one's life). Changing implicit appraisals such as these only requires that a given memory becomes objectified and set apart from the present experience. These phenomena are relevant to emotional processing because the personal meanings one attributes to life events are partly a function of context and the way in which events are retrieved from memory. This auto-editing within the recall and narrative processes is often tacit and ongoing, but it can also be the result of deliberate manipulations.[3] This chapter explores the ways in which our relationships with specific memories (i.e., the metadata) quietly influence one's emotion through the narrative.

Metadata: What Is Subject to Change?

The veridicality of a memory is constantly being reevaluated in the context of newly emerging information. Said another way, the issue here is about the truthiness of a memory. As cited in one of this chapter's epigraphs, Stephen Colbert quipped about this in another arena. In short, people systematically try to reconcile opposing sources of evidence (e.g., the memory at hand vs. any presenting evidence on the contrary). Thus, the circumstances under which one recalls an autobiographic memory will alter how that recollection is constructed and is influenced by relatively subtle changes to the soliciting cues. This is true even when the memories in question are about *life transitions*—events typically associated with important impacts to the way people perceive themselves, the way they understand the world or engage others, and consequentially, how they live their lives (Boucher & Scoboria, 2015). Even attributions of meaning that are ostensibly fixed in their relation to significant events of the past can and will change as a function of the conditions under which the memory is retrieved.

There are several major ways in which our appraisal of an autobiographical memory may change (Boucher & Scoboria, 2015; Mazzoni et al., 2010; Scoboria et al., 2014, 2015). First, our *confidence in the accuracy* of a memory (or belief) that the event occurred as one recalls it is continually being reassessed and is subject to change. Second, the degree to which one feels as if *one can easily recall vivid and perceptual features* of a memory is another evaluative process. Third, autobiographical events may have *a sense of coherence*, or they may feel disjointed and incomplete. Fourth, when we recall an autobiographical narrative, the degree to which *the event seems psychologically distant or near* will shift based on several elements including contextual features during the moment of recollection. And fifth, autobiographical events may have a *sense of closure* or they may feel open and unresolved. Lastly, *centrality*—the degree to which a narrative is considered important, emblematic, or definitive to one's identity—is also subject to change (Pals, 2006). Whereas the contents of a memory may change through other processes, the kind of appraisals described here speak to changes in the ongoing relationships we have with our memories, which nevertheless shape what the memories mean.

What Influences How We Relate to a Memory?

Two factors are inextricably linked to the recall of autobiographical narratives. They are elaborated in later chapters, but I mention them here by way of introduction. One is the role of self-concept as an overarching framework for interpreting experience (see Chapter 21). The other is the level of construal at which one examines the autobiographical content, which represents the scope or level of analysis for recollection (see Chapter 22). These are ever-present factors that inform and are informed by the moment-by-moment generation of autobiographical narratives.

However, in this chapter I explore a range of other factors that are ubiquitous to both the therapeutic process and everyday life, including "social feedback, event plausibility, alternative attributions, general memory beliefs, internal event features, consistency with external evidence, views of self/others, and personal motivation" (Scoboria et al., 2015, p. 545). These determinants are essentially metadata that influence the way people relate to their stories during the moment of recollection and the narrative construction that follows. They are critical dimensions by which we dynamically appraise the value and significance of each personal narrative.

EMOTION CHANGES WITH THE METADATA OF A MEMORY

Appraisals about one's belief in, distance from, and sense of closure regarding autobiographical memories are only somewhat independent from one another, and these judgments one makes are very much contingent on one's presiding mental frame of reference.

Belief, Accuracy, and Recollection

Believing that an event occurred and being able to recall that event are not as strongly associated as is commonly thought (Scoboria et al., 2014). This is already apparent from statements like "I don't remember much, but what I think happened was . . ." (i.e., low recollection, high belief) or other statements like, "Well, I'm not sure, but that's how I remember it!" (i.e., low belief, high recollection). However, experiments on autobiographical memory clearly show that these are indeed distinct elements of the narrative experience, and they are each influenced by their own sources of information. More specifically, the recollection of an autobiographical event was predicted by it including perceptual features, reexperiencing, and felt emotion (but those same characteristics did not predict belief in the event). In contrast, whether someone believed an autobiographical event had indeed occurred was most strongly predicted by their judgments about the event's plausibility (Scoboria et al., 2014).

This has interesting implications for understanding the deep role therapeutic enactments and imaginal dialogues have in therapeutic change. For example, particularly in humanistic–experiential approaches, clients are sometimes encouraged to introduce tacit or even new aspects of their emotional experience during a reenactment (e.g., Therapist: "Say what was left unsaid and speak your truth"). At other times, clients are guided to role play significant others with whom they have unfinished business (e.g., Therapist: "Switch chairs, be the mother you never had. What would she say if she could have responded? In her heart of hearts, if she could have heard you, what does she say?"). When this happens, clients know full well that the content is being fabricated, even if it is elaborated from some aspect of reality. Yet so long as it is perceptually vivid, emotionally meaningful, and at least somewhat plausible, it will likely impact the future recollection of events.

Frequent questions from skeptical therapists who are first learning to use therapeutic enactments are the following: (a) How can one ensure that the enactment is an accurate reflection of events?, (b) How do we know it's true?, and (c) What is the point of enacting something that can never happen? However, these questions are misplaced because such interventions are not concerned with historical accuracy; rather, their aim is to generate personal meaning in the service of health care. The critical issue is whether the embellishment of an enactment is something that seems plausible within the client's frame of understanding.

As introduced in Chapter 10, this aspect of enactments is what Moreno (1958) referred to as *surplus reality*, which are psychological experiences that extend beyond the boundaries of physical reality and recorded history. Although an enactment may not reflect something that historically occurred, it can still carry some embodied truth in much the same way metaphors, legends, or mythological stories reflect an essential truth about the core issue. In other words, the abstraction of an invariant (see Chapter 17) can be incarnated through the creation of a fictitious conversation or enactment. This may be true for the enacted rendition of a single event, but it is also true for a person's autobiographical identity, which can be construed as a personal myth continually elaborated from adolescence onward (McAdams, 2019).

In other words, as a therapist might clarify, it doesn't necessarily matter what was said; instead, what matters is the message that was sent. The experience of childhood neglect is a good case in point, because the fact that "nothing really happened" is often precisely the problem but also makes it hard to concretize or grapple with as an injury (Paivio & Pascual-Leone, 2023). That reality might be captured in an enactment, for example, if the client says, "He never said much to me, but it was always like a disdainful indifference. It was as if he was saying 'you are just clutter, like a broken chair, you have nothing to offer.'" Moreover, research suggests the plausibility of an event, such as enacted dialogue, is the essential variable that subsequently leads one to have some belief in the memory's event as such. Meanwhile, the feeling and experiential aspects of an enactment are what alter the quality with which events are subsequently recalled (Scoboria et al., 2014). Even though the client knows certain parts of what they recall are not true (in a literal sense), the client may still come to feel as if they are true—or capture truth. This can be helpful for positive emotional change, especially when the enactment symbolically captures a previously implied meaning, one that was already there but perhaps was too abstract or too nebulous to consider until the enactment made it tangible.

In contrast, historical accuracy is obviously important in forensic efforts to be used in legal proceedings. Furthermore, the malleability of memory means therapists need to be judicious about the possible impact of either embellishing or questioning past events. For example, therapists should never suggest to their clients that they may have suffered maltreatment that the client does not remember (e.g., sexual abuse as a child). Doing so substantially increases the risk of creating false memories. That is particularly a risk when therapists are using discovery-oriented approaches or experiential enactments (Patihis & Pendergrast, 2019). Suggesting something may have happened but that it has been forgotten can lead a client to doubt themselves and lose their focus on the presenting concerns, and it will destabilize memory (Muschalla & Schönborn, 2021). Whether something happened or not (historically) should not be the focus of health care interventions. What matters is how the client interpreted what they do remember and how they feel about it, irrespective of historical accuracy.

Interestingly, in autobiographical memory, separation between the processes of recollection and belief can have either an additive or a subtractive effect. The influence that enactments and exploring surplus reality might have on increasing the vividness of later recollections is an example of the additive effect. But in exceptional cases, when external evidence is to the contrary of a given memory, people may withdraw their belief altogether from something they had previously held as an autobiographical memory. Researchers refer to this phenomenon as a non-believed memory (Scoboria et al., 2015). Almost 25% of the general population reports having had some experience like this (e.g., Client: "For a long time I used to think that happened to me, and I still seem to vividly remember it, but I suppose I must have imagined it"; Mazzoni et al., 2010).

Creating a Coherent Story

Part of the benefit of disclosing personal difficulties is that it implicitly requires one to organize and synthesize complex information about the events of one's life (Angus & Greenberg, 2011; Pennebaker & Chung, 2011). However, people are notoriously bad at thinking their way around negative emotion in an unstructured way. For example, when participants were asked either to think or to write about a distressing experience, those who spent time thinking privately about their difficulties received no benefit, even though the mode of processing was the only difference (Park et al., 2016). Thinking privately lends itself to unproductive rumination, possibly because it does not demand the same level of narrative coherence as making a verbally explicit statement. Conversation, and even more so writing it down, requires the development of a structured, intelligible, and coherent narrative. Creating order and resolving internal contradictions means that, to feel complete, all stories will have a beginning, middle, and end (Bruner, 1990). Formulating a coherent story is an aspect of emotional processing that is unique to working with narrative.

The Need to Be Whole

The drive for narrative coherence is likely hardwired in the brain and ultimately rooted in very basic neurobiological processes of pattern seeking, perceptual parsimony, and the detection of discrepancy versus coherence

(J. Pascual-Leone & Johnson, 2021; D. N. Stern, 2010). Furthermore, having narrative coherence is related to reduced symptomatology. For example, when adult survivors of childhood abuse were asked to write about their personal traumas, stories that were less coherent predicted their authors' suffering higher levels of trauma (Mundorf & Paivio, 2011). Admittedly, painful emotional events are sometimes related to intrinsically incongruent, fragmented, or truncated events, and there are many reasons for why this might be the case.

Sometimes people have memory gaps or the emotion and plot of what happened may be at odds. At other times, elements of the story may seem like an assortment of bizarre juxtapositions that need to be reconciled (Carpenter et al., 2016; Paivio & Pascual-Leone, 2023). For example, a client of mine who suffered complex trauma in childhood reflected on the chaos of her early adolescence and offered an abrupt revelation:

> I don't remember too much around it, but I'm pretty sure I had sex with my brother, more than once. It's embarrassing, but we both wanted it. It's so weird to think that! It's hard to make it fit together.

For my client, this was one of several disjointed fragments from her past that did not fit well into a coherent narrative, and that was disturbing to her. Whether her patchy recollection was explained by impression management or by motivated forgetting (i.e., repression) does not change the fact that her story felt confusing to her. Furthermore, as discussed in the opening of this chapter, stories that lack coherence are inherently hard to remember—like keeping a box of assorted puzzle pieces that seem not to belong together. These stories often go untold, remaining unrehearsed and therefore even more difficult to recall.

Whatever the content, one of the implicit processes during therapeutic disclosures is that people attempt to create accounts of themselves and renditions of their life events that are internally coherent. The narrative must be made explicit and not just vaguely thought about in generalities (Park et al., 2016). When one explores the specifics, the basic psychological process of creating coherence occurs irrespective of whether one anticipates having an audience to witness one's formulation or not (Frattaroli, 2006; J. Pascual-Leone & Johnson, 2021; Pennebaker & Chung, 2011).

Narrative coherence is also relevant to the overall story of change, which will eventually relate to one's life story and sense of self. In an example from research on narrative coherence in psychotherapy (Adler et al. 2013), a client contemplates the coherence among affective process:

> I anticipate therapy with excitement and trepidation. I know from the past that I can have significant growth periods doing therapy, but I also know that it can, at times, drag me into sadness and depression. (p. 842)

Another client makes efforts to coherently integrate disparate story lines into a larger picture:

> I am feeling like I was very lost for a very long time. Everything in my life revolved around everyone else and their needs rather than my own. Therapy is giving me a chance to realize that I still have my self, and it's helping me learn how to take care of myself first, even though it's really hard. (p. 842)

Furthermore, when the stories that clients tell from one psychotherapy session to the next were observably coherent, it predicted an impending sudden treatment gain in terms of symptom reduction and improved mental health (Adler et al., 2013).

Even so, the coherence achieved within a change narrative seems to be much more prominent in retrospective accounts of experiences that are already complete as compared with stories told about events that are still playing out. For instance, when clients in psychotherapy were asked to write reflections about their life after every session, there were no systematic changes in the narrative coherence across accounts (Adler, 2012). Arguably, as one continues to negotiate, work through, and then revisit personal difficulties, some aspects of one's ongoing narrative become increasingly retrospective in their construction. It is also possible that the narrative coherence in one's story of personal change represents a longer term outcome that is only apparent after other themes have already been developed (Adler, 2012). In fact, when people were asked to reflect on a time they were in psychotherapy and give a narrative account of how they changed, those with more coherent narratives also enjoyed higher levels of socioemotional development (Adler et al., 2007).

Feeling Coherent Beats Feeling Good

The sense that one's personality stays relatively consistent and stable over time and across range of situations is an integral part of one's self-concept. When one's self concept is at odds with the personal events one recalls, it creates instability within one's sense of self. This is a distressing experience and spurs on the drive to somehow create coherence. The research on autobiographical memory and its function in shaping the self reveals the need to foster a sense of self that is both coherent and favorable (Conway, 2005; A. E. Wilson & Ross, 2003). Furthermore, cognitive dissonance (i.e., psychological tension from disharmony between one's motives) is highest and most clinically relevant when one is confronted by inconsistencies with the values one holds most dear.

On the one hand, when the memory of a certain event characterizes the self in a way that seems different from one's self concept, it threatens one's sense of coherence (i.e., self-concept coherence). Then, this threat prompts efforts to reconcile how the target event and the self from the past relate to one's current self-view (Conway & Pleydell-Pearce, 2000). On the other hand, based on a separate motivation for self-enhancement, one might disown specific aspects of a memory (or the entire event) should they reflect poorly on one's sense of self. However, if the motives to be coherent and to be favorable ever conflict, it creates an internal tension or a "cognitive–affective crossfire" (Swann et al., 1987, p. 882). Under such circumstances, people tend to choose narrative coherence by verifying their self-perceptions over making efforts toward self-enhancement, which might have otherwise made them seem more favorable. For example, a person with low self-esteem is more likely to recall a past failure, tacitly satisfying their motive for self-coherence, at the expense of recalling other events that might offer self-enhancement.

This type of misleading situation is a frequent occurrence in psychotherapy, and it is probably one reason why self-critical processes are so pernicious: all things being equal, the basic psychological need to be coherent is stronger than the need to be good, lovable, or capable. As most therapists will already have witnessed, experimental research confirms that people with low self-esteem typically ignore positive information and will instead attend to negatively valanced information so long as it remains consistent with their presiding self-view (Libby & Eibach, 2011; Swann et al., 1987). For people who have suffered abuse (especially during childhood) or are in the wake of complex trauma, the most coherent and efficient way of understanding what happened (the natural conclusion) becomes something like "It's my fault." This explains why pushing for coherence too soon in a treatment process may be harmful. It also clarifies a key problem with treatment approaches that rely too heavily on the power of positivity when working with self-doubt and feelings of shame or inadequacy because the drive for coherence is simply more fundamental.

A drive for coherence in self-concept, beliefs, and goals is a subtle yet influential force in shaping narrative. When one encounters dissonant or other information that threatens a coherent sense of self, people will alter, distort, reinterpret, and at times fabricate renditions of a memory to maintain a current self-concept (Conway, 2005). This influence can act for better or for worse, so it is useful to consider the default conditions (e.g., in this case, a client's coherent self-concept) that will influence the telling and retelling of stories. For those who are particularly high in neuroticism and suffer from mental health and emotional challenges, this drive for coherence could create increased entrenchment of unhealthy memories if enacted without appropriate guidance. I suggest this is one of the reasons why rumination has consistently been found to be related to psychopathology (e.g., Aldao et al., 2010).

But coherence is relative to a given set of elements. Even if one pursues coherence above all else, there are various levels of abstraction at which one might establish that coherence. When local inconsistencies become apparent within one's personal narrative, the threat to self-coherence might be amended by integrating the painful discrepancy into a broader life narrative. A wider lens allows one to cite a turning point or some personal development to explain why who one was in the past is different from who one is now (Gonçalves et al., 2011; Habermas, 2019; Libby & Eibach, 2011; A. E. Wilson & Ross, 2003). Thus, the question becomes, coherence of what? It turns out that the level of construal that one mentally focuses on will essentially determine the type of coherence one seeks to create. This issue regarding metal focus and the level of construal one is poised to use during meaning making is the topic of Chapter 22.

Psychological Distance: Life Was Very Different Then . . .

In his novel *Slowness*, Milan Kundera (1997) poetically described how someone wishing to forget something that recently happened walks more quickly, as if the memory could be shaken off as one rushes forward and away from what happened. Meanwhile, the person struggling to recall the details of what occurred walks slowly and pensively, trying to slow the passage of other events as they recapture what happened and keeps the memory close at hand.[4] *Psychological distance* often refers to one's perception of how remote in time or space an experience was. Broader conceptions of psychological distance include not only the perceived temporal or physical distance but also the perceived social or hypothetical distance between a past experience and the present self (Trope & Liberman, 2010).

Judgments about this perceptual frame are also closely related to emotional processing. The more intense one's emotion about an event, the shorter the perceived psychological distance (Van Boven et al., 2010). Think of expressions like "It feels like it was only yesterday" or "If our love burns bright, the ocean doesn't seem so big after all." However, presenting symptoms also have a bearing on what one recalls and how close emotional narratives may seem. As mentioned in Chapter 18, people who suffer symptoms of depression report feeling psychologically distant from positive events they remember, whereas those who report symptoms of posttraumatic stress disorder feel the negative events of their life are psychologically near (Janssen et al., 2015).

Manipulating Psychological Distance

Various factors influence psychological distance, some of which are quite easy to manipulate. For example, the use of abstract terminology when construing past experiences increases psychological distance, whereas the use of concrete terminology decreases psychological distance (Liberman & Trope, 2014; Trope & Liberman, 2010). In addition, when stimuli come to mind more easily (e.g., are more cognitively fluent), they are perceived as psychologically closer and get construed in concrete terms (Alter & Oppenheimer, 2008; Van Boven et al., 2010). To manipulate cognitive fluency, researchers have simply changed the visibility of written words (i.e., stimuli that are easier to read are more cognitively fluent); other examples include the presence or absence of a priming word related to the stimulus of interest, or the pronounceability of a chosen stimulus word (Alter & Oppenheimer, 2008). The practical implication is that people can psychologically distance themselves from an experience and reduce negative emotion by essentially impeding their ability to think about it (i.e., decreasing cognitive fluency). This happens in everyday life when someone, for example, physically removes reminders of a relationship following a breakup or when one relies on unnecessarily technical and abstract language to discuss the death of a loved one.

Experiments that use mechanical interventions for regulating psychological distance recall a procedure in eye movement desensitization and reprocessing therapy. A central technique in that approach to psychotherapy has clients recount a traumatic narrative while asking them to simultaneously attend to external sensory stimulation (e.g., Therapist: "Don't stop talking, but I want you to try to keep your eye on my finger as it moves back and forth"; R. Shapiro & Brown, 2019). Systematically dividing the client's attention in this manner seems to be one mechanism by which eye movement desensitization and reprocessing therapy reduces the intensity of a client's emotional arousal (Landin-Romero et al., 2018). In contrast, other approaches to psychotherapy intervention will purposefully focus on a client's immediate emerging experience to decrease psychological distance and correspondingly heighten the vividness of emotion. For example, the clarity, brevity, and incisiveness of a therapist's reflection will enliven a memory being recollected and make it more present (Elliott et al., 2018). So, the way a therapist interjects can either widen or shorten a client's psychological distance from the story they are telling.

The use of third-person imagery in autobiographical memory and narrative is believed to act as a generalized mechanism for self-distancing, which in turn dampens emotional arousal (Gu & Tse, 2016; Holmes & Mathews, 2010) and may even be used to avoid more vivid experience (McIsaac & Eich, 2004). The relevance of this will be obvious to psychotherapists who are attending to how much clients seem to own their emotional experiences as they recount them. For example, a client remembered when, as a child, her parents forgot her birthday, says, "It doesn't feel good when people don't remember your birthday. It's like you just don't matter." In this example, the client speaks in generalities (e.g., "It doesn't feel good") but also speaks vaguely of other people when she knows very well that they are referring to a specific incident with her parents. Finally, in a common form of distancing, the client only refers to herself indirectly by speaking in second person (i.e., "your birthday" instead of "my birthday"). By comparison, as discussed in Chapter 10 on the vividness of imagery, research has shown that using a first person-perspective and introducing imagery is more emotionally evocative (Holmes et al., 2007).

Distancing From Experience: Avoidance or Closure?

A clinical perspective observes that people might create (and then feel) distance from their distressing memories for two general reasons, and these are related to different stages in the process of change and to different symptom outcomes. On the one hand, people may be motivated to use psychological distance defensively to stave off engagement with painful emotional experience. This is mainly emotional and situational avoidance, a short-term fix to cope with immediate distress, but it has potentially long-term consequences for people who fail to eventually work through the underlying issues (Chapter 3, this volume; McIssac & Eich, 2004). Part of the complexity here is that avoidance should not be reduced in categorical terms as a universally adaptive strategy. There may be a time and place for the healthy use of exactly this short-term fix (see Chapter 3, this volume; see also Hofmann & Hay, 2018).

On the other hand, a memory may feel distant precisely because it has already been sufficiently dealt with. Thus, working through various aspects of the issue and reaching closure will also impart the memory of distress with an increasing sense of (psychological) distance. Simply put, feeling that it is far behind you is indeed part of what defines closure in the sense of resolution (Boucher et al., 2024). Moreover, while avoidance and closure are two possible moments in the developmental process of change, each lending themselves to an individual feeling psychologically distant from their emotional experience, neither are absolute. The early emotional avoidance and the eventual downstream experience of closure should both be thought of as dynamic states of functioning that entail some flux depending on the circumstances under which one revisits the experience.

Beyond this relationship between psychological distance and states of resolution (or lack thereof), in some situations, self-distancing can also be used prescriptively as a strategy for indirectly preserving engagement before one tries to promote any change. Here, keeping one's distance is a short-term strategy to avoid direct confrontation, which would preclude further work. For example, for therapists trying to secure working relationships with people who have acted violently against their partners, asking about that perpetration of violence from an outside perspective is less evocative and a less confrontational way of exploring the treatment concern. For instance, a therapist might ask, "Is this a problem you have had for a long time? Is it mostly against your partner that you use violence?" (Lømo et al., 2019). Again, forensics issues like this are an interesting case in point, because while personally admitting the truth is critical within a legal framework, it may not be as essential in the arena of emotional change. Of course, having first-person experiences of primary and adaptive guilt typically move a person toward atonement, but getting someone to admit that something happened (e.g., that one perpetrated physical abuse) can be rife with cognitive dissonance. Sometimes it is more effective to offer perpetrators some face-saving measure. So, a therapist might engage the emotional issue more obliquely (e.g., Therapist: "Regardless of what happened or didn't happen, what might it have looked like to someone from the outside?"; Marshall et al., 2011).

The Objective Onlooker: Taking a Distance From One's Story
The use of self-distancing is believed to sometimes play an important role in objectively reflecting on oneself and one's emotional experience, which might be adaptive (Liberman & Trope, 2014). For example, among people suffering depression or bipolar disorder, self-distancing was a helpful procedure for reducing emotional arousal. And just as critically, adequate self-distancing is thought to be a key aspect of what distinguishes unhealthy rumination from productive self-reflection (Gruber et al., 2017; Kross & Ayduk, 2011). A series of experiments explicitly instructed people to think about their emotional challenges using either first-person pronouns (i.e., Client: "Why do I feel this way?") or assuming a third-person perspective by using their own name (i.e., Client: "Why does [client's name] feel this way?"). Results of these studies have consistently shown the linguistic nudge of adopting a third-person perspective helps people better regulate (i.e., control) their emotion so it does not negatively interfere with stressful performance-based tasks. A meta-analysis of these studies showed that participants' levels of anxiety did not moderate the results, suggesting the potential benefits of self-distancing applies across levels of symptomatology (Kross et al., 2014).

Research on the mechanisms of expressive writing showed that a day after doing a series of writing sessions, undergraduate students spontaneously used more self-distancing and adopted a third-person perspective. This, in turn, led to them feeling slightly less emotionally reactive 1 and 6 months after the intervention. Moreover, this chain (i.e., expressive writing leading to more self-distancing and then to reduced emotional reactivity) related the task to reduced physical symptoms (Park et al., 2016).

As seen in each of these research examples, psychological distance can be facilitated through relatively easy instruction. This extends to the context being implicitly presented by therapists as they organize a client to reflect on an autobiographical narrative, often implicitly from a third-person perspective. For example, one advantage of using written thought records and homework in cognitive behavior therapy to review what happened is that it deliberately reorients a client's vantage point to that of an external observer by watching and commenting on their own documented narrative about what happened. This disembedding (i.e., retrospectively looking at homework) is important because it helps clients both down-regulate emotion while also encouraging a conceptual analysis (e.g., Therapist: "I see from what you've written, you had a relapse on Friday. Hmm, okay, so what happened just before that? What might have been an alternative for you?").

Using the more distant observer perspective when reflecting on oneself is also related to the wise mind state described for clients in dialectical behavior therapy (Linehan, 2015). This and other mindfulness-based approaches to cognitive or behavioral treatment encourages clients to hold their emotional distress at a distance and take an attitude of nonattachment when navigating personal difficulties. One of the best psychological treatments for chronic pain is precisely this mindfulness-based approach of acknowledging one's pain as an unimpassioned observer (M. C. Davis et al., 2015). In these ways, individuals can manage emotional distress and pain by increasing psychological distance and emphasizing the broader context of meaning rather than being immersed in the sensory details of a distressing experience.

Wise reasoning can be thought of as recognizing the limits of one's own knowledge, considering the viewpoints of other people, accepting the value of compromise, and acknowledging the need for changes in the future. There is a popular notion that people are wiser when reasoning through other's social problems than when working through their own, and it stands up to experimental scrutiny (I. Grossmann & Kross, 2014). Moreover, a series of studies has clarified that wise reasoning comes with adopting a psychologically distant (rather than an immersed first-person) framework of understanding. Moreover, when people were instructed to use a third-person observer's perspective or imagine it was someone else's problem, creating that psychological distance eliminated the shortcomings of being enmeshed in one's own presenting difficulties. A replication study comparing younger adults (20–40 years) with older adults (60–80 years) found age alone had no effect, but the benefit that psychological distancing had on wise reasoning held across cohorts (I. Grossmann &

Kross, 2014). The adage has been that with age comes reason, but the wisdom of elders may be explained by their ability to maintain psychological distance.

Getting Closure

The construction of some satisfying ending to a narrative creates a sense of closure. Closure in cognitive and perceptual theories has its origins in Gestalt psychology (Bühler, 1926/1965; Köhler, 1929/1969). Part of the mental hardware in thinking organisms is such that one automatically synthesizes missing units to complete a visual or auditory configuration, thereby creating a perceived whole. This perceptual operating principal for seeking out a coherent unity in meaning also extends to behavioral and conceptual phenomena (J. Pascual-Leone & Johnson, 2021). Still, the fact that this is a fundamental perceptual–experiential principal of mental processing does not necessarily mean narrative closure is always successful. So, the organismic drive makes a lack of closure particularly distressing or painful when there are obstacles to obtaining it.

The measurement of psychological closure shows it is not a unitary construct. Closed memories are perceived as entailing a sense of clarity, mental liberation, emotional release, and behavioral deactivation as compared with open memories. Still, their finality might be captured simply in the way they are more psychologically distant (Boucher et al., 2024). When people remember events with more emotional detail, both in terms of intensity and the number of emotions people recall having, it predicts a lack of closure regarding those events (Beike & Wirth-Beaumont, 2005). Furthermore, there also seems to be some sex or gender differences, in that men tend to rate their memories as having more closure than women. Most importantly, getting closure to one's story is related to subsequent improvements in both psychological and even physical health (Beike & Wirth-Beaumont, 2005).

The spontaneous framing of stories to have endings at all is not self-evident. Even so, in discourse, this process is so automatic that it is easy to overlook the fact that a story ending is somewhat arbitrary. Without imposing narrative delimitations, life moves on, and there are always subsequent events that could be added on to extend the story. Sociocultural conventions are used to demarcate an ending (e.g., take a bow, draw the curtain, say "The End"), but there are also neuropsychological parameters related to how one determines the structure of suitable endings (D. N. Stern, 2010). The most critical issue here is that having closure is not an inherent property of narrative content per se. In other words, while an autobiographical memory about some lived experience may be unresolved, that recalled content might be appraised as being either open or closed. In short, within certain margins, the appraisal of having closure is a memory-related phenomenon and might be applied to any kind of event (Beike & Wirth-Beaumont, 2005). Even so, it is not usually a simple matter of choice.

Manipulating Closure

The simple passage of time predicts better narrative closure, and this is probably due to the normative fading affect that occurs in the recollection of events over time (Beike & Wirth-Beaumont, 2005). However, the reported experience of closure turns out to also be significantly influenced by the context in which a memory is recalled. Research on the properties of autobiographical narratives and from experiments in both clinical and social research show that having an explanation renders troubling stories more benign (e.g., Pennebaker & Chung, 2011). When events are unexplained, their emotional impact is both amplified and extended. Oddly enough, depending on the issue, sometimes the explanation in question does not even have to explain anything. For example, when participants were confronted with a puzzling interpersonal event but also given some pseudo-explanatory phrases (e.g., using causation words but without real substance), it reduced their emotion and facilitated a return to baseline more quickly than when participants were given the same information without the trappings of an explanation (T. D. Wilson et al., 2005).

A small body of research has examined the relationship between psychological closure and psychological distance. Psychological distance, whether it be temporal, conceptual, or from a shift in perspective is related to getting closure of troublesome autobiographical memories (Boucher, 2024). This is because having enough psychological distance opens a clearer view of the future, one that extends beyond the internal boundaries of the problematic event and assimilates it into a larger narrative of greater significance. This is essentially what is suggested when someone says, "I've lost the battle, but not the war." Creating psychological distance from the distress of a more local issue is what allows someone to arrive at a more integrated understanding of how they relate to the world, which guides future life choices. Changing the scope of mental analysis—for example, by directing someone's mental focus or prompting them to use a certain imagery perspective—mediates both psychological distance and closure (Gu & Tse, 2016). This is because attending at the level of autobiographical narratives changes the frame of reference and therefore the interpretive context of personal meaning. Recall Figure 17.1, which described self-understanding as existing on a continuum of epistemological levels (see also Chapter 22).

Working Toward Closure

Most emotional difficulties will first require personal work before they are resolved, and longstanding interpersonal grievances (e.g., unfinished business) represent a case in point. There is no skirting around the fact that closure requires people to effortfully undertake some emotional change process, one that goes beyond how the memory is cued (L. S. Greenberg, 2021; Paivio & Pascual-Leone, 2023). In short, the issue is not to foist closure when something has yet to be resolved but rather to see when a person's manner of engagement might enhance closure. For example, resolving complex relational trauma such as abuse may first require increased emotional awareness and then a sequential transformation of emotion (as discussed in earlier parts of this book). However, when the appropriate working through has been done, it will be helpful in psychotherapy to intentionally facilitate the closure of autobiographical memories. There are at least four processes that seem to be useful as one approaches closure.

Attend to external details. First, placing a relative emphasis on external details (e.g., plot, characters, historical context) rather than subjective experience seems to potentiate closure (Beike & Wirth-Beaumont, 2005). As suggested earlier, one needs to be mindful that emphasizing psychological distance could be an avoidance strategy, where one attempts to keep problematic material out of awareness. However, when people have already worked through enough of the issue, distancing could help implement a healthy commitment not to ruminate nor to perpetually reengage past events (McIsaac & Eich, 2004).

Have an explanation. Second, it will help to focus on what one understands about a troubling event and to elaborate some explanation. Already, focusing on external details moves to a less personal and more objective level of discourse. Conceptual understanding allows what happened to make sense, which strips away its mystery. For some people this sense of a lesson learned also offers a sense of (perceived) mastery.

Demarcate the past. Third, exploring the ways in which the past event is no longer relevant to one's current situation helps create closure (Beike & Wirth-Beaumont, 2005). An example of this latter point comes from a client of mine in his mid-30s who suffered some obsessive traits. Near the end of treatment, he came across pictures of past girlfriends while he packed belongings to move in with his newly wedded wife:

> I'm glad I kept them as long as I did to remember and compare while I was dating. I had these reflective feelings, like I dodged a bullet there, close but no cigar, that one broke my heart. . . . But, yeah, once I got married it didn't make much sense to keep 'em.

These fragments of his incomplete narratives and possible unfinished business are brought together and then laid to rest by reflecting on the larger narrative and committing to a new chapter in his life.

Other examples of demarcating the past to facilitate closure are routinely found in how therapists explore with their clients the origins of certain psychodynamic themes (Luborskuy et al., 1994). A therapist might explain, "Of course, as a kid you couldn't control your circumstances, but I guess it's different now as an adult." Or when exploring a client's transference, the therapist might contrast the nature of past and present relationships: "Yes, in some ways our ending therapy might feel similar to the old abandonments you suffered in the past, but maybe there are some important differences here too." In each of these examples, framing parts of the past as no longer relevant also suggests the present is a different story.

Make a choice. Fourth, the final step in getting closure is sometimes also an existential choice. At that final stage in the process, the way a narrative is framed becomes increasingly relevant because the act of closure is essentially a summative appraisal. Although one cannot simply impose closure, even when that possibility comes within reach, it's still not over until one decides it's over

(Paivio & Pascual-Leone, 2023; A. Pascual-Leone & Greenberg, 2007b). That is where the way we choose to relate to our stories becomes increasingly pertinent.

THE CENTRALITY OF REMEMBERED EVENTS TO ONE'S SELF-CONCEPT

All other processes being equal, the narrative framework within which one cues, retrieves, and explores autobiographical memories involve several moving parts (e.g., belief, accuracy, coherence, psychological distance, closure). However, even though they are highly complex, these various appraisals, motivations, and contextual features can all be relied on to shape emergent experience in a predictable way. In summary, both memories and the emotion they elicit will change based on the meaning context in which they are recalled. These changes are subtle, but they are also ubiquitous in the way we use language to construe the story of what happened (recall Alan Scoboria's conclusion in the epigraph of this chapter that "the cue is everything"). Furthermore, some of these changes are carried forward, often silently, into the next time one recalls the memory. Thus, the memory of what happened, what it felt like, and what it means silently evolves over time. Memory reconsolidation is one of the neural mechanisms of these changes to memory (see Chapters 13 and 17; Lane & Nadel, 2020).

People's judgments of the extent to which one remembers a life transition as having been personally impactful and relevant to one's sense of self is also subject to change. Moreover, the centrality one feels a given autobiographical memory may have to one's identity can change based on relatively simple manipulations to the social and meaning context within which the memory is being cued (Boucher & Scoboria 2015). This observation is important for psychotherapeutic work because clients often hold certain memories as emblematic events, which define them as who they are, rendering a sense of self. However, the assessment that a memory being recalled is defining of who one is and in what way is a perceptual construal of the individual client. For example, construing a traumatic event as central to one's identity is an appraisal that seems to maintain the debilitating symptoms of posttraumatic stress disorder. At the same time, however, an event's centrality is also the strongest predictor of posttraumatic growth. This mixed impact highlights that how one frames negative life events in relation to oneself can be a double-edged sword (Boals & Schuettler, 2011). While one may recall powerful emotional experiences from the past, they are not necessarily as defining of a person as they may seem, and changing the context of meaning can change that appraisal.

Furthermore, when discussing the identity function of autobiographical memories and the emotional experience that comes from engaging those memories, it is important to be aware of the inherent biases and the motives that shape someone's memories about themself. These change mechanisms are often part of the normal mental operators that allow the construal of meaning while reremembering, but they can also be psychodynamically motivated to (subconsciously) manage one's distress. Research on both autobiographical memory and narrative identity in the general population has highlighted the tension between stability and change in one's self-concept (McAdams, 2019). When our self-concept is favorable, we attend to the coherence of memories and the stability of those narratives. However, when what we remember about ourselves is less palatable, we tend to perceive ourselves as having changed, grown, and improved, often disparaging past selves and distancing from who we once were (A. E. Wilson & Ross, 2003).

Finally, there are a host of methods for expanding or narrowing the mental lens through which one evaluates the significance of personal events. The belief that events occurred as well as their accuracy and plausibility are all facets of a recollection (i.e., metadata) that vary and are continually appraised when working with difficult personal memories. Lastly, the psychological distance with which one engages an emotional experience and particularly the pronouns and imagery perspective one uses are powerful tools when working with emotion.

ENDNOTES

1. I am grateful for feedback of Dr. Alan Scoboria, University of Windsor, while writing this chapter. He was a clinical psychologist and prominent researcher of autobiographical memory. Sadly, he passed away during the writing of this book. He had joked about making a conference T-shirt with the quote in the first epigraph because he thought it summed up his program of research.
2. *Metadata* is a term used to refer to information about the substantive data. For example, if one takes a photo with a smartphone, the picture is the data content itself. However, there is also additional information about the date, time, and location where a photo was taken, which represents another layer of information (i.e., metadata).
3. Part of the point here is that "memory recall" is a misnomer, still used as a vestige from an outdated understanding of what it means to remember some event (see Alberini & Ledoux, 2013; Lane & Nadel, 2020). Memory is much more dynamic that previously believed. It would be more precise to refer to memory construction and reconstruction rather than to recall, but I will keep with the convention so as not to complicate the language. In short, remembering is more of a subjective process than the word "recall" would suggest.
4. Kundera poetically suggests that a personal concern seems to influence someone's speed of movement, but this is not just allegory. As cited in Chapter 9, neuroscience has shown how fast or slow one's movement is (e.g., walking, shifting gaze) both reflects and informs the value one assigns to objects or experiences (Shadmehr & Ahmed, 2020).

20

Stepping Out of the Frame

"I Am Myself and My Circumstances"

The only people who see the whole picture are the ones who step out of the frame.

—SALMAN RUSHDIE, *THE GROUND BENEATH HER FEET*

I am myself and my circumstance.[1]

—JOSÉ ORTEGA Y GASSET, *MEDITACIONES DEL QUIJOTE*

Sometimes what is a familiar part of someone's world is not what is good for them. When that happens, the impetus for change will often come top down, through an insight and then a deliberate choice. In his maxim cited in the epigraph, the philosopher José Ortega y Gasset observes that the self cannot be detached from one's context. Making this observation represents a moment of self-awareness where one dis-embeds enough to see the bigger pictures one is part of. More profoundly, he also suggests that one plays some role in the curation, creation, and ownership of one's circumstances. In everyday life, people may or may not be fully aware of the narrative framework they use when telling their life story even as it manifests their identity. However, at key moments, people may be prompted to recognize and reflect on their own frame of reference as it is being constructed. So, whereas narrative formulation itself is a process, extracting oneself from one's initial frame of reference and then making choices about that conceptualization is another kind of process. The latter process is the focus of this chapter.

https://doi.org/10.1037/0000460-021
Principles of Emotion Change: What Works and When in Psychotherapy and Everyday Life, by A. Pascual-Leone
Copyright © 2026 by the American Psychological Association. All rights reserved.

AWARENESS VERSUS REFRAMING: CONTRASTING BUT COMPLEMENTARY

Both emotional awareness and using narrative reflection to reframe one's circumstances are forms of meaning making (see Figure 17.1). Indeed, they even share similar neural profiles: increased activation in prefrontal cortex and decreased activity in the limbic system (Torre & Lieberman, 2018). Perhaps because of these similarities, comparative discriminations in the literature often fall short in articulating how reframing and awareness are operationally distinct. Nevertheless, they are dramatically different approaches to the generation of meaning (working either top down or bottom up; see Chapter 17). This section explains the complementary relationship between reframing and emotional awareness as principles of emotion change.

Is This Meaning About the Figure or the Background?

A moment of emotional experience and its associated narrative framework can be thought of as a figure–ground grouping as discussed in Gestalt psychology (Köhler, 1929/1969). Here, the figure is emotion and stands in juxtaposition to its background, which represents the circumstances or narrative context that surround an emotion. So, from the whole structure (i.e., the Gestalt) of an emotional experience, one could explore meaning as it pertains to either the figure or its relevant background. Both a psychodynamic interpretation and cognitive reframing (hereafter simply "reframing")[2] target the perception and understanding of external narrative events as the associated background.

So, in a using narrative reflection to reframe emotion, one focuses outward on the external context to reconsider one's situation or sociopersonal history. For example,

> The way I grew up taught me that even though I was ill-equipped, I was the only one responsible for the welfare of my younger siblings. So now, I assume every problem is mine to solve. No wonder I feel so desperate and alone at work! But actually, my workplace is full of other competent adults. I could probably even let others take the lead. There is no need to get so fired up, anyway. The stakes are not so high anymore either. Everything will be fine enough, even without me. It's worth a try!

This process elaborates the background as a context of meaning. In contrast, increasing experiential awareness is a process that targets the perception of internally felt experiences (i.e., the figure itself) by exploring one's immediate feeling and identifying underlying needs or wishes (Chapters 6 and 7). So, when increasing emotional awareness, a different kind of meaning is made as one focuses inward and elaborates the immediately lived experience. For example,

> I get to this place of feeling, like, "I'm the only one holding the bag." And it's too much! I feel burdened and alone. It's like this clawing feeling inside my chest. [*sigh, pause*] And I hold my breath. But what I need is some breathing room. I

wish I could trust others to help so I could rely on them. What I've always longed for is to feel I'm part of a team, a sense of camaraderie. If I felt that, I could relax.

These processes—narrative reflection and experiential awareness—differ in at least two important ways. First, they explore different content areas. A reframe (i.e., the first example) elaborates on the meaning of external stimuli, triggers, and what happened. These represent a change to the background (i.e., perceptual field) in a figure–ground grouping, and elaborating it gives revised meaning to a given emotion by providing more context. This kind of meaning making focuses on the interpretive framework and the circumstances surrounding that emotion. In contrast, awareness (i.e., the second example) elaborates the significance of what is happening within one's internal environment. That feeling one attends to is itself the focus of attention (i.e., perceptual figure) in the figure–ground grouping, and exploring it generates meaning from within.

Second, the objectives of change are different for each kind of processing. Making a reframe (as in the first example) involves an attempt to modify emotion after an initial reaction has already occurred. The objective of that reframing is to rework one's understanding of the related events. Changing the context in this way implicitly changes the meaning of a presenting feeling (recall Figure V.1). It follows that a new sense of direction emerges from a shift in the background or framework of understanding. In contrast, when one focuses on increasing awareness (as in the second example), explanations of the feeling are given little attention and there is no attempt to interpret or modify the contextual meaning. Rather, the objective of emotional awareness is to deepen and carry forward an already existing experience until a new sense of direction emerges from that exploration (Chapter 7).

Clarifying Internal Versus External Environments: Intervention Differences

Interventions that help clients either make meaning about the figure or of the background are emphasized differently across treatment perspectives (recall Figure 17.1). Cognitive and solution-oriented approaches aim to discern the meaning of what is out there in the world, whereas experiential therapies tend to focus on identifying the meaning of what is happening in here, within one's person. A perennial but surface-level question is, what approach works best? But the full meaning of one's experience entails both.

Which part of the overall meaning most calls for elaboration will depend on the processing style of a given client and their presenting concerns (rather than a treatment's declared theory of change). For example, some clients struggle with low emotional awareness (i.e., alexithymia), and they need to elaborate that (see Chapter 6). Meanwhile, as discussed later in this chapter, other clients struggle to think rationally when they are caught up in the power of a maladaptive emotion, so they might need to revisit the context of those feelings. For instance, a client's lived experience can be eclipsed by an outdated set of assumptions at the expense of new information in their presenting circumstance.

In clinical practice, errors in rational thinking have been referred to as cognitive biases, relational transference, and so on. These reflect a person's shortcomings in using the existing context of information for generating well-balanced conclusions about what one's experience means. Such stylistic differences represent qualitatively different deficits in processing when working with emotion as figural or when working with the background of contextual meaning that surrounds an emotion. A few studies highlight these as differential pathways to change, tying them back to client characteristics (see Beutler et al., 2018; Harrington et al., 2021; Høglend et al., 2011). This distinction reveals an important point for working with emotion at large: reframing (or reappraisals) and emotional exploration are not two interventions for facilitating the same kind of emotional change; rather, they represent two interventions, each facilitating very different kinds of emotional change. In short, one intervention approach helps clarify the external environment, whereas the other clarifies one's internal environment. The rest of this chapter focuses on decentering, which is the switch point where one steps outside of one's experience in the hope of examining it more objectively.

META-PERSPECTIVE: I AM BOTH THE READER AND THE AUTHOR OF MY STORY

Using a meta-perspective to create emotional change has two essential steps. First is the mental act of shifting to a higher level of observation. Safran and Segal (1990) identified this process in clinical work as "stepping outside of one's immediate experience, thereby changing the very nature of that experience" (p. 117), which is now referred to as *decentering*. This is a different process from expanding emotional awareness or the sequential ordering of emotions. As J. Pascual-Leone and Johnson (2021) explain, there are two different acts of mental attention that can be used to change the content of what is being attended to. On one hand, a thinker might change the content they are attending to but not the level of analysis, something cognitive neuroscience has called *executive updating*. In relation to emotion, that might be changing topics within the same scope of analysis or simply a narrative elaboration. As one explores emotion in a linear or sequential fashion (e.g., emotional awareness), that flow of experience keeps unfolding, and so the content in one's mind is continually being updated. On the other hand, a thinker might change the content and often also the level of their analysis, which cognitive neuroscience has referred to as *executive switching* (when it involves a change between mental sets) or what has been called decentering (when it involves a change between levels of analysis). Decentering affords the metacognitive awareness of one's emotional state. The change in scope, zooming out to consider a broader set at a higher order of analysis, represents the first step in accomplishing a unique kind of emotional change.

The function of decentering is that it allows for change. Decentering is the attentional act that makes it possible to subsequently (a) make attempts to down-regulate one's arousal; (b) attempt a behavioral exercise or otherwise find a way to reengage the same old challenge using some new strategy; or (c) reflect, adjust, and pivot toward entirely new goals, perhaps through an existential shift in priorities. The key issue, however, is that after decentering, one must introduce a transition to new content. That new direction is not self-evident; it represents a second step. Decentering is a metacognitive operation in that it creates a window of opportunity for thinking (or acting) differently, but it does not represent the substantive new content or modification itself. Literature on decentering as a clinical intervention has largely overlooked this point. To use another analogy, decentering is like depressing the clutch in one's mental engine. It momentarily opens a space to change gears. However, decentering as such does not change emotion, so the next critical question becomes about how one can use that moment of psychological distance to engage in alternative ways of thinking, behaving, and ultimately, of feeling.

The second step in this change is to do something with the moment of self-awareness by using it as an opportunity to add new content into one's original framework of understanding (e.g., through a reappraisal of assumptions, a shift in objectives). As the epigraphs of this chapter suggest, decentering creates psychological distance, which allows one to incorporate new information about the broader context into the experience itself. That broader context could include information about the presenting situation, or it could include much more, such as an entire sociopersonal history. Thus, there are several ways in which emotion is changed through the elaboration of its context, and they differ in the content and relative scope of their reappraisal.

In cognitive approaches, reframing purposefully explores alternative frameworks for understanding distressing emotion, but it does this within a local situation. In contrast, psychodynamic insights offer a variation of reframing that aims to foster understanding of the origin and broader meaning of distress across situations. In the next section, I discuss the first step and what it means to decenter from one's subjective experience. Following that, I explore the second step, the cognitive and then dynamic approaches to reappraising the context (i.e., background narrative, or circumstances) of one's experience.

STEP 1: DECENTERING, THE ACT OF SHIFTING TO A HIGHER LEVEL

When it comes to emotional experience, separating the figure from the ground of that perceptual gestalt is a prodigious act of mental attention. During emotionally challenging events, momentarily extracting oneself from the problematic experience (i.e., bracketing out or stepping outside) allows one to gain a meta-perspective of oneself. Here the individual comes to reflexively appreciate that they are actively contributing and making choices about the imminent construal of personal events (i.e., one is both the reader and author of their own story).

Mindfulness refers to a range of practices that invariably involve trying to create a little bit of distance between oneself and the situations at hand. It might be a little distance between one's sense of self and one's busy mind or between the sense of self and one's body. Whatever the case, creating this little bit of distance is the act of decentering, or extracting oneself from the buzz of presenting worldly experiences (including that of one's body). For example, when one is mired in the congestion of a traffic jam that is stagnant in the heat, with a long row of headlights and taillights, and with horns sounding, it can be an aggravating and desperate situation. However, if one imagines looking down from an airplane at the colored snake of road at that distance and especially at night, it might be quite beautiful. Self-consciously stepping outside one's contextual frame affords one a meta-perspective where one becomes aware of the content of one's experience as well as its frame of reference. This is explicitly part of treatment perspectives that engage in top-down processes for working with emotion by working with its context of meaning.

Chapter 5 discussed a critical distinction, which contrasted two ways in which one can explore emotion: experiencing emotion from within (i.e., bottom-up emotional engagement and awareness) or observations from outside and looking upon that experience (i.e., decentering and top-down meta-reflection). This chapter discusses the latter in full as a method of working with emotion. The most studied techniques for operationalizing this process are mindfulness interventions, reframing, and reflection on a psychodynamic insight. Still, the fact that this is a human process of change means it also occurs, sometimes covertly, in any number of treatments (A. Pascual-Leone & Greenberg, 2007b). Whether the process is leveraged explicitly and didactically or through the implicit confrontation of ultimate concerns, taking a meta-perspective creates the window of opportunity for making new choices.

Using Models to Externalize a Process

Formulating working models allows one to externalize the immediate process and step outside its frame. Objectifying and working on (not working in) representations of one's experience is epitomized by the written thought record used in cognitive behavior therapy (CBT). In that approach to modeling the process of emotion, causal reasoning has primacy, and one makes meaning about emotion (i.e., target behavior) by understanding it as couched between antecedents and consequences (i.e., the context). The chief advantage of working in this way is that it creates a focus that allows one to adopt the vantage point of an outside observer. Furthermore, manipulating a model of one's reality can also have a strong affinity to the function of playful experimentation. The model might literally be toy-sized representations mechanically used in play or creative arts therapies. They could also be deeply symbolic models such as in the formulation of interpersonal themes or identifying interrelated parts of the self as modeled during the enactments of chairwork. Ultimately, models are usually problem clarifications about how one's emotion relates to meaning that has been construed from a given situation, interaction, personal history, or outside influence.

The physical process of setting up a dialogue between different voices either implicitly (as in a thought record) or explicitly (as in play therapy, chairwork, or enactments) creates a meta-awareness of the processes at hand. Using models to externalize the process allows one to better survey all the moving parts. When asked at the end of treatment what was most helpful, a client I worked with stated that it was "those exercises in which I externalized the dialogue and my shame voice." While the chairwork facilitated an emotional shift (Chapter 14), it also provided a structure that helped the client understand their own depressogenic process (for similar examples, see Pos & Greenberg, 2012). In a different example, a couples therapist often encourages clients to refer to and explore their negative interactive cycle as a sort of third (interactive) variable, a model of something that exists between partners and apart from the individuals themselves (L. S. Greenberg & Goldman, 2019; Wiebe & Johnson, 2016). At other times, external models are much more explicit, like diagrams on a whiteboard or written exercises (e.g., as in psychoeducational or behavioral treatments). Still other examples are presented to the client by using a narrative formulation or emblematic story (e.g., core conflictual relationship themes; Luborsky et al., 1994).

Working with either physical or symbolic models allows one to take the position of a more omniscient narrator and experiment with various hypothetical scenarios. In play therapy with children, one might put different toy action figures in relation to one another and speak for each character, while the child is the all-seeing narrator that looks on and makes commentary. In a cognitive approach, that may involve brainstorming the possible alternative appraisals about a given situation. In psychodynamic approaches, it may involve thoughtfully reflecting on the origins of personal themes. In experiential approaches, this is often done more implicitly through playful experimentation with the plausible elaborations of one's narrative (e.g., Client: "What if he said . . . ? What might I do? What didn't I have the words for at the time? What should have happened? What is it like to know this?"). Lightheartedly working through scenarios in this way is the very definition of play, and it helps adults and children alike gain experience and make meaning about the possible realities that would otherwise have remained beyond their grasp.

When clients gain a meta-perspective, they perceive their own personal constructs as generating a present and ongoing experience. They come to appreciate their own functioning as agents in the creation of their immediate emotional experience. In this manner, clients experience themselves as responsible for their own framework of awareness (A. Pascual-Leone & Greenberg, 2007b). With depressed clients, for example, this may appear as an awareness of how one's self-critical voice plays a role in producing an ongoing sense of hopelessness. Alternatively, clients may momentarily become aware of a self-interruptive process and the automatic ways in which they avoid painful or threatening content. Mentalizing-based treatments aim to help clients to think better about their experience (Bateman & Fonagy, 2013; Fonagy et al., 2002). When clients can conceptualize their own experience (and the experience of others) in a more complete way, that objectivity and modeling of their own experience brings choice points to light. It also likely allows them to make better informed choices about how to interact and cope.

Decentering as a Metacognitive Skill: What Is Involved?

According to a metacognitive perspective (Dimaggio et al., 2020), one of the main purposes of therapy is to facilitate emotional experiences, interpersonal encounters, or behavioral exercises simply to continually generate new content in one's life, content that in turn becomes the focus of thoughtful reflection about one's experience. That metacognitive reflection could be momentarily extricating oneself from a state of distress and then considering the chain of events or circumstances that contributed to one feeling that way. The attentional shift to reflect on one's state allows one to, for example, circumvent problematic anger or entertain alternative methods of engagement beyond one's habitual default to despair. The cognitive load for stepping outside the flow of immediate distress is inherently challenging, so a key role of therapists is to provide mental scaffolding in support of that metacognitive function (Dimaggio et al., 2020). The subprocesses involved in lifting out of one's first-person experiential perspective to contemplate that perspective itself have been formulated in a model. From a clinical perspective, Bernstein and colleagues (2015) propose that the phenomenon of decentering is an attentional act that emerges from three interrelated processes: meta-awareness, disidentification from experience, and reduced reactivity to thought content.

First, the meta-awareness about an episode of thinking is when one becomes aware of the thinking process itself rather than staying focused strictly within the boundaries of the thought's content. This is essentially an intention to decenter or to take a third-person perspective. Often, this augmented level of awareness entails some appreciation of the operative process by which one may be generating one's own experience. For example, one might come to grasp a self-critical thought as something one has internalized from an abusive history (e.g., Client: "I'm damaged goods, and nobody would want me"). The realization that a self-criticism is not necessarily true or inherent to one's sense of self is a moment of meta-awareness, even as one experiences the feelings that go with such a nasty thought. The healthy skepticism that comes with meta-awareness is captured by a quip from comedian Emo Philips, often paraphrased as follows: "I used to think my mind was my most important organ. Then I noticed which organ was telling me that!" (Groovy Flicks, 2020, 35:30). Thus, meta-awareness is the first of three interrelated processes, but it also initiates and engenders the other two processes, which are closely related and essentially capture the reduced struggle with one's inner experience (Bernstein et al., 2015).

The second process of disidentification from experience refers to the sense that one's internal states are separate from oneself. Sensations, emotions, or thoughts are regarded as experiences that dynamically occur internally but are not themselves integral aspects of the self. The authorship or ownership of these experiences becomes more incidental and less of a consequential or defining feature (e.g., statements like "I am not my thoughts"; "I don't take the critique too seriously"; "I sometimes change my mind!"; "My brain is generating this experience").

Finally, decentering involves a third process of reduced reactivity to thought content such that the thought comes to have less affective power. A thought is considered in terms of its informational or truth value and less for its emotional or vital value (e.g., Client: "I know I'm overweight, but I say that without much judgement, even if it informs my lifestyle choices"; J. Pascual-Leone & Johnson, 2021). In this reduced reactivity, thoughts themselves are less evocative, and one is less sensitive or triggered (e.g., Client: "I'm being insulted, but I'm not very angry about it. It's like water off a duck's back").

As Bernstein and colleagues (2019) explain, there are positive feedback loops between the three processes:

> Meta-awareness may engender disidentification from internal experience because observing subjective experience creates a distinction (i.e., disidentification) between the observing self or consciousness and the observed subjective experience. Likewise, meta-awareness may engender reduced reactivity to thought content by disengaging attention from thought content to present moment experiences. (p. 225)

Furthermore, disidentification and reduced reactivity are synergistic processes in reducing one's struggle with inner experience, and together they reinforce the initial shift toward meta-awareness by further concretizing the process of extracting oneself from immediate subjective experience (Bernstein et al., 2015). However, because disidentification and reduced reactivity can each occur while one is mired in a narrow scope of awareness (e.g., feeling numb, detached, depersonalized, unreal, confused), meta-awareness is not reducible to the other two processes. Meta-awareness remains the instigating moment of insight that there actually is some bigger picture, like a glimpse at the wizard or machinery behind the curtain of one's own perception. This new vantage point (meta-awareness) is what can lead thought content to now be reconstrued as an interpreted representation rather than any self-evident reality in the past, present, or future.

The components hypothesized to be part of decentering have been supported by factor analyses on self-reports about decentering in both clinical and nonclinical samples (Hadash et al., 2017; Naragon-Gainey & DeMarree, 2017). Additional evidence on the role of decentering in emotional change comes from behavioral measures, micro-intervention experiments, and intensive experience sampling as one might do during treatment research (for a review, see Bernstien et al., 2019). Meanwhile, cognitive developmental research has elaborated an understanding of the causal determinants to decentering at the levels of both cognitive resources and mental capacity (J. Pascual-Leone & Johnson, 2022).

The fact that decentering is intentional holds importance for two reasons. First, a deliberate application of effortful mental attention is key to understanding the basic mechanisms of this mental process (J. Pascual-Leone & Johnson, 2022). Second, the clinical implication of intentionality separates it from automatic processes, which may be more akin to inattention (e.g., mind-wandering) or to forms of avoidance or intellectualization (Hadash et al., 2017; A. Pascual-Leone & Greenberg, 2007b). Ultimately, intentional decentering is a higher order coordination of several subprocesses, where the individual's allocation of attention zooms out to momentarily straddle both a lived experience as well as an awareness of oneself as a participant (e.g., Client: "I am myself and my circumstances; I am both the reader and the author").

Neural Correlates of Decentering

Using labels or reframes to contemplate one's experience are semantic processes that are both related to increased activity in the executive parts of the brain (the prefrontal cortex) and decreased activity in the emotional brain (limbic system; Torre & Lieberman, 2018). But the initial act of decentering itself is special. Recall (from Chapter 17) that midline structures of the brain are essentially where affect and cognition come together to produce personal and self-referential processes, and it is precisely these regions that become less active in the act of decentering. Sometimes decentering happens unintentionally, such as during mind-wandering. When that happens, there is a decoupling of one's mental work from what would be immediate perceptual engagement. Mind-wandering occurs because of either episodic or affective events, and its regulation is a metacognitive function exercised by executive processes (Smallwood & Schooler, 2015). This gives some insight into what is going on when decentering is done purposefully and one steps back from the flow of emotional experience.

A study of mindfulness-based intervention used functional magnetic resonance imaging (fMRI) to clarify the neural substrates of two kinds of selfawareness, which the researchers termed "experiential focus" and "narrative focus" (Farb et al., 2007). The disidentification from internal experience was related to a decoupling of neural areas that support cognitive–affective representations of the self (i.e., ventromedial prefrontal cortex) from areas supporting bodily sensations (i.e., right insula). Further, although these areas of functioning are habitually integrated, an 8-week mindfulness training helped people develop the ability to decouple those areas of neural processing. Indeed, as discussed in Chapter 19, when people are instructed to use a self-distancing perspective, they show less activation in the cortical midline structures typically associated with self-referencing (i.e., medial prefrontal cortex, posterior cingulate, and precuneus; Northoff et al., 2006; St. Jacques, 2012). In addition to this separation, one observes reduced activation in other brain areas related to emotional reactivity. The immediate moment of intentional decentering is probably further aided by the involvement of brain areas that are used in switching frames of reference, specifically between first- and third-person perspectives (i.e., right angular gyrus of the inferior parietal lobe; Farb et al., 2007).

Cognitive therapy is effortful work, and the ability to decenter in a moment of distress is not something that comes easily for people suffering clinical issues. As discussed in Chapter 18, major depression is associated with several cognitive deficits in problem solving, which makes it hard to take full advantage of cognitive interventions. One attempt to address (and test) this has been the introduction of neurological interventions to support clients during psychotherapy by using an exogenous source of energy to boost their mental activity during CBT for depression. This experimental intervention adds transcranial direct current stimulation, where a client in psychotherapy wears electrodes placed on their head to run a low electrical current through certain parts of their brain, providing extra stimulation to a targeted brain area during their weekly session (Nord et al., 2019).

The dorsolateral prefrontal cortex is a brain area known to be associated with executive control functions such as switching tasks, reconfiguring the relations within a set, preventing interference, or planning out a next step. Adding activation to that brain area aims to artificially enhance cognitive control and planning. By supercharging the dorsolateral prefrontal cortex or the left prefrontal cortex more generally, clients would be able to decenter more easily and subsequently make the most of CBT. Randomized controlled trials of this additive intervention suggest that it works. However, the effects are highly variable and only benefit certain subgroups, such as those who present with cognitive decline or prefrontal cortical atrophy (Brunoni et al., 2014; Nord et al., 2019). In any case, the notion that cognitive therapy interventions help clients to decenter from an existing difficulty is highlighted by the fact that artificially boosting specific kinds of cognitive power can sometimes be of benefit over and above CBT alone.

When Might Decentering Work Best or Worst?

Deliberately and effortfully decentering assumes a person has the will to change. Being entrenched in a familiar old rut also has a certain inertia, and if anger or grumpiness is part of that, then the negative state also has some power to it. Sometimes, without fully realizing it, people actively resist the opportunity to decenter, and willfulness is a character trait that exemplifies this. However, changes of context can be useful to dislodge such a person. Although little research has detailed the contextual factors that facilitate decentering and subsequent reframing (Bernstein et al., 2015), using humor is a salient case in point.

Using Humor Helps With Decentering

Positive emotion, humor, and playfulness create a climate for a broader, less embedded, and alternative perspective on one's context and habitual patterns of feeling and thinking. In short, positive emotion allows one to broaden one's understanding of difficult emotion and then build on that in an upward spiral (Fredrickson, 2001; Chapter 13, this volume). Positive emotion either presession or early in treatment anticipate subsequent moments of insight or deeper experiencing that occur later in the session or in treatment (Stalikas et al., 2015). Experimental interventions—such as when people practiced coming up with funny reinterpretations of bad events or inventing funny solutions to problems—produced more happiness and less depressive symptoms in a community sample irrespective of their self-reported sense of humor (Wellenzohn et al., 2018). When jokes are positive, they epitomize a form of reframing in which the individual decenters and then abruptly shifts interpretive frames to get the joke. The unexpected nature of humor shakes up a change in one's cognitive set, sparking an alternative outlook that is more positive, lighthearted, and novel (Samson & Gross, 2012).

In a self-evident example, one of my clients described a personal insight he had when reading the newspaper, one that helped him momentarily shift out of his typical pessimism and ruminative disappointment with himself: "Well, my life hasn't turned out, or I haven't steered it much in the direction I've wanted, but if it's any consolation to me or others, at least I am not this guy!" He chuckled, pulling a crumpled newsprint out from his pocket. The headline read, "Burglary Suspect Kept Stolen Brain Beneath Porch and Used It to Get High, Police Say" (*Chicago Tribune*, 2016).[3] Despite my client's morbid humor, there was a simple sincerity in making this bizarre contrast. Unbeknownst to my client, his downward comparison strategy for changing emotion is described in dialectical behavior therapy (Linehan, 2015). The strategy is to change emotion by thinking about its context differently using the classic refrain, "It could be worse!" Seeing the humor in this tragedy facilitated my client's initial shift in perspective. Decentering allowed him to take a broader perspective, not just focusing on his own life but comparing it to the range of possible lives being lived by others out there. I asked whether the comparison he was making offered any consolation, to which he replied, "It helps me appreciate more of what I do have. . . . And I guess I still have some choices left to make, too."

There are very few prescriptive examples in psychotherapy for introducing humor and play. Examples include gestalt workshops such as clowning for couples, where couples in (manageable) distress are encouraged to humorously exaggerate and role play one another. Another example is disowned parts parties, where clients in gestalt group therapy show up in costume dressed to blatantly portray and caricaturize aspects of themselves that they fantasize about but otherwise typically deny, hide, and disown (e.g., acting like a baby dependent on others, an overcontrolling despot, a powerful seductress, a loafer with no goals). Another development has been teaching improvisational theater (i.e., improv) as a treatment for anxiety and depression (Felsman et al., 2019; Krueger et al., 2017). Chapter 11 also discusses playfulness in therapy.

Overwhelming Arousal Impairs Decentering

When immersed in an emotionally stressful event, decentering is a formidable task of mental effort. This is illustrated by a comically tragic account of a couple who have spent weeks learning how to communicate better and how to be attentive to one another. Nonetheless, the fights between sessions are reportedly unchanged and still seem to escalate quickly. The therapist asks, "But what happened? Did you forget the skills or lose sight of your deeper feelings?" After some introspection, one of the partners awkwardly responds,

> Honestly, it's been weeks that we've been doing this. I basically know what the right thing to say really is, and I can do the skills just fine, it's just that in the heat of the moment, I'm so mad that I just don't care about the damn skills! (L. S. Greenberg, personal communication, October 15, 2008)

The problem here is more profound than a client being stubborn or resistant to using a skills-based treatment. Any motivation to use skills is contingent on one's moment-by-moment ability to pause, just long enough to decenter and generate alternatives. However, that ability is hampered when emotional arousal is already overwhelming.

This concrete challenge to preemptively decenter before emotional problems get worse may not be as apparent from the large number of studies on cognitive reappraisal, perhaps because many of them use nonclinical samples (Wallace-Hadrill & Kamboj, 2016). When people are engulfed in or tumbled by emotions like anger or despair it creates tunnel vision, where they are no longer able to work with their surrounding context. In short, reflecting on emotion and making new contextual meaning is not easily done in states of high distress.

In support of this, a line of experimental research shows that cognitive strategies for working with emotion fail when people are under acute stress. For example, in a study discussed in Chapter 13, participants under no stress were able to use cognitive reappraisal to reduce feelings of experimentally evoked anger, but the benefit of that strategy disappeared when their arm was submerged in painfully cold water (a paradigm used in experiments to induce bodily stress or measure pain tolerance; Zhan, Wu, et al., 2017). Another study showed a participant's mastery of cognitive regulation strategies was markedly impaired for a temporary period during which they underwent an acute stress induction related to conditioned fear (Raio et al., 2013). The neuroendocrine responses (e.g., increased cortisol) that drive a participant's sharp stress reaction seem to impair executive functioning in the prefrontal cortex and thereby undermine the application of cognitive strategies which (ironically) were intended to mitigate that distress. As the title of that research paper sums up, "Cognitive emotion regulation fails the stress test" (Raio et al., 2013).

Critically, stress does not debilitate all strategies for working with emotion. In fact, it can even facilitate some other strategies. The reason is that elevated cortisol (stress hormone) is associated with impaired switching of sets, which is the essence of decentering and reframing. However, the same hormonal response will enhance the degree to which one can assimilate and incorporate new and relevant information (Goldfarb et al., 2017). The implication is that very poignant and painful moments contraindicate the use of top-down cognitive strategies or efforts to think more rationally, whereas bottom-up experiential strategies seem to be more useful (Wang et al., 2022; Zhan, Wu, et al.,

2017). Examples of experiential strategies include symbolizing the meaning of an emotion (Part II; Chapters 6 and 7) and sequential transformations (Part IV; Chapter 13).

Timing and Individual Differences Matter

Apart from when decentering may not be as effective as intended, if decentering is used at the wrong time, it may undermine other clinical efforts. For example, in exposure therapy, where the intention is to increase a person's emotional engagement by confronting them with evocative stimuli, then decentering may have a paradoxical and maladaptive effect (Bernstein et al., 2019; Foa & Kozak, 1986). First, decentering would preemptively create psychological distance from the emotional experience that one is supposed to be activated and habituating to. But second, instructing the individual to decenter at poignant moments facilitates precisely the kind of emotional avoidance most typical of anxiety, among other disorders. Indeed, studies of clinical populations show that when decentering occurs spontaneously, adopting a third-person perspective is counterproductive (Wallace-Hadrill & Kamboj, 2016).

Finally, prompting a client to decenter is usually an explicit process, and so client characteristics will also play a role in how receptive that person will be to such an influence. For example, decentering is likely to be less effective with people who are willful, stubborn, and set in their own ways regardless of consequences. Relatedly, a meta-analysis showed that client personality features have a medium to large effect in the moderation of treatment outcomes (Beutler et al., 2018). Clients who externalize (i.e., under stress they avoid, act out, or blame the environment) benefit more from symptom-focused treatments such as cognitive, behavioral, and solution-focused therapies, which typically make use of decentering. In contrast, clients who internalize (i.e., under stress they adopt an inner blaming, neurotic style) benefit most from treatments that focus on insight and awareness, such as psychodynamic or experiential approaches (Beutler et al., 2018). Potential moderators like these have not received enough attention despite their obvious implications for treatment planning.

Decentering Constructs

It is paramount to appreciate that unlike many of the other processes described in this book, decentering is necessarily a post-hoc strategy for working with emotion. This way of changing emotion is one that mostly gets applied after the initial generation of an emotion. Intentional decentering is about interrupting that flow of attentional focus. As such, by definition, it is a secondary step when working with emotion. Furthermore, although decentering can sometimes occur spontaneously (at worse as an unconscious avoidance strategy, or at best as an overlearned metacognitive strategy), it is typically a very conscious and deliberate process intended to manipulate one's current emotional experience.

With an eye for evaluating these kinds of intervention strategies across treatment approaches, a host of decentering-related constructs have been identified

(Bernstein et al., 2019). Some of these processes are fully characterized by the model of decentering discussed before, including metacognitive awareness (Dimaggio et al., 2020; Teasdale et al., 2002), cognitive distancing (Beck, 2020), metacognitive mode (Wells, 2000), and detached mindfulness (Wells, 2005). Other constructs partially capture the notion of decentering as it is defined here, including reperceiving (S. L. Shapiro et al., 2006), cognitive defusion and self-as-context (S. C. Hayes et al., 2012), and the self-distanced perspective (Kross & Ayduk, 2011; also discussed in Chapters 19 and 22, this volume). Supporting the emphasis put on this construct, a review of process research specifically in CBT shows that eight meta-analyses have examined decentering (i.e., re-framing) as a process of change in the treatment of anxiety, demonstrating positive effects that range from small to large. Two other meta-analyses have also shown small to medium effects for decentering and reframing as a process in CBT for depression (Kazantzis et al., 2018).

Decentering-related constructs are well represented in cognitive therapy, mindfulness, and third-wave cognitive behavior treatments such as acceptance and commitment therapy (ACT). In contrast, this process is not typically examined as a mechanism in humanistic–experiential therapies. That is because emotional awareness and exploring from within a first-person perspective are mainstays of experiential work but are also antithetical to decentering and stepping out of the flow. This is an example wherein using different ways to work with emotion simultaneously or within the same envelope of time would work at cross-purposes with one another.

Whatever the case, a fundamental technique in all cognitively oriented therapies is (a) to step out from the flow of one's feelings to reflect on the process (i.e., decentering) and then (b) to modify those cognitive processes top-down (i.e., adding or attending to new information). The initial process is decentering, but its operationalization and implementation has been referred to using various terms (e.g., reappraisal, reframing, diffusion, restructuring). Furthermore, the popularity of decentering as a mechanism in cognitive approaches is that it can easily be embedded within the Socratic method (i.e., asking questions to lead the client toward rational conclusions). Indeed, a strength of such approaches is the very explicit instruction they give clients on how to position themselves in relation to a presenting problem.

Mindfulness and Decentering

As discussed in Chapter 2, the practice of mindfulness involves a host of processes, many of which are undeclared in the account of how mindfulness facilitates positive change. However, the most specific mechanism of mindfulness is practice and training in focusing one's attention and the capacity to sustain a meta-perspective when observing one's immediate experience. Decentering is argued to be the central psychological process at work in mindfulness-based therapies (Bernstein et al., 2019). This is especially relevant to working with emotion, given that a key property of emotion is that, like a tractor beam, it automatically orients one to problematic content and primes one for action. Put plainly, mindfulness is a trainable skill that essentially increases one's traction in a range of cognitive efforts, allowing one to better focus on some content or resist the automatic engagement of other (emotional) content.

Mindfulness is a process whereby one positions oneself in relation to the flow of experience in a way that actively prevents one from slipping down the many rabbit holes (i.e., attractor states) of emotion or being less vulnerable to passing cognitive distractions. In this way mindfulness is the de-automatization of reactive (i.e., mindless) responding (Kang et al., 2013). While various acts of decentering (e.g., pausing to reframe an immediate problem situation) are concrete instances of changing an emotional state, mindfulness is not typically intended as a one-off or case-by-case intervention. The aim of a mindfulness-based practice is an ongoing effort to develop a trait-like capacity for maintaining that little bit of separation between oneself and one's circumstances.

A meta-analysis of over 170 studies that examined the impact of mindfulness on various psychological disorders showed that mindfulness-based interventions had a moderate effect over no treatment, but did not differ from the effect of established evidence-based treatments. Self-selection likely plays an important role in the findings of many studies on mindfulness, which should be better controlled for and reported on. However, the most consistent benefits of mindfulness were observed in the treatment of depression, pain conditions, smoking, and other addictive disorders (Goldberg et al., 2018). Adding to this list, another meta-analysis demonstrated the moderate effect of mindfulness in reducing aggression and anger, specifically among children and adolescents (which is a markedly larger effect than most behaviorally oriented violence prevention programs; Tao et al., 2021).

Although the impact of mindfulness is astonishingly broad, mindfulness is most impactful in working with depression, pain, addiction, and problematic anger (for more on this, see Chapter 2 in this volume and the meta-analysis by van Agteren et al., 2021). It is worth noting that these areas of suffering are also cited in original Buddhist teachings as chief targets of mindfulness. More critically, these are domains where decentering seems most important for preventing an individual from slipping more deeply into maladaptive feelings and behaviors.

The reason why cognitive approaches to therapy and mindfulness-based therapies marry so well is because they share the view that emotional processing is the product of mental discipline. One must practice detaching from the throws of emotional distress to think more clearly or more rationally. Decentering from the flow of one's thoughts and feelings has become a central tenant of several third-wave forms of cognitive behavior therapies, including dialectical behavior therapy, mindfulness-based cognitive therapy, and ACT, among others. Research also supports decentering and meta-awareness as a central mechanism in these treatments (Yasinski et al., 2016).

Trials of mindfulness-based cognitive therapy have explicitly highlighted the role of decentering as a key mechanism in the treatment of depression.

Participants who increased in their ability to decenter during treatment (compared with those who did not) were less likely to suffer a depressive relapse over the 4 months after treatment had ended (M. T. Moore et al., 2022). This research, along with other clinical trials using similar designs (e.g., Teasdale et al., 2002) concluded that decentering seems to be a mechanism in preventing relapse into depression, an effect that held irrespective of the prescribed treatment approach (i.e., cognitive therapy, treatment as usual, or mindfulness-based cognitive therapy).

ACT has some unique differences from its predecessor, CBT. Nevertheless, the former continues to rely on (a) decentering and (b) behavioral interventions, albeit motivated by a mindful consideration of personal values in the context of a reality that needs to be accepted for what it is, which contrasts with reframing one's thoughts about the local context. The major process mechanisms in this therapy are probably decentering, so that one can reflect on life narratives and values, as well as the behavioral and experiential work that follows in the pursuit of narrative congruence. An experiment compared cognitive reappraisal (i.e., modifying one's thoughts about a negative experience) and acceptance (i.e., accepting one's feelings without trying to change them; Troy et al., 2018). Findings show reappraisal (CBT's approach to decentering) and acceptance (ACT's mindfulness-based strategy for decentering) each had large effects on the nonclinical participants. However, the two processes may work for different reasons: Evidence suggested that acceptance was less difficult to deploy and was associated with less physiological arousal, which contrasts with the effortful reframe of how one was interpreting an experience.

Third-wave cognitive therapies are not the only treatments to incorporate mindfulness. Psychotherapy researchers have also elaborated how mindfulness bears a resemblance to engagement in experiential mechanisms of change as well as the psychodynamic process (e.g., Geller & Greenberg, 2012; Safran, 2003). The observation that decentering may be a process in emotional change irrespective of the treatment approach is in keeping with a core argument presented in this book. Namely, the processes of emotional change are endorsed and deployed by clients, and they are not unilaterally implemented by therapists nor proprietary to treatments.

STEP 2: INTRODUCING NEW INFORMATION ABOUT THE CONTEXT OF EMOTION

Decentering is the first step for reflecting upon one's emotional experience. The second step that changes the presenting experience is the introduction of some new information, insight, or experience before reengaging the original emotion. The issue is that without actively making use of Step 1 (decentering) as a window of opportunity, the individual does not have anything but their original default trajectory to go back to. It would be as if their train of thought were, "Wait a minute! What day is it? I've been stuck in this rut for a long time.

Maybe I should do something different . . . or not. . . . Oh well, back to the usual." Because of this, a second step is needed to insert new interpretive context, which changes one's experience in some way, setting one up to engage an alternative. However, the scope of context (i.e., the size of the frame) matters. The experiencer can ask, what does my emotion mean in this situation? or, what does it mean in the context of my life and personhood? That is a critical distinction, with implications for the kind of treatment intervention that follows.

Generating New Context: The Short Game Versus the Long Game

Sometimes, as in reframing, the shift in meaning is done using a local cognitive change, while at other times, the shift in meaning could be one that refers to a broader set of life goals. I refer to "local" cognitive change because although a core dysfunctional belief (i.e., "I am a failure" or "the glass is half empty") has deep personal meanings, cognitive approaches to therapy tend to focus on specific and concrete situations as the sources of empirical evidence. We see this when cognitive therapists encourage clients to consider the evidence against some core dysfunctional belief. For example,

CLIENT: I'm such a loser because Olivia didn't say yes when I asked her out on a date to that new coffee shop downtown.

THERAPIST: That's disappointing. But let's look at the facts too. This rejection is one specific event. Does one person's response determine your worth? Maybe there's other relevant evidence. Can you think of times when you've connected well with others or had positive relationships? What about when you were making plans with your close friend Alex?

Cognitive interventions like this are about decentering and reinterpreting the present situation and local events (Beck, 2020). One can think of this as the short game, and it is a specific strategy when using cognition to work with emotion.

But there are other ways of elaborating the context of meaning. As such, elaborating a local situation contrasts with the long game, which would be to consider themes and reevaluate one's overall goals in life. The long game generates the requisite new information quite differently. Acknowledging relational themes that one participates in, as done in psychodynamic treatments (Luborsky et al., 1994), or clarifying one's personal values, as done in ACT (S. C. Hayes et al., 2012), are kinds of evidence that are epistemologically different from anything that would typically be observed in a specific situation. For example,

THERAPIST: You're really wanting to connect with Olivia but it feels like rejection, and that leaves you feel unworthy. It reminds me of

> what it was like for you when I rescheduled the sessions. . . .
> Maybe it even echoes a bit of the dismissiveness you felt growing
> up . . . and yet pursuing connection is really important to you
> too; it always has been.

I will first explore the role of local cognitive change as exemplified in cognitive therapy and CBT at large. Then I will return to the epistemologically different strategy (the long game) that is typical of psychodynamic and values-oriented work.

Reinterpreting the Present Situation: How the Short Game Works

Reframing a situation so as to think differently about one's emotional concerns or working rationally to correct a dysfunctional belief are intuitive ideas for overcoming distress and have been championed over decades of psychotherapy research. Unfortunately, empirical support for this mechanism in working with clinical samples has been less than conclusive, and still there is something important about the impact of thoughts on feeling.

Cognitive Change May Not Cause Symptom Change

The cognitive mediation hypothesis is a fundamental pillar of cognitively oriented treatment in all its incarnations. This is the idea that changing one's thoughts will change how one feels. Although well over 500 meta-analyses have been conducted on the various effects of CBT, only about 2% of these reviews have produced findings about process-to-outcome relationships that support the role of reframing as a change process (Kazantzis et al., 2018). Interestingly, those eight meta-analyses showed positive effects for the role of cognitive change, although mostly only in context of working with anxiety. Still, the directionality of the hypothesized effect remains a critical issue.

Longitudinal mediation analyses are incisive methods for clarifying the direction of relationships between process and outcome. Even so, several such studies on depression have now shown that cognitive changes occur concurrently with symptom change. They do not precede symptom change, nor do they mediate the effect treatment has on symptom change. This has held true whether the hypothesized mediator was cognitive content (e.g., negative automatic thoughts, dysfunctional beliefs, cognitive distortions) or higher order cognitive structures (e.g., low self-esteem, hopelessness, cognitive schemes; Lemmens et al., 2017; Quigley et al., 2019). Moreover, when treatments in randomized trials for adult depression have been compared, cognitive changes have not proven to be discriminating process predictors as one would expect. Cognitive processes did not mediate the effects of cognitive therapy any more than they did for interpersonal therapy (Lemmens et al., 2017). Going further, antidepressant medication produces just as much reduction in depression-relevant cognitions as CBT, which again suggests cognitive interventions might not make a direct difference (Quigley et al., 2019).

A study using ecological momentary assessments tracked the temporal order of people's mood, cognition, and behavioral gains by taking measurements five times a day for 4 months during the treatment of their depression (Snippe et al., 2024). Analyses examined whether the earliest alleviation of sad mood (i.e., a symptom gain) occurred before, after, or during the same week as cognitive or behavioral changes. Contrary to cognitive theory, change in someone's negative way of thinking (i.e., cognitive gains) typically occurred during the same week as their alleviation of sad mood (58% of the time) as compared with preceding (18% of the time) or following that target symptom gain (24% of the time). The fact that changes to negative thinking and mood both occurred around the same time explains why prior research on cognitive change has been unable to predict the alleviation of emotional symptoms (Snippe et al., 2024).[4]

Summing up, cognitive change at various levels of abstraction appears to be a correlate, not a mediator, of symptom improvement. Findings from high-quality process-to-outcome studies as well as ecological momentary assessments do not support a cognitive mechanism of change as put forth in cognitive theory. Even so, several meta-analyses on treatment as well as experimental research continue to show using cognitive reappraisals can be helpful when working with emotional distress.

Inconsistency in the literature may be the result of several possibilities I have suggested. First, many of the experiments supporting cognitive reappraisal have used healthy or subclinical samples (e.g., Wallace-Hadrill & Kamboj, 2016) and may not generalize to working through clinical concerns. Second, the cognitive and attentional demands of this type of intervention are substantially compromised in moments of acute distress (Goldfarb et al., 2017; Zhan, Wu, et al., 2017). And third, whether working with cognition has an impact on symptom change may depend on whether one is negotiating primary maladaptive emotions (e.g., deep-seated shame that often underpins depression) or secondary symptomatic emotion (e.g., anxiety). And while the studies on depression cited previously do not support the cognitive mediation hypothesis, this critical issue calls for longitudinal mediations to be conducted on CBT for anxiety.

Finally, using cognition to change emotion may be much less linear, more complex, and perhaps an adjunct to other processes (Lemmens et al., 2017; Quigley et al., 2019). Recall from Chapter 7 that a longitudinal mediation on the role of client experiencing (i.e., awareness) over time also showed an interdependent relationship with the unfolding of symptom change—very similar to the role of cognition being reported here (Pinheiro et al., 2021). A major premise of this book is that certain processes work best for certain emotions, rather than being universal facilitators of change. However, for research designs to show those complex relationships, they must consider both processes and their moment-by-moment targets.

New Hypotheses on the Role of Cognition

It is implausible that what one thinks about one's situation has no bearing on how one works with what one is feeling. So, if evidence suggests that cognitive work is not a direct mediator, how might a process like reframing still be relevant to working with emotion? In what follows, I suggest three compatible hypotheses.

Cognition is a modifier. Cognition may or may not function as a direct cause (i.e., mediator) of emotional change, but it serves as a modifying variable, influencing the amplitude or direction of change when working with emotion. The best example of this is the role of rumination in psychopathology. Rumination and the mental rehearsal of feared scenarios is a maintaining factor in anxiety (Borkovec et al., 2004; Fresco et al., 2002). Similarly, when people who are depressed focus on their symptoms and ruminate on the possible causes or consequences of their symptomatology, they suffer depressive episodes of longer durations (Nolen-Hoeksema, 1991). Also, people with body dissatisfaction are more likely to become depressed, but that relationship is moderated by rumination (Forward, 2023). Experiments also show that thinking vengeful thoughts about someone while hitting a punching bag increases the angry feelings one had toward that person (Bushman, 2002). Even the physiological sensation of hunger can be modified into negative affective experiences (e.g., feeling hangry [hungry + angry]) by adding meaning cues that were unrelated to the hunger (MacCormack & Lindquist, 2019). Cognition is clearly a modifier that can exacerbate negative emotional experiences. Thus, the treatment idea of correcting a bias in negative thinking may speak to the attenuation of unhealthy emotion, or at least it may hedge against the emotion getting worse.

Mind over mood changes secondary emotion. I suggest that attempts to rationally change one's belief are only going to impact secondary emotion, but they will not impact the deeply seated meanings of identity embodied by primary maladaptive emotion. Secondary emotions (e.g., global distress, anxiety, hopelessness, helplessness) are a major reason for avoidance behavior, the most prominent obstacle in anxiety disorders as compared with major depression (Hofmann & Hay, 2018). If one is fearful of a situation, asking oneself, "What's the worst-case scenario? How might I cope?" are rationalized bids to promote agency and decrease helplessness. One can sometimes convince oneself that an immediate experience is not so scary, at least long enough to test that out.

Experiments of everyday life examples (e.g., karaoke singing, public speaking, math performance) show that people who have performance anxiety can reappraise their emotion as excitement by using simple self-talk strategies (e.g., saying out loud "I'm excited!" or "This is going to be exciting!"). Doing this prompts them to adopt an opportunity mindset and can change the behavioral performance that follows (Brooks, 2014). This observation also highlights the importance of having emotions that are somewhat congruent with an intended reappraisal (e.g., anxiety can be reappraised as excitement but not as tranquility).

Findings like these are valuable, but it is important to notice that the emotions being changed in such examples tend to be secondary symptomatic emotions. In contrast, when the presenting emotion is a reprise of the same old story and a maladaptive identity narrative about being unlovable or inherently inadequate, changing that core maladaptive shame using rational arguments will not be enough. In clinical practice, CBT for anxiety tends to make reappraisals about secondary symptomatic distress, and these seem more compelling than reappraisals made in CBT treatments for depression, which tend to target primary maladaptive emotion. This hypothesis is supported by the fact that most meta-analyses supporting cognitive reappraisal are in the treatment of anxiety, not for depression (Kazantzis et al., 2018).

In short, I argue that cognitive modifications are not enough to change primary maladaptive emotion but may be enough to change secondary symptomatic emotion. The clinical implication of this is that although cognitive reappraisals may not create the deep substantive changes that it is often claimed to do, it may simply get the person to temporarily rally forth from a given slump of distress. Cognitive reframing is used in small cumulative increments, like helping someone caught in a rainstorm dash from one dry patch to another. A key point is that although the idea of mind over mood may not be the chief mechanism of change, it may be enough to encourage behavioral engagement. Still, behavior is a subsequent and separate change process, the effects of which are sometimes misattributed to cognitive reframing.

Cognitive reframing provides a rationale for behavioral engagement. Unlike viscerally experiencing one's emotional needs, the verbal elaborations produced by reframing are not directly wired into affective change. Decentering involves disidentification from experience and reduced reactivity to thought content. However, that metacognitive moment is transitory unless clients follow through with some behavioral commitment and new engagement.

This begs for a careful comparison across the process components of CBT. Direct comparisons have shown that behavioral activation significantly outperforms cognitive therapy in the treatment of depression (Dimidjian et al., 2006). Meanwhile, dismantling studies demonstrate that in combined treatments, behavioral components alone can sufficiently account for the treatment effects of cognitive therapy. In fact, some authors have concluded that, at least for posttraumatic stress disorder, the beneficial effect of behavioral exposure is diminished when the treatment is diluted by attempts to augment it with cognitive procedures (Foa et al., 2003). This is compelling evidence that the behavioral components in CBT are the primary agents of change.

There is a powerful simplicity in imposing a behavioral schedule top down, such as lifestyle changes for self-care (Linehan, 2015) or just increasing the raw number of hours of social contact within a relationship to address marital distress (Minuchin, 2012). A review of meta-analyses on the active processes in CBT shows that engaging in behavioral processes (e.g., activity scheduling, activation, exposure, contingency management) has consistently positive effects in the prediction of treatment outcomes (Kazantzis et al., 2018). Of course, all this presumes that people will engage in behavioral tasks at all. As the notorious attrition rates of behavior therapy can attest (i.e., 40%), asking clients to engage in exposure or prescribing other behavioral interventions is a tall order for clients (Gros et al., 2017). These are interventions that could be committed to if based on a thoughtful decision. Thus, getting people to engage in behavioral change often requires some convincing and the fostering of positive expectations. I suggest the cognitive components of cognitive and behavioral therapies contribute to change by providing clients with a clear rationale for why anyone might attempt and persist with the arduous work of unpleasant behavioral interventions. Cognitive work is what sells clients on the more central (behavioral) mechanism of such treatments, after which behavioral adherence becomes the challenge.

A key function of working with and changing cognitions is problem clarification and problem solving, both of which clearly usher one toward some new behavioral engagement (Grosse Holtforth et al., 2006). In short, decentering and then generating a reframe (reappraisal) is what provides both (a) the choice point and (b) the rationale that prepares and motivates people for behavioral exercises. Therefore, I suggest the role of cognitive interventions is as an upstream mediator, one that prepares and facilitates the engagement of behavioral work that will follow. This hypothesis, which remains to be tested, is that cognition does not have a direct impact on lasting emotional change, but that it acts upstream, the first in a series of two mediators. Cognition prepares the ground as needed, paving the way for commitment to behavioral change, which is the primary causal process. Supporting this, research on exposure-based CBT for depression has led authors to suggest an early and rapid treatment response might be primarily related to cognitive changes, whereas symptom changes that occurs later may be explained by behavioral exposure (A. M. Hayes et al., 2007).

Cognition as a change process: Future research directions. There is uncertainty about evidence for the cognitive mediation model and a growing need for alternative explanations of how cognitive changes might be affecting emotion. I have put forth five testable hypotheses about cognition as a process for facilitating emotion change:

Hypothesis 1: Working with cognition acts as a modifier of painful emotion even if it cannot eliminate it.

Hypothesis 2: A more novel hypothesis is that cognitive modifications may impact secondary symptomatic emotions (e.g., feelings of anxiety, reactive anger, hopelessness, helplessness), but they are not likely to have meaningful impact on primary maladaptive emotion (e.g., feeling incompetent, shamefully unworthy, lonely, abandoned).

Hypothesis 3: When they are useful, the key function of cognitive modifications is to prepare clients and entreat them to engage in exposure and behavioral activation, which are the more active ingredients in CBT and its third wave treatments.

Hypothesis 4: The function of modifying cognition in emotional change is limited to (a) problem clarification and (b) building motivation, organizing the client toward a particular set of strategies for engagement.

Hypothesis 5: If hypothesis 3 and 4 are taken together, it suggests that cognition may be part of a serial mediation model, where working rationally to change cognition may serve as an upstream mediator in psychotherapy. As such, rational–cognitive work offers one of several potential pathways to initiate or to maximize the more primary mechanisms of emotional change.

Convincing people to engage is a cognitive process akin to building motivation, commitment, self-efficacy, or other preparatory work that clears the way for a primary mediator. Regrettably, primary mediators in CBT are often lumped under the nonspecific banner of exposure, which is an intervention, not a change process. Nevertheless, the term "exposure" is used as a conceptual shorthand among some authors to point at processes like behavioral action, emotional engagement, and experiential work (Chapter 3). These hypotheses need to be empirically examined in what would be a serious revision to the cognitive theory of emotional change. Such a revision would open a more nuanced perspective on the integration of psychotherapy theories.

A Deeper Understanding of the Present: How the Long Game Works

In the short game, the way one interprets a local situation may be rapidly reappraised with small adjustments to information, which results in reinterpreting one's external reality. For example, a feared situation can be reframed as a much-needed opportunity, or, if one feels outraged about the email sent by a colleague, one might find alternative ways to explain its seemingly negative tone. These insights are about understanding a specific situation.

By contrast, in the long game, reframing is done by reconsidering personal narratives and themes. Psychodynamic insights, for example, are often about understanding oneself in terms of what one wishes for, how one typically responds, and how one generally expects others to respond (Luborsky et al., 1994; Figure 17.1, this volume). Identifying personal themes and clarifying one's identity or values adds a deeper self-understanding about what one has been participating in (or enacting). These narrative aspects of one's life shift one's interpretation of an internal reality, but typically the change is neither rapid nor dramatic. A psychodynamic insight might not abruptly stop one from having the same old concern, but it could lead to those concerns being experienced more softly, thoughtfully, or in a way that better relates to the present context rather than with the rigidness or forcefulness reminiscent of past injuries or traumas. The psychodynamic insight allows one to distance from the assumptions of there and then to better see how they are different from what is happening in the here and now.

As a final contrast, cognitive reframing is often a short game strategy for reinterpreting the present situation. It creates horizontal breadth on experience in the sense that although one had certain assumptions, the reframe broadens the array of alternative interpretations one could use to reconsider that single presenting situation. In contrast, psychodynamic interventions use a longer term strategy that involves a deeper understanding of the present. By creating vertical depth, one gains a more complete understanding of the sociohistorical reasons why one may have a certain perspective (i.e., bias). This illuminates what having that perspective across situations might mean, even as one engages in it, and it highlights the existential choice.

The Psychodynamic Insight: Will It Be About Love or About Work?
Chapter 17 discussed top-down processing as the abstraction of an invariant across several situations (see Figure 17.1). This conceptual linking is privileged by psychodynamic approaches and goes beyond the immediate experience of a new perspective (Messer & McWilliams, 2006). Here, self-knowledge is construed at a high-level of abstraction to extract a personal theme. When clients arrive at conclusions like "I feel persecuted because of the following autobiographical reasons," they reach a better self-understanding. Linking insights of this kind are most often experience-distant because the thematization of experience requires a broader level of analysis or a connection between elements, which takes precedence over the client's actual moment-by-moment experience of any individual element (A. Pascual-Leone & Greenberg, 2007b).

Although one could observe any number of constants across a set of situations (i.e., invariants), only some will be clinically meaningful. Treatment approaches have converged on two chief themes that are typically used to cultivate new overarching meanings regarding one's life narrative (Bakan, 1966). On one hand, treatments have focused on themes related to a client's sense of self as agent in its various capacities. This is done by linking different psychological components to one another (e.g., emotion + anxiety + defenses; Malan, 1979; Messer & McWilliams, 2006). On the other hand, treatments may focus on themes about a person's interpersonal dynamics, linking temporal relationship events to one another (e.g., a past significant other + a current other + the therapist; Luborsky et al., 1994; Malan, 1979). These represent two distinct lenses for formulating an interpretation of one's emotional experience. A practical consequence of this is that insights in psychodynamic therapy are either emotional or relational in nature. More accurately, the theme of a psychodynamic insight is typically either about self-definition and agency or about connection to others and communion (i.e., work or love). I return to these two avenues of thematic meaning making in Chapter 21.

Importantly, irrespective of how emotional or evocative these insights might be, the realization that one is living a certain type of narrative theme will not and cannot come from only exploring one's experience from a first-person perspective. Other processes like emerging awareness and emotional expression are about unpacking the meaning within a single and immediate moment, but conflictual themes in one's life can only be observed when looking across situations (i.e., they are invariants abstracted across situations; Chapter 17). Looking at oneself across various life situations necessarily requires a third-person perspective. This can be done through decentering and then critically examining a collection of one's own stories, or it can occur through an interpretation offered by a therapist, who literally holds a third-person outside perspective on one's experience.

In the following example from A. Pascual-Leone and Greenberg (2007b), a client suffering depression first reflects on her marital distress and then on her relationships with her children before discovering a theme.

THERAPIST: Oh, so you can't accept love just for being who you are?

CLIENT: [*Talking rapidly*] No. I owe them. Somebody . . . I owe my children when they do something nice for me. I owe them so big I could never buy them enough gifts. I am so touched that somebody bothers to love me. It's so big for me. I think . . . I'm starting to formulate something here in my mind. [*Her speech slows*] Give me a second. . . . I think I turn people off so I don't have to owe. I'm just realizing that at this moment in time. . . . because I turn a lot of people off. And it seems to me—Why would I do that? I mean, that's like shooting yourself in the foot. . . . But I think I do that simply for the purpose of not having to owe them. I just discovered that. (p. 43)

An understanding like this about how a repetition of dysfunctional patterns in one's life may be related to one's life history is an example of reflecting on the larger narrative that contextualizes one's presenting emotional experience. A meta-analysis of 23 studies has shown a moderate association between clients having this kind of insight and the outcomes of their psychotherapy (Jennissen et al., 2018). Furthermore, the study found no difference in the role of insight between psychodynamic therapy, CBT, or other established approaches to psychotherapy. This underscores the pantheoretical nature of the process, despite the fact that it is typically associated with psychodynamic theory.

A large study included in the previously cited meta-analysis followed clients for 3 years after treatment and showed increases in the quality of client insight mediated their relief from presenting symptoms (Johansson et al., 2010). Moreover, contrary to what is commonly believed, clients who had more troubled interpersonal histories and poorer interpersonal relationships were the ones who benefited the most when therapists identified their relational themes (i.e., made transference interpretations), as compared with clients who already had better relationship histories. This finding highlights that people suffering personality disorders and longstanding relational trauma may especially benefit from reflecting on the relational themes that contextualize their problematic emotion. Later research on the same sample showed both these (third-person) insights and (first-person) emotional awareness are likely mechanisms of change in the long-term outcomes of psychodynamic therapy (Høglend & Hagtvet, 2019).

Finally, analyses have not yet been conducted to explore the temporal relationship between psychodynamic insight and symptom change within the course of ongoing treatment. Such analyses have already been done in the study of cognitive change (Quigley et al., 2019; cited earlier this chapter) as well as experiential processing (Pinheiro et al., 2021; Chapter 7, this volume). A longitudinal mediation analysis of psychodynamic insight is an important future research direction.

Identifying a Theme Is a Call to Action

The purpose of a psychodynamic interpretation is to generate insight into one's problem but that also implies a charge of responsibility—one that incites existential choice. Psychodynamic insights typically involve drawing upon the sociohistorical context to help explain the nature of one's personal difficulties. A meta-analysis of 16 studies examined therapists' use of interpretations during psychodynamic therapy and showed that providing clients with this sort of additional context for understanding their own experience had a small to medium effect size in the prediction of better symptom outcomes posttreatment (Zilcha-Man et al., 2023).

The delivery of a psychodynamic case formulation to a client typically comes with some acknowledgment or validation that what one has suffered (e.g., perhaps abuse or neglect as a child) was not their own fault and not a choice the client was responsible for. Indeed, the origins of such maladaptive themes are usually a tragedy due to forces that were beyond the client's control. Doing this contextualizes one's personal difficulty in a developmental landscape, and critically, it often highlights the moment currently being lived as an existential choice (e.g., Therapist: "Although the past was not your choice, the future is. Will you choose to continue along the old familiar path? Or will you risk trying something different?"). Thus, the client is ultimately faced with a choice to either remain within the cycle of a familiar but chronically unhealthy pattern or to find the courage to begin behaving and responding in new ways. This confronts the individual with an existential choice to reinvent themselves. In sum, the psychodynamic insight is a call to action.

There are other approaches that also use the long game strategy to bring choice to the foreground. Some treatments like ACT (S. C. Hayes et al., 2012) or motivational interviewing (Miller & Rollnick, 2013) similarly use decentering to shift the client's interpretive framework to a broader scope of analysis, one that highlights an individual's personal values and life goals. Bringing attention to and articulating one's personal values creates a point of implicit comparison with one's life as it is. Like a psychodynamic insight, examining one's personal values implicitly imposes the task of making more congruent choices in one's life. Becoming mindful of the choice one has and is taking in the present changes the way one perceives life events and highlights opportunities for being more congruent.

This recalls the adage that ignorance is bliss. But as the themes one is living, the values one holds, and the opportunity for change becomes more explicit, one can no longer shake the burden of responsibility to which one was previously ignorant. However, if it all stays in the person's head (cognitive reframing or dynamic insight alike), that is not going to make the person feel substantively different. Theorizing from the safety of one's armchair is not emotional change. And yet, the insight that there is a theme and that one is unhappy about it is a thought one cannot unthink. As such, it often looms or nags on until one decides to act and try something different. That becomes the real choice, an existential choice, one that involves action.

ENDNOTES

1. "Yo soy yo y mi circunstancia," translated by author.
2. "Cognitive reframing" is often used interchangeably with "cognitive reappraisal." In this book I use "reframing" because it more clearly captures working with the surrounding context of meaning. And that is the means for achieving some reappraisal. As an aside, the term "cognitive" is too often added in psychotherapy theory without much careful consideration of what the term really contributes. I suspect authors do this in an effort to appear more scientifically precise—particularly if they view "emotion" as messier and more nebulous than "cognition." Nevertheless, typically what is being referred to as "cognitive" (reframing, restructuring, etc.) is as much a rational process as an affective one. A more candid term might be "psychological" (reframing, restructuring, etc.), but in a paper on psychology, that would be stating the obvious. In any case, "reframing" (alone) will often suffice.
3. For the reader who is as perplexed as I was, according to reports the real human brain was most likely a stolen teaching specimen. The individual kept the brain wrapped in a department store bag and used embalming fluid drawn from the specimen to spray on his marijuana before smoking it.
4. Interestingly, behavioral gains overwhelmingly followed emotional gains (70% of the time) and only occasionally preceded emotional change (8% of the time; Snippe et al., 2024). This finding points to the role of emotion in daily life as a pivotal motivational factor for behavioral changes.

21

Life Narrative and Identity

The Story Itself Is an Agent of Change

The universe is made up of stories, not of atoms.

—MURIEL RUKEYSER, *THE SPEED OF DARKNESS*

Freud (1910) suggested that his "patients suffer from reminiscences" (p. 187). From an autobiographical memory perspective, this idea is that some memories are threatening to the current self because when attended to, they "destabilize the goals of the working self and cast the whole system into turmoil" (Conway & Pleydell-Pearce, 2000, p. 282). Both the content and structure of a client's stories provide their therapist with insight into that client's emotional processing, their perspectives on the self and others, and their ability to make meaning out of experiences (Boritz et al., 2013). The contrast to highly elaborative stories is having stories that are either empty or highly repetitive. Moreover, it is when those narratives become disjointed or misaligned that a client tends to seek out therapy. At the same time, the hackneyed imperative that to feel better, one must tell one's story follows from the belief that narrative is an effective tool for working with emotion to produce positive health changes (Pasupathi et al., 2017).

In Chapter 18, I presented narrative modes that might be observed at any given moment in the stories told during psychotherapy, namely, problematic narratives (e.g., same old story), transition narratives (e.g., completing plotlines), innovative moments, and change narratives (e.g., a discovery narrative; Angus et al., 2017; Gonçalves et al., 2011). Those processes are local narrative devices, revealing how someone engages in their story's construction. Sometimes they

https://doi.org/10.1037/0000460-022
Principles of Emotion Change: What Works and When in Psychotherapy and Everyday Life, by A. Pascual-Leone
Copyright © 2026 by the American Psychological Association. All rights reserved.

are even observable from just one or two phrases and predict a person's level of symptom distress (A. Pascual-Leone et al., 2023). However, such narrative passages also aggregate at a much broader level to create the story of someone's identity. That is the topic of this chapter.

STORYTELLING

Research on the prevalence with which people tell stories suggests that married couples will bring up 9 to 15 specific past events within 15 minutes of open conversation, whereas a discussion over family dinner will bring up a different story about every 5 minutes (McLean et al., 2007). Irrespective of the type of emotion that they entail, 90% of emotional experiences are disclosed to other people as stories within a few days of their occurrence. Moreover, this observation holds true across both cultures and genders (Rimé et al., 1991). As suggested by the epigraph to this chapter, although emotional experience and its processing occur moment by moment, individual experiences are always nested in some story. As introduced in Chapter 17, those stories are the medium through which we contemplate emotional changes. Indeed, the findings speak to how common it is to formulate emotion within a narrative framework not only to communicate it but as a means of contextualizing and understanding it.

Situated stories are about the personal past or imagined future as well as its impact on the self, and they are formulated for some private or interpersonal purpose (Libby & Eibach, 2011; McLean, et al., 2007). Moreover, stories people tell about negative events are more likely to have the search for meaning as an ongoing theme with compared with stories about positive or neutral events (McLean & Pratt, 2006). However, even when they are stressful, it is easier to tell stories about common life experience—like leaving home, looking for job, or getting over a relationship—than unconventional events. What happened, why one feels the way one does, and the search for meaning is simply easier to formulate for stories that conform to social templates and expected trajectories than for stories about unexpected and difficult change events, particularly when those experiences are highly personal and idiosyncratic (Adler et al., 2007). This is the work involved in a narrative process, and it reflects, in part, that complexities of emotional change may unfold across time and across situations. Putting together the story of emotional change seems especially important to maintain treatment gains resulting from psychotherapy (Adler et al., 2007; Frank, 1961). That story offers both some conclusion as well as some functional handle as a referent for what happened and how one feels about it.

The Development of Narrative as an Influence of Change

Although small children can recognize and recall events from their personal past, they do not tell coherent stories about the things that happened to them until they reach the age of 3 or 4 years old (Conway, 2005). Of course, an attentive listener can use questions and prompts to draw out the story of what happened.[1] That mental scaffolding helps buttress a child's story with context, coherence, and requisite themes to co-construct a meaningful narrative. Several studies on parent–child dialogue and the emergence of autobiographical narrative reveals that some parents use a highly elaborative style: They ask evaluative questions, make comments to support the developing narrative, and elicit more information, doing so in a manner that supports the child's point of view. Other parents who use a low elaborative style do not make inquiries to elaborate the details of an event; instead, they tend to repeat the same question and then change topics quickly (McLean et al., 2007). Over time, this mentorship in how to tell meaningful, rich, and searching narratives (or how not to do so) shapes how children tell their stories. There is also reason to believe that this socialization continues later in life.

Such observations have been tested using intervention research. One study trained mothers of 3- or 4-year-olds to be more elaborative in their narrative style when talking to their children. Following up 2 years later when the children were invited by an experimenter into a discussion, those whose mothers received the training had since developed more complex narratives as compared with children of mothers who were in a control condition (Peterson et al., 1999). This is reminiscent of psychotherapy research in which clients have been trained to use more autobiographical specificity (see Chapter 18). When a client's stories are empty, repetitive, or relatively entrenched, they are typically related to problematic processes such as rumination and the same old story, which are related to psychopathology (Aldao et al., 2010; Angus, 2012). Thus, the mentorship of one's narrative style is not only part of early development but may also be extended into adulthood as part of a corrective therapeutic experience.

The socialization of narrative style also points to several sociocultural issues. Parents tend to encourage girls more than boys to emotionally elaborate their stories, an impact that can later be observed in adulthood (McLean et al., 2007). This is consistent with the more micro-level observation made among college students that both cultural and gender differences in emotional awareness are partly explained by the emotion socialization that was offered by one's parents (Le et al., 2002; Chapter 6, this volume). Largely, the opportunities for narrative to act in shaping the self depends on one's social context. For example, working-class mothers tend to be more challenging when their children tell stories about autonomy, whereas middle-class mothers tend to allow their children more leeway (Wiley et al., 1998). This difference in narrative style across social class is related to views on whether autonomy is taken as something to be earned or whether it is a gift that is bestowed. The socialization that follows from each framework of understanding shapes the stories one tells about oneself and likely the experience of autonomy itself. As such, there are also systemic frames of influence on how emotional experiences can and will be narrated.

Cultural Influences and Master Narratives

The focus and content of freely recalled autobiographical memories turn out to be profoundly different across North American, Northern European, and Asian countries. For example, when participants are asked to recall memories from early childhood, North Americans are more likely to generate memories that are oriented toward the individual, are more specific, and are more emotional as compared with Chinese participants, whose memories are more likely to capture social themes and be less emotional (Conway, 2005). In addition to being influenced by their country of origin, the kinds of autobiographical narrative people tell also appear to be socialized in culture-specific ways by the context in which they grow up (McLean et al., 2007; see also Ryder et al., 2018). Stories also evolve as they search to anchor one's personal experience to social and cultural frameworks of understanding. Layered on top of those cultural frames of references are the specific narrative devices typically used for telling such stories.

Master Narratives Provide Ready-Made Frameworks

A personal story is influenced by archetypal narratives that are culturally familiar. *Master narrative* describes the overarching norms and expectations that relate a story to its given cultural and social framework. They are typically gendered and hold other implicit biases around ethnicity, economic class, and so on (McLean et al., 2007). The implication is that positive master narratives are culturally relative but also that they can act as off-the-shelf stories to support one's personal narrative construction.

A *redemption narrative* is one of the most studied constructs in the field of narrative identity, and it is the classic story in North American culture in which a protagonist suffers but then confronts adversity, triumphs, and experiences the positive outcomes of agency and freedom (McAdams, 2013; McLean et al., 2020).[2] The *recuperative narrative* is a contrasting example from the United Kingdom that tells the story of a gradual attenuation of suffering as a person effortfully develops their ability to cope with the scars of trauma-related hardship (Blackie et al., 2020). Iconic examples of Chinese narratives frequently entail more emphasis on social morality, with fewer details about the individual (McLean et al., 2007). Master narratives like these are socially valued scripts that offer a structure for someone to both interpret and scaffold a story onto their lived experience. In short, the way we formulate our life stories is in accordance with (or in reaction to) culturally informed templates that are familiar to us through the accounts shared in books, television, movies, and even in the reporting of world news. The act of reflecting on one's life story is done in a cultural milieu of expectations about what the narrative of a healthy person "usually" looks like.

Familiar stories and culturally loaded tropes are models of change that often facilitate an individual through healthy emotional transitions. They do this by acting as a narrative scaffolding and implicitly proposing a default in life direction. Easy examples of this are coming-of-age or boy-meets-girl stories that are celebrated within a given society. This is useful for facilitating conventional trajectories and shaping the personal identities most compatible with such narratives. For example, when a young person joins the military, this offers a narrative template with a set of values, behavioral guidelines, and expected outcomes, which cultivates a specific identity. So, within some range, adopting a readily available narrative helps model the emergence of a corresponding identity. However, as seen in extremist hate groups, when they are shared and rehearsed within an esoteric community, assuming a narrative can also facilitate identities of destruction (Simi et al., 2017).

The Dark Side of Master Narratives

If one's life follows a less conventional path, master narratives will rigidly model a framework for understanding one's emotional experience that could actively hinder personal development. This is striking in the stories of people structurally marginalized in society (e.g., cultural or sexual minorities), such that working against presiding master narratives becomes a genuine struggle for identity (McLean et al., 2018). For example, the happy love story of my transgender client deviated markedly from mainstream romances, but after forging a unique story, it became their anchor for identity and a beacon of hope.

Master narratives also work against those who must make less celebrated life choices. When a woman came to me for therapy after having an abortion, she was overwhelmed with confused grief: "I made that choice. So, I don't know if I get to grieve what happened or what it means." Almost 50% of women who have abortions report having grief experiences similar to that of my client (Curley & Johnston, 2013). Even so, sadly, the most familiar narratives that might have applied to my client's situation would actively villainize her and offer no solace. This highlights how frameworks offered by cultural and master narratives are not always representative of our collectively lived experiences but are also shaped top down by historical antecedents and social values. Most critically, the cultural narratives available to my client offered no guidance on how she might move on with her life.

People whose emotional experiences are more idiosyncratic and do not conform with master narratives will often need help working with their story in at least two ways. First, they need help extracting themselves and distancing from the dominant narrative and values they may have internalized (e.g., a gay man with internalized homophobia). Second, they need to search out examples of counter-narratives that support their emerging story (e.g., the bookish girl in a country that prohibits the education of women). For better or worse, master narratives are readymade tools to make meaning about emotional events. They shape how an individual initially formulates their life story and which kinds of stories will be experienced as most emblematic.

The Social Influence on Narratives

Privately formulating covert stories to oneself will indeed shape experience, but that formulation is still subject to both master narratives as well as social expectations even before one's narratives are shared openly. Stories shared publicly are further influenced by social reinforcement and the behavior of listeners. Listeners prefer to hear certain kinds of stories over others, and this direct feedback either encourages or hinders the formulation by which one understands one's experience (McLean et al., 2007). Concretely, a listener's behavior influences how much elaboration the storyteller will offer, and the effect of having made that accommodation is apparent later in how one remembers the same event. For example, experiments show that telling one's story to a distracted or unresponsive listener can deteriorate one's recollection of the event later (Pasupathi & Hoyt, 2010). The neurological underpinning of this potentially harmful effect is explained by memory reconsolidation, in which a memory can become obfuscated or muddied (Lane & Nadel, 2020).[3] In summary, emotional experience is embedded within stories about how one grapples with reality, but stories themselves are crafted within a culturally informed framework that bears on one's understanding of oneself.

THE SELF IS THE ULTIMATE CONTEXT FOR UNDERSTANDING EMOTION

Socialization and culture are external factors shaping our stories of emotion, but they also have an important internal counterpoint. Even as identity itself is influenced by sociocultural factors, one's subjective sense of self and the overarching story of who one is emerges as the ultimate reference—one that lends context to any immediate feeling. This is at play when people experience themselves as interacting with culture or when they conclude, for example, "But that's not me!" or "It feels right for me." Narrative identity is a high level of epistemological abstraction, and it highlights that an individual's experience is deeply contextualized (Adler, 2016).

A study on the impact of 4 days of diary writing after the difficult end of a relationship showed similar degrees of effectiveness when participants were instructed to either use cognitive reframing or to formulate a redemptive narrative of what had happened (Slotter & Ward, 2015). Moreover, these processes had a lagged effect, so when participants used either process on earlier days, it predicted they would have less distress on later days. However, unlike cognitive reframing, the elaboration of a redemptive narrative remained a significant predictor of reduced distress over time (Slotter & Ward, 2015). While cognitive reframing offers alternative interpretations for a given event (external), a redemptive narrative redefines the self (internal). This is an important distinction between the processes and may explain the enduring effect of working with narrative identity over reframing the local situation or events (for more on cognitive reframing, see Chapter 20).

One's immediate experience of emotion is always nested within some presenting situation (i.e., a set of external or internal cues). That situation is the local context (e.g., a cognitive frame) or proximal trigger of change. But moment-by-moment situations themselves are further nested in a much larger sociohistorical arch, which we can call a life narrative—as in, ([{immediate emotion} Local Situational Context] OVERARCHING LIFE NARRATIVE). These layers of context cumulatively inform the experience of any given moment. For example, in an uncertain situation, if my preverbal experience is of anxious tension mixed with frustration but the broader self-perception is that I am a brave, strong, and forceful person, then that context of identity will shape my emotional response, making it more likely that I will feel anger rather than intimidation. In this way, a reflection on one's emotion is ultimately a reflection (to some degree) about the self.

Autobiographical memory, fictional events, and fantasies about the future collectively form a narrative fabric for interpreting one's moment-by-moment experience, but they also help discern the self. The memory of an event is simultaneously a triangulation of the self:

> An *event memory* is a mental construction of a scene. . . . The construction need not come with a sense of reliving or be made by a participant in the event, and it can be a summary of occurrences from more than one encoding. The mental construction, or physical rendering, of any scene must be done from a specific location and time; this introduces a "self" located in space and time. (Rubin & Umanath, 2015, p. 1, italics in original)

Both emotional and nonemotional memories help one conceptualize a sense of self (Beike et al., 2004; Conway & Pleydell-Pearce, 2000). A narrative is also an effective way of modeling intersubjective as well as interpersonal dialogue. Furthermore, the formulation of the self is confluent with a felt sense of one's immediately emergent experience (Gendlin, 1996; Chapter 6, this volume). In this way, as we contemplate our emotional experiences, we contemplate who we are.

A striking feature of self-related memories is that recalling an autobiographical memory takes considerably more time to formulate than the access and retrieval of other kinds of knowledge from memory, including even when one remembers factual knowledge about oneself (Conway, 2005). This delay in processing reflects the computational challenge of abstracting a representation of the self from a vast horizon of one's concrete experiences (Gilead et al., 2020). Understanding the self as a dynamic psychological construction means that having certain memories about oneself, what happened, and what it meant are factors that shape one's sense of self and identity (e.g., Client: "So, that's what happened, and it makes me who I am today!" [at least according to this instance of remembering[4]]). Part of the way our sense of self interacts with affective content has to do with what I referred to as the metadata of memory or how we relate to our personal narratives (see Chapter 19), whereas another part has to do with shaping the content of memory itself (Chapters 18 and 22). Whatever the mechanism, as one considers an increasingly wider scope of analysis (i.e., from perceptual–affective moments to personal–social encounters to identity-based values), the episodic processes of meaning making start to coalesce into a much more overarching process of what could be called self-making (Pals, 2006b).

NARRATIVE IDENTITY: "SELVES CREATING STORIES, CREATING SELVES"

The concept of one's narrative identity[5] has been examined since the mid-1980s as a potential mechanism of personality change and lifespan development (Adler, 2019). Telling one's story is inherently validating and it affirms the ownership of personal experiences, and these are in addition to the social role of sharing stories. From a longitudinal study on how identity is shaped through narrative, a middle-aged woman tells her story about a difficult time in her life:

> I knew I reached an emotional bottom that year . . . but I began making a stable life again, as a more stable, independent person. . . . It was a period full of pain, experimentation, and growth, but in retrospect it was necessary for me to become anything like the woman I am today. (Pals, 2006a, p. 1080)

Before the quote even begins, this woman decenters from her lived experience to reflect upon what it might mean as part of an overarching story (Chapter 20). She then draws causal connections between her falling to an emotional bottom and her resilience, as well as the function that a redemption sequence played in shaping her current identity. Statements like this are common if one asks adults to reflect on difficult life events that challenged their sense of identity. Reflecting on this example, Adler and colleagues (2016) highlight the most critical issue for appreciating how narrative informs emotional change:

> *This was not the only narrative option available to this woman.* She could have resolved the negative chapter without finding any redeeming value in it, a scene in which negative beginnings have negative endings. She could have described the stability and independence she found, which characterize her present self, as the start of a new chapter, one that began with this positivity that has endured to today. Instead, she makes temporal and causal connections between the depth of her pain and her growth into a new, valued self, narratively redeeming the experience in a way that data suggest was more likely to support her well-being. *There is nothing historically objective about this sequence; it represents a narrative reconstruction, one vital to this woman's well-being.* (p. 163, italics added)

The example illustrates how aspects of narrative identity represent a level of meaning making that is neither reducible to bottom-up visceral experience nor better explained by individual differences when predicting well-being.

People's behavior can vary dramatically across different local situations, and the course of anyone's life will be full of hazards and chaotic influences, but nevertheless, we seek to bring it all together and make meaning in the form of a narrative. This story of who one was, who one is, and who one hopes to become represents one of the largest frameworks for understanding oneself and one's emotional experience within a given event (McAdams, 2019). This is one's self concept in narrative form, and it is a layer of personality superimposed onto dispositional traits as an implicit part of personal development. Narrative identity is a process model of self-development, where personal memories, articulated through stories, are anchored in an existing sense of self. The creation of that story subsequently contributes to the self-development and lived experience in an iterative manner (Conway, 2005; McLean et al., 2007).

A narrative process of this kind is not an exclusively descriptive tool for reminiscence; it also serves as a prospective lens for perceiving and interpreting future emotional experiences (see also Chapter 18).[6] So in the grand scheme, narrative identity serves two important functions. First, one's autobiography acts as a framework for integrating together various events, feelings, and meanings about one's life. Second, it creates a sense of purpose as one looks toward (and acts on) the horizon of one's life. Both these functions are implicit; their influence is embedded in the assumptions of one's story. (At the end of Chapter 20, I also highlighted that decentering and becoming consciously aware of one's life themes or values creates an explicit sense of intentional commitment to then fulfill any identified wishes or aspirations.) Finally, the formulation of a narrative identity by integrating meaning and creating a sense of purpose impacts an individual's well-being and mental health.

Cognitive Factors in How Narrative Identity Shapes Emotion

Before further exploring the ultimate factors by which narrative identity is believed to influence emotional experience, there is the question of how narrative identity bears on one's moment-by-moment formulations of experiences. At least three cognitive factors explain how life narratives could offer a unique influence on shaping and changing emotion. Each of these factors point to the context of information that is drawn upon when processing an emergent feeling, and they show the importance of stories as a point of reference when working with emotion (see also Chapter 4).

First, not all aspects of self-knowledge can be summarized or abstracted semantically; some are singular and emblematic. We all have significant life events, momentous scenes, and self-defining memories. They may represent high points, low points, or pivotal episodes of transition. Whatever the case, as highly emotional one-time events, many of these are uniquely captured by specific autobiographical episodes (Adler et al., 2016; Boucher & Scoboria, 2015; McLean et al., 2020).

Second, these personal and specific narrative accounts are frequently recalled, reactivated, and purposefully rehearsed when cued by relevant issues encountered in one's life. For better or for worse, such reactivations lend immediate contextual information to a presenting situation (e.g., "This relationship is souring just like my marriage did, here I am again"; or "I did it before, I can do it again"). Over time, the impact of repeated activations accumulates to render a broader and stable influence or theme, shaping how one perceives oneself vis-à-vis one's circumstances. This formulation is supported by the neuroscience of how memories literally change (Lane & Nadel, 2020). The result is a sense of unity within the self, implicitly offering a blueprint for how one might respond to life's challenges.

Third, narratives also embody unconscious wishes in a way that cannot be afforded through either cognitive reflection or the purposeful labeling of emotion. Whereas people can readily respond to questions about their explicit wishes, implicit wishes cannot be elaborated through direct inquiry even as they shape one's motives and behavior. They are, however, often embedded within the personal narratives one constructs (Woike, 2008). So, the more time one spends elaborating narratives, the more implicit motives and unconscious wishes will come to manifest themselves. This, of course, is a central tenant of psychodynamic approaches because it offers a unique entry point to emotional processing (Luborsky et al., 1994; Messer & McWilliams, 2006; D. B. Stern, 1997). These three factors are means by which narrative identity likely serves as an integrative framework and imparts a sense of purpose.

Autobiography as an Integrative Framework

Elaborating one's experience into a story has been proposed as a central process for achieving the highest level of self-integration (McLean et al., 2007). Narrative identity is critical in this process because it becomes the integrative framework for interpreting events and relating emotional experiences to one's sense of self. The result is increased *identity clarity*, which is "when a person describes a past event's impact as bringing about increased clarity regarding self-definition and purpose or meaning in life" (Lilgendahl & McAdams, 2011, p. 406). As a story becomes clearer, so does the person; the process renders emotional coherence and self-clarity.

Narrating Emotion, Formulating Identity

The tools one uses for autobiographical reasoning are modeled early on in life. For example, a study of middle-class families in New Zealand looked at the everyday conversations that parents had with their 4- to 6-year-old children (Bird & Reese, 2006). When conversations focused on explaining the causes and consequences of the child's negative emotions as well as on evaluating positive emotions, it was moderately related to the child having a more consistent sense of self. In contrast, during those same conversations, processes like awareness and labeling emotion were unrelated to a child's consistent self-view (Bird & Reese, 2006). This contrast supports the notion that explaining emotion (top down) is closely related to how one understands oneself and is a process distinct from (bottom up) emotional awareness.

Another study of ethnically diverse middle-class American families showed that when mothers were emotionally expressive and explained emotion while recounting negative family events, it predicted their 9- to 11-year-old children would have higher self-esteem 2 years later. Mothers also expressed and explained emotion more than fathers, which is probably good, because unfortunately, fathers' narrated emotion had the inverse effect, predicting lower self-esteem in their preadolescent children (Bohanek et al., 2008). Narratives are used to evaluate and elaborate emotion, fleshing out the meaning of past events and articulating their relevance to one's life. The narrative becomes a conceptual anchor or point of reference, linking what something feels like to what it might mean in one's life.

Narrative identity starts to get formulated in early adolescence and continues to develop throughout one's lifespan with the same strengths and weaknesses as any oral history (McAdams, 2019; also see Chapter 19, this volume). Erikson (1968) argued that identity emerges in early adolescence because a young person discovers themselves as being significantly different in some way from when they were a child. That transformation is explained in the form of a personal story. People develop their life narratives as a sort of drawstring to help pull everything together. An observation made across studies and cultures is that the prevalence of autobiographical memories people recall are unevenly distributed over the lifespan. People remember more personal events that occurred between the ages of 10 and 30 as compared with any other life period, a phenomenon referred to as the reminiscence bump. The most compelling explanation of this is that during adolescence and young adulthood, experiences are more self-defining and play a role in stabilizing the formation of one's identity and sense of self (Conway, 2005).

Trajectories of Meaning
The reminiscence bump also suggests palpable implications for emotional experiences that may unfold in the future (Conway, 2005). For instance, if a story is construed as having a happy ending, it could come to represent the emergence of an affective theme. Such narrative resolution (as a process) is complex and applies teleologically. In other words, when we generate narratives about the possible resolution of existing challenges it is either (a) a wishful fantasy—which broadens the horizon of actual possibilities—or it is (b) a goal statement, or both.[7] For example, consider that "I yearn to feel special" (a wish) or "I strive to be special" (a goal) hold the same intentionality. Particularly when the self is located within a hopeful narrative, the drive for narrative coherence and closure offers a concrete sense of meaning and purpose. All stories have a beginning, middle, and end (Chapter 19), so coherent stories that reflect narrative identity often lay out compelling trajectories for one's sense of direction in life.

In short, personal narratives serve a very different epistemological purpose than rational arguments, truth claims, or the recollection of (presumably) factual knowledge. The aim of storying one's experience is to capture a rich description of personal experience and locate that vector of experience within a sociohistorical frame of reference (Adler, 2011). Sitting at the intersection of cognitive development, autobiographical memory, and narrative work is a process referred to as *autobiographical reasoning*, which is what one does while both making use of and building on one's life story (Habermas, 2019). Meaningful personal events involve more than the relatively sterile truth value or historical facts that they entail. They need to also capture an account of one's vital values, which are explained and contextualized through the life narrative itself (J. Pascual-Leone & Johnson, 2021). These events are not only linked by their chronological order but also by the construction of arguments based on causal and motivational implications as well as themes, consequences, and the personal relevance of events.

Thus, the role of autobiographical reasoning is as an overarching constructive process that goes beyond the mere computation of remembering (Conway & Pleydell-Pearce, 2000; Habermas, 2019). This requires more mental effort than a laundry list of one's personal history; it represents a form of meaning making which then lends service to emotional processing (Angus & Greenberg, 2011; J. Pascual-Leone & Johnson, 2021). The extraction of themes and knowingly reflecting on those themes pertains to another process, which is decentering from one's narrative context. (I explored that mechanism in Chapter 20, and its clinical implications are picked up in Chapters 22 and 23.) In relation to narrative identity, it is enough to recognize there are pivotal moments when people become aware of their role in the narrative construction and how that forthcoming act of meaning creation will shape them.

NARRATIVE IDENTITY'S ASSOCIATION WITH EMOTIONAL HEALTH

The ultimate role of narrative identity is as an integrative framework, providing a wellspring of meaning and purpose. The implication of these two functions, one immediate and the other prospective, is that narrative identity comes to play a central role in one's personality. The hermeneutic process of exercising and expressing one's personality informs our lived experience, so much so that it also impacts our mental health and well-being.

What Are the Critical Features of Narrative Identity?

Personal narratives can be examined using an infinite number of themes and qualitatively rich descriptions, but both reviews of critical theory (e.g., Adler, 2016) and factor analyses (McLean et al., 2020) have identified core overarching dimensions or latent factors in research to date. Their conclusions are largely in agreement with each other as well as with various panels of experts in the field. McLean and colleagues (2020) identify three to four kinds of factors—narrative structure, autobiographical reasoning, and motivational or affective themes—wherein the last two dimensions are conceptually distinct but remain fundamentally intertwined in practice.

Reviews of the evidence suggest the structural elements (e.g., coherence, complexity) of one's narrative identity do not consistently predict well-being, although they are probably prerequisites to rendering the pertinent features of other dimensions that are critical to well-being (Adler et al., 2016; McLean et al., 2020). I suggest a variation of this hypothesis, which is that the degree of complexity and coherence may be a moderator of narrative's effects. Consider, for example, that one may have a negative self-view that is either vague and poorly formulated or detailed and highly coherent; the latter would represent a more entrenched threat to mental health. Similarly, positive narratives that are well structured and highly coherent promise more emotional resilience than if they were unelaborated.[8]

The structure of narratives aside, a review of 30 studies concluded that two sets of variables predict well-being: autobiographical reasoning and motivational–affective themes (Adler et al., 2016). This conclusion was also supported by a large-scale factor analysis (McLean et al., 2020). I explore these variables in the corresponding sections that follow.

Autobiographical Reasoning Predicts Emotional Health

Autobiographical reasoning has been operationalized using various measures including integrative meaning, accommodating or navigating change, actively synthesizing closure, and gaining insight through a narrative's construction. Examples of this are found when a person identifies their storying of a past event as having affected how they generally think about their own personal issues (Lilgendahl & McAdams, 2011; McLean et al., 2020). It is common in everyday life that people candidly identify moments when the way they construed their narrative led to a presenting state of emotional health. When people spontaneously offer up these instances of autobiographical reasoning, it represents an analysis of subjective causality that should be given some serious consideration. Pals (2006b) documents vivid examples of this self-making. In the following excerpt, she discusses how autobiographical reasoning seems to have shaped a person's life:

> Asked to tell his life story, a middle-aged man begins by making a causal connection between his sense of himself in the present—his identity—and a significant piece of his past. With his opening statement, this man makes his volatile childhood a central lens of interpretation through which he makes sense of his life and constructs his story. The magnitude of the positive impact of this man's marriage on his sense of growth—something he vividly refers to as a "springboard effect"—can only be fully appreciated within the context of the pattern of interconnected causal connections he makes leading up to it, beginning with the acknowledgment of his painful childhood and his interpretation of its initially very growth-limiting impact. (p. 175)

As highlighted in this example, autobiographical reasoning often involves stepping out of the plot-and-characters narrative account to comment on the story itself (Chapter 20). That pause in the external narrative creates room for a reflective narrative about the deeper significance that the episode may have for one's identity and life story (Adler et al., 2016; Angus & Greenberg, 2011). As in the previous account, weaving a life story with its reflexive commentary gives narrative identity a sense of purpose and unity.

Several research examples illustrate how autobiographical reasoning of this kind predicts well-being (Adler et al., 2016). In one study, parents who found out their child had Down syndrome were asked to write narratives about the experience and then were followed up 2 years later. Foreshadowing and conjecturing on happy endings are narrative devices that anticipate resolution. For instance, well before the end of their story, one participant stated, "I knew everything would be alright" (L. A. King et al., 2000, p. 523). Statements of faith in a happy ending also implicitly frame the narrative within a grand design or hidden purpose, which often carries a spiritual undertone (whether that be secular or religious).[9] When parents used such formulations, it predicted a high level of closure and subjective well-being both concurrently and longitudinally, even when controlling for a host of family-level and temporal variables.

Another finding from the same study pertained to stories that revealed a paradigmatic shift in how the parent lived life upon learning their child had Down syndrome, such as the following account:

> I was surprised how much I totally suppressed the information. Total denial for 3 weeks. I was shocked at my own inability to deal with such an unexpected event. I cried a lot. The pain was so deep. I felt cheated—I could hardly function. I was so absorbed with my own fears. But I did regroup. I did grow. And I did learn to accept the situation. That opened the door for me to bond and love my child. But it took time. (L. A. King et al., 2000, p. 521)

Narratives such as this go beyond a happy resolution by suggesting a deeper restructuring (e.g., "That opened the door for me"). In similar examples, parents actively accommodated the disruptive turn of events. The narrative formulation about a change in worldview is what predicted the greatest stress-related growth as well as increases in a narrator's emotional development over time (L. A. King et al., 2000). The two findings from this early study reveal a pattern that later studies have converged on: The kind of change that follows depends on the way a narrator construes and presents new personal meaning (Adler et al., 2016). I detail each of these different approaches to autobiographical reasoning in the two sections that follow.

Positive Meaning Making: Narrative Assimilation of New Meaning

On one hand, a narrator might assimilate new meaning, often with a positive valence (e.g., optimism, gratefulness, pleasant feelings), by connecting it to their (pre)existing identity (Adler et al., 2016). Authors working with narrative identity have highlighted the emotional tone of this process and refer to it as positive processing (Lilgendahl & McAdams, 2011). However, this is essentially *positive meaning making* as discussed in Chapter 18, where certain narratives are elaborated to add and assimilate positive content into one's stories—although here the narratives are about identity. The narrator treats the content as personally important but also as somewhat resolved, and there is no break from existing meaning structures. Integrating meaning in this way strengthens one's sense of personal coherence and purpose, which seems related to more contentment, enjoyment of life, and being free of distress (i.e., hedonic well-being and everyday pleasure).

For example, when a representative sample of adults in the United States wrote about the September 11, 2001, terrorist attacks in New York City, stories that revealed a sense of satisfactory personal closure about the events concurrently predicted an author's lower psychological distress, improved affect, and life satisfaction (Adler & Poulin, 2009). In a different study, when middle-aged Chinese participants wrote about the loss of a parent and could be observed to connect their sense of self to past positive events, engaging that process predicted that they would suffer a shorter period of grief (Huang et al., 2020). Another study invited adults to tell stories about both the high points and low points of their lives, examined the affective valence of those stories, and then followed up 2 years later. Participants who had included positive meaning in both kinds of stories reported better emotion regulation at follow up. However, when the narratives about low points included negative meaning making, it predicted that the authors would be struggling with poorer emotion regulation 2 years later (K. Cox & McAdams, 2014).

Notice that incorporating positively valenced content into one's existing narrative does not signal any major reconfigurations in identity or worldview. Still, this assimilative integration of positive and often-optimistic meaning predicts the reduction of distress as well as an increase in everyday pleasure and a general satisfaction with life. Considering the five relevant studies reviewed by Adler and colleagues (2016), I estimate that positive meaning making has a large overall effect in the prediction of well-being.[10]

Differentiated Processing: Narrative Accommodation of New Meaning

On the other hand, sometimes narrators accommodate new meaning, which involves partly reconfiguring the story of their identity (Adler et al., 2016). Here, the person explores the meaning of an event to new ends, often puzzling, questioning, and searching before reaching a more radical integration.[11] Some authors have referred to this as differentiated processing (Lilgendahl & McAdams, 2011). Narratives that capture this paradigm shift in meaning and identity often describe a storyline of destabilization followed by a categorically new personal growth, which seems related to existential maturation, happiness, and personal fulfillment (i.e., eudaimonic or existential well-being; Adler et al., 2016; see also Gelo & Salvatore, 2016, on destabilization). Furthermore, there is some evidence that this kind of differentiated processing is an important predictor of well-being when working through negative emotional events but is less so for positive events (Lilgendahl & McAdams, 2011). Although there are different ways to operationalize existential or emotional maturity as an outcome, the fact that it can be anticipated by how meaning was integrated is consistent with Erikson's (1968) theory of identity development.

Some studies have prompted the integration of new and more differentiated meaning by asking participants to narrate possible future selves when they imagined if their life conditions had been different. For example, divorced women were asked to write two fictional narratives about the future. Stories were about their best possible selves in one of two scenarios: where the divorce had happened or if it had never occurred. The sense of self observed in these stories predicted psychosocial maturity 2 years later (L. A. King & Raspin, 2004).

In a now seminal study by Pals (2006a), adults at age 21 were first asked to describe themselves, and then, at age 52, the same participants were asked to reflect on the difficult events of their life. For people who initially described themselves as being open and flexible, over 30 years later, the stories they told were more exploratory than those of adults who had not described themselves as open and flexible earlier in life. This shows personality as a static predictor of narrative style. But narrative identity also adds a dynamic role, which was observed when participants were followed up yet another decade later. The narrative's exploratory style at age 52 subsequently mediated the influence of personality traits such that it predicted more emotional maturity at age 61. These outcomes illustrate very long-term change in a normal population.

In psychotherapy with a clinical population, some individuals experience dramatic symptom improvements (i.e., sudden gains) that occur abruptly between two consecutive sessions over the course of treatment. These sudden gains have been predicted by the narrative meaning making in a preceding session (Adler et al., 2013). In short, from one session to the next, it was possible to assess the narrative changes that anticipated an abrupt improvement in mental health during routine clinical care. It is important to note that what predicted sudden gains was not the content of narratives (e.g., a given self-appraisal, revealing hopefulness) but rather the qualitative process, variables that tapped emergent autobiographical reasoning and coherence (This is in keeping with the observed effect of the much more specific narrative modes reviewed in Chapters 17 and 18.) Moreover, the nonlinear development of the narrative processes echoed the pattern of sudden gains and had a medium to large effect in the prediction of imminent treatment gains (Adler et al., 2013). Observing this exact tipping point between sessions, where narrative change anticipates targeted symptom change, adds support to the autobiographical reasoning in identity narratives as a possible mechanism of therapeutic change.

Exploring the existential meaning of an event in relation to a new identity or worldview is the differentiation of new meaning, which then gets accommodated in one's life narrative. This way of integrating new meaning into a narrative is predictive of psychosocial maturity, and it has an effect that reaches over and above the role of various personal characteristics, cognitive styles, or situational variables. Based on 10 studies reviewed by Adler and colleagues (2016), I estimate that differentiated processing has a medium to large overall effect in the prospective prediction of emotional well-being.

Motivational–Affective Themes Predict Emotional Health

There is evidence that when personal narratives reveal themes about their motivation toward agency or communion, or an affective theme of either redemption or contamination, those features are associated with emotional well-being. A narrator's implicit decision in how to parse the flow of time, what events or details should be included, or what is central to the account of events are revealed by their formulation of personal themes (see also Chapter 19).

Agency and Communion

In a landmark work, psychologist David Bakan (1966) identified *agency* and *communion* as "two fundamental modalities in the existence of living forms. . . . Agency manifests itself in self-protection, self-assertion, and self-expansion; communion manifests itself in the sense of being at one with other organisms" (pp. 14–15). Thus, when people tell stories about their drive to master or about coping with isolation, they touch upon themes of agency. Tales of openness, contact, noncontractual cooperation, and union signal themes of communion. As Bakan (1966) observes, one aspect of agency is separation, such that agency itself can entail the repression of communion, which creates a tension between these two overarching motivations. The integration of these, however, points to the higher motivational theme of generativity particularly in midlife (Erikson, 1986; McAdams, 2019) and is an important focus of religion (Bakan, 1966). Thematic meaning within autobiographical narratives represents a level of self-knowledge that is distinct from a person's semantically based self-reports about their agency and communion and explains unique variance in well-being (Philippe et al., 2011; see also Libby et al., 2014; Woike, 2008).

In psychotherapy, the theme of personal agency has been discussed as not only heralding in but manifesting a new sense of the self (e.g., Yalom, 1981). For example, writing narratives about their change process in psychotherapy, one client formulated the agency theme as follows:

> Being on my own is a scary place. At times, I feel like a little kid going somewhere for the first time—exciting, frustrating, wonderful, and scary all at once. These are a lot of changes in my life. I was feeling completely at their mercy, but now I see that I do have control. It's up to me to be able to stick with it, and I will rise. (Adler et al., 2013, p. 842)

This excerpt comes from a study of psychotherapy clients asked to write weekly about their experience in treatment and its impact on their sense of self over 12 separate weeks. When controlling for neuroticism, personal demographic, and the treatment approach itself, analyses revealed that the theme of agency progressively increased over time and that those narrative changes systematically preceded a client's incremental improvements in mental health (Adler, 2012). In another study with longer term outcomes, when college students were asked to write about major life events, narratives that depicted personal goals for growth in either agency or communion predicted participants' well-being over the following 3.5 years. Themes of agency predicted changes to psychosocial maturity, whereas communion predicted changes to subjective well-being, with both effects holding beyond the impact of personality traits (Bauer & McAdam, 2010).

Overall, there has been more empirical support for the role of emerging themes of agency and relatively less on communion. Yet the influence of a cultural framework is ubiquitous here. Narrative identity and agency have been a North American focus of research, and that may be why the role of communion has not yet shown itself to be as critical in studies to date. Furthermore, gender differences have been observed in the kinds of themes people express through their stories. For whatever reason, women are more likely to tell stories about feeling fear and sadness as compared with men, and they are also more likely to tell stories that have a theme of communion and relational experiences with others (McAdams et al., 2006). It remains unclear whether such differences are fundamentally tied to biological factors or to the impact of gender role socialization (other sex or gender differences in narrative were reported in Chapter 18).

Redemption and Contamination

Affective themes represent a higher level of complexity than a story's affective tone (e.g., its positivity or negativity). They manifest temporal and causal connection in a narrative arc, discerning purposeful shifts in direction, often with implications for one's identity.[12] The most studied affective themes either move from negative to positive in what are known as stories of *redemption* (i.e., when bad things turn good), or from positive to negative in stories of *contamination* (i.e., when good things turn bad; McAdams et al., 2001; see also Maruna, 2001, on scripts of generativity vs. condemnation). The dynamic shift within such themes has a stronger relationship with well-being than the simple valence of a narrative (Adler et al., 2016; McLean et al., 2020).

Contamination themes observed in narratives from a diverse group of midlife adults was unrelated to a global and depressogenic attributional style, often a focus in cognitive behavior therapy. Although both were related to depression, low self-esteem and low life satisfaction formulating one's narrative around themes of contamination was a predictor above a range of personality and cognitive traits (Adler et al., 2006). In another study, when narratives of psychotherapy clients showed concurrent experiences of happiness alongside sadness (i.e., mixed emotion), it systematically preceded their successive session-by-session improvements. Furthermore, the temporal precedence of a narrative's emerging emotional complexity and its association with well-being explained change more than the passage of time or individual indices of affective valence (Adler & Hershfield, 2012).

In self-help groups such as Alcoholics Anonymous, members repeatedly share their stories, and that becomes a central framework for understanding their difficulties and in making interventions (McAdams, 2019). Participants enrolled in Alcoholics Anonymous who had recently given up drinking were indistinguishable based on an initial assessment of personal and situational variables, but they were then asked to write about the last time they took a drink. After 4 months, those who had spontaneously formulated redemption themes in their narratives were almost twice as likely to have maintained their sobriety (i.e., a rate of 83% sobriety among those with redemption themes vs. 44% among those without; Dunlop & Tracy, 2013). After controlling for a host of relevant variables (e.g., trait affect, anxiety, controllability attributions), the authors concluded that the theme of redemption in these identity narratives played a causal role in prolonging healthy behavioral changes and maintained recovery from addiction.

Motivational themes such as agency and communion or dynamic affective themes such as redemption and contamination are predictive of healthy changes in psychological distress, self-esteem, and subjective well-being. These are the same kind of (hedonic) outcomes related to everyday enjoyments that were also predicted by positive meaning making (cited in the previous section). Furthermore, the abstraction of these also reveals the sense of purpose an individual has formulated for their life (for more on sense of purpose, see Chapter 23).[13] The effect of these themes on well-being is not better explained by affective valence, individual differences, or situational variables. Reviewing 19 studies (in Adler et al., 2016), I estimate the overall effect of these motivational–affective themes on well-being is of a small to medium size.

STABILITY OR CHANGE: WHICH NARRATIVE DYNAMIC ANTICIPATES WELL-BEING?

Longitudinal studies on narrative identity as a layer of personality has mostly focused on nonclinical samples, often examining personality change over periods of 2 years or more. Most of the research reviewed in the current chapter takes this approach and has been published in studies on personality and social psychology. In that context, holding to one's narrative identity is taken to indicate healthy stability in one's sense of self and good adjustment across life's circumstances.

However, health care research has taken a different perspective. In treatment studies of psychotherapy, narrative process is usually examined within a framework of event-based research, identifying the precise moment of a narrative innovation or shifts between successive episodes of storytelling. In-session events are then used as predictors of symptom outcome at the end of what is typically just a few months of treatment (for examples from clinical research, see Chapter 18). Thus, in the treatment context, stability in one's narrative style is often a reflection of ongoing symptoms, a sign of intractable difficulties (e.g., the same old story of feeling trapped or a story of trauma are narrative expressions of emotional difficulties; Chapter 17).

There is also an open-endedness to the study of personality and identity at large, with innumerable possibilities for different lateral shifts in life as one explores qualitatively different selves, which might be equally healthy or viable. In contrast, in treatment research, the target for change is less ambiguous: Narratives that specifically lead to improved emotional health and symptom reduction are better. The difference between these two conceptualizations is highlighted by comparing constructs from the two fields of research (Habermas et al., 2021). *Innovative moments*, as discussed in psychotherapy research (see Chapter 18), are statements elaborating the emerging narrative of change—the hinge point—with respect to some previous personal problem. This narrative explores that pivotal moment where one tried something new in thought, feeling, or action. In contrast, *autobiographical reasoning* (this chapter) draws connections between past events and other parts of the narrator's existing life or identity. It captures making sense of the past to create a more integrated context, coherence, and sometimes closure. In narratives from a large subclinical sample of students, innovative moments were more typical among those with a trait-like tendency toward adaptive reflection but not among those with a tendency toward unhealthy rumination. Autobiographical reasoning, however, captured meaning making more broadly and with a less functional lens without discriminating between an author's tendency toward productive reflection versus harmful rumination (Habermas et al., 2021).

It follows that the influences of narrative identity in shaping emotional experience can be adaptive or maladaptive. Some clients in psychotherapy identify deeply with their own pathology (e.g., "I've always been alone [or alien, depressed, awkward, etc.], that's who I am!"). Unfortunately, this can create ambivalence toward healthy change. One might strongly identify as the lone wolf, rebellious outsider, or brooding and heartbroken poet. Tragically, even when there is an opportunity for that person to feel effective or included and enjoy love or camaraderie with others, it might be at odds with maintaining their stable sense of identity. As explained in a section from Chapter 19, feeling coherent beats feeling good (see Swann et al., 1987). So, although there may be opportunities to satisfy an unmet existential need (Chapter 14), embracing that change can also create a new crisis of identity (e.g., "If I'm not lonely and forsaken, then who am I? I am not myself!").

Thus, narrative stability can be construed as either healthy continuity or stagnation, whereas change can be understood, likewise, as either personal growth or idle flux. A review of personality research shows as much evidence for people's narrative identity as being mired by unhealthy stagnation or lost in aimless flux as it does for fostering healthy continuity or positive growth (McAdams, 2019). Thus, neither stability nor change in one's narrative has been consistently related to well-being—that is, at least as far as personality research is concerned. The indices of narrative identity are also often too broad to have clear clinical implications for brief intervention, although they should be used to enrich case formulation in longer term treatments.

In contrast, the evidence from intervention-based research suggests that narratives about a client's initial ways of being are first destabilized before leading to a new order within the self (Angus, 2012; Ecker et al., 2012; Gelo & Salvatore, 2016; Gonçalves et al., 2017). In short, whether healthy narrative process is expected to be stable or to change has everything to do with the point of departure, how much one is suffering, and the risks versus benefits of further elaborating one's narrative. Thus, change and stability will serve different functions for narrative identity depending on one's level of well-being. Still, in the end, the story of navigating change may be more fundamental. As McAdams (2019) observes, "Without the perception that I have changed in some way, or the perception that my life has changed, I would not need to construct a story in the first place" (p. 207).

STORIES PEOPLE LIVE BY: CAVEATS AND CONCLUSIONS

Several points deserve consideration when theorizing about the role of narrative identity in emotional change, and these should guide future research. First, people have highly personal and characteristic ways of construing their stories, but they also get older and more experienced. Research designs that are cross-sectional or use a limited number of time points will never yield findings that adequately distinguish individual differences (i.e., relatively stable characteristics and abilities) from developmental stages (i.e., typical growth-related changes). These two sorts of observations will only be disentangled by following people over time. This field needs causal models based on longitudinal data to tease personal characteristics apart from maturational stages.

Second, when people are asked to explain their understanding of themselves, they often draw from the same set of theories and assumptions about human experience that researchers themselves generated as part of ongoing inquiry. In social science, this has been referred to as the *double hermeneutic* (i.e., the double interpretation or two-way understanding), and it can produce confirmatory findings as an artifact of broader psychological and sociocultural theories (Giddens, 1982). In other words, researchers are sometimes unwitting contributors to the same sources of self-understanding (i.e., research dissemination, self-help, popular culture) that their own participants are drawing from. When researchers ask participants about their life stories, the findings risk reflecting that circularity. Third, stories are developed within a range of cultural contexts and exemplified by master narratives. Thus, how broad cultural and social factors shape the formulation and function of narrative identity also needs further attention.

As we remember what we have lived in story form, those personal experiences accumulate layers of added meaning. Over time, the broader significance of one's story is honed as a lens for interpreting the next round of life experiences. All things considered, autobiographical reasoning in a way that leads to positive implications for the self (e.g., themes of redemption, increased agency) represents a narrative package that is reliably associated with well-being. Furthermore, there are different ways of integrating that meaning. On one hand, assimilating new positive meaning into one's narrative involves making amendments to improve one's narrative, and doing so is associated with more enjoyment and satisfaction in life. On the other hand, accommodating new meaning through the differentiation of what are typically negative events represents a more radical change that is associated with existential development and more psychosocial maturity. Thus, the method by which one reconciles one's story will become an implicit choice toward either psychological comfort or wisdom.

Whatever the case, the way someone parses their experience—by demarcating episodes in time but also selecting them as pertinent and then connecting those episodes into causal theories about themselves—is a powerful tool for working with emotion. This is a hypothesized engine of change, both as a direct mechanism and as a mediator of other personality factors that predict emotional well-being. Of course, there is more than one side to every story: Distinct modes of mental construal contribute to narrating one's life story. The next chapter unravels the mechanism of that dialectic between different narrative perspectives.

ENDNOTES

1. Anyone who has interviewed small children by asking, "What happened?" has discovered how impressionable and vulnerable to confabulation these narrative constructions are. Even so, although discerning the truth on what really happened is critical in forensic interviews (or in figuring out how the toaster got filled with Legos), it is less relevant to the development of narrative structures. Even when the story is untrue, the elaboration of that narrative remains an education in how to tell a story.

2. The emotional trajectory implied by this narrative structure also speaks to certain sequential shifts in emotional experience (McLean et al., 2020). Again, we find a parallel between the higher epistemological level of narrative meaning and the moment-by-moment level of sequential emotional transformations (cf. Chapter 14).

3. Here, I only refer to the impact on one's autobiographical memory as such. When there is a relational impact of not being attended to, that would stand as an additional but separate issue and has its own implications.

4. The inverse is also true: Various lines of research show that how one perceives and understands oneself also influences what one recalls from memory or not, as discussed in Chapter 19.

5. The heading of this section is borrowed from the poetic title of a summative paper by McLean and colleagues (2007, p. 262).

6. As I argue in Chapter 18, the issue of whether narratives are descriptive accounts or causal agents of change has not been fully addressed in psychotherapy process research. To be fair, that issue is also harder to disentangle in the short time frame available to treatment research as compared to the lifespan research discussed in this chapter.

7. Chapter 18 explored the role of positive emotional elaborations in creating hopefulness and concretizing the possibility of good outcomes.

8. This is an important consideration for psychotherapy theory because authors on psychotherapy have often identified developing a coherent narrative as a key process. Yet coherence on its own has not been a reliable predictor of healthy change, either in clinical or general populations. As indicated in the body of the chapter, coherence is more likely a prerequisite or a modifier of other narrative variables.

9. Using foreshadowing to suggest a benevolent grand design is akin to the role of surrender in many spiritual traditions. For example, when people have the faith to proclaim, "There is a reason for everything," "It is the will of God," or "Trust the process," they make statements of blind faith in a forthcoming positive resolution. Surrender of this kind is a theme in various spiritual traditions including Buddhism and Christianity as well as secular mindfulness and mediation practices. See also Chapter 18, on grateful surrender, and Chapter 23, for the role of mantras and prayer.

10. The various summary effects of relationships between narrative identity and well-being that I report in this chapter are based on my own review and calculations from studies already compiled by Adler et al. (2016). However, the effects I report are not a based on a complete set of formal meta-analyses.

11. Differential processing (as a process) in narrative identity has an affinity to level 5 on the depth of experiencing scale, which has been discussed on a smaller scale in the context of moment-by-moment awareness (see Chapter 7).

12. Using affective themes to predict emotional change may seem tautological. The issue is addressed in Chapter 18 (see the section "Is the Story a Description or an Agent of Change?").

13. Thematic abstraction was defined and discussed in Chapters 17 and 20 (see also Figure 17.1).

22

Storying the Self

It's a Matter of Perspective

The only true voyage of discovery . . . would be not to visit strange lands but to possess other eyes, to behold the universe through the eyes of another, of a hundred others, to behold the hundred universes that each of them beholds.

—MARCEL PROUST, *REMEMBRANCE OF THINGS PAST*

We cannot perceive the world and at the same time apprehend a look fastened upon us; it must be either one or the other.

—JEAN-PAUL SARTRE, *BEING AND NOTHINGNESS*

When an autobiographical narrative is constructed from the memory of what happened, it is always authored from some perspective. Typically, the stories are implicitly constructed using either a first-person actor perspective or a third-person observer perspective. There is a wealth of literature on autobiographical narratives demonstrating a relationship between emotional functioning and the imagery perspective with which one elaborates the story of what happened. This observation has a long history in philosophical traditions and pioneers of psychology. William James (1890) referred to the "I" as a first-person experiential perspective of the self as subject, which is essentially the operative self and a procedural expression of the will (as elaborated by J. Pascual-Leone & Johnson, 2021). James distinguished this from the "me," a third-person conceptual perspective of the self as object, which is the figurative self (J. Pascual-Leone & Johnson, 2021).

I am grateful to Dr. Chantal Boucher, University of Windsor, for our discussions on the issues presented in this chapter.

https://doi.org/10.1037/0000460-023
Principles of Emotion Change: What Works and When in Psychotherapy and Everyday Life, by A. Pascual-Leone
Copyright © 2026 by the American Psychological Association. All rights reserved.

This chapter highlights the role of a third-person conceptual perspective (i.e., the Jamesian "me" as figurative) in working with emotion, but part of that is done by contrasting it with the impact of an experiential first-person perspective (the Jamesian "I" as operative). Readers will notice this point of contrast is connected to observations I already made in Chapter 4 on how labeling an emotion can either bolster or truncate emotional awareness. In that chapter, I argued that a singular emotional experience can be approached in two ways: (a) from an external perspective, observing emotion as an object (common in cognitive behavior therapy) or (b) from a subjective, internal perspective, experiencing emotion from within (typical of experiential approaches). The specific impact on the process of awareness and a treatment's bias in regard to emotional experience from one or another vantage point are theoretical formulations that I proposed based on clinical observation.

In the field of autobiographical memory, however, this issue has garnered considerable research attention. In short, reflecting on narrative context can be done from at least two meaningfully distinct perspectives, and how one chooses to do this has implications for the process at both psychological and neurological levels (reviewed later in this chapter). Moreover, experimental findings on the use of visual imagery or field of view when recalling the past (or imagining the future) parallels research on the use of personal pronouns when people either write or speak about personal events. The perspective one takes in mental imagery, whether manifested in pronouns or visual imagery, is essentially a representational tool. But that representational tool also imparts an epistemological loading to the kind of meaning it will help facilitate. In short, how one tells the story has a bearing on the emotional experience that it will evoke and that will ensue. It does this by influencing the level of analysis one uses and by prescribing a certain evaluative lens to reflect on the self (Libby & Eibach, 2011).

LEVELS OF MENTAL CONSTRUAL: EXPERIENTIALLY HOW OR CONCEPTUALLY WHY

Meaning making is a term often used to discuss what happens in psychotherapy and is referenced within a range of treatment approaches, but what gets referred to as meaning making varies quite a bit. (For operational definitions and discussions of meaning making, see the introduction to Part II of this book as well as Chapters 4 and 17.) However, the kind of meaning one generates has largely to do with the type of mental construal that takes place. Specifically, it depends on what one focuses on.

"How I Feel" Versus "Why I Feel"

An *experiential focus* involves looking for the feelings and meanings that were lived in each autobiographical memory. This is making meaning about the process of an event, as in, "how I feel the way I do." It typically happens by way of small strokes and details in the lived moment, producing small but critical felt shifts. At this scope of analysis, new knowledge is generated bottom up about what it means to be in the here and now. Experiential meaning involves attention to the contents of emotional awareness by recalling and mentally attending to (a) perceptual and affective cues as if they were occurring in the present and (b) experiences that flow from recalling a memory. To borrow a phrase from Laura Rice, an experiential focus is when one "turns one's eyeballs inward and attends to what's happening."[1]

In contrast, a focus on *conceptual coherence* involves searching for continuity and coherence in a memory about oneself. This is meaning making by reflecting on an event's place within the story of one's life and "why I feel the way I do." New knowledge typically speaks to the big picture, is created top down, and begins with big strokes. In practical terms, this includes surveying the range of implications related to a given event that one recalls and how it relates to the larger context of one's life (or beyond). The elements of a coherence focus when working with autobiographical memories tend to involve the consideration of life themes, personal traits, and superordinate goals that coalesce into a sense of self that continues to develop over time.

Imagery Perspective Is a Representational Tool

When people recall past events or when they mentally simulate a future event, they tend to visualize it from either a first-person actor's perspective or a third-person observer's perspective. However, as is often the case, the tool one selects impacts the nature of the work that gets done. In this case, the representational framework one uses to explore personal stories will subsequently shape how those stories are to be elaborated. The use of third-person perspective and focusing on conceptual coherence go hand in hand, facilitating a reflective framework for understanding oneself and one's emotion. Moreover, this holds true for positive as much as negative events and for whether that event is being recalled from the past or imagined in the future (Libby & Eibach, 2011). In short, imagery perspective is a representational tool that potentiates a given level of construal.

The expressive writing paradigm asks people to record their deepest thoughts and feelings about an upsetting event, which recruits various narrative processes.[2] Common instructions for this task tell people to choose a difficult personal event to write about and then *"link this event to* your past, present, or future; or to who they have been, who they would like to be, or who they are now." Instructions often also suggest, *"you might tie it to* your relationships with others, including parents, lovers, friends, or relatives" (see Park et al., 2016; A. Pascual-Leone, Herpertz, & Kramer, 2016; Pennebaker & Chung, 2011). These prompts in italics encourage the author to adopt an observer's perspective on their own life, and they also emphasize conceptual coherence (Park et al., 2016). Instructions like these usher the writer into taking the broad perspective of an outside observer and contemplate the way disparate aspects of one's life might all fit together and perhaps why.

Using a third-person perspective may not directly foster psychological distance, but it cues a more abstract and less concrete level of analysis (A. Pascual-Leone & Greenberg, 2007b; recall Figure 17.1, this volume). In turn, abstract or hypothetical constructs are typically experienced as more subjectively distant (Trope & Liberman, 2010). Although the notion of explicitly adopting a third-person perspective—for example, through pronoun use—might seem unnatural at times, that vantage point is used implicitly much more often than one might realize. For example, after thinking about the difficulty she was having with her husband, a client of mine put together a playlist of songs that spoke to the journey of their relationship: "Songs that remind me of . . . when we first met, when we fell in love, when we made life plans, when I felt him getting distant." Through the lyrics, the ordered songs tacitly offered this client a third-person perspective of the larger love story that was underfoot. This was like reading (or listening to) a story about someone else's life, but a story very similar to one's own. Moreover, physical mementos, spiritual symbols, and keepsakes are often used explicitly as prompts to help one to take pause and adopt an observer's perspective. Such prompts are reminders to act in the prescribed interest of a broader life narrative (see also Chapters 21 and 23). Similarly, assuming a third-person perspective on one's emotional difficulty becomes quite literal when someone asks themselves, "What would my mother say?" or "What would my late husband do?"

It is important to appreciate the magnitude of effects that are possible from meaning making that come from simply focusing on the conceptual coherence of a difficult personal event, even without a therapist's offering thoughtful challenges to help guide a client in a well-balanced formulation of events. Cognitive processing therapy is a widely recognized and empirically supported trauma-focused therapy. It teaches clients to recognize and challenge their dysfunctional beliefs about thoughts regarding traumatic events, themselves, others, and the world (Chard, 2005). Even so, when a randomized clinical trial on the treatment of war veterans with posttraumatic stress disorder compared 5 sessions of expressive writing with 12 sessions of cognitive processing therapy, the much simpler task of expressive writing showed noninferior effects to the established treatment. Moreover, the comparable impacts of the two treatments were maintained 9 months later (Sloan et al., 2018).

Instructions written in third-person also set up an external frame of reference, modeling the lens though which the one will complete that task (e.g., "What could someone do if they start to feel discouraged? Make a list of enjoyable activities!"). Although it may seem natural for instructions to be written this way, it is in stark contrast with other possible modes of engagement. Among humanistic–experiential therapists, it is common to couch empathic reflections to client in first-person, where the therapist speaks as if they were the client (e.g., L. S. Greenberg, 2021; Paivio & Pascual-Leone, 2023; Watson & Greenberg, 2017). A therapist might empathically conjecture, "So when you think of your loss, it's like, 'I have this sinking feeling inside, and maybe I can't handle it all on my own.' Is that right? Does that fit for you?" This frame of reference is paradigmatically different from inviting a client in cognitive therapy to discuss their thought record. In short, imagery perspective is foremost a reflection of the level of construal and the kind of meaning analysis that an author is engaged in (Libby & Eibach, 2011).

When one commits a story to paper, it helps externalize the issue even more dramatically by creating a document to reflect upon. A body of research, primarily based on the expressive writing paradigm, shows specific linguistic patterns are related to positive change. This research tends to be very granular, using computer programs to count the frequency of specific word usages and relate them to health benefits (Pennebaker & Chung, 2011). Rather than specific word usages being salubrious, I suggest that these linguistic patterns are concrete manifestations (i.e., markers) indicating that the mental construal being made is about conceptual coherence with its corresponding imagery perspective. For example, one study showed that the increased use of causation words (e.g., reason, why, because) but a decrease in both negative emotion words (e.g., sad, upset) as well as a decrease in first-person pronouns (e.g., I, me) together predicted more self-distancing, which expressive writing seems poised to promote through a focus on conceptual coherence (Park et al., 2016). Moreover, these are among the linguistic patterns that reviews have consistently found to be related to the benefits of expressive writing (Pennebaker & Chung, 2011). The message to take from this is that types of word usage by clients are concrete indicators of the client taking a certain imagery perspective. Furthermore, when used by therapists, similar kinds of word usage may serve as prompts to the client toward a given mental focus.

THE PERSPECTIVE EFFECT: HOW FIRST-PERSON AND THIRD-PERSON VIEWS SHAPE MEANING

When one shifts between first- and third-person perspectives, several aspects in the process of meaning making are implicated. First, the type of processing can shift from perceptual–emotional to more conceptual–rational or vice versa. Second, the change in perspective moderates the psychological distance from which one engages personal material. Third, the change in perspective facilitates access to different kinds of information.

Between Emotion and Reason: Shifts in Type of Processing

A body of experimental research has explored the implications of using first-person or third-person perspectives. This work has also progressively revealed the impact of meaning construal at correspondingly different levels (experiential states vs. conceptual coherence, respectively; that epistemological distinction was also represented in Figure 17.1). The most salient processing difference related to imagery perspectives is the degree to which people access and make use of their emotional experience. For example, people instructed to recall past events from a first-person perspective will have more detailed recollections of past emotions, sensory perceptions, and mental states than if they are instructed to use third-person imagery. Moreover, when participants are free to spontaneously use either imagery perspective, those who adopted a first-person perspective also report more experiential detail. Meanwhile, participants who spontaneously used a third-person perspective are more likely to describe external and conceptual features such the spatial layout of a scene. The evidence for these relationships comes from both clinical samples (e.g., people with posttraumatic stress disorder) and nonclinical samples (e.g., undergraduates; McIsaac & Eibach, 2002, 2004). These differences in type of processing are also supported by neural imaging research (reviewed later).

In an everyday example, when people decide to end close interpersonal relationships (e.g., romances, friendships), they typically do so for acute emotional reasons. Namely, being in the relationship is too painful or feels unhealthy. Breaking up creates distance, but then with that distance, one sometimes starts to miss the lost relationship. However, the internal emotional yearning can be eased if one shifts to an outside perspective. Then, when people feel resolved to stay apart, that is no longer motivated by immediate emotional reasons but rather by cooler cognitive reasons. These cognitive reasons involve thinking more objectively about oneself and making decisions about what is best for one's future.

Close Up or Far Away: Shifts in Psychological Distance

A review of experimental manipulations that asked people to use either a first-person perspective or a third-person perspective shows that using the latter engenders a more psychologically distant perspective. Furthermore, shifting to a third-person perspective lowers the intensity of one's emotion when the focus was on why the event happened rather than on what happened (particularly for anger; Wallace-Hadrill & Kamboj, 2016). This has functional implications: When people adopted a third-person perspective of either themselves or the task they were doing, it helped control their emotion such that it did not negatively interfere with performance (Kross et al., 2014). This effect that a third-person perspective has in down-regulating emotion through psychological distance applies across a range of discrete emotions and situational domains (Orvell et al., 2021; Wallace-Hadrill & Kamboj, 2016). It also seems not to be moderated by the severity of one's clinical symptoms (Kross et al., 2014).

The level of construal put into practice by way of a given imagery perspective has implications for how one organizes toward the future. A first-person focus on experiential elaboration is the kind of meaning construal needed to find out what one's idiosyncratic values and endogenous needs are (e.g., "What do I feel about this?"). An existential need is something one can only taste in the now. Feeling the lived poignancy of an unmet need creates an affective-meaning state that is procedural as much as it is representational, and it immediately orients one to act on the felt need (A. Pascual-Leone & Greenberg, 2007b; Watson & Rennie, 1994).

Meanwhile, mental simulations where one imagines future or hypothetical scenarios offer a context of possibilities to guide future behavior. For this reason, third-person imagery implicitly facilitates conceptually coherent planning and can be especially useful in situations where people are at risk of failures in self-control. People continually negotiate concrete temptations in the here and now, which might be in the form of short-term diversions, the pressure of an angry (instrumental) outburst, or urges toward addictive behavior. When people lapse in these moments, they essentially lose sight of the more abstract values and personal goals that they otherwise hold dear. Using a third-person perspective to mentally focus on the abstract levels of conceptual coherence highlights why one might resist temptation, and doing so helps prevent one's derailment by short-term impulses (Fujita & Carnevale, 2012). For example, motivational interviewing is a treatment approach to address decisional ambivalence, and it does this by systematically leveraging psychological distance to consider the larger picture (e.g., weighing pros and cons, considering long-term goals; Miller & Rollnick, 2013).

Subjective or Objective Knowledge: Accessing Different Information

Higher cognition is also guided by the imagery one uses because it potentiates different kinds of self-knowledge. In a real-world example, when people were anxious about an impending pandemic, reflecting on the reality of their personal situation using a third-person perspective helped them access objective facts that bear on the rational assessment of their risk. The strategy enhanced rational thinking and reduced worry, whereas people engaged in a first-person process did not access the same kind of information as easily (Kross et al., 2017).

Using first-person facilitates access to associative evaluations (i.e., subjective knowledge) about people, objects, or situations. These implicit judgments are the affective and operational biases that are usually outside one's full awareness (Libby et al., 2014). This is one reason why exploring moment-by-moment experience from a first-person perspective can lead one to serendipitously discover or recognize genuine aspects of oneself during an experientially rich retelling of a narrative event (e.g., Client: "I never really thought of myself that way, but if I take an honest look at what I find myself saying here, I guess it tells me something about where I really stand"). Sometimes this Aha! experience happens when a client is groping toward some experiential meaning and then suddenly formulates a meaning bridge. In short, what one feels gets connected to its contextual circumstances, accessing a different kind of knowledge (Watson & Rennie, 1994; Chapter 7, this volume).

In contrast, using third-person facilitates access to declarative self-beliefs about one's conscious preferences, propositions about personal values, and self-knowledge that is deliberately used to inform one's explicit choices (Libby et al.

2014). Consequentially, a third-person perspective facilitates psychodynamic or cognitive insights, a click that comes from assembling newly considered aspects of one's life into a much larger meaning structure. This is integrative meaning making starts with the pieces of "what I know about myself" and "how this could make sense in the bigger picture." Thus, "what I feel" gets connected to "why I feel this way."

NEURAL SUBSTRATES OF IMAGERY PERSPECTIVES

Developing emotional awareness through a first-person construal of experiential states or reflecting on emotion from a third-person construal of conceptual coherence are distinct forms of emotional work. There is reason to believe that these two imagery perspectives are each supported by different patterns of neural activity. For example, functional magnetic resonance imaging (fMRI) of the brain has shown that when people imagined doing simple hand or foot actions from a first-person perspective (i.e., from the visual field of the actor), their sensorimotor cortex became more active when compared with the same actions being imaged from a third-person perspective (i.e., as if watching someone else). Meanwhile, using third-person imagery involved more visuospatial transformations and was supported by areas of the brain that carry both visual processing and the logical ordering of events (e.g., lingual gyrus; Jackson et al., 2006).

Going beyond simple actions, presenting movies of complex and sequenced imagery can render a first-person versus third-person perspective on the narrative of events. A study did this by inviting participants to watch a slideshow of images from either their own life (i.e., self or first-person perspective) or someone else's life (i.e., other or third-person perspective) and instructed them to emotionally engage with these movies by trying to reexperience or understand them from the corresponding self- or other-perspective (St. Jacques et al., 2011). Again, brain imaging (using fMRI) showed that exploring either the self-perspective or the other-perspective during this task recruited distinct regions of the brain. When participants adopted a self-perspective and reimagined their personal past, it involved areas of the brain related to making inferences about oneself (i.e., ventral medial prefrontal cortex). Adopting another person's (other) perspective recruited brain areas that have been related to reflecting on the mental state of others, or theory of mind (i.e., dorsal medial prefrontal cortex). In a subsequent step, functional connectivity in these brain activations showed that the self-perspective also contributed to regions linked with memory processing (in the medial temporal network), whereas activations related to the other-perspective contributed to control processes (in the frontoparietal network; St. Jacques et al., 2011).

Furthermore, the role of different neural substates goes beyond imagining physical actions by extending to the subjective experiences of emotion. Using a first-person perspective to generate an emotional experience originates through the recruitment of more medial parts of the brain (Berthoz et al., 2002; Holzel et al. 2011). This neural activation is then believed to blend with other patterns of lesser activity that connect affect to higher levels of meaning and action in the brain's dorsolateral and frontal areas (see also Chapters 5 and 6). In contrast, when one adopts a third-person perspective while contemplating the significance of one's emotional experience, the principal neural regions being recruited include the dorsolateral, parietal temporal, and frontal areas of the brain (Davidson, 2000; Holzel et al., 2011; J. Pascual-Leone & Johnson, 2021).

Autobiographical memories of specific events in one's life (i.e., first-person experiences) can also be constructed from a visual perspective that was never experienced. This would be imagining what it might have been like to witness one's own lived experience from a third-person perspective, that is, as if a fly on the wall had been watching what happened. Doing so represents a reconstrual rather than a retrieval per se. That process of shifting perspectives has been studied using neuroimaging (i.e., fMRI; St. Jacques et al., 2017). When participants were explicitly asked to shift their recollection of autobiographical memory from an original first-person perspective to the alternative perspective of an imagined or hypothetical outside observer, the precuneus played a critical role in supporting the modulation of that perspective shift. Other analyses showed the role of the precuneus contributed to both immediate and longer term changes in how the memory was subsequently recalled. Shifting to an outside perspective attenuates a memory's emotional intensity, but the act of changing perspective itself also introduces newly imagined information. These observations suggest that the manipulation of mental imagery over time can bias what one recalls (St. Jacques et al., 2017).

IMPLICATIONS FOR FACILITATING EMOTIONAL CHANGE

Treatment approaches differ in the way they leverage these distinct kinds of self-knowledge. For instance, a rational–cognitive approach is more likely to emphasize a third-person perspective when working with a client's hostile self-criticism (e.g., Therapist: "What is the evidence for this [dysfunctional] belief?"). Here, an observer's perspective is used to introduce a rational discussion about declarative beliefs. In contrast, in an emotion-focused approach, the central issue is not about objective truth at all, but rather its devastating emotional impact (e.g., Therapist: "Well, I don't know if it's true or not, but I guess the important part is, what does it feel like to be on the receiving end of that self-contempt?"). In the latter intervention strategy, a first-person experiential perspective seeks to access associative evaluations and any of the recalcitrant emotions that subsequently emerge. These are imagery perspectives in action, and they are each leveraged by different treatment strategies.

Facilitating change in this way is possible because the language in which an intervention is framed has ramifications for how one engages and vice versa. Moreover, as I have argued, therapeutic meaning making typically involves psychological elaboration along several epistemological levels (recall Figure 17.1). This means that sophisticated forms of emotional processing involve toggling between different levels of mental construal.

The Influence Goes Both Ways

The imagery perspective during a narrative exploration depends on whether the speaker is attending to an event's meaning in terms of who they are (i.e., coherent self-concept; third-person) or to what it was like and the lived experience of the event (i.e., experiential; first-person). However, although the imagery perspective that people spontaneously choose is influenced by their level of meaning making, that corresponding focus can also be manipulated. As a seminal paper by Libby and Eibach (2011) concludes,

> Alone, this variation in imagery perspective might be interpreted as epiphenomenal, and thus as serving no purpose in psychological processes. However, given that the effect also works in the opposite causal direction . . . variation in the use of first-person versus third-person perspectives reflects their representational function. According to this account, first-person images define an event in terms of the experience of acting on and reacting to the environment whereas third-person images define an event in terms of its meaning in a broader context. . . . When people picture life events as they think about them, the visual perspective of those images may play a role in maintaining a certain construal of the event. (p. 724)

In short, the specific words and imagery one chooses are not purely an expressive product; rather, their influence is bidirectional. Imagery and pronouns use will express, but they can also evoke, a given level of mental construal and the processes that are subsequently associated with that.

For example, an experiment manipulated the narrative perspective that people took as they recalled autobiographical memories, using first-person pronouns (I, me) to cue a subjective–experiential perspective and third-person pronouns (she, he, they) to cue the observer's perspective (Gu & Tse, 2016). When narrative perspective was shifted using these cues, it served as a linguistic nudge that changed the emotional intensity that people felt in relation to their memories. The memory recall experience was less intense when people shifted from first- to third-person pronouns but not when the shift in perspective was the other way around. Mediation analyses showed that shifting to a third-person perspective was dampening the emotional intensity of personal memories by creating more psychological distance and reducing the vividness of mental imagery (Gu & Tse, 2016; Park et al., 2016). Meanwhile, process research on a clients' emotional engagement during psychotherapy suggests that prompting clients to use first-person pronouns can activate emotion and will signal increased engagement, which represents a different intervention objective (Paivio et al., 2001; see Chapter 5, this volume).

For therapists who are attentive to the imagery perspective a client spontaneously uses, noticing the frame of reference will offer an immediately recognizable marker for the kind of meaning making a client is poised to elaborate on. This process diagnosis can also help therapists recognize when a client is stuck in a particular mode of mental construal. For example, a client might consistently theorize about the self rather than attending to their feeling, or alternatively, they may habitually focus on the details of their emotional pain at the expense of relating it to the broader context. However, the most significant practical implication for psychotherapy and emotion change is that when a therapist offers a given imagery perspective to their client as a representational tool, it will facilitate the client's focus on either experiential meaning or on conceptual meaning depending on the perspective that therapist offers. In the search to create overarching meaning, a simple act of picturing one's life event from a more distant third-person perspective causes one to analyze the deeper narrative meaning of those events and connect them to general knowledge about oneself and the story of one's life.

Toggling Between Levels of Mental Construal

What is the best imagery perspective or construal level to process emotion? The answer will depend very much on the task at hand. Reflections on the big picture and the story of one's life go with the grain of taking a third-person perspective and facilitate a mental construal about conceptual coherence in the larger narrative. In contrast, exploring and deepening one's immediate experience to making meaning about "what it is like to be me in this lived moment" demands an immersed first-person perspective.

Complementary Processes, but Timing Matters

It is possible that a third-person perspective and a survey of the context of emotional experience at hand will provide an easier and more natural point of entry when starting to work with emotion. The need for narrative coherence often prescribes that people begin exploring their difficulties by explaining some overview of the plot and characters, and that is how most first sessions will begin (e.g., "Once upon a time . . ." or "It all started with . . ."; Angus, 2012). When there is a solid understanding of the broader context, people can more easily zoom in, shifting their focus to elaborate the experiential narrative of a specific moment from a first-person perspective. For example, a client might transition from a third-person observer perspective to a first-person experiencer perspective: "So, while all that was going on between my parents, I guess inside I was feeling . . . ."

However, at other times, after having elaborated on fragmented first-person experiences, it is common for individuals to need to step back (i.e., zoom out) and take a broader perspective. This wider vantage point allows them to examine how disparate pockets of experiential meaning might fit together to form a larger narrative. For example, a client might shift into a third-person observer perspective, focusing on broader coherence: "So, I guess I'm the type of person who . . . and the role I want to play in all this is . . . ." Thus, rather than there being a single best approach, the most productive examples of emotional processing involve shifting between imagery perspectives to help toggle between the corresponding levels of mental construal. In short, each perspective (or mode of processing) is complementary, and when they occur in sequence, each will provide a context of meaning for the other.

However, these two forms of emotional processing, though both valuable, are dialectically opposed and cannot be used simultaneously, as Sartre's epigraph to this chapter suggests. For example, when participants are asked to reflect on the causes of their feelings and thoughts (e.g., exploring why) from a distance, third-person perspective has consistently been shown to help with emotional processing. However, when the participants were explicitly instructed to use an immersive first-person perspective but nevertheless still asked to explore why they felt the way they did, it was unproductive, and rumination and negative affect increased (Yasinski et al., 2016). This highlights that one's level of construal needs to be congruent with one's imagery perspective. Thus, creating conceptual coherence and reflecting on causality is best done from a third-person imagery perspective. In contrast, attempting to do it from a first-person perspective goes against the natural grain and undermines the potential benefits of making narrative reflections about one's emotion.

Treatment Differences and Clinical Implications

I have suggested that cognitive therapy interventions lend themselves to a construal of meaning about conceptual coherence (best facilitated through a third-person perspective), whereas experiential interventions lend themselves to a construal of meaning about experiential states of feeling (best facilitated through a first-person perspective). But this categorization is only a matter of predisposition insofar as different therapies emphasize different levels of discourse and therefore processes. These are primarily client processes, and they will both periodically occur in any therapy, whether spontaneously or following the nudge of therapist interventions.

For example, although experiential approaches tend to give preference to first-person experiencing, the same therapists may also prompt a third-person perspective when encouraging the client to imagine themself in the past or when attempting to activate self-soothing. Chairwork is an interesting example of this. In emotion-focused therapy, clients will be encouraged to explore emotion from a deeply felt first-person perspective. However, at later stages of a chairwork task, clients are often encouraged to respond to their emergent emotion as if they were the other (e.g., Therapist: "Switch chairs. Okay, what might your father say if he could take in what you are saying? I know this is a conversation you could never have, but imagine. . . . Speak as if you are him. . . . What do you want [client's name] to know? Tell [client's name]").

In another example, when exploring the experience of past childhood abuse, an experiential therapist might ask a client to imagine themself as a child sitting in an empty chair (e.g., Therapist: "Can you imagine little [client's name] sitting over here in this chair? What's going on for her? What do you think she needs from you right now?";[3] i.e., prompting a third-person observer's perspective;

Paivio & Pascual-Leone, 2023). Although the purpose of this is to help activate emotion and elaborate the untold story of childhood experience, prompting a third-person perspective also activates something else: The client's reflection on their life story and the subsequent search for coherence. Assuming the adult client is no longer at risk, imagining oneself as a child during periods of abuse obviates a discrepancy: One is no longer as vulnerable as before, and one now has new adult resources, which highlights how far one has come since those desperate times. The observer's perspective is what allows the client to relate to themselves differently, perhaps assuming the role of an older, wiser adult who speaks to a younger, more vulnerable version of oneself (e.g., Client: "I want to tell her that it's going to be okay"). Psychological distance here facilitates a wise frame of mind (Grossmann & Kross, 2014; Chapter 19, this volume).

The third-person shift to reflecting on the self is often used transitorily to highlight a view of the self as changed (to some degree). Doing this activates an emotional reaction from that new perspective (e.g., the client begins to tear up). Then, following this spark of insight, an experiential approach would typically shift back to a first-person perspective to activate and explore from within that new view of self (e.g., Therapist: "Okay, and I see this brings up a lot of feeling for you. Can you switch chairs and speak from that position? What's happening inside right now? Let the tears speak"). In this use of enactment, external prompts such reflecting on old photographs will literally put a client in the observer's perspective. However, a therapist might then guide the client to shift and speak from a first-person perspective. For example, a therapist might say, "It's a nice picture. Such a long time ago. . . . What's life like for the child in this picture? How does she see the world? What would she say about what she needs as a little girl? Speak as if you were her: 'I'm only 12 but . . .' What would she say?"

One finds a similar dialectic between third-person conceptual coherence and first-person focus on experience in productive segments of cognitive and behavioral therapies, although through different interventions. Exposure-based tasks often implicitly ask clients to immerse themselves in a highly arousing experience and then periodically offer a metacognitive assessment of how they are handling the experience. For example, a client might say, "My anxiety is at about an 8 out of 10 right now, and this is freaking me out, but okay, I'm okay, I'm good"—and then begin diaphragmic breathing as per skills training. Self-appraisal and self-management in this way comes from an observer's perspective.

In practice, the most productive use of imagery perspective (and levels of construal) is not in one or the other but in toggling between these modes of engagement. In a treatment like eye movement desensitization and reprocessing therapy, the therapist provides external sensory stimulation (e.g., directing a client's gaze or bilateral tapping on the client's knees to alternate rapidly from side to side), and they do this while a client recalls and recounts a traumatic experience (R. Shapiro & Brown, 2019). Although several mechanisms have been proposed for this treatment, some evidence suggests that it capitalizes on switching between the different levels of mental construal (Landin-Romero et al., 2018). The initial task of telling one's story creates a demand for narrative coherence from a third-person perspective. Meanwhile, first-person experiential engagement is prescriptively focused on physical stimulation, which tethers the client's attention to the present moment. Doing this displaces or switches out the contents of experience, mitigating against a client's first-person reentry into what could be overwhelming. Toggling this way prevents emotional arousal from capturing attentional resources and makes sure narrative continuity is not derailed.

What Matters Is Whether You Shift at All!

Lexical analyses on the most productive examples of pronoun use in expressive writing further support the idea that optimal processing involves shifting between perspectives and their associated levels of construal:

> The more that people oscillated in their use of 1st person singular pronouns (I, me, my) and all other personal pronouns (e.g., we, you, she, they), the more people's health improved. If individuals wrote about emotional upheavals across the 3–4 days of writing but they approached the topic in a consistent way as measured by pronoun use, they were least likely to show health improvements. The findings suggest that the switching of pronouns reflect a change in perspective from one writing day to the next. Interestingly, it doesn't matter if people oscillate between an I-focus to a we- or them-focus or vice versa. Rather, health improvements merely reflect a change in the orientation and personal attention of the writer. (Pennebaker & Chung, 2011, p. 277)

This description also has a remarkable affinity to what psychotherapy researchers have described as the assimilation of experiential voices that are conflicting at first but then converge through a back and forth into a gradual consensus in the overarching meaning (Brinegar et al., 2006; see also Chapter 7, this volume). Similarly, cognitive neuroscience has identified toggling between different levels of analysis as cognitive shifting between tasks. More precisely, shifting between higher and lower levels of analysis has also been referred to as *decentering* (see Chapter 20), which is when the thematic content could remain the same but what changes is the scope of elements under consideration (J. Pascual-Leone & Johnson, 2021).

In the end, what matters most may be whether one shifts at all. Not making use of different perspectives suggests a rigid or entrenched approach to working with emotion. Just as creative problem solving requires decentering, working with emotion will benefit from alternative frameworks: sometimes exploring the first-person details, at other times contemplating the bigger picture using an outside, third-person perspective.

What Instructions, When, and for Whom?

Both third-person reflections on why and first-person internal explorations on what are important as complementary modes of meaning construction, but these processes are woven into the fabric of working with emotion. People periodically engage in them spontaneously, and they are peppered throughout clinical work. To be as incisive as possible, one needs to consider how directive one should be in facilitating a shift in perspective (if at all), when it might be most useful, and for whom.

Shifting Perspectives: How Much Direction Do People Need?

Making a narrative reflection about conceptual coherence can be a powerful form of emotional processing, but it is not without limitations. For example, when participants who felt sad were asked simply to generate narrative accounts about their personal loss, not all attempts at meaning making were successful. In the absence of any guiding structure, prompting people to consider their larger narrative may be setting some people up for failure (Huang et al., 2020). The *spectator critique* highlights that identifying a change process helps explain outcomes, but that does not necessarily mean one can implement the process through intervention (A. Pascual-Leone, Yeryomenko, et al., 2016). In other words, some processes are related to personal characteristics or tendencies, and although they might be observed and are predictive of positive outcome, whether that target process can be facilitated is an altogether separate question.

Various studies suggest that some people have a trait-like tendency to use reappraisal (Memedovic et al., 2010) or that they more spontaneously engage in reappraisal from either a self-distanced perspective (Kross & Ayduk, 2011) or a positive reframing of events (Denson et al., 2012). Moreover, most people who tend to systematically engage in this third-person perspective experience both decreased emotional arousal and decreased cardiovascular activity while recalling provocatively negative interpersonal experiences. Some people seem to default to a more conceptual manner of engagement with emotional content (i.e., using narrative reflection to work with emotion), whereas others tend to be more feeling-oriented and experiential (i.e., using awareness to work through emotion). These observations on cognitive style may also be related to the individual differences on arousal discussed in Chapter 9, where some people rely more heavily on contextual cues to interpret their physical arousal.

Research on treatment has also shown that clients are more likely to spontaneously shift into reflective narrative (e.g., an interpretive and coherence focus on why and what this all means) but are less likely to spontaneously shift into internal narratives (e.g., an experiential focus on what it feels like in one's body right now; Angus & Greenberg, 2011). Other research has underscored that being instructed to shift to more psychologically distanced reflection on why is more helpful than spontaneous shifts to the exploration of why as a stylistic default, which may be related to avoidance (Wallace-Hadrill & Kamboj, 2016). So, although people will spontaneously engage in either narrative reflection from a third-person perspective or experiential work from a first-person perspective, it seems the shifting should be more systematic or purposeful to be as useful as possible.

A study of experiential psychotherapy for depression examined the frequency of shifts between narrative modes from one talk turn to the next and showed that when therapists facilitated a higher proportion of shifts from conceptual reflection to emotional experience, it predicted good outcomes as compared with when therapists made relatively fewer prompts for that shift (Angus, 2012). Thus, when a client has sufficiently elaborated the conceptual coherence of events, it becomes particularly critical for a therapist to then prompt the client to shift out of their third-person observer's focus in favor of turning their focus inward to adopt a first-person experiential perspective. Of course, the critical issue here is not that one level of elaboration is more useful than the other. Rather, focusing on the differentiation of emotional experience is most productive when it is done in the context of narrative reflection and conceptual coherence (Angus, 2012; Angus & Greenberg, 2011).

Perhaps using a conceptual framework to reflect on personal difficulties has a more intuitive and self-explanatory objective, such that clients require fewer prompts to do it. Meanwhile, the objective of emotional exploration is less obvious. Indeed, clients often ask, "What's the use in bringing up all those bad feelings?" but they almost never ask, "How is thinking about my life and my problems going to help me feel better?" As a case in point, interventions like expressive writing or journaling are helpful to many people, even when they are relatively unstructured. Those are also tasks bent toward making observations from a third-person perspective. In contrast, using a first-person perspective to productively explore emotion seems to require that participants receive more moment-by-moment guidance (i.e., structure) during the process than standard journaling can typically offer (Nardone et al., 2024; cf. Yasinski et al., 2016).

Shifting to a Third-Person Perspective: Who Benefits and When?

There probably are several clinical factors that serve as moderators and mediators for the benefit of narrative reflection from a third-person perspective. For example, when people are excessively self-focused, as in cases of worry and depressive rumination, it may be harmful to foster general self-distancing through a third-person perspective. For such people, doing so in an expressive writing task predicted maladaptive thinking and increased their negative emotion (Finnbogadottir & Berntsen, 2014). Furthermore, interventions that promote taking a third-person perspective among emotionally vulnerable people might increase their depressive symptoms (Giovanetti et al., 2019). One might anticipate similar deleterious effects among people who intellectualize defensively.

Pushing people to integrative meaning can sometimes be associated with worse well-being—an iatrogenic effect—although evidence for this is still new. For example, among younger adults (i.e., 18–28 years), those whose narratives were high on content related to identity yet low on coherence reported the lowest levels of purpose and meaning in life as compared with those with high coherence in their narrative identity who also enjoyed correspondingly high levels in well-being (Waters & Fivush, 2015). This suggests that when young people are struggling with their identity, it may be harmful to prematurely push them toward coherence (e.g., questioning, challenging). Meaning making is a monumental feat of cognitive processing, and autobiographical reasoning about how past events relate to one's current self can be distressing, especially if one does not have the resources (cognitive or otherwise) to pull together a coherent narrative (Adler et al., 2016). The critical issue here is that some young people will not give much consideration to how coherent their narrative identity is until some personal challenge in life prompts them to do so.

Unsurprisingly, variables such as age, maturity, and years of education increase the odds that people will be able to successfully grapple with this challenge in emotional processing (Huang et al., 2020). Looking for the bigger pictures may also only be more beneficial after the passage of time. For example, the narrative elaboration about a lost self following a divorce predicted women's psychosocial maturity. However, that positive relationship only came to emerge several years after the divorce in what could be described as a sleeper effect (L. A. King & Raspin, 2004). Thus, distress related to the initial engagement with narrative meaning making may simply be the beginning of a longer process, one that may only come to fruition years later.

In sum, not everyone will benefit from an invitation to take a step back to reflect on the conceptual coherence of their life. The challenge for clinical work is that a predisposition in information processing may be more influential than a therapist's prompts to elicit a targeted kind of emotional processing. Thus, toggling between perspectives may involve developing new ways of engaging, which change how an individual typically does emotional work.

CHANGING PERSPECTIVES: IMPLICATIONS FOR INTERVENTION

When people tell stories, they use a narrative perspective that authors the story from either a first-person perspective (i.e., "I" as the knower of experience) or from a third-person perspective (i.e., "me" as the known experience). That narrative perspective one takes has implications for the level of mental construal and kind of emotional processing to follow. Using a first-person perspective in the construction of a personal story brings experience into the here and now and activates more relevant emotion. In turn, this facilitates emotional engagement, awareness, and expressive arousal. These forms of emotional processing often yield more immediate and dramatic impacts, particularly in the early phase of treatment or when emotional processing has become stagnant or lost its direction. Thus, the impact of first-person perspectives on emotional change tends to be more immediately apparent. Even so, considering emotional processing longitudinally, there are other process moments where people need to take a step back (i.e., to increase psychological distance) and assume the vantage point of an outside observer. Stepping outside the immediate experience helps one make construals that focus on conceptual coherence and explore how the many individual pieces of meaning might all come together.

The type of problem emotion that a person needs to work through will often require multiple strategies for healthy processing. Early on, a coherence focus may promote good outcomes. For example, when just starting to grapple with personal difficulties, a third-person perspective can help people gain psychological distance and clarify problems. However, promoting a focus on self-coherence may be unhelpful or even harmful when people understand the events in a maladaptive and self-disparaging way (Libby & Eibach, 2011). For example, when someone suffers a maladaptive emotion, pushing for coherence can be risky because if one has been mistreated or abused, then the most direct route to narrative coherence is for the person to simply conclude that it is their own fault or that they deserved the abuse. Ultimately, it is a first-person perspective that will help generate the new adaptive emotion, which then acts as an antidote to maladaptive emotion. Consistent with this, promoting awareness and facilitating transformational sequences are key forms of emotional processing that use a first-person experiential framework (e.g., Chapter 7 and 15). Searching for coherence from a third-person perspective becomes important again in the late stage of a personal change process, when people have developed an adaptive response to their difficulties but still need to integrate them into their self-understanding.

An experiment comparing the benefits of self-distancing for various emotions showed that it reduced the intensity of anger and sadness over an interpersonal difficulty but had little impact on feelings of guilt and shame (Katzir & Eyal, 2013). The authors explained this by pointing at the self-evaluative nature of guilt and shame. However, I suggest the sharper contrast here is that self-distancing pulls for coherence seeking and that this process helps with the contextualization of primary adaptive emotions (i.e., in this case, anger and sadness) but offers less benefit for resolving primary maladaptive emotions (i.e., in this case, guilt and shame). The reason is that maladaptive emotions are often already experienced as instantiations of a same old story, and simply reflecting on that does not change it. These hypotheses should be empirically explored, but they suggest an optimal matching between type of emotion and different forms of processing.

For case formulation, one must consider the client's original spontaneous perspective, how much time the client already spent elaborating a given perspective, and how much structure or direction that client needs to make use of each imagery perspective. Finally, although each narrative perspective and its corresponding level of mental construal could be useful, transitioning between perspectives is also a unique experience. Engaging in multiple narrative perspectives, particularly in a reasonably brief time frame, can sometimes create a sharp contrast through those different scopes of analysis. The brevity of that time frame is related to the role of memory reconsolidation, which suggests it could be from 10 minutes up to several hours (see Chapter 13, this volume; Ekert et al., 2024; Lane & Nadel, 2020). In any case, such a contrast highlights for people the possibility of engaging old problems in varying ways, which is an important metacognitive insight (Dimaggio et al., 2020). Experiencing the contrast between modes of engagement might pull them out of a rut or could offer a novel perspective, thereby opening new possibilities to old problems.

I have argued that differentiation and integrations are two prongs of development (Chapter 7), and that is as true for the moment-by-moment unfolding of awareness as it is for narrative elaboration. For this reason, productive work with narrative construction will involve some oscillation between imagery perspectives. While the third-person perspective offers a bird's eye view and a survey of narrative themes, it also highlights and brings attention to discrepancies. To further explore these discrepancies, it is helpful to zoom in on specific experiences using a first-person perspective. This allows for differentiation and depth, enabling a more nuanced understanding of problematic points. As new facets of experience emerge, they can be integrated back into the broader narrative context, connecting the immediate feelings and sensations of the lived moment to the larger story of one's life.

By taking different perspectives in storytelling, we can develop a deeper and richer understanding of the narrative's meaning. This process often reveals a crucial turning point: the possibility of some existential choice. That choice point is the topic of the next chapter.

ENDNOTES

1. I am grateful to Dr. Les Greenberg and Dr. Jeanne Watson for sharing this marvelous and strange phrase from their mentor.
2. The open-endedness of the instructions for expressive writing tasks means the processes that ensue could involve narrative as well as other processes discussed in this book such as emotional engagement, labeling emotion (Chapters 5 and 6), and emotional expression (Chapter 8).
3. Although the passages related to this example have not previously been published, the example comes from a case of emotion-focused therapy described at length in A. Pascual-Leone and colleagues (2019).

23

Existential Meaning

Having Purpose and Making Choices

I wonder if I've been changed in the night. Let me think. Was I the same when I got up this morning? I almost think I can remember feeling a little different. But if I'm not the same, the next question is, "Who in the world am I?" Ah, that's the great puzzle!
—LEWIS CARROLL, *THE ADVENTURES OF ALICE IN WONDERLAND*

Viktor E. Frankl (1963), an Austrian psychiatrist, argued that people suffered a widespread affliction that was "the feeling of the total and ultimate meaninglessness of their lives. They lack the awareness of a meaning worth living for. They are haunted by the experience of their inner emptiness, a void within themselves" (p. 128). His book, which introduced logotherapy, explored this concern, selling over 16 million copies and being named (in the United States) one of the most influential books of all time (Fein, 1991). More than half a century later, his observation is still so astute that the quote could have been posted today on X (formerly Twitter). Indeed, having meaning in life and a sense of purpose is a fundamental protective factor for people grappling with adversity. Several studies have shown that meaning in life is negatively associated with the severity of psychopathology across a range of clinical diagnoses (Steger, 2022). This holds true even for those who endure long-term mental health challenges. For example, a study of 60 inpatients with schizophrenia whose psychiatric histories dated back 5 or more years showed that meaning in life was positively related to these patients' quality of life and their maintaining treatment adherence and was inversely related to depressive symptoms (Stolovy et al., 2009).

https://doi.org/10.1037/0000460-024
Principles of Emotion Change: What Works and When in Psychotherapy and Everyday Life, by A. Pascual-Leone
Copyright © 2026 by the American Psychological Association. All rights reserved.

Research also points to meaning in life as serving a protective role (Hamby et al., 2018). A Swiss study showed that among patients presenting to a psychiatric emergency department, those who reported having higher meaning in life were less likely to report suicidal ideation (Costanza et al., 2020). In contrast, if patients reported that they were searching for meaning, this alone offered no protection and did not even mediate having meaning. When Chinese college students were followed for 7 weeks spanning the outbreak of COVID-19, it gave longitudinal evidence for the protective role of meaning in life. Having meaning in life before the pandemic predicted both higher life satisfaction after the outbreak and healthier psychosocial adjustment (Lin, 2021).

EXISTENTIAL INSIGHTS ARE ABOUT INTENTIONALITY

According to existentially oriented therapists and philosophers, existential insight is achieved by grappling with ultimate concerns such as death, isolation, meaninglessness, and freedom.[1] However, these realities cannot be understood in an abstract and detached way. Confrontation with such nonnegotiable aspects of life are visceral and emotional experiences that are lived within a given moment. The "I am" is an experience of reality as such (i.e., an ontological experience) and is the central concern of an existential therapy (May & Yalom, 1989). This existential awareness of one's own freedom, connectedness, or disconnectedness is an emotionally rooted perspective of life and living. It is an insight that engenders a higher order perspective and an experiential meta-awareness (A. Pascual-Leone & Greenberg, 2007b).

Moments of Existential Clarity

Existential insights are reflexive in nature. The prototypical *existential insights* described by Yalom (1981) are essential reflections that recontextualize distressing emotion, offering a new interpretive framework: (a) "Only I can change the world I have created"; (b) "There is no danger in change"; (c) "To get what I want I must change"; and (d) "I have the power to change" (pp. 340–342). Reflexive experiential states such as these are simple yet profound. These are not only beliefs that hold some truth value; rather, they are complex and emotional meaning states, and they capture vital values abstracted from across the living of life in various concrete situations. These reflections are often entertained from an experience-distant position as philosophical possibilities (recall Figure 17.1). One does this, for example, when acknowledging the plausibility of one's own mortality. But the full impact of such existential observations are only appreciated when they are lived moments of awareness rather than items of conceptual or behavioral learning. Existential insights provide the client with an experience of empowerment, agency, and sensing the possibility of change (Perls, 1969; Yalom, 1981). For instance, when clients tell stories about unexpected outcomes, the formulation of such stories heightens an individual's sense of personal agency, particularly in the challenge of older expectations about what hereto had been the same old story (Chapter 18, this volume; Khattra et al., 2017).

An *existential moment* is when one grasps in self-awareness that a specific event being lived embodies a larger significance, one which then suggests some intentionality going forward. A moment like this earmarks a particular situation or manifest action because it will also serve as a symbol of change. This is why an existential moment can be a simple and mundane act but as a gesture represents something much more profound. It carries a self-aware truth about some theme or change in theme across situations. An act as simple as getting a haircut can be more than just routine grooming—it could signal a pivot point (e.g., in one's identity, life narrative, relationship). Similarly, enactments may serve as existential moments because they are much more than a behavioral rehearsal or practice for real life, particularly when they capture a new way of being that is yet to be fully manifested (Chapter 10). This is what makes the enactment a therapeutic experience, whether it be enacting transference in a self-aware way, enacting a new way of communicating with one's partner in couples therapy, or enacting an imaginary conversation with another person. The content is newly explored, but the doing of it is symbolic in and of itself.

Intentionality

Innovative moments signal a new direction (Gonçalves et al., 2017). But intentionality is what gives the existential insight its substance. May (1983) has argued that decision precedes knowledge and insight if decision is taken to mean a decisive attitude toward existence—an attitude of commitment. This is also something discussed earlier with respect to expressive arousal (Chapter 9) and therapeutic enactments (Chapter 10), which both engender a commitment to the momentum of budding meaning. Rogers (1942) referred to the embodiment of choice and action as the true indicator of insight. An immediate and lived self-understanding is when a client says, "I never realized how deeply these feelings affected me and how strongly I want to experience them again in my life" (Schneider & May, 1995, p. 171). A client statement like this indicates a new self-understanding within the context of both their worldview and their usual manner of processing such feelings. It also embodies intentionality toward new goals for a lived experience. In another example, a client in dialectical behavior therapy for borderline personality disorder described the pivotal insight that helped her more fully engage with treatment:

> I realized therapy was like a plate of food in front of me, and why am I not eating? I'm going to take advantage of this opportunity. This is what they do here. This is the moment. So, I allowed myself to be vulnerable and get involved. (Cristoffanini et al., 2023)

Admittedly, the four insights described previously by Yalom are realities that any client will need to contend with in order to exercise personal change, irrespective of the approach to treatment. As explored later in this chapter, some treatments bring out existential issues more readily and make them a more deliberate focus. It often has to do with using emerging experience in the here and now as a viscerally felt instantiation of some overarching theme. This kind of work highlights the distinction between knowing something versus feeling it and owning it.

HAVING PURPOSE

Conceptually, "meaning in life" and having "life purpose" are very close cousins. Although hope is also an oft-cited positive emotion, the issue of change is not simply about hope and positivity; the mediator of health is probably more about having meaning and purpose (Ryff & Keyes, 1995). *Hope* is about having a vision of the possible and seeing a light at the end of the tunnel, which then affords one a sense of direction and something worth striving for.

Purpose in Life and Mortality

Having a sense of *life purpose* is the degree to which people experience their lives as having a sense of direction and being motivated by life goals. When reporting on the focus of their life purpose, people typically list targets such as family and relationships, community, helping others, cultivating new skills, contributing to a larger effort, or even participating in hobbies that align with valued life goals. A national sample of close to 7,000 people in the United States has shown that the strength in one's life purpose is an important predictor of mortality after adjusting for an extensive array of health care predictors including personal demographics, medical history, health characteristics, lifestyle choices, and psychological well-being. The hazard ratio for someone with strong versus weak life purpose was over 2.4:1 for all causes of death (Alimujiang et al., 2019). This means, all things being equal, people who have a strong sense of purpose in life were two to three times more likely to survive almost anything as compared with those who had only a weak sense of purpose. Regarding specific causes of death, this effect was strongest for heart, circulatory, blood, and digestive tract conditions. However, in these analyses, life purpose did not seem to affect mortality associated with cancer, tumors, or respiratory conditions (Alimujiang et al., 2019). The overall message from these findings is stark: When people have no purpose, they tend to die.

The fact that purpose in life was measured with a 7-item self-report should also encourage all frontline health care practitioners to pause. Although physicians typically prescribe medication, if a patient has low purpose in life, there are virtually no pharmaceuticals that can have an impact comparable to increasing that patient's purpose in life (except in cases such as life-threatening infections or severe endocrine problems). Health practitioners of all stripes should ask people about their "[a] sense of whether their lives have purpose, [b] whether they are realizing their given potential, [c] what is the quality of their ties to others, and [d] if they feel in charge of their own lives" (Ryff & Keyes, 1995, p. 725).

The Paradox of Having Purpose: "All Joy and No Fun"[2]

There are many illustrations of how purpose supports both health and emotional change. However, an interesting observation is that having meaning in one's life is often more important for our well-being than having happiness. This has direct implications for understanding what healthy emotional change really is—and how to facilitate it—because a great number of situations in life (not only parenting) ask people to choose between what they find meaningful and what they find pleasurable. In short, the satisfaction or even joy of having purpose in life may not actually mean less emotional pain, which presents a paradox. Indeed, it is often overlooked that finding a higher purpose usually offers no immediate moment-by-moment payoff in the relief of quotidian suffering. Notice that bottom-up experiencing, central to emotional awareness (Chapters 4–7), becomes secondary here, and that is precisely the point. Having a sense of larger purpose puts one's life on an unwavering trajectory where the top-down mission one has dedicated oneself to becomes more important than the bottom-up moment of some unpleasant experience.

In short, having purpose creates a superordinate context within which all other experiences then unfold and are interpreted through. While spiritual, humanitarian, or cultural pursuits can be dramatic examples, dedicating oneself to a life project is often more about everyday commitment than grand spiritual endeavors. Believing in the value of one's daily work or raising children are good examples. The latter also gives a clear illustration of the paradox in which having purpose may or may not actually increase everyday (hedonic) happiness. In fact, because this example has been studied so much, it has been referred to as the "parenthood happiness puzzle" (Kohler & Mencarini, 2016, p. 327).

Research has triangulated the remarkable contradiction between the joy of having children and parents' ratings of their own happiness within a given day and across their life. It is well documented that happiness ratings drop precipitously for young parents such that their daily experience is reported to be relatively miserable (Glass et al., 2016; Kahneman et al., 2004; Twenge et al., 2003). Furthermore, although there are hills and valleys in any person's daily reports of happiness, the ratings of parents generally do not recover to their pre-parenting days until after their children leave home (Gilbert, 2006). That said, when asked to consider a much broader lifespan perspective, most parents report feeling life is better and happier since they had children (Baumeister et al., 2013; Gilbert, 2006). The contradiction is remarkable and likely has to do with key moments in one's life as a parent, which take on more importance and eclipse the grind of day-to-day challenges.[3]

The deeper issue is one of figure versus ground, but it can also be understood as a measurement issue of immediate experience versus overall satisfaction and how contradictory findings can result when trying to assess top-down processes using bottom-up metrics (Kahneman et al., 2004; Kohler & Mencarini, 2016). The point here is that having a strong sense of purpose allows one to endure a tremendous amount of misery because one sees beyond the horizon of one's daily existence. This produces healthy emotional change even though it may not decrease one's level of daily suffering. The misery itself is not qualitatively different, it just has trivial importance when placed in the context of a higher purpose. Higher purpose is experienced as more central than one's emotional distress at any given moment.

FOSTERING PURPOSE AND HIGHER MEANING

Having low meaning in life is a modifiable risk factor for mental illness, physical illness, and death (Alimujiang et al., 2019; Steger, 2022). Furthermore, the question of purpose and a search for meaning are frequent reasons that ultimately bring people to seek therapy, even if the initial issues of concern are related to symptom management.

Treatments for Generating Meaning in Life

Although all psychological treatments generate some level of meaning, there are approaches specifically aimed at helping people in their quest for existential meaning. Furthermore, there is reason to believe some approaches are more effective at this than others.

Clinical Research Evidence

One meta-analysis considered 60 treatments, each targeting specific psychological problems (i.e., not just self-discovery, religious development, or philosophical practices) and focused primarily on search for meaning in a systematic treatment approach (e.g., meaning-focused treatments, existentially oriented treatments; Vos & Vitali, 2018). The findings showed large pre- to posttreatment effects. A further meta-analysis of 33 randomized clinical trials examined the effect various interventions had on increasing a client's meaning in life. Again, formal active treatments showed a large effect in generating meaning in life over a waitlist or passive support in controlled studies. This suggests using systematic efforts to develop meaning in one's life can help, and they work better than when people are left to their own devices.

Findings also showed that purposeful interventions aimed at generating meaning in life had a small to medium effect, even when compared with active treatments with similar contact time (Manco & Hamby, 2021). The most effective approaches were narrative methods, such as life review and autobiographical approaches (see Chapter 18), which showed a medium to large effect in increasing a client's sense of meaning. Other treatments, including conventional psychotherapy, mindfulness techniques, and psychoeducation, also demonstrated a small but significant advantage over active comparisons. However, compared with active controls, there seemed to be no more benefit to the use of prosocial interventions or spiritual reminiscence (i.e., clarifying one's spiritual journey and relationship with a higher power; Manco & Hamby, 2021). Summing up, a number of systematic approaches offer a benefit over having people mill around for meaning. Still, it is noteworthy that evidence-based interventions, including narrative methods, mindfulness, and psychoeducation, are relatively brief, do not require licensed professionals, and may even be done online.

Some Treatments Are More Existential Than Others

In the landscape of contemporary psychotherapy, almost any treatment approach could help generate existential meaning, but not all treatments do. That will be a matter of emphasis and depends on both the focus of a treatment as well as its implementation in practice. Existential issues usually present an emotional confrontation with a nonnegotiable reality. As a case in point, the primary cause of cancer death among women is breast cancer, and over 20% of those patients also suffer major depression (Beutel et al., 2014).

Cognitive behavior therapy (CBT) is commonly the default approach in health psychology settings across North America and is particularly effective when dealing with health care procrastination, managing distress over physical symptoms, or lifestyle adjustment. However, while CBT is typically associated with large effects in the treatment of depression, a Cochrane review and meta-analysis of randomized clinical trials revealed that the treatment's efficacy is notably reduced in alleviating depression among breast cancer patients, yielding only small to medium effects (Jassim et al., 2023). This may be due to the limited comfort offered by standard cognitive reframes when confronting one's mortality and possibly impending death.

Such a dark reality requires the broadest frame of reference. Psychodynamic psychotherapy typically tends to use a much broader frame of reference than traditional CBT (see Chapter 20, "Generating New Context: The Short Game Versus the Long Game"). This is an epistemological difference in the kind of new meaning each treatment seeks to facilitate (recall Figure 17.1). Although direct comparisons have not yet been made with CBT, a randomized controlled trial of psychodynamic psychotherapy for the treatment of depression in breast cancer patients has shown a remarkably large effect compared with a treatment-as-usual control group (Beutel et al., 2014). Rather than focusing on symptom management and behavioral activation when working with this population, the psychodynamic approach aims to reconcile one's existential needs with one's interpersonal role and to negotiate one's place in a sociohistorical narrative.

Mechanisms Explaining the Impact on Health

Having purpose and meaning in life sets a framework for interpreting and understanding personal events whereby life is fundamentally valued for reasons that go beyond immediate personal difficulties (or pleasures; Baumeister et al., 2013). The salubrious impact these processes have likely occurs through several pathways. First, one's sense of purpose might be more likely to protect one's health. For example, keeping one's purpose in mind underscores the importance of keeping healthy and able, therefore motivating a person to exercise more, eat better, and use preventive health services.

Second, several studies suggest having life purpose and meaning in life reduces stress such that people with purpose are less troubled by hassles and recover better when they are stressed. For instance, the common refrain of "Don't sweat the small stuff" is predicated on a sense of priorities (e.g., P. L. Hill et al., 2018). In other words, having purpose clarifies someone's priorities and therefore their allocation of attention and resources. In this way, clear purpose and higher meaning entail an unencumbered forward directionality, allowing one to better weather the ups and downs of life.

The third role life purpose may play in buffering against stress is that it seems to reduce inflammation. When one's immune system responds to an irritant, it produces inflammation, which deteriorates the body and is itself associated with higher rates of illness and death. However, purpose and higher meaning in life is associated with lower levels of inflammation and inflammatory markers (e.g., certain levels of gene expression, hormones, proteins; Alimujiang et al., 2019). These three pathways are important psychobiological explanations that help us understand how someone's sense of purpose may impact their physical and psychological health.

IMPLEMENTING PURPOSE AND HIGHER MEANING

While purpose and meaning in life may improve health, generating and consistently implementing that purpose over the lifespan cannot be taken for granted. The undertaking is more like a marathon than a sprint. People also often need reminders to keep their purpose and higher meaning salient. However, priorities can also shift over the lifespan, and the underlying reason for making any such existential choices still requires explanation.

The Role of Mantras, Prayer, and Physical Mementos

Developing meaning in life and a sense of purpose has clear benefits, but doing so requires periodic decentering from the flow of experience to reorient and focus on that meaning (Chapter 20). One cannot be spiritual without decentering. This is because spirituality always encompasses more than the present moment. In *spiritual moments*, the envelope for one's focus extends beyond the mundane or painful present toward a promising future, which is tied to some higher purpose. In the face of enduring difficulties, tolerance for misery may be the deeper meaning of serenity. However, the reality of present suffering is compelling and demands attention (Pessoa, 2013). Thus, mindful decentering is an ongoing and familiar struggle in the pursuit of spirituality. See also Chapters 18 on grateful surrender and Chapter 21 on the use of a grand design in autobiographical reasoning.

Remembering to be mindful of a larger existential meaning that awaits beyond the immediate horizon of experience is a technical challenge for carrying out enduring emotional change. Practical solutions to this problem often involve everyday reminders, automatized habits, or lifestyle practices (e.g., morning yoga). Personal mantras (e.g., "Seize the day!"), rituals (e.g., burning incense in the garden), scripted prayer (e.g., giving thanks, surrendering to a higher power), and physical mementos (e.g., a wedding ring, keepsake, or special tattoo) are all common tools that efficiently reference and affirm existential choices that people have made through prior reflection.

These covert tools serve at least three functions. First, they offer something palpable to do or say when affirming commitment to one's chosen purpose, since embodiment and enactment of existential choices are not always self-apparent. Second, mantras or ritualized practices provide an immediately accessible scaffold during times of distress, helping orient and focus a person on their values and choices. They act as concrete references and simple scripted procedures for engaging with abstract intentions, allowing one to toggle between first-person and third-person perspectives (Chapters 17 and 22). Third, these concrete aids are quick handles that provide continuity over time, folding existential intention into one's narrative identity (Chapter 21). Additionally, rituals, symbols, and mementos that stand the test of time are often rooted in personal or cultural narratives and may even rouse a supportive network of like-minded others.

In fostering emotional change, the most essential aspect of mantras, prayer, and physical mementos is that they are associated with a moral imperative, leveraging existing meanings and values to guide action. These tools carry explicit references to the personal life goals and spiritual aspirations by which one is trying to live. Without deeper personal anchors, however, the procedures or words may become trite or naively hopeful expressions that lack true meaning. Still, even going through the motions can offer comfort and a familiar structure during periods of distress (e.g., see Chapter 2 on mindfulness, "An Example of Many Processes Overdetermining Outcome").

Keeping a firm hold on fragile and tentative constructions of personal meaning is an ongoing challenge, one that becomes especially hard in the face of increasing arousal, which is when one needs it most! This practical issue is pervasive across approaches to emotion change (Chapter 20). Reflection on emotion (Chapter 17) and, specifically, on existential meaning (this chapter) requires one to maintain well-differentiated meaning despite rising emotional arousal. Formal rituals and reflective practices help anchor a person during swells of emotional pain that might otherwise be disorienting. Such practices provide a mental bookmark to help one focus and reconnect to one's purpose (Chapter 18, this volume; Bakan, 1966).

Meaning in Life Over the Lifespan

Clients in psychotherapy report that focusing on their meaning in life is of especially high value when they find themselves at transitional moments in life, such as when confronted with life-threatening or chronic physical illness (Vos & Vitali, 2018). Research with a nonclinical rural sample of over 2,500 participants from the United States echoes that finding. Generally, meaning in life increased from adolescence to middle adulthood, but there were identifiable turning points as well as plateaus in meaning over the lifespan (Hamby et al., 2017). For example, men in rural parts of the United States typically have a crisis in their sense of purpose around age 27 to 30. Although gender effects were small, the same study showed that women tend to enjoy higher levels of meaning in life than men across the lifespan.

Such findings suggest moderators and clinical opportunities to leverage existential work for emotional change. However, there are also risks in introducing existential confrontations too early. For example, when an individual is not yet able to make a necessary choice, a confrontation with the question of higher purpose can be overwhelming and can also set them up for failure. For instance, in Chapter 18 I cited an example where teens with low self-identity deteriorated when they were pressed to reflect on the purpose of their life. Similarly, in treating clients with complex trauma, clients need to have worked through certain issues before they can reasonably be confronted with the choice to move on and let go of their painful past (Paivio & Pascual-Leone, 2023).

Developing life purpose is largely an issue of existential choice and commitment to contributing or building forward in almost any domain. When asked what gives them meaning or purpose in life, people often cited a connection to something much larger than themselves (Hamby et al., 2017, 2018). Notable themes included

- dedication to some cause,

- commitment to social roles (e.g., relationships, family, community),

- adherence to some code of values or ethics (e.g., religious traditions, military), and

- mastery-oriented meaning making (e.g., developing competence, expertise, a personal practice).

The first three of these typically became increasingly important sources of meaning over the lifespan. In contrast, however, the last one (self-oriented mastery) was the only domain that decreased as a source of meaning, dropping between adolescence and the mid-30s (Hamby et al., 2017). By the same token, when people rely too heavily on commitment to social roles as their source of meaning in life, it often carries an associated cost of caregiver burden (Hamby et al., 2018). At a higher order, all these can be thought of as commitments to some manifestation of agency or communion in one's narrative identity (see Chapter 21, this volume; Bakan, 1966).

Making Choices With Hope and Courage

Confrontations with existential reality can be pivotal moments for change. Karl Jaspers, a German Swiss psychiatrist and philosopher, described a *limit situation* as when an individual's life circumstances become so unbearable that they force a choice point (Fuchs et al., 2014). Examples include everyday situations that evoke fright, guilt, a sense of finality, or suffering. At these moments, the individual either succumbs to despair and depression or confronts the challenge and emerges transformed. Limit situations are encounters with reality that unsettle us. They push us to break from conventional and routine solutions, requiring us to choose or act in ways that often have us questioning our identities.

Perhaps the most important aspect of a limit situation is that the criteria of relevance become sharper in the face of an existential threat. Simply put, when under pressure, the individual sees much more clearly what is important, what is not, and what now needs to be done. The following example comes from a study that interviewed men with histories of using intimate partner violence and who were then confronted with the prospect of fatherhood:

> I had to make a choice when he came, and that was either the kid or the people I was with. That changed me. I cut them out and started to take care of him. God knows where I would be today if I hadn't got a kid. . . . I feel I have learned to handle problems. Before, I drank, and the alcohol made me do bad things. (Mohaupt et al., 2020, p. 866)

As illustrated in this excerpt, in a limit situation, an individual sees their future laid out in front of them, and that creates both a challenge and opportunity for growth.

The existential choices that follow are pivotal moments in which the figure and ground are essentially switched. The content of a distressing emotional experience is not just interpreted through an existing framework (e.g., Chapter 20), but rather it becomes the inspiration for an altogether new context of meaning that is projected into the future. *Hope* is being able to imagine something better; it is contingent on the vision of some future possibility that one sees as both realistic and feasible. *Courage* is the feeling that some cause (or purpose) is worth accepting the inherent risks in committing oneself to it. Some people have their purpose thrust upon them (e.g., "I didn't ask for this responsibility! But now I accept it."). Meanwhile, others make conscious decisions to choose their purpose (e.g., "I promise to dedicate myself to this effort"). Shirking or avoiding these choices prolongs ambiguity and typically leaves the person to live with resentment and despair tied to an uncertain future. Whatever the case, the person who feels resolved has always made an active choice about their circumstances, sometimes by deciding and other times by explicitly accepting.

IS THIS MYSELF AT BEST OR AT WORST?

Irrespective of age and processing capacity, people do not always apply all their mental resources (affective and cognitive) to working on personal problems. Research shows that this is partly a function of how difficult a given task appears to be and what the minimum level of passable exertion will be (J. Pascual-Leone & Johnson, 2021). Motivation, fatigue, and divided efforts are other reasons for underperformance in emotional as much as cognitive work. When one's capacity for emotional processing becomes a focal point, individuals reflect on their current performance, evaluating its maturity and effort against past experiences or idealized standards (DiMaggio, 2020). This metacognitive reflection involves considering these questions: Am I bringing my best self to this? Is this my best game, or am I underperforming? And do I know better?

The question, "Is this myself at best or myself at worst?" is a formulation developed in interpersonal psychodynamic models (Benjamin, 2000), but it also parallels a framework in dialectical behavior therapy that asks clients whether they are in "wise mind" (vs. "emotional mind" or "rational mind"; Linehan, 2015). Self-at-best and self-at-worst are also conceptualized extensively in accelerated experiential dynamic psychotherapy (Fosha, 2021). These are embodied states, but referring to them as versions of oneself facilitates decentering by objectifying one's current functioning, monitoring it, and then considering alternatives (see Chapter 20, "Step 1: Decentering, the Act of Shifting to a Higher Level," and Chapter 22, "Toggling Between Levels of Mental Construal"). Psychodynamic, behavioral, and humanistic–experiential perspectives all emphasize the role of conscious choice in exercising one's best self and present this choice to clients as an existential confrontation. The consideration of alternative selves is key to working with instrumental emotion and changing unhealthy strategies of emotion regulation.

Working With Instrumental Emotion

Sometimes the expression of emotion, though a genuine personal experience of feeling, is also highly instrumental in eliciting a particular response from others (Introduction). Categorizing this kind of emotional expression as manipulative is misleading because it often suggests the client's experience is not authentic or is contrived in some way, which is an oversimplification. The deeper question here is to what extent the manner or intensity of an emotional communication has been shaped or reinforced by social factors. For example, the businessman who habitually expresses grave disappointment as soon as others disagree with him (i.e., pursing lips, clenching teeth, shaking head) is indeed upset, but his exaggerated expression may also offer some advantage to him in the ensuing negotiations.

Similarly, an elderly woman whom I saw in psychotherapy would routinely get angry and yell on the phone when service providers did not comply with her demands. She also sheepishly prided herself on the effectiveness with which she executed this. However, when she used the same approach to get more visits from her grandchildren, it backfired, and her son hung up on her. On another occasion, when she was verbally abusive to staff in the office of her pain specialist, the staff canceled the upcoming appointment. As we considered the larger narrative context and what mattered to her, contrasting it with her short-term wins over service providers, the misery and social hardship of her go-to style became increasingly obvious. This bad habit robbed her of relief and longer term joys. As a lived experience, instrumental emotion is itself trying for clients, like being tossed about on emotional waves. Reflecting on the social function of these emotions increases one's motivation for change (e.g., Client: "If I didn't have to put other people through this to get what I need, maybe I don't have to weather these emotional storms myself either!").

Changing instrumental emotion involves a process of narrative reflection. The therapist initiates a conversation about the impact of these emotional experiences, focusing on two key considerations. Firstly, they collaboratively explore the effectiveness of the instrumental emotion in meeting the client's needs. Secondly, they reflect on what this socioemotional process might be like for others to endure, particularly those with whom the client has significant relationships.

Next, reflecting instrumental emotions in social interactions aims to explore alternative, more adaptive ways of meeting one's needs. However, the motivation for developing social skills hinges on a client's ability to decenter and gain insight into the issue (Chapter 20). Sustained change also depends on the client's ability to gain sufficient psychological distance from the heated moment or to receive feedback without too much shame. I suggest that this formulation for changing instrumental emotion converges with case formulations from humanistic, behavioral, and dynamic perspectives (see Kramer, 2019).

Unhealthy Strategies for Regulating Emotion

As discussed in Chapter 3, down-regulating emotion can be a functional and adaptive process in certain situations. I also cautioned that overreliance on strategies for reducing emotion, such as excessive avoidance, was unhealthy. Moreover, certain strategies, such as substance abuse, are inherently unhealthy from the outset. In this section, I highlight the importance of existential choice in emotion regulation. Notably, various chronic problematic behaviors, often operating outside awareness, can serve as implicit forms of affect regulation and may take on an addictive quality. Prime examples of this include

- self-injury (e.g., cutting, burning; Linehan, 2015),

- problematic anger and hate (e.g., chronic reactive anger, hate-based identities; A. Pascual-Leone et al., 2013; Simi et al., 2017),

- problematic sexual behavior (e.g., pornography and sex addictions, some perpetration of sexual abuse[4]), and

- procrastination (Sirois & Pychyl, 2013).

All these acts provide short-term emotional repair to immediate emotional discomfort ranging from boredom to intense distress.

At best, these are unhealthy diversions from painful emotion. For example, as a client bluntly explained to me, "I try to f*ck the pain away." However, the habitual nature of these behaviors often worsens as behaviors become part of entrenched feedback loops. Beyond their social or external functions, these problematic emotion-based behaviors have a powerful automatic or internal component. Like substance abuse, behaviors such as reactive anger, problematic sexual behaviors, and self-injurious behaviors produce rapid and fundamental shifts in one's affective state. The swift and implicit nature of these changes can be attributed to their biological underpinnings (Nock & Prinstein, 2004). These biologically driven changes often operate outside of awareness, as they are less mediated by reflective processes like interpretation and meaning making. Behaviors such as anger, sex addiction, and self-injury can provide both negative reinforcement (i.e., the relief of displacing an unpleasant feeling) and positive reinforcement (i.e., providing a more pleasurable experience), with both mechanisms contributing to the behaviors' persistence (Nock & Prinstein, 2004). Although ultimately unhealthy, these behaviors provide a sense of focus and control, countering feelings of being overwhelmed and disorganized. They also allow one to feel powerful, given a sense of thrilling escape from the emotional pain of shame and disappointment.

Gaining insight into this link involves narrative reflection, a crucial first step toward change when working with instrumental emotion. A common strategy is to help clients become aware of the behavioral chain of antecedents-behaviors-consequences through narrative elaboration (Beck, 2020; Linehan, 2015). As clients reflect on the true function of these behaviors, they can also identify healthier alternatives. This reflection creates an opportunity for existential choice, marking the second step toward change. By recognizing the long-term consequences of their actions, clients can move beyond the immediate escape and relief these behaviors provide, acknowledging that the future self ultimately bears the costs (Sirois & Pychyl, 2013). In a very real way, the dialogue here on existential choice circles back to the topic of down-regulation discussed at the beginning of this book (Chapter 2).

THE FUTURE SELF: WHO DO YOU WANT TO BE?

Reinventing the self is a process of identity elaboration. For most people, this occurs very incrementally as a developmental process. However, there are also some dramatic examples of people who decidedly choose to assume a new kind of self with a new kind of life. Case examples are celebrated in psychotherapy literature, but as a group, their commonalities are not typically considered. Nevertheless, the curious occurrence of prisoners who experience religious conversion while behind bars is a possible illustration of certain mechanisms by which people might reinvent themselves (Maruna, 2001; Maruna et al., 2006). Many features of these life narratives have been discussed in Chapter 21.

There are at least four specific features that seem to be part of reinventing oneself through a story of conversion, redemption, or generativity (Maruna et al., 2006). First, as seen with master narratives, the narrative draws on a framework of *sociocultural scripts*, and that language offers a medium for elaborating one's intentions, purpose, and existential meaning. Second, the story delineates a *new social identity*, one that can now replace the older label of self as bad, broken, or disconnected. In some sense, the story of conversion is a tool for managing shame and compartmentalizing "myself then" from "myself now." Third, such narratives highlight the *empowerment* of an individual as a new agent. Fourth, the new story explains the past but also projects an intention into the future, a mission that offers a sense of *control over an unknown future.* These general features fit with many of the anecdotes from clinical work, and they also recall the existential insights of Yalom (1981) that I cited at the beginning of this chapter.

Interventions involving creative construction and projection of oneself into future realities can take various forms depending on the treatment approach. Constructing a future self could even begin with behavioral goal setting, where the personal narrative is framed as a story that has yet to be completed (Chapter 18). Simple questions about an alternative and better future also help orient a client to actively construct their future self—as seen, for example, in the hallmark intervention of solution-focused therapy, which asks, "If you woke up tomorrow and this was somehow better, what's the first thing you would notice? What would be different for you?" (Chapter 20). Furthermore, research on sudden gains suggests that this source of inspiration may occur differently across treatment approaches. For example, in CBT, the inspirational experience is often thought to be a discovery during the behavioral homework that occurs between sessions, where clients test their beliefs against the world out there. However, in experiential treatments, the inspiration for new life direction comes from emotional experiences that take place within the session itself (Singh et al., 2021; reviewed in Chapter 16, this volume).

Specificity is a key issue here. Free choice is only viscerally experienced in the clarity of a constructed possibility. Rather than general hopefulness or vague positive wishes, this requires concrete possible plans for oneself in a specific future. Enactments, for instance, are opportunities for fleshing out a future possibility. Whereas focusing on present experiences generates emotion, imagining an alternate future is equally crucial for driving change (Chapter 10). During chairwork and imaginal dialogues with abusive others, an emotion-focused therapist asks their client, "What do you wish you had said? Say it now"; or "What would a good parent have done? Can you imagine doing that for yourself? What do you need to hear when you feel like that?" (Chapters 14 and 15, this volume; Paivio & Pascual-Leone, 2023).

Ultimately, after all the insights and new experiences someone may have (e.g., relational, emotional, conceptual), a successful change still requires that person to take action. This involves exercising free will to deliberately choose to engage with the world—both internally and externally—in a way that breaks from problematic, habitual patterns. This last step is what separates armchair psychologizing from true existential change (A. Pascual-Leone & Greenberg, 2007b). For some individuals, the shift is already implicit as they begin to reframe their situation and themselves and are motivated to adopt a new way of being. However, others require a more explicit moment of existential choice to bridge the gap between insight and lasting change. Without this, new understanding may not translate into meaningful action.

Figuring out how to leverage choice and intentionality is where people need to exercise creativity (see also Chapter 11 on playfulness and spontaneity). Decentering is essentially thinking outside the original framework, so some effortful creativity is needed for people to generate alternatives, consider other explanations, or bring about innovative moments. The creative reinvention of the self, whether in a local context or in terms of one's broader life script, is an effortful and deliberate process. Interventions that do this best will invite a client to envision themselves in the future and develop practical plans. By doing so, clients concretely experience their agency in making an existential choice in the present, deciding whether to pursue or reject an imagined future.

When a client is ambivalent about committing to some action, it is a marker for their therapist to introduce an existential confrontation. This intensifies the limit situation, revealing a client's potential reservations about taking action. Articulating a specific goal, wish, or need can also prompt existential confrontations with one's current trajectory in life and the implications of inaction. This helps highlight the cost of not choosing. For example, a therapist could ask, "And when you die one day, what will they write on your tombstone? Will it say, 'Here lies [client's name]. They never had the courage to risk making a change, and their life went on always the same. So many years and they never even really asked for what they wanted.'?"

There are everyday choices—sometimes thoughtful, sometimes less so—but then there are existential choices made with full awareness of the implications one's action could have for one's identity and life trajectory. A client of mine gave a remarkably candid account of defining their future self. Notice the critical role that reflecting on emotion plays in shaping their future self-concept and in driving personal change:

> I was driving to work today and . . . I hit a squirrel. There were two lanes of traffic, and it ran out between passing cars. . . . I was the unlucky one who hit it. It just ran right in front of me, I heard it rattle under the car [*grimaces*]. There was nothing I could do! I . . . I kept driving for about half a block and was looking in the rearview mirror. I thought, "What if it's not dead? What if there's still a chance?" And then I was like, "Even if there's nothing to do, what kind of person would I be if I just turned on the radio and pretended it was a normal everyday thing?" I've never killed anything before; I mean, not a mammal. . . . I guess it was like, "Who do I want to be?" I realized, even though I was afraid to see what I had done, it was a choice point: There are people who don't care, and then there are people who do. . . . So, I felt like I was going to have to do something, if I wanted to be in that second group, you know? . . . I made a U-turn, parked, and I walked back. . . . It was pretty gross. I moved it to the ditch. Too bad. But at least I gave it the dignity of not getting mushed into the road. . . . I think, in a small way, it was important how I handled that respect for life. . . . I'd just never crossed that bridge before. But I did it right.

While my client's example encapsulates the process, everyday life offers similar moments where the way one chooses to cope with adversity becomes a deliberate choice to define oneself. In the face of limit situations, we are reshaped by the conscious decision to meet challenges with an act of compassion, courage, or grace.

ENDNOTES

1. Parts of this section are adapted from "Insight and Awareness in Experiential Therapy," by A. Pascual-Leone and L. S. Greenberg, in L. G. Castonguay and C. E. Hill (Eds.), *Insight in Psychotherapy* (pp. 31–56), 2007b, American Psychological Association. Copyright 2007 by the American Psychological Association.
2. Senior's (2010) article in the *New York Times* uses this phrase (i.e., "All joy and no fun") to refer to the parenting puzzle.
3. To be clear, a drop in parents' life satisfaction is not only a matter of outlook and the figure–ground construal. Concrete social issues matter too! Glass and colleagues (2016) showed that a country's social policy in support of parents is also a critically objective factor. Countries like the United States have the lowest life satisfaction for parents, whereas the highest is among Scandinavian countries.
4. Some sexual offenders report using both consenting and nonconsenting sexual activities as strategies for coping with negative affect when they face stressful and difficult personal situation (Gunst et al., 2017).

VI

**CONCLUSIONS:
A NEW PARADIGM**

CONCLUSIONS: A NEW PARADIGM

The classic work of Alexander and French (1946) was an early seminal contribution focused on principles of psychotherapy, and it highlighted the importance of a corrective emotional experience. Since then, valuable elaborations have emphasized the interpersonal aspect of this curative process. While interpersonal relationships are an important mechanism of change, an emotion change itself must ultimately register within the individual client. This book focuses on change at the intrapersonal levels of information processing, self-organization, and personal meaning. Theories often offer up labels for phenomena that acknowledge some kind of change has happened within the client (e.g., corrective experience, emotion regulation, processing), but such labels often fail to explain the underlying process.

This book has clarified key concepts in emotion change literature and provided an integrative review of supporting evidence across various treatment perspectives. As outlined in Chapter 1, the objective has been to present a general theory that describes and organizes our understanding of emotional change. This theory offers three main contributions:

- It presents a coherent set of explanations for how five distinct kinds of change happen by attending to their functional differences.

- It identifies observable features (i.e., unique markers) that signal when a given change process is called for (summarized in Chapter 24).

- It explores how the five overarching kinds of change manifest and are facilitated through very different approaches to treatment.

In short, the general theory laid out in this book addresses how change happens, under what circumstances, and for whom.

EMOTION REVISITED

In rudimentary and often purely behavioral accounts, emotional distress is seen as a symptom to be reduced. However, emotional arousal can be more than a symptom; it also often plays a role as a process, one that might facilitate positive change. Different emotions serve as distinct tools for navigating experience. Rather than narrowly understanding emotion as a disorganizing state that derails one's cognitive efforts, a process perspective recognizes discrete emotional states as unique mental sets or frameworks of engagement.

The most critical aspect of emotion is not that it is representational (e.g., signaling some negative attribution or belief). Instead, much more importantly, emotion is procedural, organizing a person to engage in certain ways with their world, with others, and sometimes most importantly, with themselves. Emotion implicitly sets one on a trajectory of action, and it also primes our perceptual expectations and recruits cognitive resources. Emotion is about doing, and different emotions facilitate engagement in distinct ways. Discrete emotions also serve as different tools that may (or may not) be at someone's disposal to address personal issues. It follows that an important aspect of mental health is emotional flexibility, the ability to engage and explore new and different approaches to feeling one's way through an old problem.

In summary, although many negative emotions are aversive experiences, emotions are also states that offer different ways of engaging an experience. Those states then call for corresponding change strategies (i.e., operations) to resolve personal and emotional difficulties. Still, the question of which emotion requires which change principle has been a great puzzle for theory and research.

SYNTHESIZING THEORY AND RESEARCH

If emotions are taken as the target, then principles of emotion change are the operations being applied to work with those states. Currently, different schools of psychotherapy champion distinct processes, both in their interventions and in their corresponding lines of research. A general theory of emotional change is desperately needed to coherently distinguish between various ways of working with emotion. Without it, research will continue to yield mixed findings and ongoing debates due to inconsistent process formulations. Many treatment theories oversimplify emotional change, typically reducing it to just a few isolated processes. Ultimately, it is the client who chooses the process that will be embarked on—not the therapist and much less the researcher.

In this general theory of emotional change, I have described five distinct ways of working with emotion (summarized in Chapter 24). The synthesis was based on converging lines of evidence drawn across subdisciplines and levels of analysis, namely

- phenomenological evidence,

- psychological measurement,

- psychotherapy and change process research,

- basic research in psychology (e.g., cognitive, developmental, social areas),

- neuroscience, and

- existing clinical interventions.

These lines of evidence support my formulation of a limited number of distinct processes by which emotion will change. Moreover, the treatment literature offers specific interventions to target each of these using methods from different approaches.

The final point on clinical intervention was an important touchstone. Both scientific parsimony and clinical pragmatism determined the concise number of principles I have presented. Despite overgeneralizations in treatment theories about how a given intervention works to foster client change, specific interventions work in distinct ways. The mechanisms of client changes then occur through separate causal pathways, each reflecting one of the five forms of emotional processing. This is the sort of formulation that matters most for practice. The final chapter of this book summarizes the clinical implications for each kind of change.

24

The Five Principles of Emotion Change

As for me my bed is made: I am against bigness and greatness in all their forms, and with the invisible molecular moral forces that work from individual to individual, stealing in through crannies of the world like so many soft rootlets, or like the capillary oozing of water, and yet rendering the hardest moments of [human] pride if you give them time. The bigger the unit you deal with, the hollower, the more brutal, and the more mendacious is the life displayed. So, I am . . . against all big successes and big results; and in favor of the eternal forces of truth which always work in the individual and immediately unsuccessful ways, underdogs always, till history comes, after they are long dead, and puts them on the top.

—WILLIAM JAMES, *THE LETTERS OF WILLIAM JAMES*

As I have affirmed throughout this book, emotional change typically does not occur through isolated mechanisms. Treatment theories often suggest a one-to-one correspondence between interventions and mechanisms, with different psychotherapies celebrating their preferred mechanism. (The reasons for that partiality are as much tied to a treatment's fundamental view on human functioning as they are to issues of branding and promotion.) However, whether an intervention facilitates, for example, labeling affect, enactments, cognitive reframing, or narrative work is not as straightforward as treatment manuals may suggest; it could serve multiple purposes depending on the underlying mechanism. Sometimes an intervention facilitates a given process, but at other times, the same intervention might be used to facilitate some other process. This does not mean that all kinds of emotional

https://doi.org/10.1037/0000460-025
Principles of Emotion Change: What Works and When in Psychotherapy and Everyday Life, by A. Pascual-Leone
Copyright © 2026 by the American Psychological Association. All rights reserved.

processing are the same but rather that the therapist and treatment theory do not unilaterally determine which process will ensue. The skillful therapist potentiates an optimal process based on how they present an intervention. Then, what determines the functional role of a given process is a combination of the client's own intention and their internal (psychological) circumstances at that moment. In all instances, there are multiple potential entry points (i.e., markers) to facilitate a given process.

Furthermore, I have argued that five overarching principles leverage the lion's share of emotion change. This is a general theory that acknowledges the independent value of existing theories while putting them together in an integrated framework, delineating their limits of applicability, and resolving contradictions. Research on potential mechanisms of change shows that the five ways of working with emotion (i.e., down-regulation, awareness, expression, sequences, and narrative reflection) have varying effect sizes depending on research design and context. Each type of emotional work typically has a small to medium effect on symptom change when studied in isolation. However, this poses a methodological puzzle for researchers because change processes rarely operate alone (see Chapter 1, this volume; A. Pascual-Leone & Kramer, 2023). In reality, people undergo tremendous emotional change at key moments and also over time. When those large effects are observed, they are often driven by synergies among multiple processes that affect a client—at just the right time and in just the right way.

Disentangling the mechanisms of emotion change is also crucial for therapists who want to get the most purchase from their interventions. Therapists who better understand what is happening within the session will have a clearer sense of what needs to be done to facilitate change. Meanwhile, clients and other people suffering emotional distress are squarely concerned with obtaining the outcomes of immediately incremental change. To that end, people in distress are active agents who will make use of any and all possible mechanisms, sometimes blindly but often with synergistic effects. Even so, a general theory like this could eventually provide laypeople with insights for navigating emotional challenges.

A common question is, what is the best or most important type of processing? However, there is no single tool that can accomplish all aspects of emotional processing. Any complex task with many different aspects (whether building a house or resolving personal difficulties) requires the use of different tools at different times. A more incisive question is, what type of processing is best for a specific emotional difficulty and when? The following sections summarize when each kind of emotional change is most helpful. The chapter then concludes with future directions in understanding emotion change.

DOWN-REGULATING EMOTION

Down-regulation of emotion is defined as the process of calming down or reducing arousal at a moment when the intensity of one's feelings is too high. Relatedly, *distress tolerance* refers to an individual's upper limit in their capacity for enduring and functioning despite the high intensity or duration of painful emotion. There are markers for when therapists should or should not facilitate the down-regulation of emotional arousal. These include both specific kinds of emotions as well as moment-by-moment clinical observations (discussed in Chapters 2 and 3).

When to Promote Down-Regulation

Emotion regulation is often broadly defined, encompassing almost any form of working with emotion. When it has also been paired with the behaviorist view of emotion as symptomatic, this breadth has led to overemphasizing down-regulation in clinical manuals. More narrowly, down-regulation or reduction of emotional arousal is called for in 11 specific scenarios. Markers for reducing the emotional intensity include target states as well as certain clinical observations that may be made within the session or as part of case formulation.

Emotion Markers

Several kinds of emotion signal that down-regulating arousal will be necessary. Generally, these are emotional states that interfere with processing meaning more deeply, or they could be emotions that are simply activated beyond an individual's window of tolerance.

- *Secondary emotion and symptom distress* can be addressed through down-regulation, and that should be the primary target for this kind of emotional processing.

- *Primary maladaptive emotion* (e.g., feeling shamefully unlovable, feeling worthless, traumatic fear, terror) may need to be down-regulated, but only at moments when the feelings are overwhelming or disorganizing. The activation of maladaptive emotion may be a rich opportunity to facilitate deeper changes, but sometimes an individual will need temporary reprieve from the intensity of such experiences. At other times, clients may need help reigning in their emotional arousal to keep it within a safe and functional range. However, it is important to note that exposure alone to primary maladaptive emotions cannot extinguish the causal determinants of that dysfunctional experience.

- *Instrumental emotion* should be down-regulated because of its socially and personally dysfunctional nature. Reducing the intensity of these emotions also makes them more amenable to being reflected on from a less reactive or disengaged state. In facilitating this, clinicians should be mindful that clients may be (often unconsciously) ambivalent about curtailing the arousal of instrumental emotion because it is inherently motivated and reinforced by social contingencies.

Moment-by-Moment Markers

Down-regulating emotion is a critical process at times of crisis. There are a few scenarios where this is the only process of choice, namely in the following:

- *An emotional response carries imminent risk,* such as suicidality, self-harm, danger to others, addiction relapse, and so on.

- *The intensity of an emotional experience is disorienting or disorganizing,* such that the individual is unable to productively process information or generate useful meaning. Examples of this include panic, sobbing uncontrollably, unchecked rage, and dissociation.

- *A situation needs concentration and high performance* that also require calming down before a difficult or complex performance that demands a clear and undistracted mind (e.g., taking an exam, a job interview, an athletic competition, during an emergency). The situation may not be a crisis, but it represents a decisive moment of effort that could be derailed by excessive emotional arousal.

Client Characteristics

Clients who are very reactive or prone to feeling overwhelmed will benefit from the immediate down-regulation of their emotion or developing a better overall capacity to calm down. There are also clinical observations about a client that suggest practicing the down-regulation of emotion would be a useful process. These include the following:

- *Consistent hyperarousal when confronted with certain cues* and being unable to function on account of that overarousal. Here, exposure, desensitization, and coping skills are indicated.

- *Suffering specific problems that put the person at risk,* such as anger, a history of aggression, substance abuse, impulsive risky behavior, and so on. For people at risk, it will be useful to use adaptive avoidance, develop a repertoire of behavioral coping skills, and make lifestyle changes that reduce their vulnerability to dysregulation.

- *Suffering problems related to chronic hyperarousal.* Desensitization and behavioral skills coping may be particularly useful for people who are frequently highly aroused. This includes people suffering problems with anger and aggression, borderline personality disorder, substance abuse, panic disorder, other anxiety disorders, obsessive–compulsive disorder, dissociation, and sometimes trauma. However, down-regulation is a process indicated first and foremost by identifiable moments of high and dysfunctional or dangerous arousal, not by diagnostic category per se.

- *If people suffering dementia become agitated,* they will need help with down-regulating their arousal through sensorimotor soothing such as touch, massage, or calm music.

In addition,

- *Adolescents, middle aged, and older adults suffering from mild to moderate depression* are better able to regulate their emotions when they exercise regularly. Walking, lifting weights, and other resistance exercise training (e.g., for less than 45 minutes) has a large effect on reducing distress, improving mental health, and increasing resilience.

When in Treatment: Phase-Based Markers

Down-regulating emotion is called for according to immediate moment-by-moment markers (e.g., the client is overwhelmed), which would override any considerations of the treatment's phase. For this reason, down-regulation might be applied at any time. The critical issue is whether emotional arousal exceeds the individual's level of tolerance. Markers that signal someone is beyond their tolerance for arousal include when they become disorganized or have trouble with cognitively processing new information.

Before entering the middle or working phase of treatment, clinicians should assess a client's capacity for down-regulation and coping. Early appraisal should consider a client's history of risky behavior to escape distress (e.g., self-harm, substance use, violence). For clients with poor emotion regulation, the early phase of therapy may require special attention to skills training and perhaps exposure to enhance their capacity for down-regulation.

When Not to Use Down-Regulation

Down-regulation is an essential process that temporarily staves off an emotional experience, although emotion typically signals that something is wrong and needs attention. Thus, although it may be useful in times of crisis, this way of working with emotion will be problematic if used habitually or when other processes could apply. Do not use down-regulation when managing everyday life situations

- for extended periods of time;

- when solving significant life concerns;

- when trying to make meaning of one's life;

- when searching for purpose; or

- if the primary emotion is tolerable to the client, even if that emotion is maladaptive.

Using distraction or changing the topic to down-regulate maladaptive emotion removes the opportunity for that painful emotion to be worked with and changed. Furthermore, people will not habituate to maladaptive emotions, in which getting used to, for example, the same old story of shame and inadequacy would likely be unhealthy. Similarly, down-regulating primary adaptive emotions might leave clients (and sometimes also therapists) feeling temporarily less disturbed by the presenting concerns, but it will also prevent the opportunity to make use of the information and healthy direction embodied in such experiences. Thus, primary adaptive emotion will not typically be targeted for significant down-regulation, with the exception that one may need to help modulate engagement for clients who are prone to becoming derailed by their arousal.

Finally, exposure and desensitization involve a temporary activation of high arousal as a means of decreasing reactivity over time (through habituation or inhibition). However, an important contextual factor for this process to be therapeutic is that the client is willing to engage and feels it is their choice to participate. Pressuring or coercion to participate in such interventions is unethical and could be traumatic.

Mechanisms of Change Related to Down-Regulation

There are three mechanisms of change by which down-regulation can change one's state of emotion (discussed in Chapter 3). They are

- adaptive avoidance,

- desensitization (through habituation or inhibition), and

- using behavioral coping skills.

In addition, lifestyle factors such as adequate sleep, exercise, nutrition, and reducing substance use (e.g., alcohol) are critical in reducing one's overall vulnerability to dysregulated affect. In some cases, lifestyle factors have even been effectively used as treatments for emotional disorders.

EMOTIONAL AWARENESS

I have used emotional awareness as a general term to refer to a range of processes related to engagement and the moment-by-moment experience of emotion. In this definition, *emotional engagement* is purposefully approaching and accepting the significance of some emotional experience. Once engaged, *emotional awareness* can be more narrowly defined as the process of exploring somatic sensations, thoughts, action tendencies, and needs associated with an emotional experience to label it and clarify its meaning as an immediately lived feeling (i.e., symbolization). There are markers for when one should facilitate engagement or deepen the awareness of emotion, and they are related to specific types of emotions as well as certain clinical presentations (discussed in Chapter 4).

When to Promote Emotional Awareness

Promoting emotional awareness through engaging, labeling, and symbolizing a feeling is almost always helpful, although there are a few specific exceptions. There are six specific scenarios in which promoting emotional awareness is explicitly called for. The markers for increasing emotional awareness are certain emergent emotional states as well as other moment-by-moment observations.

Emotion Markers

Engagement with emotional poignancy of any kind is a process that can efficiently orient one to the most important content in a presenting concern. Therefore, both primary and secondary emotion alike will serve as markers for further engagement and for labeling affect. Once the person has a handle or initial label for their feeling(s), then primary emotions (either adaptive or maladaptive) are the chief targets for deepening emotional awareness, symbolizing the experience, and then generating bottom-up meaning (e.g., as with a meaning bridge).

Moment-by-Moment Markers

Various moment-by-moment clinical observations can also serve as markers for increasing emotional awareness. These reflect specific moments in which increased engagement will help people work with their feelings, namely the following:

- *Feeling uncertain* about one's preferences, values, needs, or identity, which are all instances that signal emotional awareness is the process of choice.

- *A visceral gut feeling about something that is still vague* (e.g., feeling uncomfortable, uneasy, irritable). In short, the experience lacks clarity and has yet to be elaborated into a meaningful focus or direction. That unclear felt sense is a classic marker for emotional awareness (either affect labeling alone or labeling plus deepening and exploration).

- *Feeling puzzled by one's own reaction* to a situation or confused by its meaning. This could include feeling puzzled by the content of one's dreams while also having some inkling of their emotional significance. Feeling unsure of what emotional experiences mean or what they relate to is another marker for working on emotional awareness so that deepening and symbolizing the experience can lead to some larger coherent meaning.

- *Seeking more creative or artistic direction.* Emotion is a wellspring for artistic inspiration. When people need to be more creative, either in their work or in how they grapple with a personal problem, increasing emotional awareness helps inspire a sense of direction.

When in Treatment: Phase-Based Markers

Emotional engagement is particularly critical at the beginning of treatment both to initiate any kind of emotional processing and because it sets a precedent for the client's future levels of engagement. Part of that is believed to be an issue of individual differences, in that some clients are more disposed to explore emotion than others. Another part of the initial level of engagement is about socialization and setting expectations because some interactional styles or treatment approaches stress emotional exploration more than others. Emotional awareness will continue to be important over therapy, although the largest gains in this process seem to be from the beginning to the middle phase of treatment, after which it may plateau. Nevertheless, engaging emotion and symbolizing complex experiences are useful throughout treatment.

When Not to Use Emotional Awareness

There are specific emotions and states that are contraindications, signaling that one should not promote further emotional awareness. These include the following:

- *Instrumental emotion* should not be the target of heightened awareness and symbolizing because it would be unproductive and could be harmful.

- *When the experience is too intense.* In this case, lingering any longer on evocative content is fruitless and will only disorganize the client as it moves beyond the client's window of tolerance. Even if the client would benefit from more awareness related to the issue at hand, pushing at that moment is not helpful and would likely be harmful. The process should be aborted and can be reengaged some other time.

- *When time is of the essence* and more meaning about one's current feeling will not help. Consider, for instance, that the client is called to immediate external action (e.g., an emergency, a competitive performance, writing an exam) or needs to focus on a task. In these circumstances, bringing attention to awareness may take attentional resources away from the task at hand.

- *When clients are better served by an incompatible process.* Awareness from a first-person perspective will undermine or derail other kinds of emotional processing such as reframing one's experience, formulating goals, or reflecting on their purpose in life.

Mechanisms of Change Related to Emotional Awareness

There are four pathways by which engagement, emotional awareness, and symbolizing one's emerging experience facilitates therapeutic change (discussed in Chapters 5–7).

- Engagement opens a new source of information.

- Labeling emotion turns it into a point of reference, which can either regulate or focus it.

- Deepening the experience of emotional awareness enriches its meaning.

- Symbolizing emotion changes the feeling and generates a new sense of direction.

EXPRESSIVE AROUSAL

Emotional arousal is the bodily and psychological experience of an emotion state being activated and heightened. Relatedly, *emotional expression* is when one externalizes that emotion in verbal and nonverbal forms to vividly portray the affective tone associated with one's internal experience. I have introduced the term *expressive arousal,* which involves some overt action or enactment that captures a lived moment of feeling and supports some emotional trajectory. There are markers for when it is most useful (or not) for a therapist to encourage the arousal, expression, and enactment of emotion. These markers are related to the kinds of emotion being experienced as well as clinical observations about what is happening (Chapter 8).

When to Promote Expressive Arousal

Generally, when emotion is flat and not active enough to inform the meaning of one's experience, then increasing arousal and promoting expression will likely be helpful. This may be done just to get a process started, for example, when initiating enactments or an experiential exploration. Sometimes doing this requires interpersonal or contextual support so an individual can feel comfortable enough to express their covert feelings. There is evidence for at least 16 scenarios that signal promoting expressive arousal will be helpful. These markers include emergent emotional states, clinical observations made during the session, and an individual's personal characteristics.

Emotion Markers
Several kinds of emotions signal that expressive arousal is indicated as a change process:

- *Complex or vague emotional distress.* When clients have unclear feelings, then promoting expressive arousal fosters emotional exploration through the physicality of engagement. This use of expressive arousal creates momentum in a discovery-oriented process. As emotion comes to be expressed, what emerges could turn out to be secondary symptomatic, primary maladaptive, or primary adaptive emotion. (If the emotion turns out to be secondary or instrumental, optimal processing would then shift to some other way of working with the emotion.)

- *Primary adaptive emotion* will always be the most important target for expressive arousal. The objective in doing this is to facilitate adaptive action tendencies, elaborate embodied meaning, and complete the emotional experience, whether through a lived or imaginary experience. When people begin to express primary adaptive emotion, it should be engaged and fully expressed in all its facets and meanings. Doing this, the client will organize in some new and healthy way, and at the conclusion of that experience, arousal will subside.

- *Primary maladaptive emotion* can also be modestly aroused and expressed as a way to foster awareness of unmet needs. When people are stuck in the same old story of maladaptive emotion, they will often eventually collapse back into secondary symptomatic emotion. Neither of these kinds of emotion allow for the completion of an emotional experience through enacting their action tendencies—which are to withdraw or collapse. However, primary maladaptive emotion embodies an essential meaning related to the pain of one's unmet need. A moderate amount of expressive arousal when someone is in a state of maladaptive emotion will help focus them on what is most painful and what the emotion is calling for to feel better. Using expressive arousal to extract that meaning from maladaptive emotion will reorient the client, and it often sows the seeds of forthcoming adaptive emotion. However, the expressive arousal of maladaptive emotion should be limited in time and circumscribed in scope.

Moment-by-Moment Markers

Clinical observations within the session may serve as indicators for promoting expressive arousal. These indicators could be the client

- feeling stuck, blocked, numb, or distant;

- having a lack of agency or a poor sense of direction or needs;

- acknowledging their own self-interruption or suppressed emotion;

- feeling that their emotion is forbidden;

- displaying ambivalence about emotion and difficulty activating it; or

- wanting to engage and feel more.

Client Characteristics

Clients who rarely express their feelings benefit more from interventions that encourage expressive arousal as compared with clients who are typically highly expressive. There are several specific observations about the client or their processing style that suggest expressive arousal could be useful:

- *Clients who do not yet feel understood by their therapist* could benefit from expressive arousal.

- *Clients in treatment* for depression, certain anxiety disorders (i.e., social anxiety or generalized anxiety disorder), eating disorders, complex relational trauma, and somatization, as well as those with personality disorders typified by anxiety and avoidance (i.e., Cluster C) will often benefit from complex enactments.

- *Somatic symptoms of client mental health distress* can be effectively worked with using expressive arousal and enactments. This kind of processing is more suitable for body-based symptoms rather than thought-based symptoms, which are mainly cognitive or verbal in nature.

- *Loss of a previous level of functioning* is a problem that calls for the arousal and expression of grief. Examples of this health concern may not initially present for psychotherapy but include reproductive losses (e.g., miscarriage, termination of pregnancy), certain neurological problems (e.g., loss of speech), physical illness (e.g., recent amputees, when someone starts going for dialysis), or after someone has their first episode of acute psychosis.

- *Negative symptoms of psychoticism* have been suggested as indicators for working on expressive arousal.

- *People higher in alexithymia* and anyone who has general difficulty with the verbal elaboration of emotion will benefit from using expressive arousal and enactments. Some evidence suggests that men (as compared with women) will also benefit more from this process than from more verbally mediated explorations of emotion.

- *The mechanism may depend on cognitive style.* Some individuals' emotion is more influenced by the structuring of their physical expressiveness (peripheral theory of emotion), which is often accompanied by a cognitive style that characteristically uses an internal frame of reference. In contrast, other people are more influenced by situational context and social cues (attributional hypothesis), which is believed to be linked to a cognitive style that uses an external frame of reference.

When in Treatment: Phase-Based Markers

In the early phase of treatment, expressive arousal is helpful to boost the initial engagement and awareness of emotion, whether the emotion be secondary, primary maladaptive, or primary adaptive. Across treatment approaches, there is some convergence on the observation that when using enactments, these interventions are best introduced as soon as the therapeutic relationship will allow, which is typically by the fourth session if not earlier. Expressive arousal is a process that is most important during the middle or working phase of treatment, which is when clients struggle with conflicting primary emotions—wrestling between adaptive and maladaptive self-organizations.

As one enters the later phase of treatment, the main target of expressive arousal should be primary adaptive emotion. Finally, the function of promoting expressive arousal seems to shift over the course of treatment. Early on in treatment, expressive arousal is often a means for promoting emotional awareness and exploration. However, in the latter half of treatment, aroused emotional expression likely comes to be more about affirming one's self-identity.

When Not to Use Expressive Arousal

There are certain kinds of emotion as well as certain scenarios with respect to clinical process that should never be facilitated through expressive arousal:

- *Instrumental emotions* are motivated (often unconsciously) by the social impact they tend to have. Encouraging the expression of these emotional maneuvers (or manipulations) is not helpful in working with emotion and may exacerbate unhealthy emotional and social patterns.

- *When emotion (of any kind) is too intense*, it should never be worked with using expressive arousal because that can exacerbate distress and raise the level of clinical risk. This is especially the case when exploring the meaning of primary maladaptive or secondary symptomatic emotions and those emotions are already highly aroused.

- *The individual feels overwhelmed.* Related to the intensity marker, this process should not be used when a person may be too aroused to function well, when they are cognitively overloaded, or when they are showing signs of dissociation.

- *If the individual is unwilling* to enter intense experiences and the exploration of their feelings, then more expressive arousal is inappropriate and may be harmful (e.g., retraumatizing). This is because a key aspect of the process is that the individual is willing and feels that being involved in the process is their own choice.

- *The individual is already engaged in a meaningful narrative reflection.* Conceptualizing the larger meaning of an emotional experience and integrating it into a story is a different process that works best at lower arousal levels. High arousal can derail that process, so it is best not to disturb a client's efforts at making meaning in this way unless the treatment plan specifically calls for that.

With respect to timing of interventions, heightening arousal in the last 10–15 minutes of a session—particularly when one is uncertain about the client's ability to manage high distress, when the client does not have a reliable social support network, or when the client has no immediate plans for after the therapy session—is contraindicated. Doing so would create a situation where risks cannot be adequately managed. Similarly, heightening expressive arousal in the final session(s) of therapy is not necessarily contraindicated, but it should only be done judiciously and strategically.

Mechanisms of Change Related to Expressive Arousal

There are five pathways by which arousal, expression, and enactment facilitate therapeutic change (discussed in Chapters 9–11).

- Arousal is a form of genetic impetus (particularly for high arousal emotions such as anger, fear, or romantic attraction, but it is less effective in this way for low arousal emotions such as grief).

- Physical expression can generate experience.

- Arousal increases awareness.

- Enactment creates commitment to meaning.

- Active expression affirms the self.

SEQUENTIAL TRANSFORMATION OF EMOTION

When working with emotion, a *sequential transformation* is an ordered pattern of discrete emotional states where the meanings and action tendencies of the first emotion are modified through the subsequent experience of a second and often opposing emotion. This change process helps generate new experiences that are not reducible to either of the contributing feelings on their own, which increases one's emotional repertoire (i.e., range). Several such sequences can also be chained together. Relatedly, *emotional flexibility* refers to someone's capacity to both experience and make use of a range of discrete emotional states by shifting fluidly between them to resolve personal concerns. Markers for the transformation of emotion include both specific kinds of emotions as well as clinical observations (discussed in Chapter 12).

When to Promote the Sequential Transformation of Emotion

There are at least seven process moments that indicate promoting a sequential transformation is called for. These markers include either emergent emotion or clinical observations during the moment-by-moment process.

Emotion Markers

This process is for working with primary maladaptive emotions of fear, shame, guilt, or irreconcilable loneliness. When these emotions are maladaptive, they contribute to a sense of being incompetent, bad, or unlovable. There is convergent evidence supporting several specific sequences of productive transformation:

- *Antidotes to maladaptive shame and sadness* include the subsequent experience of assertive anger, pride, and self-compassion as primary adaptive emotions.

- *Antidotes to maladaptive fear* include the subsequent experience of self-compassion, curiosity, or, when possible, courageous assertion as primary adaptive emotions.

- *Antidotes to problematic anger* include the subsequent experience of primary adaptive sadness and grief. Feelings of anger can also be countered by love, compassion, sympathy for others, and forgiveness. Furthermore, these positive emotions may be used preemptively as a sort of inoculation against potentially angering events that may follow.

Moment-by-Moment Markers

Clinical observations about the client indicating a sequential transformation are useful when the client expresses

- negative self-treatment (e.g., harsh self-criticism, self-blame),

- a lack of integration of the self (e.g., feeling torn, indecisive, disempowered),

- feeling haunted by unresolved interpersonal problems, or

- feeling stuck and with little direction or personal agency.

When in Treatment: Phase-Based Markers

Maladaptive emotion typically emerges after exploring presenting concerns. This means that opportunities for sequential transformation often arise in the middle or working phase of treatment, when clients deeply explore their core issues. Sequential transformations are most indicated when emotion is active, specifically when clients feel primary maladaptive emotion. Once maladaptive emotion becomes highly activated, there are a limited number of ways for working with it. When a person is highly distressed, cognitive strategies often fail, while sequential transformations become increasingly more feasible. (The only other option at such a point is to down-regulate emotion by disengaging from it and trying again later.)

When Not to Use Sequential Transformations

Primary maladaptive emotion often underlies chronic symptom distress, but sequential transformations cannot be applied directly to symptomatic distress because undifferentiated distress does not (yet) afford deeper meaning. Additionally, sequential transformations involve increasing arousal as one shifts between emotional states. That makes this process unsuitable for clients when they are struggling to manage high emotional intensity.

- *Secondary emotions* (e.g., anxiety, global distress) are not useful sources of deeper meaning and are not core. Therefore, attempting to transform these feelings will be a superficial process that does not address the deeper concern.

- *When the client is dysregulated and overwhelmed*, then the sequential transformation of emotion should not be promoted, even if the presenting state is maladaptive emotion.

- *When the client is already engaged in a new and meaningful reflection* about their context or how core issues relate to their social and personal history, then a sequential transformation should not be facilitated. Productive narrative reflection is a distinct process that requires some psychological distance, and it is compromised by high arousal, making it incompatible with a sequential transformation in the same instant.

Mechanisms of Change Related to Sequential Transformations

There are five pathways by which sequences of emotion facilitate therapeutic change (discussed in Chapters 13 and 14):

- One emotion can serve as the antidote to another (e.g., positive, activating, or adaptive emotions have an undoing effect on negative, inhibitory, or maladaptive emotions).

- Coactivation of emotions creates higher order schemes for integrating meaning and feeling.

- New emotion developmentally expands one's emotional repertoire.

- Emotional flexibility creates more dynamic responding.

- Existential needs drive the direction of transformations.

REFLECTION ON EMOTION AND THE NARRATIVE CONTEXT

I have introduced the term *narrative reflection* to capture several interrelated processes for reworking one's frame of understanding, which could also be done at varying scopes of analysis. *Narrative elaboration* is a process of developing and adding details to either the story or the contextual circumstances that surround some experience. *Decentering* is defined as stepping outside the framework of one's immediate experience to consider broader or alternative perspectives. *Narrative identity* is the formulation of a story about oneself as a protagonist, which extends from one's personal past to the present and into one's anticipated future. Finally, *purpose and meaning in life* are existential processes that refer to a higher order framework of understanding, offering an overarching perspective on the significance of one's present experience. There are both emotion and clinical markers to indicate when clients will most benefit from more narrative reflection on their emotional experience (introduced in Chapter 17).

When to Promote Narrative Reflection

Whenever an individual could gain from a new perspective on their emotional life, taking a step back and reflecting on the narrative framework of that experience will help. Research supports at least 24 specific scenarios in which promoting narrative reflection is likely of benefit. The markers are emergent emotional states or within-session clinical observations, or may be indicated more generally by client characteristics. Because of the very different ways narrative reflection may be deployed (e.g., straight psychological elaboration vs. decentering and reflecting on the story itself), the specific processes may vary in effectiveness across subgroups of clients. Therefore, not all forms of narrative reflection are indicated based on a single marker.

Emotion Markers

There are a large number of markers for this process, which corresponds to the multiple ways one can work with storytelling, autobiographical memories, and decentering. All of these markers are moments of emotion that call one to take a third-person perspective on the presenting experience.

- *After the experience of primary adaptive emotion*, promoting narrative elaboration can help consolidate changes by incorporating them into the story of one's life and who one is.

- *When maladaptive emotion is being formulated in terms of patterns or themes,* shifting into a deliberate reflection on narrative will be helpful. Once unhealthy experiences have become entrenched in a rigid lifestyle or interpersonal theme, they frequently eclipse the current reality, making it difficult for individuals to recognize the disconnect between their frame of narrative reference (e.g., assumptions, expectations, overall understanding) and their actual circumstances. If this is the case, decentering from the situation or one's self-concept can help create space for new perspectives and experiences.

- *Secondary symptomatic emotions* (e.g., feelings of anxiety, depressive feelings of hopelessness or helplessness, reactive anger) may be temporarily managed or attenuated through cognitive reframing. The purpose of reframing secondary emotions is to provide a rationale for subsequently engaging behaviorally with experiences that are emotionally uncomfortable.

- *Instrumental emotions* are key targets for reflecting on emotion because understanding their role in social influence and one's impact on others is a prerequisite to modifying such feelings.

- *Problematic anger and hate* are critical examples of secondary emotional reactions and instrumental emotion, which need to be managed by de-escalation and taking psychological distance to consider the broader context. Decentering through mindfulness has proven to be useful for managing anger. Then, reflecting on the larger context involves examining one's social impact as well as personal values or goals.

- *Chronic hardship or physical pain* can be coped with to some degree through decentering and becoming mindful of one's larger purpose in life. This offers the individual some relief in an ongoing struggle while maintaining a sense of direction.

- *Unhealthy emotion regulation strategies* are another set of emotion-related indicators for decentering and then reflecting on one's broader life narrative. Examples of this include
  - substance or psychological addictions,
  - self-injury,
  - sex addiction–related behaviors (e.g., pornography use), and
  - procrastination.

These short-term strategies often have strongly implicit functions for down-regulating or managing emotional distress, which typically is unrelated at first. Decentering to mindfully attend to urges in the moment is a useful coping process. Further, reflecting on the underlying function of these automatic and often biological processes is another process of narrative formulation that helps people make different choices.

Moment-by-Moment Markers

Clinical observations within the session are another type of indicator for when decentering and narrative reflections about emotion are useful.

- *When a client is mystified by their symptoms* or their lack of clarity about the problem, those are key markers for reflecting on emotion. Developing a narrative understanding of the relevant emotional problems is a priority. Insight into one's overarching problem (i.e., problem clarification) takes a narrative form and is an important prognostic indicator.

- *Unstoried emotion* is when clients report or express emotion that lacks sufficient context and is often missing relevant pieces of the story's plot and characters. This is a marker that the circumstances surrounding emotion need to be elaborated.

- *Problematic reaction points and dreams* often signal the need to connect these preverbal and often visceral emotional experiences to the bigger picture about one's circumstances or sense of self.

- *Overgeneralized autobiographical memories or superficial stories* are vague and lack detail, which calls for psychological elaboration to increase one's narrative specificity.

- *When the client refuses exposure-based or enactment-based interventions*, emotional engagement through narrative specificity and psychological elaboration can be a more palatable alternative than interventions that feel too intense, evocative, or confrontational.

- *When personal narratives are socially undesirable, self-incriminating, or condemning* (e.g., as in a forensic setting), then exploring those experiences from the perspective of a third-person observer can offer an easier point of entry for building an alliance and working with emotional content.

Client Characteristics

People of all ages, from children to older adults, benefit from telling and exploring personally significant stories. However, the intersection of client's characteristics and individual processing style suggests certain kinds of narrative reflection are most relevant.

- Narrative elaboration
    - *For older adults suffering from depression, chronic physical disease, or early dementia,* the reminiscence of life events may be particularly useful.

- *For women, memory specificity seems to be more prominent than for men,* suggesting sex or gender may mediate the effect of psychological elaboration on emotional change.

• Positive meaning

- *In the treatment of depression, anxiety, and perhaps schizophrenia,* the elaboration of positive emotional experiences seems to be especially useful.

- *When a person's identity is threatened,* positive self-affirmation helps draw on a broader personal context and prompt their readiness to engage adverse circumstances. This process seems to have a greater impact on children and adolescents who are socially or economically disadvantaged compared with those with more resources.

• Decentering

- *Clients who characteristically externalize under stress* (i.e., they avoid, act out, or blame the environment) benefit most from treatments that encourage them to think about their symptoms more objectively (e.g., decentering and then choosing alternatives).

- *People who suffer more severe or entrenched interpersonal difficulties* (e.g., have poor quality object relations) benefit more from reflecting on the thematic nature of their interpersonal experiences as compared with those who have healthier relationship histories.

- *Self-selection impacts the effectiveness of mindfulness.* Mindfulness training fosters a capacity for decentering. However, personal attributes shape adoption and adherence to this disciplined practice.

• Life meaning and purpose

- *When people are undergoing life transitions,* having a sense of purpose and higher meaning helps them navigate immediate emotional difficulties. Relatedly, when people are confronted with chronic physical illness or end-of-life issues, they report that it is especially valuable to explore meaning in life and purpose.

When in Treatment: Phase-Based Markers

In the early phase of therapy, narrative reflection is especially important because it lays the initial foundation for understanding existing and forthcoming emotions (e.g., the story of what someone thinks their problems and challenges are). This initial narrative sets the stage for a shared framework that will be collaboratively explored while the relationship between client and therapist is first established. It is also the point of departure for an initial case formulation. When the risk of social undesirability or being too evocative is a pressing concern, processing from a distanced perspective helps broach emotional content without eliciting too much vulnerability. Top-down cognitive strategies or dynamic formulations are most effective when a client recognizes that some aspect of their life is not working and expresses the desire to improve their life.

The middle or working phase of therapy will be punctuated by various ways of working with emotion, such as practicing skills for down-regulation, enhancing emotional awareness to clarify unmet needs, sequential transformations to address maladaptive emotion, and expressive arousal to activate primary adaptive emotion. Throughout that work, however, periodic shifts into narrative reflection will help integrate these distinct kinds of insights into the formulation of a new or revised story. Whenever a new bout of emotional work is completed, narrative reflections update and adjust the sociohistorical context. This reshapes one's understanding of the past and interpretations of the future. Fostering either third-person or first-person perspectives should be related to an evolving case formulation that considers a client's default perspective, time already spent in each perspective, and the amount of structure or directiveness that a client needs.

Narrative reflection is also critical later in treatment and in the termination phase. Reflecting on emotion from a third-person perspective helps clients create psychological distance, facilitating closure. Because reflecting on life narratives pulls for increased coherence, this process is often beneficial in the later stages of treatment, but only after people have already made headway in working through difficulties such as self-doubt and self-criticism. Facilitating reflection at the end of therapy enables clients to take stock of their progress, celebrate their accomplishments, and clarify what remains to be resolved. Crafting a coherent narrative is important for consolidating treatment gains as well as formulating new goals. Finally, increasing one's capacity for decentering and metacognition seems to guard against future depressive relapses.

When Not to Use Narrative Reflection

Certain moments should not involve facilitating a narrative reflection on emotion:

- *When clients are under acute physical or emotional stress,* it undermines the flexibility with which they might otherwise engage top-down cognitive strategies. This means that calls to think rationally are unpromising in the face of high distress.

- *Secondary symptomatic emotions* are contraindicated as the targets for developing elaborate narratives, and doing so often resembles unhealthy rumination and brooding.

- *An empty story* is a highly external narrative about the plot and characters of an event that is missing details about emotions and motives. This marker contraindicates further narrative elaboration of contextual circumstances because it would reinforce the external focus, typically at the expense of emotional awareness and expression—which are needed to enrich the meaning of an experience.

- *When attempting to increase emotional engagement,* decentering can undermine the intended process and work at cross-purposes. Decentering during exposure-based interventions, for example, will facilitate psychological avoidance rather than emotional engagement.

- When clients are *actively expanding emotional awareness* (e.g., symbolizing the concrete experience of a presenting emotion), that first-person process will often be derailed by a more abstract level of reflection or a third-person perspective.

Client characteristics can also signal that one should be judicious in facilitating this process.

- *For people very high in alexithymia,* it is uncertain whether promoting reflection on emotion is more beneficial than developing emotional awareness. Some evidence suggests they may struggle with abstract, psychodynamic reflections about emotion because they lack the basic emotional awareness necessary for such reflections to be meaningful.

- *When their construal of life events is self-disparaging and excessively self-focused* (e.g., ruminative depression, social anxiety, intellectualization), then having clients reflect on the causal factors related to their personal difficulties may be harmful. A client's tendency to self-blame can also undermine the effectiveness of treatments that typically encourage one to reflect on symptoms more rationally or objectively.

- *Prematurely seeking narrative coherence when people suffer maladaptive emotion* (e.g., shame, guilt, loneliness) will risk driving them toward conclusions that are self-condemning. This is because when people are forced to choose between the centrality of an autobiographical narrative that either offers self-verification or offers self-enhancement, they often choose self-verification, even if it disparages the self.

- *Dissociative identity disorder* entails the narrative of a fragmented and discontinuous identity. Although more research is needed, narrative elaborations about each self-part's story may inadvertently foster the reification and further segregation between parts of the self.

Mechanisms of Change Related to Narrative Reflection

The broad scope of these mechanisms involves additional, detailed change processes in mental functioning. These are not intervention processes per se, but fundamental mental operations influencing change. Examples include seeking closure, a drive for integration, coherence, and task or narrative completion. Narrative perspective also plays a role, affecting mental focus (e.g., subjective experience vs. narrative coherence).

Returning to the level of clinical or personal work, there are five pathways by which contextual elaboration, telling one's story, reframing, and reflection on meaning can facilitate therapeutic change (discussed in Chapters 18, 20, 22, and 23):

- Psychological elaboration gives one more to feel about (including increased specificity, positive meaning making, and emotion–narrative elaboration).

- Positive meaning making and self-affirmation prompts an internal readiness to respond adaptively to threat.

- The story itself can drive change by offering an interpretive framework, which then shapes the direction of one's emotional growth.

- Decentering from one's frame of reference gives new perspective and existential insights.

- Reinventing the self opens new avenues for feeling and motivation.

FUTURE DIRECTIONS FOR RESEARCH AND THEORY

The study of emotional change, particularly from a clinical perspective, has almost invariably examined process through the lens of specific treatment interventions. This has yielded an array of different frameworks for understanding emotion change, each one tied to a particular treatment perspective. The problem is that principles of emotion change, as discussed here, do not originate from any given treatment perspective; rather, they spring from the organism itself.

The Puzzle of Studying Emotion Change: A New Paradigm

Most often, interventions have been designed based on some clinical intuition and pragmatism. This characterizes the strategy of early traditions of psychodynamic, behavioral, cognitive, and humanistic–experiential treatments. Treatment interventions have been largely shaped by the practical experience of clinicians and what seemed to work in helping clients. While the science of emotion change now uses these intervention perspectives to study change, the frameworks themselves were developed without a deep understanding of how individuals functionally process emotion and its meaning. To better study emotional change, we need to consider process from an organismic perspective rather than through specific intervention perspectives. Essentially, to better understand treatment interventions, we need to reinterpret them through the eyes of the person undergoing change (J. Pascual-Leone et al., 2015). Research should focus on how the organism, as a functional whole, generates change.

Alternative Formulations and Multiple Interactions

Emotional processing occurs in multiple ways, but the different ways of working with emotion are sometimes incompatible with one another (A. Pascual-Leone & Kramer, 2024). When distinct processes occur simultaneously, they often operate synergistically. However, at other times, distinct processes can conflict within a given moment and then they work at cross-purposes. A comprehensive understanding of emotion change requires considering the many mechanisms that overdetermine it, unfolding either simultaneously or ordered in time.

Each of the five forms of emotional processing facilitates change through multiple pathways, with several submechanisms for each. These pathways represent functional descriptions of general process trajectories for working with emotion (e.g., awareness, expression, narrative reflection). The exact number of pathways is debatable, as some overlap, many blend into one another, and most (but not all) occur synergistically.

My goal in identifying emotional processes and the mechanisms by which they promote change is rooted in clinical utility: Therapists (and clients) need precise intentions for the kind of processing they aim to leverage. When mechanisms are described too broadly (as treatment theories are prone to do) or with more specificity than practice will allow (as research sometimes does), the usefulness for therapists gets lost. My contribution has been to translate available research and theory into a manageable number of principles—balancing comprehensiveness and applicability—to optimize the implications for practice. I hope the theoretical developments in this book will help therapists focus their interventions more effectively, leading to increasingly precise and targeted interventions.

Deeper Causal Mechanisms

The causal descriptions of change I present should eventually be further explained using a model of cognitive–affective development. This would entail describing individual psychological units and the organismic principles by which those units interact. Emotions and their meanings can already be understood as schemes: neurologically represented networks that are cofunctional and coactivated. However, clinical theory still needs to develop a clearer understanding of mental functioning, integrating that with progress made in cognitive science (e.g., J. Pascual-Leone & Johnson, 2021).

WHAT IS THE FUTURE OF PSYCHOTHERAPY?

The future of psychotherapy hinges on process research, a perspective long championed by pioneers (e.g., Elliott, 2010; L. S. Greenberg & Safran, 1987) and reinforced by more recent calls for process-based therapy (Hoffman & Hayes, 2019). Research shows that well-grounded approaches to treatment have large effect sizes in their impact on health, whereas the differences between treatments are often minimal. Client factors like individual differences, motivation, and the intended use of a given process far outweigh the impact of either therapist or treatment factors. While proprietary treatment branding has some rationale, it too often becomes an impediment to science and innovation. The implication for science and practice is thus: "Debates that concern principles of change, rather than specific trademarked therapies, will return our attention to what psychology is about" (Rosen & Davidson, 2003, p. 308).

Therapists use interventions from various treatment approaches because they believe the techniques will facilitate one or another process. However, even if all therapies are effective, integrative therapists know that one cannot deliver treatment in the abstract—specific treatment strategies still need to be selected and used. Adding to the complexity, while therapists may intend to facilitate a certain process, it is often less clear whether interventions work only as the corresponding theory suggests. So, unexpectedly, process research has become the integrative forum. Irrespective of treatment, it is ultimately the client who chooses which process to engage at a given moment. The most useful process research is about what clients do when they improve rather than what therapists were hoping clients might do.

In the end, it is not a specific therapy that drives client change but rather key processes. As process research articulates the various ways clients change, the differences between treatment theories will dissolve and become less important. Cutting across treatment approaches, this book has presented a theory with five general principles of emotion change. Research should aim to better identify and clarify those processes. In doing so, process research will emerge as a unifying substrate for treatment perspectives. In the future, psychotherapy will increasingly shift to facilitating specific processes rather than delivering prescribed therapies. In this way, identifying and developing interventions to best facilitate a given process is the new frontier of inquiry.

REFERENCES

Abbass, A. A., Nowoweiski, S. J., Bernier, D., Tarzwell, R., & Beutel, M. E. (2014). Review of psychodynamic psychotherapy neuroimaging studies. *Psychotherapy and Psychosomatics, 83*(3), 142–147. https://doi.org/10.1159/000358841

Abbass, A. A., & Town, J. M. (2013). Key clinical processes in intensive short-term dynamic psychotherapy. *Psychotherapy: Theory, Research, & Practice, 50*(3), 433–437. https://doi.org/10.1037/a0032166

Abbass, A., Town, J., & Driessen, E. (2012). Intensive short-term dynamic psychotherapy: A systematic review and meta-analysis of outcome research. *Harvard Review of Psychiatry, 20*(2), 97–108. https://doi.org/10.3109/10673229.2012.677347

Abbass, A., Town, J., Ogrodniczuk, J., Joffres, M., & Lilliengren, P. (2017). Intensive short-term dynamic psychotherapy trial therapy: Effectiveness and role of "unlocking the unconscious." *Journal of Nervous and Mental Disease, 205*(6), 453–457. https://doi.org/10.1097/NMD.0000000000000684

Adams, K. E. (2010). *Therapist influence on depressed clients' therapeutic experiencing and outcome* [Unpublished doctoral dissertation]. York University.

Adler, J. M. (2012). Living into the story: Agency and coherence in a longitudinal study of narrative identity development and mental health over the course of psychotherapy. *Journal of Personality and Social Psychology, 102*(2), 367–389. https://doi.org/10.1037/a0025289

Adler, J. M., Harmeling, L. H., & Walder-Biesanz, I. (2013). Narrative meaning making is associated with sudden gains in psychotherapy clients' mental health under routine clinical conditions. *Journal of Consulting and Clinical Psychology, 81*(5), 839–845. https://doi.org/10.1037/a0033774

Adler, J. M., & Hershfield, H. E. (2012). Mixed emotional experience is associated with and precedes improvements in psychological well-being. *PLOS One, 7*(4), Article e35633. https://doi.org/10.1371/journal.pone.0035633

Adler, J. M., Kissel, E. C., & McAdams, D. P. (2006). Emerging from the CAVE: Attributional style and the narrative study of identity in midlife adults. *Cognitive Therapy and Research, 30*(1), 39–51. https://doi.org/10.1007/s10608-006-9005-1

Adler, J. M., Lodi-Smith, J., Philippe, F. L., & Houle, I. (2016). The incremental validity of narrative identity in predicting well-being: A review of the field and recommendations for the future. *Personality and Social Psychology Review, 20*(2), 142–175. https://doi.org/10.1177/1088868315585068

Adler, J. M., & Poulin, M. J. (2009). The political is personal: Narrating 9/11 and psychological well-being. *Journal of Personality, 77*(4), 903–932. https://doi.org/10.1111/j.1467-6494.2009.00569.x

Adler, J. M., Wagner, J. W., & McAdams, D. P. (2007). Personality and the coherence of psychotherapy narratives. *Journal of Research in Personality, 41*(6), 1179–1198. https://doi.org/10.1016/j.jrp.2007.02.006

Adolphs, R., Gosselin, F., Buchanan, T. W., Tranel, D., Schyns, P., & Damasio, A. R. (2005). A mechanism for impaired fear recognition after amygdala damage. *Nature, 433*(7021), 68–72. https://doi.org/10.1038/nature03086

Adolphs, R., Tranel, D., & Buchanan, T. W. (2005). Amygdala damage impairs emotional memory for gist but not details of complex stimuli. *Nature Neuroscience, 8*(4), 512–518. https://doi.org/10.1038/nn1413

Akbari, M., Hosseini, Z. S., Seydavi, M., Zegel, M., Zvolensky, M. J., & Vujanovic, A. A. (2022). Distress tolerance and posttraumatic stress disorder: A systematic review and meta-analysis. *Cognitive Behaviour Therapy, 51*(1), 42–71. https://doi.org/10.1080/16506073.2021.1942541

Alberini, C. M., & Ledoux, J. E. (2013). Memory reconsolidation. *Current Biology, 23*(17), R746–R750. https://doi.org/10.1016/j.cub.2013.06.046

Aldao, A., Nolen-Hoeksema, S., & Schweizer, S. (2010). Emotion-regulation strategies across psychopathology: A meta-analytic review. *Clinical Psychology Review, 30*(2), 217–237. https://doi.org/10.1016/j.cpr.2009.11.004

Aleixo, A., Pires, A. P., Angus, L., Neto, D., & Vaz, A. (2021). A review of empirical studies investigating narrative, emotion and meaning-making modes and client process markers in psychotherapy. *Journal of Contemporary Psychotherapy, 51*(1), 31–40. https://doi.org/10.1007/s10879-020-09472-6

Alexander, F., & French, T. M. (1946). *Psychoanalytic therapy: Principles and application.* Ronald Press.

Alimujiang, A., Wiensch, A., Boss, J., Fleischer, N. L., Mondul, A. M., McLean, K., Mukherjee, B., & Pearce, C. L. (2019). Association between life purpose and mortality among US adults older than 50 years. *JAMA Network Open, 2*(5), e194270. https://doi.org/10.1001/jamanetworkopen.2019.4270

Alter, A. L., & Oppenheimer, D. M. (2008). Effects of fluency on psychological distance and mental construal (or why New York is a large city, but New York is a civilized jungle). *Psychological Science, 19*(2), 161–167. https://doi.org/10.1111/j.1467-9280.2008.02062.x

Andersson, L. G., Butler, M. H., & Seedall, R. B. (2006). Couples' experience of enactments and softening in marital therapy. *The American Journal of Family Therapy, 34*(4), 301–315. https://doi.org/10.1080/01926180600553837

Angus, L. (2012). Toward an integrative understanding of narrative and emotion processes in emotion-focused therapy of depression: Implications for theory, research and practice. *Psychotherapy Research, 22*(4), 367–380. https://doi.org/10.1080/10503307.2012.683988

Angus, L., Boritz, T., Bryntwick, E., Carpender, N., Macaulay, C., & Khattra, J. (2015). *Narrative-emotion process coding system manual: NEPCS version 2.0.* York University.

Angus, L. E., Boritz, T., Bryntwick, E., Carpenter, N., Macaulay, C., & Khattra, J. (2017). The Narrative-Emotion Process Coding System 2.0: A multi-methodological approach to identifying and assessing narrative-emotion process markers in psychotherapy. *Psychotherapy Research, 27*(3), 253–269. https://doi.org/10.1080/10503307.2016.1238525

Angus, L. E., & Greenberg, L. S. (2011). *Working with narrative in emotion-focused therapy: Changing stories, healing lives.* American Psychology Association. https://doi.org/10.1037/12325-000

Angus, L. E., Lewin, J., Bouffard, B., & Rotondi-Trevisan, D. (2004). "What's the story?" working with narrative in experiential psychotherapy. In L. E. Angus & J. McLeod (Eds.), *The handbook of narrative and psychotherapy: Practice, theory, and research* (pp. 86–101). Sage Publications. https://doi.org/10.4135/9781412973496.d8

Angus, L. E., & Rennie, D. L. (1989). Envisioning the representational world: The client's experience of metaphoric expression in psychotherapy. *Psychotherapy: Theory, Research, & Practice, 26*(3), 372–379. https://doi.org/10.1037/h0085448

Aristotle. (1996). *Poetics* (M. Heath, Trans.). Penguin Classics. (Original work published ca. 330 B.C.E.)

Armstrong, C. R., Rozenberg, M., Powell, M. A., Honce, J., Bronstein, L., Gingras, G., & Han, E. (2016). A step toward empirical evidence: Operationalizing and uncovering drama therapy change processes. *The Arts in Psychotherapy, 49*, 27–33. https://doi.org/10.1016/j.aip.2016.05.007

Armstrong, C. R., Tanaka, S., Reoch, L., Bronstein, L., Honce, J., Rozenberg, M., & Powell, M. A. (2015). Emotional arousal in two drama therapy core processes: Dramatic embodiment and dramatic projection. *Drama Therapy Review, 1*(2), 147–160. https://doi.org/10.1386/dtr.1.2.147_1

Arnott, P. (1959). *An introduction to the Greek theatre*. Palgrave Macmillan. https://doi.org/10.1007/978-1-349-00529-1

Austenfeld, J. L., & Stanton, A. L. (2004). Coping through emotional approach: A new look at emotion, coping, and health-related outcomes. *Journal of Personality, 72*(6), 1335–1364. https://doi.org/10.1111/j.1467-6494.2004.00299.x

Auszra, L., Greenberg, L. S., & Herrmann, I. (2013). Client emotional productivity—Optimal client in-session emotional processing in experiential therapy. *Psychotherapy Research, 23*(6), 732–746. https://doi.org/10.1080/10503307.2013.816882

Bagby, R. M., Parker, J. D., & Taylor, G. J. (1994). The twenty-item Toronto Alexithymia Scale–I: Item selection and cross-validation of the factor structure. *Journal of Psychosomatic Research, 38*(1), 23–32. https://doi.org/10.1016/0022-3999(94)90005-1

Bakan, D. (1966). *The duality of human existence: An essay on psychology and religion*. Rand McNally.

Baldwin, J. M. (1891). *Feeling and will: Handbook of psychology*. Henry Holt.

Balfour, M., Westwood, M., & Buchanan, M. J. (2014). Protecting into emotion: Therapeutic enactments with military veterans transitioning back into civilian life. *Research in Drama Education, 19*(2), 165–181. https://doi.org/10.1080/13569783.2014.911806

Ball, T. M., & Gunaydin, L. A. (2022). Measuring maladaptive avoidance: From animal models to clinical anxiety. *Neuropsychopharmacology, 47*(5), 978–986. https://doi.org/10.1038/s41386-021-01263-4

Barlow, D. H., Allen, L. B., & Choate, M. L. (2004). Toward a unified treatment for emotional disorders. *Behavior Therapy, 35*(2), 205–230. https://doi.org/10.1016/S0005-7894(04)80036-4

Barrett, L. F., Robin, L., Pietromonaco, P. R., & Eyssell, K. M. (1998). Are women the "more emotional" sex? Evidence from emotional experiences in social context. *Cognition and Emotion, 12*(4), 555–578. https://doi.org/10.1080/026999398379565

Barry, T. J., Hallford, D. J., Hitchcock, C., Takano, K., & Raes, F. (2021). The current state of memory specificity training (MeST) for emotional disorders. *Current Opinion in Psychology, 41*, 28–33. https://doi.org/10.1016/j.copsyc.2021.02.002

Barry, T. J., Sze, W. Y., & Raes, F. (2019). A meta-analysis and systematic review of memory specificity training (MeST) in the treatment of emotional disorders. *Behaviour Research and Therapy, 116*, 36–51. https://doi.org/10.1016/j.brat.2019.02.001

Bartolic, E. I., Basso, M. R., Schefft, B. K., Glauser, T., & Titanic-Schefft, M. (1999). Effects of experimentally-induced emotional states on frontal lobe cognitive task performance. *Neuropsychologia, 37*, 677–683. https://doi.org/10.1016/S0028-3932(98)00123

Bateman, A., & Fonagy, P. (2013). Mentalization-based treatment. *Psychoanalytic Inquiry, 33*(6), 595–613. https://doi.org/10.1080/07351690.2013.835170

Bauer, J., Rottler, V., & Brodner, J. (2008). Emotional crying: Frequency and effects on mood in a sample of psychosomatic outpatients—Evidence for different types of emotional crying. *Psychotherapie, Psychosomatik, Medizinische Psychologie, 58*(2), S10. https://doi.org/10.1055/s-2008-1061516

Bauer, J. J., & McAdams, D. P. (2010). Eudaimonic growth: Narrative growth goals predict increases in ego development and subjective well-being 3 years later. *Developmental Psychology, 46*(4), 761–772. https://doi.org/10.1037/a0019654

Baumeister, R. F., Vohs, K. D., Aaker, J. L., & Garbinsky, E. N. (2013). Some key differences between a happy life and a meaningful life. *The Journal of Positive Psychology, 8*(6), 505–516. https://doi.org/10.1080/17439760.2013.830764

Bechara A. (2004). The role of emotion in decision-making: Evidence from neurological patients with orbitofrontal damage. *Brain and Cognition, 55*(1), 30–40. https://doi.org/10.1016/j.bandc.2003.04.001

Becht, M. C., & Vingerhoets, A. J. J. M. (2002). Crying and mood change: A cross-cultural study. *Cognition and Emotion, 16*(1), 87–101. https://doi.org/10.1080/02699930143000149

Beck, J. S. (2020). *Cognitive behavior therapy: Basics and beyond* (3rd ed.). Guilford Press.

Beike, D. R., Kleinknecht, E., & Wirth-Beaumont, E. T. (2004). How emotional and nonemotional memories define the self. In D. R. Beike, J. M. Lampinen, & D. A. Behrend (Eds.), *Studies in self and identity: The self and memory* (pp. 141–159). Psychology Press. https://doi.org/10.4324/9780203337974

Beike, D. R., & Wirth-Beaumont, E. T. (2005). Psychological closure as a memory phenomenon. *Memory, 13*(6), 574–593. https://doi.org/10.1080/09658210444000241

Benjamin, L. S. (2000). *INTREX user's manual.* Interpersonal Reconstructive Therapy Institute. (Original work published 1983)

Benoit, R. G., Szpunar, K. K., & Schacter, D. L. (2014). Ventromedial prefrontal cortex supports affective future simulation by integrating distributed knowledge. *Proceedings of the National Academy of Sciences of the United States of America, 111*(46), 16550–16555. https://doi.org/10.1073/pnas.1419274111

Beresnevaite, M. (2000). Exploring the benefits of group psychotherapy in reducing alexithymia in coronary heart disease patients: A preliminary study. *Psychotherapy and Psychosomatics, 69*(3), 117–122. https://doi.org/10.1159/000012378

Berggraf, L., Ulvenes, P. G., Oktedalen, T., Hoffart, A., Stiles, T., McCullough, L., & Wampold, B. E. (2014). Experience of affects predicting sense of self and others in short-term dynamic and cognitive therapy. *Psychotherapy: Theory, Research, & Practice, 51*(2), 246–257. https://doi.org/10.1037/a0036581

Bergomi, C., Tschacher, W., & Kupper, Z. (2013). Measuring mindfulness: First steps towards the development of a comprehensive mindfulness scale. *Mindfulness, 4*(1), 18–32. https://doi.org/10.1007/s12671-012-0102-9

Berkowitz, L. (2000). *Causes and consequences of feelings.* Cambridge University Press. https://doi.org/10.1017/CBO9780511606106

Bernstein, A., Hadash, Y., & Fresco, D. M. (2019). Metacognitive processes model of decentering: Emerging methods and insights. *Current Opinion in Psychology, 28*, 245–251. https://doi.org/10.1016/j.copsyc.2019.01.019

Bernstein, A., Hadash, Y., Lichtash, Y., Tanay, G., Shepherd, K., & Fresco, D. M. (2015). Decentering and related constructs: A critical review and metacognitive processes model. *Perspectives on Psychological Science, 10*(5), 599–617. https://doi.org/10.1177/1745691615594577

Bernstein, A., Marshall, E. C., & Zvolensky, M. J. (2011). Multi-method evaluation of distress tolerance measures and construct(s): Concurrent relations to mood and anxiety psychopathology and quality of life. *Journal of Experimental Psychopathology, 2*(3), 386–399. https://doi.org/10.5127/jep.006610

Berthoud, L., Kramer, U., Caspar, F., & Pascual-Leone, A. (2015). Emotional processing in a ten-session general psychiatric treatment for borderline personality disorder: A case study. *Personality and Mental Health, 9*(1), 73–78. https://doi.org/10.1002/pmh.1287

Berthoud, L., Pascual-Leone, A., Caspar, F., Tissot, H., Keller, S., Rohde, K. B., de Roten, Y., Despland, J.-N., & Kramer, U. (2017). Leaving distress behind: A randomized controlled study on change in emotional processing in borderline personality disorder. *Psychiatry, 80*(2), 139–154. https://doi.org/10.1080/00332747.2016.1220230

Berthoz, S., Artiges, E., Van De Moortele, P. F., Poline, J. B., Rouquette, S., Consoli, S. M., & Martinot, J. L. (2002). Effect of impaired recognition and expression of emotions on frontocingulate cortices: An fMRI study of men with alexithymia. *The American Journal of Psychiatry, 159*(6), 961–967. https://doi.org/10.1176/appi.ajp.159.6.961

Beuchat, H., Grandjean, L., Junod, N., Despland, J.-N., Pascual-Leone, A., Martin-Sölch, C., & Kramer, U. (2024). Evaluation of expressed self-contempt in psychotherapy: An exploratory study. *Counselling Psychology Quarterly, 37*(2), 216–231. https://doi.org/10.1080/09515070.2023.2201417

Beutel, M. E., Scheurich, V., Knebel, A., Michal, M., Wiltink, J., Graf-Morgenstern, M., Tschan, R., Milrod, B., Wellek, S., & Subic-Wrana, C. (2013). Implementing panic-focused psychodynamic psychotherapy into clinical practice. *Canadian Journal of Psychiatry, 58*(6), 326–334. https://doi.org/10.1177/070674371305800604

Beutel, M. E., Weißflog, G., Leuteritz, K., Wiltink, J., Haselbacher, A., Ruckes, C., Kuhnt, S., Barthel, Y., Imruck, B. H., Zwerenz, R., & Brähler, E. (2014). Efficacy of short-term psychodynamic psychotherapy (STPP) with depressed breast cancer patients: Results of a randomized controlled multicenter trial. *Annals of Oncology, 25*(2), 378–384. https://doi.org/10.1093/annonc/mdt526

Beutler, L. E., Engle, D., Mohr, D., Daldrup, R. J., Bergan, J., Meredith, K., & Merry, W. (1991). Predictors of differential response to cognitive, experiential, and self-directed psychotherapeutic procedures. *Journal of Consulting and Clinical Psychology, 59*(2), 333–340. https://doi.org/10.1037/0022-006X.59.2.333

Beutler, L. E., Kimpara, S., Edwards, C. J., & Miller, K. D. (2018). Fitting psychotherapy to patient coping style: A meta-analysis. *Journal of Clinical Psychology, 74*(11), 1980–1995. https://doi.org/10.1002/jclp.22684

Bhagat, R. S., Segovis, J., & Nelson, T. (2012). *Work stress and coping in the era of globalization.* Routledge.

Bhatia, M., Rodriguez, M. G., Fowler, D. M., Godin, J. E., Drapeau, M., & McCullough, L. (2009). Desensitization of conflicted feelings: Using the ATOS to measure early change in a single case affect phobia therapy treatment. *Archives of Psychiatry and Psychotherapy, 11*, 31–38.

Bird, A., & Reese, E. (2006). Emotional reminiscing and the development of an autobiographical self. *Developmental Psychology, 42*(4), 613–626. https://doi.org/10.1037/0012-1649.42.4.613

Bjureberg, J., Ojala, O., Berg, A., Edvardsson, E., Kolbeinsson, Ö., Molander, O., Morin, E., Nordgren, L., Palme, K., Särnholm, J., Wedin, L., Rück, C., Gross, J. J., & Hesser, H. (2023). Targeting maladaptive anger with brief therapist-supported internet-delivered emotion regulation treatments: A randomized controlled trial. *Journal of Consulting and Clinical Psychology, 91*(5), 254–266. https://doi.org/10.1037/ccp0000769

Blackie, L. E. R., Colgan, J. E. V., McDonald, S., & McLean, K. C. (2020). A qualitative investigation into the cultural master narrative for overcoming trauma and adversity in the United Kingdom. *Qualitative Psychology, 10*(1), 154–170. https://doi.org/10.1037/qup0000163

Blatner, A. (2000). *Foundations of psychodrama: History, theory, and practice* (4th ed.). Springer.

Boals, A., & Schuettler, D. (2011). A double-edged sword: Event centrality, PTSD and posttraumatic growth. *Applied Cognitive Psychology, 25*(5), 817–822. https://doi.org/10.1002/acp.1753

Bohanek, J. G., Marin, K. A., & Fivush, R. (2008). Family narratives, self, and gender in early adolescence. *The Journal of Early Adolescence, 28*(1), 153–176. https://doi.org/10.1177/0272431607308673

Bohart, A. C. (1977). Role playing and interpersonal-conflict reduction. *Journal of Counseling Psychology, 24*, 15–24.

Bohart, A. C. (1980). Toward a cognitive theory of catharsis. *Psychotherapy: Theory, Research, & Practice, 17*(2), 192–201. https://doi.org/10.1037/h0085911

Bonanno, G. A. (2004). Loss, trauma, and human resilience: Have we underestimated the human capacity to thrive after extremely aversive events? *American Psychologist, 59*(1), 20–28. https://doi.org/10.1037/0003-066X.59.1.20

Bonanno, G. A. (2010). *The other side of sadness: What the new science of bereavement tells us about life after a loss.* Basic Books.

Boritz, T., Barnhart, R., Angus, L., & Constantino, M. J. (2017). Narrative flexibility in brief psychotherapy for depression. *Psychotherapy Research, 27*(6), 666–676. https://doi.org/10.1080/10503307.2016.1152410

Boritz, T. Z., Angus, L., Monette, G., & Hollis-Walker, L. (2008). An empirical analysis of autobiographical memory specificity subtypes in brief emotion-focused and client-centered treatments of depression. *Psychotherapy Research, 18*(5), 584–593. https://doi.org/10.1080/10503300802123245

Boritz, T. Z., Angus, L., Monette, G., Hollis-Walker, L., & Warwar, S. (2011). Narrative and emotion integration in psychotherapy: Investigating the relationship between autobiographical memory specificity and expressed emotional arousal in brief emotion-focused and client-centred treatments of depression. *Psychotherapy Research, 21*(1), 16–26. https://doi.org/10.1080/10503307.2010.504240

Boritz, T. Z., Bryntwick, E., Angus, L., Greenberg, L. S., & Constantino, M. J. (2014). Narrative and emotion process in psychotherapy: An empirical test of the Narrative-Emotion Process Coding System (NEPCS). *Psychotherapy Research, 24*(5), 594–607. https://doi.org/10.1080/10503307.2013.851426

Borkovec, T. D., Alcaine, O., & Behar, E. (2004). Avoidance theory of worry and generalized anxiety disorder. In R. G. Heimberg, C. L. Turk, & D. S. Mennin (Eds.), *Generalized anxiety disorder: Advances in research and practice* (pp. 77–108). Guilford Press.

Borkovec, T. D., & Sides, J. K. (1979). The contribution of relaxation and expectancy to fear reduction via graded, imaginal exposure to feared stimuli. *Behaviour Research and Therapy, 17*(6), 529–540. https://doi.org/10.1016/0005-7967(79)90096-2

Bornemann, B., & Singer, T. (2017). Taking time to feel our body: Steady increases in heartbeat perception accuracy and decreases in alexithymia over 9 months of contemplative mental training. *Psychophysiology, 54*(3), 469–482. https://doi.org/10.1111/psyp.12790

Bornovalova, M. A., Gratz, K. L., Daughters, S. B., Hunt, E. D., & Lejuez, C. W. (2012). Initial RCT of a distress tolerance treatment for individuals with substance use disorders. *Drug and Alcohol Dependence, 122*(1-2), 70–76. https://doi.org/10.1016/j.drugalcdep.2011.09.012

Bornovalova, M. A., Matusiewicz, A., & Rojas, E. (2011). Distress tolerance moderates the relationship between negative affect intensity with borderline personality disorder levels. *Comprehensive Psychiatry, 52*(6), 744–753. https://doi.org/10.1016/j.comppsych.2010.11.005

Boucher, C. M., & Scoboria, A. (2015). Reappraising past and future transitional events: The effects of mental focus on present perceptions of personal impact and self-relevance. *Journal of Personality, 83*(4), 361–375. https://doi.org/10.1111/jopy.12109

Boucher, C. M., Scoboria, A., Soucie, K., & Pascual-Leone, A. (2024). Development and validation of the Closure and Resolution Scale (CRS): A measure of event resolution. *Memory, 33*(2), 205–222. https://doi.org/10.1080/09658211.2024.2427666

Bower, G. H., & Clark, C. M. (1969). Narrative stories as mediators of serial learning. *Psychonomic Science, 14*(4), 181–182. https://doi.org/10.3758/BF03332778

Bradley, B., & Furrow, J. L. (2004). Toward a mini-theory of the blamer softening event: Tracking the moment-by-moment process. *Journal of Marital and Family Therapy, 30*(2), 233–246. https://doi.org/10.1111/j.1752-0606.2004.tb01236.x

Bräuninger, I. (2014). Specific dance movement therapy interventions—Which are successful? An intervention and correlation study. *The Arts in Psychotherapy, 41*(5), 445–457. https://doi.org/10.1016/j.aip.2014.08.002

Breuer, J., & Freud, S. (1966). *Studies on hysteria* (J. Strachey & A. Freud, Eds. & Trans.). Avon Books. (Original work published 1895)

Bridges, M. R. (2006). Activating the corrective emotional experience. *Journal of Clinical Psychology, 62*(5), 551–568. https://doi.org/10.1002/jclp.20248

Brinegar, M. G., Salvi, L. M., Stiles, W. B., & Greenberg, L. S. (2006). Building a meaning bridge: Therapeutic progress from problem formulation to understanding. *Journal of Counseling Psychology, 53*(2), 165–180. https://doi.org/10.1037/0022-0167.53.2.165

Broadhurst, P. L. (1957). Emotionality and the Yerkes–Dodson law. *Journal of Experimental Psychology, 54*(5), 345–352. https://doi.org/10.1037/h0049114

Brooks, A. W. (2014). Get excited: Reappraising pre-performance anxiety as excitement. *Journal of Experimental Psychology: General, 143*(3), 1144–1158. https://doi.org/10.1037/a0035325

Brookshire, G., & Casasanto, D. (2018). Approach motivation in human cerebral cortex. *Philosophical Transactions of the Royal Society of London: Series B. Biological Sciences, 373*(1752), Article 20170141. https://doi.org/10.1098/rstb.2017.0141

Brown, M. Z., Linehan, M. M., Comtois, K. A., Murray, A., & Chapman, A. L. (2009). Shame as a prospective predictor of self-inflicted injury in borderline personality disorder: A multi-modal analysis. *Behaviour Research and Therapy, 47*(10), 815–822. https://doi.org/10.1016/j.brat.2009.06.008

Bruner, J. (1990). *Acts of meaning*. Harvard University Press.

Brunoni, A. R., Boggio, P. S., De Raedt, R., Benseñor, I. M., Lotufo, P. A., Namur, V., Valiengo, L. C., & Vanderhasselt, M. A. (2014). Cognitive control therapy and transcranial direct current stimulation for depression: A randomized, double-blinded, controlled trial. *Journal of Affective Disorders, 162*, 43–49. https://doi.org/10.1016/j.jad.2014.03.026

Brunoni, A. R., Moffa, A. H., Fregni, F., Palm, U., Padberg, F., Blumberger, D. M., Daskalakis, Z. J., Bennabi, D., Haffen, E., Alonzo, A., & Loo, C. K. (2016). Transcranial direct current stimulation for acute major depressive episodes: Meta-analysis of individual patient data. *The British Journal of Psychiatry, 208*(6), 522–531. https://doi.org/10.1192/bjp.bp.115.164715

Bryntwick, E. (2016). *An examination of the interrelationship of narrative and emotion processes in emotion-focused therapy for trauma* [Unpublished doctoral thesis]. York University.

Bühler, K. (1965). *The crisis of psychology*. Gustav Fischer. (Original work published 1926)

Burlingham, A., Denton, H., Massey, H., Vides, N., & Harper, C. M. (2022). Sea swimming as a novel intervention for depression and anxiety: A feasibility study exploring engagement and acceptability. *Mental Health and Physical Activity, 23*, Article 100472. https://doi.org/10.1016/j.mhpa.2022.100472

Burton, A. L., Brown, R., & Abbott, M. J. (2022). Overcoming difficulties in measuring emotional regulation: Assessing and comparing the psychometric properties of the DERS long and short forms. *Cogent Psychology, 9*(1), 2060629. https://doi.org/10.1080/23311908.2022.2060629

Bushman, B. J. (2002). Does venting anger feed or extinguish the flame? Catharsis, rumination, distraction, anger, aggressive responding. *Personality and Social Psychology Bulletin, 28*(6), 724–731. https://doi.org/10.1177/0146167202289002

Butler, M. H., Harper, J. M., & Mitchell, C. B. (2011). A comparison of attachment outcomes in enactment-based versus therapist-centered therapy process modalities in couple therapy. *Family Process, 50*(2), 203–220. https://doi.org/10.1111/j.1545-5300.2011.01355.x

Butti, C., Santos, M., Uppal, N., & Hof, P. R. (2013). Von Economo neurons: Clinical and evolutionary perspectives. *Cortex, 49*(1), 312–326. https://doi.org/10.1016/j.cortex.2011.10.004

Bylsma, L. M., Vingerhoets, A. J. J. M., & Rottenberg, J. (2008). When is crying cathartic? An international study. *Journal of Social and Clinical Psychology, 27*(10), 1165–1187. https://doi.org/10.1521/jscp.2008.27.10.1165

Cabeza, R. (2008). Role of parietal regions in episodic memory retrieval: The dual attentional processes hypothesis. *Neuropsychologia, 46*(7), 1813–1827. https://doi.org/10.1016/j.neuropsychologia.2008.03.019

Callahan, J. L., Maxwell, K., & Janis, B. M. (2019). The role of overgeneral memories in PTSD and implications for treatment. *Journal of Psychotherapy Integration, 29*(1), 32–41. https://doi.org/10.1037/int0000116

Cameron, K., Ogrodniczuk, J., & Hadjipavlou, G. (2014). Changes in alexithymia following psychological intervention: A review. *Harvard Review of Psychiatry, 22*(3), 162–178. https://doi.org/10.1097/HRP.0000000000000036

Cannon, W. B. (1927). The James–Lange theory of emotion: A critical examination and an alternative theory. *The American Journal of Psychology, 39*(1/4), 106–124. https://doi.org/10.2307/1415404

Cantril, H., & Hunt, W. A. (1932). Emotional effects produced by the injection of adrenalin. *The American Journal of Psychology, 44*(2), 300–307. https://doi.org/10.2307/1414829

Carey, T. A. (2011). Exposure and reorganization: The what and how of effective psychotherapy. *Clinical Psychology Review, 31*(2), 236–248. https://doi.org/10.1016/j.cpr.2010.04.004

Carpenter, N., Angus, L., Paivio, S., & Bryntwick, E. (2016). Narrative and emotion integration processes in emotion-focused therapy for complex trauma: An exploratory process-outcome analysis. *Person-Centered and Experiential Psychotherapies, 15*(2), 67–94. https://doi.org/10.1080/14779757.2015.1132756

Carr, E. H. (1961). *What is history?* Penguin Books.

Carryer, J. R., & Greenberg, L. S. (2010). Optimal levels of emotional arousal in experiential therapy of depression. *Journal of Consulting and Clinical Psychology, 78*(2), 190–199. https://doi.org/10.1037/a0018401

Cavicchioli, M., Rugi, C., & Maffei, C. (2015). Inability to withstand present moment experience in borderline personality disorder: A meta-analytic review. *Clinical Neuropsychiatry, 12*(4), 101–110.

Chagigiorgis, H. (2010). *The contributions of emotional engagement with trauma material to outcome in two versions of emotion focused trauma therapy (EFTT)* [Unpublished doctoral dissertation]. University of Windsor.

Chekroud, S. R., Gueorguieva, R., Zheutlin, A. B., Paulus, M., Krumholz, H. M., Krystal, J. H., & Chekroud, A. M. (2018). Association between physical exercise and mental health in 1.2 million individuals in the USA between 2011 and 2015: A cross-sectional study. *The Lancet Psychiatry, 5*(9), 739–746. https://doi.org/10.1016/S2215-0366(18)30227-X

Chen, B. K., Murawski, N. J., Cincotta, C., McKissick, O., Finkelstein, A., Hamidi, A. B., Merfeld, E., Doucette, E., Grella, S. L., Shpokayte, M., Zaki, Y., Fortin, A., & Ramirez, S. (2019). Artificially enhancing and suppressing hippocampus-mediated memories. *Current Biology, 29*(11), 1885–1894.e4. https://doi.org/10.1016/j.cub.2019.04.065

Chen, Q., Beaty, R. E., Cui, Z., Sun, J., He, H., Zhuang, K., Ren, Z., Liu, G., & Qiu, J. (2019). Brain hemispheric involvement in visuospatial and verbal divergent thinking. *NeuroImage, 202,* Article 116065. https://doi.org/10.1016/j.neuroimage.2019.116065

Choi, B. H., Pos, A. E., & Magnusson, M. S. (2016). Emotional change process in resolving self-criticism during experiential treatment of depression. *Psychotherapy Research, 26*(4), 484–499. https://doi.org/10.1080/10503307.2015.1041433

Cohen, G. L., & Sherman, D. K. (2014). The psychology of change: Self-affirmation and social psychological intervention. *Annual Review of Psychology, 65,* 333–371. https://doi.org/10.1146/annurev-psych-010213-115137

Coles, N. A., Larsen, J. T., Kuribayashi, J., & Kuelz, A. (2019). Does blocking facial feedback via botulinum toxin injections decrease depression? A critical review and meta-analysis. *Emotion Review, 11*(4), 294–309. https://doi.org/10.1177/1754073919868762

Colwill, R. M., Lattal, K. M., Whitlow, J. W., Jr., & Delamater, A. R. (2023). Habituation: It's not what you think it is. *Behavioural Processes, 207,* Article 104845. https://doi.org/10.1016/j.beproc.2023.104845

Conway, M. A. (2005). Memory and the self. *Journal of Memory and Language, 53*(4), 594–628. https://doi.org/10.1016/j.jml.2005.08.005

Conway, M. A., & Pleydell-Pearce, C. W. (2000). The construction of autobiographical memories in the self-memory system. *Psychological Review, 107*(2), 261–288. https://doi.org/10.1037/0033-295X.107.2.261

Coombs, M. M., Coleman, D., & Jones, E. E. (2002). Working with feelings: The importance of emotion in both cognitive-behavioral and interpersonal therapy in the NIMH Treatment of Depression Collaborative Research Program. *Psychotherapy: Theory, Research, Practice, Training, 39*(3), 233–244. https://doi.org/10.1037/0033-3204.39.3.233

Cooper, A. A., Clifton, E. G., & Feeny, N. C. (2017). An empirical review of potential mediators and mechanisms of prolonged exposure therapy. *Clinical Psychology Review, 56,* 106–121. https://doi.org/10.1016/j.cpr.2017.07.003

Corcoran, C. D., Thomas, P., Phillips, J., & O'Keane, V. (2006). Vagus nerve stimulation in chronic treatment-resistant depression: Preliminary findings of an open-label study. *The British Journal of Psychiatry, 189*(3), 282–283. https://doi.org/10.1192/bjp.bp.105.018689

Costafreda, S. G., Brammer, M. J., David, A. S., & Fu, C. H. Y. (2008). Predictors of amygdala activation during the processing of emotional stimuli: A meta-analysis of 385 PET and fMRI studies. *Brain Research Reviews, 58*(1), 57–70. https://doi.org/10.1016/j.brainresrev.2007.10.012

Costanza, A., Baertschi, M., Richard-Lepouriel, H., Weber, K., Pompili, M., & Canuto, A. (2020). The presence and the search constructs of meaning in life in suicidal patients attending a psychiatric emergency department. *Frontiers in Psychiatry, 11,* Article 327. https://doi.org/10.3389/fpsyt.2020.00327

Cox, D. W., Buchanan, M. J., Hoover, S. M., & Westwood, M. J. (2014). Re-experiencing military trauma in groups: A veteran's case study. *Canadian Journal of Counselling and Psychotherapy, 48*(4), 441–453.

Cox, D. W., Kealy, D., Kahn, J. H., McCloskey, K. D., Joyce, A. S., & Ogrodniczuk, J. S. (2020). Depression symptoms' impact on personality disorder treatment: Depression symptoms amplifying the interpersonal benefits of negative-affect expression. *Journal of Affective Disorders, 272,* 318–325. https://doi.org/10.1016/j.jad.2020.03.133

Cox, D. W., Kealy, D., Kahn, J. H., Wojcik, K. D., Joyce, A. S., & Ogrodniczuk, J. S. (2019). The attenuating effect of depression symptoms on negative-affect expression: Individual and group effects in group psychotherapy for personality disorders. *Journal of Counseling Psychology, 66*(3), 351–361. https://doi.org/10.1037/cou0000335

Cox, D. W., Westwood, M. J., Hoover, S. M., Chan, E. K., Kivari, C. A., Dadson, M. R., & Zumbo, B. D. (2014). Evaluation of a group intervention for veterans who experienced military-related trauma. *International Journal of Group Psychotherapy, 64*(3), 367–380. https://doi.org/10.1521/ijgp.2014.64.3.367

Cox, K., & McAdams, D. P. (2014). Meaning making during high and low point life story episodes predicts emotion regulation two years later: How the past informs the future. *Journal of Research in Personality, 50*, 66–70. https://doi.org/10.1016/j.jrp.2014.03.004

Craig, A. D. (2009). How do you feel—Now? The anterior insula and human awareness. *Nature Reviews Neuroscience, 10*(1), 59–70. https://doi.org/10.1038/nrn2555

Creswell, J. D., Way, B. M., Eisenberger, N. I., & Lieberman, M. D. (2007). Neural correlates of dispositional mindfulness during affect labeling. *Psychosomatic Medicine, 69*(6), 560–565. https://doi.org/10.1097/PSY.0b013e3180f6171f

Cristoffanini, F., Pascual-Leone, A., Kramer, U., Nardone, S., McMain, S., Grandjean, L., & Culina, I. (2023, May). *Early session observations of emotion anticipate outcome in dialectical behavior therapy for personality disorder* [Paper presentation]. The Society for Exploration of Psychotherapy Integration, Vancouver, BC, Canada.

Critchley, H. D., Wiens, S., Rotshtein, P., Öhman, A., & Dolan, R. J. (2004). Neural systems supporting interoceptive awareness. *Nature Neuroscience, 7*(2), 189–195. https://doi.org/10.1038/nn1176

Cui, X., Jeter, C. B., Yang, D., Montague, P. R., & Eagleman, D. M. (2007). Vividness of mental imagery: Individual variability can be measured objectively. *Vision Research, 47*(4), 474–478. https://doi.org/10.1016/j.visres.2006.11.013

Curley, M., & Johnston, C. (2013). The characteristics and severity of psychological distress after abortion among university students. *The Journal of Behavioral Health Services & Research, 40*(3), 279–293. https://doi.org/10.1007/s11414-013-9328-0

Dailey, J., Timulak, L., Goldman, R. S., & Greenberg, L. S. (2023). Capturing the change: A case study investigation of emotional and interactional transformation in emotion-focused therapy for couples. *Person-Centered and Experiential Psychotherapies, 23*(1), 1–19. https://doi.org/10.1080/14779757.2023.2204480

Dalgleish, T., Williams, J. M. G., Golden, A. M. J., Perkins, N., Barrett, L. F., Barnard, P. J., Au Yeung, C., Murphy, V., Elward, R., Tchanturia, K., & Watkins, E. (2007). Reduced specificity of autobiographical memory and depression: The role of executive control. *Journal of Experimental Psychology: General, 136*(1), 23–42. https://doi.org/10.1037/0096-3445.136.1.23

Damasio, A. (1999). *The feeling of what happens: Body and emotion in the making of consciousness.* Harcourt College Publishers.

Daros, A. R., Haefner, S. A., Asadi, S., Kazi, S., Rodak, T., & Quilty, L. C. (2021). A meta-analysis of emotional regulation outcomes in psychological interventions for youth with depression and anxiety. *Nature Human Behaviour, 5*(10), 1443–1457. https://doi.org/10.1038/s41562-021-01191-9

Darwin, C. (1965). *The expression of the emotions in man and animals.* University of Chicago Press. https://doi.org/10.7208/chicago/9780226220802.001.0001 (Original work published 1872)

Daselaar, S. M., Rice, H. J., Greenberg, D. L., Cabeza, R., LaBar, K. S., & Rubin, D. C. (2008). The spatiotemporal dynamics of autobiographical memory: Neural correlates of recall, emotional intensity, and reliving. *Cerebral Cortex, 18*(1), 217–229. https://doi.org/10.1093/cercor/bhm048

Davanloo, H. (2005). Intensive short-term dynamic psychotherapy. In B J. Sadock, V A. Sadock, & H. I. Kaplon (Eds.), *Kaplan and Sadock's comprehensive textbook of psychiatry* (8th ed., pp. 2628–2652). Lippincot Williams & Wilkins.

Davidson, R. J. (2000). Affective style, mood, and anxiety disorders: An affective neuroscience approach. In R. J. Davidson (Ed.), *Anxiety, depression, and emotion* (pp. 88–108). Oxford University Press. https://doi.org/10.1093/acprof:oso/9780195133585.003.0005

Davidson, R. J., & Irwin, W. (1999). The functional neuroanatomy of emotion and affective style. *Trends in Cognitive Sciences, 3*(1), 11–21. https://doi.org/10.1016/S1364-6613(98)01265-0

Davis, J. I., Senghas, A., Brandt, F., & Ochsner, K. N. (2010). The effects of Botox injections on emotional experience. *Emotion, 10*(3), 433–440. https://doi.org/10.1037/a0018690

Davis, J. I., Senghas, A., & Ochsner, K. N. (2009). How does facial feedback modulate emotional experience? *Journal of Research in Personality, 43*(5), 822–829. https://doi.org/10.1016/j.jrp.2009.06.005

Davis, M. C., Zautra, A. J., Wolf, L. D., Tennen, H., & Yeung, E. W. (2015). Mindfulness and cognitive-behavioral interventions for chronic pain: Differential effects on daily pain reactivity and stress reactivity. *Journal of Consulting and Clinical Psychology, 83*(1), 24–35. https://doi.org/10.1037/a0038200

Delatraba, A., Jódar, R., López-Cavada, C. & Pascual-Leone, A. (2025). Emotion cascade: Harnessing emotional sequences to enhance chair work interventions and reduce self-criticism. *Psychotherapy Research*. Advance online publication. https://doi.org/10.1080/10503307.2025.2460535

Denson, T. F., Moulds, M. L., & Grisham, J. R. (2012). The effects of analytical rumination, reappraisal, and distraction on anger experience. *Behavior Therapy, 43*(2), 355–364. https://doi.org/10.1016/j.beth.2011.08.001

De Panfilis, C., Ossola, P., Tonna, P., Catania, L., & Marchesi, C. (2015). Finding words for feelings: The relationship between personality disorders and alexithymia. *Personality and Individual Differences, 74*, 285–291. https://doi.org/10.1016/j.paid.2014.10.050

Diamond, G. M., Rochman, D., & Amir, O. (2010). Arousing primary vulnerable emotions in the context of unresolved anger: "Speaking about" versus "speaking to." *Journal of Counseling Psychology, 57*(4), 402–410. https://doi.org/10.1037/a0021115

Diamond, G. M., Shahar, B., Sabo, D., & Tsvieli, N. (2016). Attachment-based family therapy and emotion-focused therapy for unresolved anger: The role of productive emotional processing. *Psychotherapy: Theory, Research, & Practice, 53*(1), 34–44. https://doi.org/10.1037/pst0000025

Di Bartolomeo, A. A., Varma, S., Fulham, L., & Fitzpatrick, S. (2022). The moderating role of interpersonal problems on baseline emotional intensity and emotional reactivity in individuals with borderline personality disorder and healthy controls. *Journal of Experimental Psychopathology, 13*(4), 1–14. https://doi.org/10.1177/20438087221142481

Dickens, C. (1843). *A Christmas carol: Being a ghost story of Christmas* (J. Leech, Illus.). Chapman and Hall.

Dimaggio, G., Ottavi, P., Popolo, R., & Salvatore, G. (2020). *Metacognitive interpersonal therapy: Body, imagery and change*. Routledge. https://doi.org/10.4324/9780429350894

Dimidjian, S., Hollon, S. D., Dobson, K. S., Schmaling, K. B., Kohlenberg, R. J., Addis, M. E., Gallop, R., McGlinchey, J. B., Markley, D. K., Gollan, J. K., Atkins, D. C., Dunner, D. L., & Jacobson, N. S. (2006). Randomized trial of behavioral activation, cognitive therapy, and antidepressant medication in the acute treatment of adults with major depression. *Journal of Consulting and Clinical Psychology, 74*(4), 658–670. https://doi.org/10.1037/0022-006X.74.4.658

Doidge, N. (2007). *The brain that changes itself: Stories of personal triumph from the frontiers of brain science*. Viking.

Dunlop, W. L., & Tracy, J. L. (2013). Sobering stories: Narratives of self-redemption predict behavioral change and improved health among recovering alcoholics. *Journal of Personality and Social Psychology, 104*(3), 576–590. https://doi.org/10.1037/a0031185

Dutton, D. G., & Aron, A. P. (1974). Some evidence for heightened sexual attraction under conditions of high anxiety. *Journal of Personality and Social Psychology, 30*(4), 510–517. https://doi.org/10.1037/h0037031

Ecker, B., Ticic, R., & Hulley, L. (2024). *Unlocking the emotional brain: Memory reconsolidation and the psychotherapy of transformational change* (2nd ed.). Routledge. https://doi.org/10.4324/9781003231431

Elliott, R. (2010). Psychotherapy change process research: Realizing the promise. *Psychotherapy Research, 20*(2), 123–135. https://doi.org/10.1080/10503300903470743

Elliott, R., Bohart, A. C., Watson, J. C., & Murphy, D. (2018). Therapist empathy and client outcome: An updated meta-analysis. *Psychotherapy: Theory, Research, & Practice, 55*(4), 399–410. https://doi.org/10.1037/pst0000175

Ellison, J. A., Greenberg, L. S., Goldman, R. N., & Angus, L. (2009). Maintenance of gains following experiential therapies for depression. *Journal of Consulting and Clinical Psychology, 77*(1), 103–112. https://doi.org/10.1037/a0014653

Erikson, E. (1968). *Identity: Youth and crisis.* W. W. Norton & Company.

Esteves, M., & Conceição, N. (2022). Hear what you feel, feel what you hear: The effect of musical sequences on emotional processing. *Complementary Therapies in Clinical Practice, 48*, Article 101603. https://doi.org/10.1016/j.ctcp.2022.101603

Farb, N. A., Segal, Z. V., Mayberg, H., Bean, J., McKeon, D., Fatima, Z., & Anderson, A. K. (2007). Attending to the present: Mindfulness meditation reveals distinct neural modes of self-reference. *Social Cognitive and Affective Neuroscience, 2*(4), 313–322. https://doi.org/10.1093/scan/nsm030

Fein, E. B. (1991, November 20). Book notes. *The New York Times*, C26. https://www.nytimes.com/1991/11/20/books/book-notes-059091.html

Feinstein, J. S., Adolphs, R., Damasio, A., & Tranel, D. (2011). The human amygdala and the induction and experience of fear. *Current Biology, 21*(1), 34–38. https://doi.org/10.1016/j.cub.2010.11.042

Feldman-Barratt, L. (2017). *How emotions are made: The secret life of the brain.* Houghton-Mifflin Harcourt.

Felsman, P., Seifert, C. M., & Himle, J. A. (2019). The use of improvisational theater training to reduce social anxiety in adolescents. *The Arts in Psychotherapy, 63*, 111–117. https://doi.org/10.1016/j.aip.2018.12.001

Finnbogadóttir, H., & Berntsen, D. (2014). Looking at life from different angles: Observer perspective during remembering and imagining distinct emotional events. *Psychology of Consciousness: Theory, Research, and Practice, 1*(4), 387–406. https://doi.org/10.1037/cns0000029

Fisher, H., Atzil-Slonim, D., Bar-Kalifa, E., Rafaeli, E., & Peri, T. (2016). Emotional experience and alliance contribute to therapeutic change in psychodynamic therapy. *Psychotherapy: Theory, Research, & Practice, 53*(1), 105–116. https://doi.org/10.1037/pst0000041

Fitzpatrick, M. R., & Stalikas, A. (2008). Positive emotions as generators of therapeutic change. *Journal of Psychotherapy Integration, 18*(2), 137–154. https://doi.org/10.1037/1053-0479.18.2.137

Flack, W. F., Jr., Laird, J. D., & Cavallaro, L. A. (1999). Separate and combined effects of facial expressions and bodily postures on emotional feelings. *European Journal of Social Psychology, 29*(2–3), 203–217. https://doi.org/fdbq85

Fleet, R. P., Lavoie, K. L., Martel, J. P., Dupuis, G., Marchand, A., & Beitman, B. D. (2003). Two-year follow-up status of emergency department patients with chest pain: Was it panic disorder? *Canadian Journal of Emergency Medical Care, 5*(4), 247–254. https://doi.org/10.1017/S1481803500008447

Fleury, G., Fortin-Langelier, B., & Ben-Cheikh, I. (2016). The cardiac rhythm of the unconscious in a case of panic disorder. *American Journal of Psychotherapy, 70*(3), 277–300. https://doi.org/10.1176/appi.psychotherapy.2016.70.3.277

Flückiger, C., Del Re, A. C., Wlodasch, D., Horvath, A. O., Solomonov, N., & Wampold, B. E. (2020). Assessing the alliance-outcome association adjusted for patient characteristics and treatment processes: A meta-analytic summary of direct comparisons. *Journal of Counseling Psychology, 67*(6), 706–711. https://doi.org/10.1037/cou0000424

Foa, E., Hembree, E., & Rothbaum, B. O. (2007). *Prolonged exposure therapy for PTSD: Emotional processing of traumatic experiences therapist guide.* Oxford University Press. https://doi.org/10.1093/med:psych/9780195308501.001.0001

Foa, E. B., Huppert, J. D., & Cahill, S. P. (2006). Emotional processing theory: An update. In B. O. Rothbaum (Ed.), *Pathological anxiety: Emotional processing in etiology and treatment* (pp. 3–24). Guilford Press.

Foa, E. B., & Kozak, M. J. (1986). Emotional processing of fear: Exposure to corrective information. *Psychological Bulletin, 99*(1), 20–35. https://doi.org/10.1037/0033-2909.99.1.20

Foa, E. B., Rothbaum, B. O., & Furr, J. M. (2003). Augmenting exposure therapy with other CBT procedures. *Psychiatric Annals, 33*(1), 47–53. https://doi.org/10.3928/0048-5713-20030101-08

Fonagy, P., Gergely, G., & Jurist, E. L. (Eds.). (2002). *Affect regulation, mentalization and the development of the self.* Routledge. https://doi.org/10.4324/9780429471643

Foroughe, M. (2018). *Emotion focused family therapy with children and caregivers: A trauma-informed approach.* Routledge. https://doi.org/10.4324/9781315161105

Forward, M. (2023). *Body dissatisfaction and depression: Investigating the moderating roles of maladaptive investment in appearance and rumination* (Publication No. 9270) [Master's thesis, University of Windsor]. Electronic Theses and Dissertations. https://scholar.uwindsor.ca/etd/9270

Fosha, D. (Ed.). (2021). *Undoing aloneness and the transformation of suffering into flourishing: AEDP 2.0.* American Psychological Association. https://doi.org/10.1037/0000232-000

Frank, J. D. (1961). *Persuasion and healing: A comprehensive study of psychotherapy.* Johns Hopkins University Press.

Frankl, V. E. (1963). *Man's search for meaning: An introduction to logotherapy.* Washington Square Press.

Franzoni, E., Gualandi, S., Caretti, V., Schimmenti, A., Di Pietro, E., Pellegrini, G., Craparo, G., Franchi, A., Verrotti, A., & Pellicciari, A. (2013). The relationship between alexithymia, shame, trauma, and body image disorders: Investigation over a large clinical sample. *Neuropsychiatric Disease and Treatment, 9,* 185–193. https://doi.org/10.2147/NDT.S34822

Frattaroli, J. (2006). Experimental disclosure and its moderators: A meta-analysis. *Psychological Bulletin, 132*(6), 823–865. https://doi.org/10.1037/0033-2909.132.6.823

Fredrickson, B. L. (2001). The role of positive emotions in positive psychology: The broaden-and-build theory of positive emotions. *American Psychologist, 56*(3), 218–226. https://doi.org/10.1037/0003-066X.56.3.218

Fredrickson, B. L., & Levenson, R. W. (1998). Positive emotions speed recovery from the cardiovascular sequelae of negative emotions. *Cognition and Emotion, 12*(2), 191–220. https://doi.org/10.1080/026999398379718

Fredrickson, B. L., & Losada, M. F. (2005). Positive affect and the complex dynamics of human flourishing. *American Psychologist, 60*(7), 678–686. https://doi.org/10.1037/0003-066X.60.7.678

Fredrickson, B. L., Mancuso, R. A., Branigan, C., & Tugade, M. M. (2000). The undoing effect of positive emotions. *Motivation and Emotion, 24*(4), 237–258. https://doi.org/10.1023/A:1010796329158

Fresco, D. M., Frankel, A. N., Mennin, D. S., Turk, C. L., & Heimberg, R. G. (2002). Distinct and overlapping features of rumination and worry: The relationship of cognitive production to negative affective states. *Cognitive Therapy and Research, 26*(2), 179–188. https://doi.org/10.1023/A:1014517718949

Freud, S. (1910). The origin and development of psychoanalysis. *The American Journal of Psychology, 21*(2), 181–218. https://doi.org/10.2307/1413001

Freud, S. (1926). Inhibitions, symptoms and anxiety. In J. Strachey & A. Freud (Eds.), *The standard edition of the complete psychological works of Sigmund Freud* (pp. 77–175). Hogarth Press.

Fuchs, T., Breyer, T., & Mundt, C. (Eds.). (2014). *Karl Jaspers' philosophy and psychopathology.* Springer. https://doi.org/10.1007/978-1-4614-8878-1

Fujita, K., & Carnevale, J. J. (2012). Transcending temptation through abstraction: The role of construal level in self-control. *Current Directions in Psychological Science, 21*(4), 248–252. https://doi.org/10.1177/0963721412449169

Gaher, R. M., Hofman, N. L., Simons, J. S., & Hunsaker, R. (2013). Emotion regulation deficits as mediators between trauma exposure and borderline symptoms. *Cognitive Therapy and Research, 37*(3), 466–475. https://doi.org/10.1007/s10608-012-9515-y

Gallagher, I. (2000). Philosophical conceptions of the self: Implications for cognitive science. *Trends in Cognitive Sciences, 4*(1), 14–21. https://doi.org/10.1016/S1364-6613(99)01417-5

Gallistel, C. R., & Gibbon, J. (2000). Time, rate, and conditioning. *Psychological Review, 107*(2), 289–344. https://doi.org/10.1037/0033-295X.107.2.289

Gamoneda, J., Jódar, R., & Caro, C. (2023, June 30). *Existential Need Processing Model in complicated grief and empty chair for unfinished business* [Conference presentation]. International Society for Emotion-Focused Therapy Conference, Porto, Portugal.

Garland, E. L., Fredrickson, B., Kring, A. M., Johnson, D. P., Meyer, P. S., & Penn, D. L. (2010). Upward spirals of positive emotions counter downward spirals of negativity: Insights from the broaden-and-build theory and affective neuroscience on the treatment of emotion dysfunctions and deficits in psychopathology. *Clinical Psychology Review, 30*(7), 849–864. https://doi.org/10.1016/j.cpr.2010.03.002

Gauthier, L., Stollak, G., Messé, L., & Aronoff, J. (1996). Recall of childhood neglect and physical abuse as differential predictors of current psychological functioning. *Child Abuse & Neglect, 20*(7), 549–559. https://doi.org/10.1016/0145-2134(96)00043-9

Geller, S. M., & Greenberg, L. S. (2012). *Therapeutic presence: A mindful approach to effective therapy.* American Psychological Association. https://doi.org/10.1037/13485-000

Gelo, O. C. G., & Salvatore, S. (2016). A dynamic systems approach to psychotherapy: A meta-theoretical framework for explaining psychotherapy change processes. *Journal of Counseling Psychology, 63*(4), 379–395. https://doi.org/10.1037/cou0000150

Gendlin, E. T. (1964). A theory of personality change. In P. Worchel & D. Byrne (Eds.), *Personality change* (pp. 129–173). John Wiley & Sons.

Gendlin, E. T. (1981). *Focusing* (2nd, new rev. instructions ed.). Bantam Books.

Gendlin, E. T. (1996). *The practicing professional: Focusing-oriented psychotherapy: A manual of the experiential method.* Guilford Press.

Geyer, D., Lam, V., Gilbert, H., & Cooper, M. (2024). Depth of emotional experiencing and outcome in therapy with young people. *Psychology and Psychotherapy: Theory, Research and Practice, 98*(2), 308–321. https://doi.org/10.1111/papt.12537

Giddens, A. (1990). *The consequences of modernity.* Polity.

Gilam, G., Maron-Katz, A., Kliper, E., Lin, T., Fruchter, E., Shamir, R., & Hendler, T. (2017). Tracing the neural carryover effects of interpersonal anger on resting-state fMRI in men and their relation to traumatic stress symptoms in a subsample of soldiers. *Frontiers in Behavioral Neuroscience, 11,* Article 252. https://doi.org/10.3389/fnbeh.2017.00252

Gilbert, D. T. (2006). *Stumbling on happiness.* Knopf.

Gilboa-Schechtman, E., & Foa, E. B. (2001). Patterns of recovery from trauma: The use of intraindividual analysis. *Journal of Abnormal Psychology, 110*(3), 392–400. https://doi.org/10.1037/0021-843X.110.3.392

Gilead, M., Trope, Y., & Liberman, N. (2019). Above and beyond the concrete: The diverse representational substrates of the predictive brain. *Behavioral and Brain Sciences, 43,* Article e121. https://doi.org/10.1017/S0140525X19002000

Giovanetti, A. K., Revord, J. C., Sasso, M. P., & Haeffel, G. J. (2019). Self-distancing may be harmful: Third-person writing increases levels of depressive symptoms compared to traditional expressive writing and no writing. *Journal of Social and Clinical Psychology, 38*(1), 50–69. https://doi.org/10.1521/jscp.2019.38.1.50

Glass, J., Simon, R. W., & Andersson, M. A. (2016). Parenthood and happiness: Effects of work–family reconciliation policies in 22 OECD countries. *American Journal of Sociology, 122*(3), 886–929. https://doi.org/10.1086/688892

Goerlich-Dobre, K. S., Votinov, M., Habel, U., Pripfl, J., & Lamm, C. (2015). Neuroanatomical profiles of alexithymia dimensions and subtypes. *Human Brain Mapping, 36*(10), 3805–3818. https://doi.org/10.1002/hbm.22879

Goerlich-Dobre, K. S., Witteman, J., Schiller, N. O., van Heuven, V. J., Aleman, A., & Martens, S. (2014). Blunted feelings: Alexithymia is associated with a diminished neural response to speech prosody. *Social Cognitive and Affective Neuroscience, 9*(8), 1108–1117. https://doi.org/10.1093/scan/nst075

Goethe, J. W. von, & Hecker, M. (2015). *Goethes briefe an Auguste zu Stolberg* [Goethe's letters to Auguste zu Stolberg]. Project Gutenberg. https://www.gutenberg.org/ebooks/49024 (Original work published 1777)

Goldberg, S. B., Tucker, R. P., Greene, P. A., Davidson, R. J., Wampold, B. E., Kearney, D. J., & Simpson, T. L. (2018). Mindfulness-based interventions for psychiatric disorders: A systematic review and meta-analysis. *Clinical Psychology Review, 59*, 52–60. https://doi.org/10.1016/j.cpr.2017.10.011

Goldfarb, E. V., Fröböse, M. I., Cools, R., & Phelps, E. A. (2017). Stress and cognitive flexibility: Cortisol increases are associated with enhanced updating but impaired switching. *Journal of Cognitive Neuroscience, 29*(1), 14–24. https://doi.org/10.1162/jocn_a_01029

Goldman, N., Khanna, D., El Asmar, M. L., Qualter, P., & El-Osta, A. (2024). Addressing loneliness and social isolation in 52 countries: A scoping review of national policies. *BMC Public Health, 24*, Article 1207. https://doi.org/10.1186/s12889-024-18370-8

Goldman, R. N., & Greenberg, L. S. (2015). *Case formulation in emotion-focused therapy: Co-creating clinical maps for change.* American Psychological Association. https://doi.org/10.1037/14523-000

Goldman, R. N., Greenberg, L. S., & Angus, L. (2006). The effects of adding emotion focused interventions to the client-centered relationship conditions in the treatment of depression. *Psychotherapy Research, 16*(5), 537–549. https://doi.org/10.1080/10503300600589456

Golkar, A., Bellander, M., & Öhman, A. (2013). Temporal properties of fear extinction—Does time matter? *Behavioral Neuroscience, 127*(1), 59–69. https://doi.org/10.1037/a0030892

Gonçalves, M. M., Ribeiro, A. P., Mendes, I., Alves, D., Silva, J., Rosa, C., Braga, C., Batista, J., Fernández-Navarro, P., & Oliveira, J. T. (2017). Three narrative-based coding systems: Innovative moments, ambivalence and ambivalence resolution. *Psychotherapy Research, 27*(3), 270–282. https://doi.org/10.1080/10503307.2016.1247216

Gonçalves, M. M., Ribeiro, A. P., Mendes, I., Matos, M., & Santos, A. (2011). Tracking novelties in psychotherapy process research: The innovative moments coding system. *Psychotherapy Research, 21*(5), 497–509. https://doi.org/10.1080/10503307.2011.560207

Gordon, B. R., McDowell, C. P., Hallgren, M., Meyer, J. D., Lyons, M., & Herring, M. P. (2018). Association of efficacy of resistance exercise training with depressive symptoms: Meta-analysis and meta-regression analysis of randomized clinical trials. *JAMA Psychiatry, 75*(6), 566–576. https://doi.org/10.1001/jamapsychiatry.2018.0572

Gračanin, A., Vingerhoets, A. J. J. M., Kardum, I., Zupčić, M., Šantek, M., & Šimić, M. (2015). Why crying does and sometimes does not seem to alleviate mood: A quasi-experimental study. *Motivation and Emotion, 39*(6), 953–960. https://doi.org/10.1007/s11031-015-9507-9

Gratz, K. L., & Roemer, L. (2004). Multidimensional assessment of emotion regulation and dysregulation: Development, factor structure, and initial validation of the difficulties in emotion regulation scale. *Journal of Psychopathology and Behavioral Assessment, 26*(1), 41–54. https://doi.org/10.1023/B:JOBA.0000007455.08539.94

Greenberg, L. S. (2021). *Changing emotion with emotion: A practitioner's guide.* American Psychological Association. https://doi.org/10.1037/0000248-000

Greenberg, L. S., Auszra, L., & Herrmann, I. R. (2007). The relationship among emotional productivity, emotional arousal and outcome in experiential therapy of depression. *Psychotherapy Research, 17*(4), 482–493. https://doi.org/10.1080/10503300701667433

Greenberg, L. S., & Foerster, F. S. (1996). Task analysis exemplified: The process of resolving unfinished business. *Journal of Consulting and Clinical Psychology, 64*(3), 439–446. https://doi.org/10.1037/0022-006X.64.3.439

Greenberg, L. S., & Goldman, R. N. (Eds.). (2019). *Clinical handbook of emotion focused therapy*. American Psychological Association. https://doi.org/10.1037/0000112-000

Greenberg, L. S., & Korman, L. M. (1993). Assimilating emotion into psychotherapy integration. *Journal of Psychotherapy Integration, 3*(3), 249–265. https://doi.org/10.1037/h0101172

Greenberg, L. S., & Malcolm, W. (2002). Resolving unfinished business: Relating process to outcome. *Journal of Consulting and Clinical Psychology, 70*(2), 406–416. https://doi.org/10.1037/0022-006X.70.2.406

Greenberg, L. S., & Paivio, S. C. (1997). *Working with emotions in psychotherapy*. Guilford Press.

Greenberg, L. S., & Pascual-Leone, J. (1995). A dialectical constructivist approach to experiential change. In R. A. Neimeyer & M. J. Mahoney (Eds.), *Constructivism in psychotherapy* (pp. 169–191). American Psychological Association. https://doi.org/10.1037/10170-008

Greenberg, L. S., & Safran, J. D. (1987). *Emotion in psychotherapy: Affect, cognition, and the process of change*. Guilford Press.

Greenberg, L. S., Warwar, S. H., & Malcolm, W. M. (2008). Differential effects of emotion-focused therapy and psychoeducation in facilitating forgiveness and letting go of emotional injuries. *Journal of Counseling Psychology, 55*(2), 185–196. https://doi.org/10.1037/0022-0167.55.2.185

Greenberg, L. S., & Watson, J. C. (1998). Experiential therapy of depression: Differential effects of client-centered relationship conditions and process experiential interventions. *Psychotherapy Research, 8*(2), 210–224. https://doi.org/10.1093/ptr/8.2.210

Greenberg, L. S., & Watson, J. C. (2006). *Emotion-focused therapy for depression*. American Psychological Association. https://doi.org/10.1037/11286-000

Greenberg, M. A., Wortman, C. B., & Stone, A. A. (1996). Emotional expression and physical health: Revising traumatic memories or fostering self-regulation? *Journal of Personality and Social Psychology, 71*(3), 588–602. https://doi.org/10.1037/0022-3514.71.3.588

Groovy Flicks. (2020, January 1). *Emo Phillips HBO Comedy Special 1987* [Video]. YouTube. https://youtu.be/izH3zpAuDUs

Gros, D. F., Allan, N. P., Lancaster, C. L., Szafranski, D. D., & Acierno, R. (2018). Predictors of treatment discontinuation during prolonged exposure for PTSD. *Behavioural and Cognitive Psychotherapy, 46*(1), 35–49. https://doi.org/10.1017/S135246581700039X

Gross, J. J. (2015). Emotion regulation: Current status and future prospects. *Psychological Inquiry, 26*(1), 1–26. https://doi.org/10.1080/1047840X.2014.940781

Grosse Holtforth, M., Grawe, K., & Castonguay, L. G. (2006). Predicting a reduction of avoidance motivation in psychotherapy: Toward the delineation of differential processes of change operating at different phases of treatment. *Psychotherapy Research, 16*(5), 639–644. https://doi.org/10.1080/10503300600608215

Grossman, P. (2023). Fundamental challenges and likely refutations of the five basic premises of the polyvagal theory. *Biological Psychology, 180*, Article 108589. https://doi.org/10.1016/j.biopsycho.2023.108589

Grossmann, I., & Kross, E. (2014). Exploring Solomon's paradox: Self-distancing eliminates the self-other asymmetry in wise reasoning about close relationships in younger and older adults. *Psychological Science, 25*(8), 1571–1580. https://doi.org/10.1177/0956797614535400

Gruber, J., Harvey, A. G., & Johnson, S. L. (2009). Reflective and ruminative processing of positive emotional memories in bipolar disorder and healthy controls. *Behaviour Research and Therapy, 47*(8), 697–704. https://doi.org/10.1016/j.brat.2009.05.005

Grynberg, D., Chang, B., Corneille, O., Maurage, P., Vermeulen, N., Berthoz, S., & Luminet, O. (2012). Alexithymia and the processing of emotional facial expressions (EFEs): Systematic review, unanswered questions and further perspectives. *PLOS One, 7*(8), Article e42429. https://doi.org/10.1371/journal.pone.0042429

Gu, X., & Tse, C. S. (2016). Narrative perspective shift at retrieval: The psychological-distance-mediated-effect on emotional intensity of positive and negative autobiographical memory. *Consciousness and Cognition, 45,* 159–173. https://doi.org/10.1016/j.concog.2016.09.001

Gunst, E., Watson, J. C., Desmet, M., & Willemsen, J. (2017). Affect regulation as a factor in sex offenders. *Aggression and Violent Behavior, 37,* 210–219. https://doi.org/10.1016/j.avb.2017.10.007

Haas, H. L., Sergeeva, O. A., & Selbach, O. (2008). Histamine in the nervous system. *Physiological Reviews, 88*(3), 1183–1241. https://doi.org/10.1152/physrev.00043.2007

Haberman, A., Shahar, B., Bar-Kalifa, E., Zilcha-Mano, S., & Diamond, G. M. (2019). Exploring the process of change in emotion-focused therapy for social anxiety. *Psychotherapy Research, 29*(7), 908–918. https://doi.org/10.1080/10503307.2018.1426896

Habermas, T. (2019). *Emotion and narrative: Perspectives in autobiographical storytelling.* Cambridge University Press.

Habermas, T., Delarue, I., Eiswirth, P., Glanz, S., Krämer, C., Landertinger, A., Krainhöfner, M., Batista, J., & Gonçalves, M. M. (2021). Differences between subclinical ruminators and reflectors in narrating autobiographical memories: Innovative moments and autobiographical reasoning. *Frontiers in Psychology, 12,* Article 624644. https://doi.org/10.3389/fpsyg.2021.624644

Hadash, Y., Lichtash, Y., & Bernstein, A. (2017). Measuring decentering and related constructs: Capacity and limitations of extant assessment scales. *Mindfulness, 8*(6), 1674–1688. https://doi.org/10.1007/s12671-017-0743-9

Haeffel, G. J. (2011). Motion as motivation: Using repetitive flexion movements to stimulate the approach system. *Behavior Therapy, 42*(4), 667–675. https://doi.org/10.1016/j.beth.2011.02.006

Hakim, L. Z. (2010). *A comparative analysis of the qualities of therapists' communications in three empirically-supported psychotherapies* [Unpublished doctoral dissertation]. York University.

Hall, S. A., Rubin, D. C., Miles, A., Davis, S. W., Wing, E. A., Cabeza, R., & Berntsen, D. (2014). The neural basis of involuntary episodic memories. *Journal of Cognitive Neuroscience, 26*(10), 2385–2399. https://doi.org/10.1162/jocn_a_00633

Hallion, L. S., Steinman, S. A., Tolin, D. F., & Diefenbach, G. J. (2018). Psychometric properties of the Difficulties in Emotion Regulation Scale (DERS) and its short forms in adults with emotional disorders. *Frontiers in Psychology, 9,* Article 539. https://doi.org/10.3389/fpsyg.2018.00539

Hamby, S., Grych, J., & Banyard, V. (2018). Resilience portfolios and poly-strengths: Identifying protective factors associated with thriving after adversity. *Psychology of Violence, 8*(2), 172–183. https://doi.org/10.1037/vio0000135

Hamby, S., Segura, A., Taylor, E., Grych, J., & Banyard, V. (2017). Meaning making in rural Appalachia: Age and gender patterns in seven measures of meaning. *Journal of Happiness and Well-Being, 5*(2), 168–186.

Hamlat, E. J., & Alloy, L. B. (2018). Autobiographical memory as a target of intervention: Increasing specificity for therapeutic gain. *Practice Innovations, 3*(4), 227–241. https://doi.org/10.1037/pri0000075

Harmon-Jones, E., Gable, P. A., & Peterson, C. K. (2010). The role of asymmetric frontal cortical activity in emotion-related phenomena: A review and update. *Biological Psychology, 84*(3), 451–462. https://doi.org/10.1016/j.biopsycho.2009.08.010

Harmon-Jones, E., Vaughn-Scott, K., Mohr, S., Sigelman, J., & Harmon-Jones, C. (2004). The effect of manipulated sympathy and anger on left and right frontal cortical activity. *Emotion, 4*(1), 95–101. https://doi.org/10.1037/1528-3542.4.1.95

Harrington, S. J., Morrison, O. P., & Pascual-Leone, A. (2018). Emotional processing in an expressive writing task on trauma. *Complementary Therapies in Clinical Practice, 32,* 116–122. https://doi.org/10.1016/j.ctcp.2018.06.001

Harrington, S. J., Pascual-Leone, A., Paivio, S., Edmondstone, C., & Baher, T. (2021). Depth of experiencing and therapeutic alliance: What predicts outcome for whom in emotion-focused therapy for trauma? *Psychology and Psychotherapy: Theory, Research and Practice, 94*(4), 895–914. https://doi.org/10.1111/papt.12342

Harrison, T. (2021). *Of bridges: A poetic and philosophical account.* Chicago University Press.

Hatfield, E., Hsee, C. K., Costello, J., Weisman, M. S., & Denney, C. (1995). The impact of vocal feedback on emotional experience and expression. *Journal of Social Behavior and Personality, 10,* 293–313.

Hayes, A. M., Feldman, G. C., Beevers, C. G., Laurenceau, J.-P., Cardaciotto, L., & Lewis-Smith, J. (2007). Discontinuities and cognitive changes in an exposure-based cognitive therapy for depression. *Journal of Consulting and Clinical Psychology, 75*(3), 409–421. https://doi.org/10.1037/0022-006X.75.3.409

Hayes, S. C., Strosahl, K. D., & Wilson, K. G. (2012). *Acceptance and commitment therapy: The process and practice of mindful change.* Guilford Press. https://doi.org/10.1037/17335-000

Hebb, D. O. (1949). *The organization of behavior.* John Wiley & Sons.

Heller, M. C. (2012). *Body psychotherapy: History, concepts, and methods* (M. Duclos, Trans.). W. W. Norton & Company.

Hendricks (2009) Experiencing level: An instance of developing a variable from a first-person process so it can be reliably measured and taught. *Journal of Consciousness Studies, 16*(10–12), 129–155.

Herrmann, I. R., Greenberg, L. S., & Auszra, L. (2016). Emotion categories and patterns of change in experiential therapy for depression. *Psychotherapy Research, 26*(2), 178–195. https://doi.org/10.1080/10503307.2014.958597

Hershfield, H. E., Scheibe, S., Sims, T. L., & Carstensen, L. L. (2013). When feeling bad can be good: Mixed emotions benefit physical health across adulthood. *Social Psychological and Personality Science, 4*(1), 54–61. https://doi.org/10.1177/1948550612444616

Hill, C. E., Helms, J. E., Tichenor, V., Spiegel, S. B., O'Grady, K. E., & Perry, E. S. (2004). Effects of therapist response modes in brief psychotherapy. In C. E. Hill (Ed.), *Helping skills: Facilitating, exploration, insight, and action* (2nd ed., pp. 61–86). American Psychological Association.

Hill, P. L., Sin, N. L., Turiano, N. A., Burrow, A. L., & Almeida, D. M. (2018). Sense of purpose moderates the associations between daily stressors and daily well-being. *Annals of Behavioral Medicine, 52*(8), 724–729. https://doi.org/10.1093/abm/kax039

Hinkle, M. S., Radomski, J. G., & Decker, K. M. (2015). Creative experiential interventions to heighten emotion and process in emotionally focused couples therapy. *The Family Journal, 23*(3), 239–246. https://doi.org/10.1177/1066480715572964

Hitz, L. C. (1994). *Effects of changes in experiencing level of therapist responses on client experiencing* [Unpublished doctoral dissertation]. University of Arkansas.

Hoehn-Saric, R., Liberman, B., Imber, S. D., Stone, A. R., Frank, J. D., & Ribich, F. D. (1974). Attitude change and attribution of arousal in psychotherapy. *Journal of Nervous and Mental Disease, 159*(4), 234–243. https://doi.org/10.1097/00005053-197410000-00002

Hoehn-Saric, R., Liberman, B., Imber, S. D., Stone, A. R., Pande, S. K., & Frank, J. D. (1972). Arousal and attitude change in neurotic patients. *Archives of General Psychiatry, 26*(1), 51–56. https://doi.org/10.1001/archpsyc.1972.01750190053010

Hofmann, S. G., & Hay, A. C. (2018). Rethinking avoidance: Toward a balanced approach to avoidance in treating anxiety disorders. *Journal of Anxiety Disorders, 55,* 14–21. https://doi.org/10.1016/j.janxdis.2018.03.004

Hofmann, S. G., & Hayes, S. C. (2019). The future of intervention science: Process-based therapy. *Clinical Psychological Science, 7*(1), 37–50. https://doi.org/10.1177/2167702618772296

Høglend, P., Bøgwald, K.-P., Amlo, S., Marble, A., Ulberg, R., Sjaastad, M. C., Sørbye, O., Heyerdahl, O., & Johansson, P. (2008). Transference interpretations in dynamic psychotherapy: Do they really yield sustained effects? *The American Journal of Psychiatry, 165*(6), 763–771. https://doi.org/10.1176/appi.ajp.2008.07061028

Høglend, P., & Hagtvet, K. (2019). Change mechanisms in psychotherapy: Both improved insight and improved affective awareness are necessary. *Journal of Consulting and Clinical Psychology, 87*(4), 332–344. https://doi.org/10.1037/ccp0000381

Høglend, P., Hersoug, A. G., Bøgwald, K.-P., Amlo, S., Marble, A., Sørbye, Ø., Røssberg, J. I., Ulberg, R., Gabbard, G. O., & Crits-Christoph, P. (2011). Effects of transference work in the context of therapeutic alliance and quality of object relations. *Journal of Consulting and Clinical Psychology, 79*(5), 697–706. https://doi.org/10.1037/a0024863

Holland, J. M., & Neimeyer, R. A. (2010). An examination of stage theory of grief among individuals bereaved by natural and violent causes: A meaning-oriented contribution. *Omega: Journal of Death and Dying, 61*(2), 103–120. https://doi.org/10.2190/OM.61.2.b

Holmes, E. A., Arntz, A., & Smucker, M. R. (2007). Imagery rescripting in cognitive behaviour therapy: Images, treatment techniques and outcomes. *Journal of Behavior Therapy and Experimental Psychiatry, 38*(4), 297–305. https://doi.org/10.1016/j.jbtep.2007.10.007

Holmes, E. A., & Mathews, A. (2010). Mental imagery in emotion and emotional disorders. *Clinical Psychology Review, 30*(3), 349–362. https://doi.org/10.1016/j.cpr.2010.01.001

Holowaty, K. A. M., & Paivio, S. C. (2012). Characteristics of client-identified helpful events in emotion-focused therapy for child abuse trauma. *Psychotherapy Research, 22*(1), 56–66. https://doi.org/10.1080/10503307.2011.622727

Hölzel, B. K., Lazar, S. W., Gard, T., Schuman-Olivier, Z., Vago, D. R., & Ott, U. (2011). How does mindfulness meditation work? Proposing mechanisms of action from a conceptual and neural perspective. *Perspectives on Psychological Science, 6*(6), 537–559. https://doi.org/10.1177/1745691611419671

Honos-Webb, L., Stiles, W. B., & Greenberg, L. S. (2003). A method of rating assimilation in psychotherapy based on markers of change. *Journal of Counseling Psychology, 50*(2), 189–198. https://doi.org/10.1037/0022-0167.50.2.189

Huang, M., Schmiedek, F., & Habermas, T. (2020). Only some attempts at meaning making are successful: The role of change-relatedness and positive implications for the self. *Journal of Personality, 89*(2), 175–187. https://doi.org/10.1111/jopy.12573

Hunt, M. G. (1998). The only way out is through: Emotional processing and recovery after a depressing life event. *Behaviour Research and Therapy, 36*(4), 361–384. https://doi.org/10.1016/S0005-7967(98)00017-5

Hyett, M. P., Bank, S. R., Lipp, O. V., Erceg-Hurn, D. M., Alvares, G. A., Maclaine, E., Puckridge, E., Hayes, S., & McEvoy, P. M. (2018). Attenuated psychophysiological reactivity following single-session group imagery rescripting versus verbal restructuring in social anxiety disorder: Results from a randomized controlled trial. *Psychotherapy and Psychosomatics, 87*(6), 340–349. https://doi.org/10.1159/000493897

Ioannou, S., Ebisch, S., Aureli, T., Bafunno, D., Ioannides, H. A., Cardone, D., Manini, B., Romani, G. L., Gallese, V., & Merla, A. (2013). The autonomic signature of guilt in children: A thermal infrared imaging study. *PLOS One, 8*(11), Article e79440. https://doi.org/10.1371/journal.pone.0079440

Jackson, P. L., Meltzoff, A. N., & Decety, J. (2006). Neural circuits involved in imitation and perspective-taking. *NeuroImage, 31*(1), 429–439. https://doi.org/10.1016/j.neuroimage.2005.11.026

James, W. (1950). *The principles of psychology* (Vol. 1). Dover. (Original work published 1890)

James, W. (1969). Letter to Mrs. Henry Whitman, June 7th 1899. In H. James (Ed.), *The letters of William James*. Kraus Reprints.

Janov, A. (1970). *The primal scream*. Putnam's Sons.

Janssen, S. M. J., Hearne, T. L., & Takarangi, M. K. T. (2015). The relation between self-reported PTSD and depression symptoms and the psychological distance of positive and negative events. *Journal of Behavior Therapy and Experimental Psychiatry, 48*, 177–184. https://doi.org/10.1016/j.jbtep.2015.04.002

Jassim, G. A., Doherty, S., Whitford, D. L., & Khashan, A. S. (2023). Psychological interventions for women with non-metastatic breast cancer. *Cochrane Database of Systematic Reviews, 2023*(1), Article CD008729. https://doi.org/10.1002/14651858.CD008729.pub3

Jaycox, L. H., Foa, E. B., & Morral, A. R. (1998). Influence of emotional engagement and habituation on exposure therapy for PTSD. *Journal of Consulting and Clinical Psychology, 66*(1), 185–192. https://doi.org/10.1037/0022-006X.66.1.185

Jennissen, S., Huber, J., Ehrenthal, J. C., Schauenburg, H., & Dinger, U. (2018). Association between insight and outcome of psychotherapy: Systematic review and meta-analysis. *The American Journal of Psychiatry, 175*(10), 961–969. https://doi.org/10.1176/appi.ajp.2018.17080847

Johansson, P., Høglend, P., Ulberg, R., Amlo, S., Marble, A., Bøgwald, K. P., Sørbye, O., Sjaastad, M. C., & Heyerdahl, O. (2010). The mediating role of insight for long-term improvements in psychodynamic therapy. *Journal of Consulting and Clinical Psychology, 78*(3), 438–448. https://doi.org/10.1037/a0019245

Johnson, J. (1999). *Minor characters: A beat memoir*. Penguin.

Johnson, M. W., Hendricks, P. S., Barrett, F. S., & Griffiths, R. R. (2019). Classic psychedelics: An integrative review of epidemiology, therapeutics, mystical experience, and brain network function. *Pharmacology & Therapeutics, 197*, 83–102. https://doi.org/10.1016/j.pharmthera.2018.11.010

Jones, G., Hanton, S., & Connaughton, D. (2007). A framework of mental toughness in the world's best performers. *The Sport Psychologist, 21*(2), 243–264. https://doi.org/10.1123/tsp.21.2.243

Julien, D., & O'Connor, K. P. (2017). Recasting psychodynamics into a behavioral framework: A review of the theory of psychopathology, treatment efficacy, and process of change of the affect phobia model. *Journal of Contemporary Psychotherapy, 47*(1), 1–10. https://doi.org/10.1007/s10879-016-9324-9

Kabat-Zinn, J. (2013). *Full catastrophe living: Using the wisdom of your body and mind to face stress, pain, and illness*. Bantam Dell.

Kahneman, D., Krueger, A. B., Schkade, D. A., Schwarz, N., & Stone, A. A. (2004). A survey method for characterizing daily life experience: The day reconstruction method. *Science, 306*(5702), 1776–1780. https://doi.org/10.1126/science.1103572

Kailanko, S., Wiebe, S. A., Tasca, G. A., & Laitila, A. A. (2022). Somatic interventions and depth of experiencing in emotionally focused couple therapy. *International Journal of Systemic Therapy, 33*(2), 109–128. https://doi.org/10.1080/2692398X.2022.2041346

Kalpakci, A., Venta, A., & Sharp, C. (2014). Beliefs about unmet interpersonal needs mediate the relation between conflictual family relations and borderline personality features in young adult females. *Borderline Personality Disorder and Emotion Dysregulation, 1*(1), Article 11. https://doi.org/10.1186/2051-6673-1-11

Kang, Y., Gruber, J., & Gray, J. R. (2013). Mindfulness and de-automatization. *Emotion Review, 5*(2), 192–201. https://doi.org/10.1177/1754073912451629

Kaplan, B. J., Crawford, S. G., Field, C. J., & Simpson, J. S. A. (2007). Vitamins, minerals, and mood. *Psychological Bulletin, 133*(5), 747–760. https://doi.org/10.1037/0033-2909.133.5.747

Kaplan, B. J., Rucklidge, J. J., Romijn, A., & McLeod, K. (2015). The emerging field of nutritional mental health: Inflammation, the microbiome, oxidative stress, and mitochondrial function. *Clinical Psychological Science, 3*(6), 964–980. https://doi.org/10.1177/2167702614555413

Karle, W., Corriere, R., & Hart, J. (1973). Psychophysiological changes in abreactive therapy: I. Primal therapy. *Psychotherapy: Theory, Research, & Practice, 10*(2), 117–122. https://doi.org/10.1037/h0087554

Kassam, K. S., & Mendes, W. B. (2013). The effects of measuring emotion: Physiological reactions to emotional situations depend on whether someone is asking. *PLOS One, 8*(6), Article e64959. https://doi.org/10.1371/journal.pone.0064959

Katzir, M., & Eyal, T. (2013). When stepping outside the self is not enough: A self-distancing perspective reduces the experience of basic but not of self-conscious emotions. *Journal of Experimental Social Psychology, 49*(6), 1089–1092. https://doi.org/10.1016/j.jesp.2013.07.006

Kazantzis, N., Luong, H. K., Usatoff, A. S., Impala, T., Yew, R. Y., & Hofmann, S. G. (2018). The processes of cognitive behavioral therapy: A review of meta-analyses. *Cognitive Therapy and Research, 42*(4), 349–357. https://doi.org/10.1007/s10608-018-9920-y

Kazdin, A. E. (2009). Understanding how and why psychotherapy leads to change. *Psychotherapy Research, 19*(4-5), 418–428. https://doi.org/10.1080/10503300802448899

Kennedy, M., & Franklin, J. (2002). Skills-based treatment for alexithymia: An exploratory case series. *Behaviour Change, 19*(3), 158–171. https://doi.org/10.1375/bech.19.3.158

Kennedy-Moore, E., & Watson, J. C. (2001). How and when does emotional expression help? *Review of General Psychology, 5*(3), 187–212. https://doi.org/10.1037/1089-2680.5.3.187

Khattra, J., Angus, L., Macaulay, C. B., & Carpenter, N. (2020). Narrative-emotion process markers in cognitive behavioral therapy for generalized anxiety disorder. *Journal of Constructivist Psychology, 33*(1), 89–102. https://doi.org/10.1080/10720537.2018.1546155

Khayyat-Abuaita, U., Paivio, S., Pascual-Leone, A., & Harrington, S. J. (2019). Emotional processing of trauma narratives is a predictor of outcome in emotion-focused therapy for complex trauma. *Psychotherapy: Theory, Research, & Practice, 56*(4), 526–536. https://doi.org/10.1037/pst0000238

King, L. A., & Raspin, C. (2004). Lost and found possible selves, subjective well-being, and ego development in divorced women. *Journal of Personality, 72*(3), 603–632. https://doi.org/10.1111/j.0022-3506.2004.00274.x

King, L. A., Scollon, C. K., Ramsey, C., & Williams, T. (2000). Stories of life transition: Subjective well-being and ego development in parents of children with Down syndrome. *Journal of Research in Personality, 34*(4), 509–536. https://doi.org/10.1006/jrpe.2000.2285

King, L. A., & Smith, N. G. (2004). Gay and straight possible selves: Goals, identity, subjective well-being, and personality development. *Journal of Personality, 72*(5), 967–994. https://doi.org/10.1111/j.0022-3506.2004.00287.x

King, M. L., Jr. (1977). *Strength to love.* Collins & Word.

Kipper, D. A., & Ritchie, T. D. (2003). The effectiveness of psychodramatic techniques: A meta-analysis. *Group Dynamics, 7*(1), 13–25. https://doi.org/10.1037/1089-2699.7.1.13

Kirby, L. A. J., & Robinson, J. L. (2017). Affective mapping: An activation likelihood estimation (ALE) meta-analysis. *Brain and Cognition, 118*, 137–148. https://doi.org/10.1016/j.bandc.2015.04.006

Kircanski, K., Lieberman, M. D., & Craske, M. G. (2012). Feelings into words: Contributions of language to exposure therapy. *Psychological Science, 23*(10), 1086–1091. https://doi.org/10.1177/0956797612443830

Klein, M. H., Mathieu-Coughlan, P., & Kiesler, D. J. (1986). The experiencing scales. In L. S. Greenberg & W. M. Pinsof (Eds.), *The psychotherapeutic process: A research handbook* (pp. 21–71). Guilford Press.

Klug, G., Seybert, C., Ratzek, M., Grimm, I., Zimmermann, J., & Huber, D. (2022). Insight and outcome in long-term psychotherapies of depression. *Zeitschrift für Psychosomatische Medizin und Psychotherapie, 68*(1), 54–73. https://doi.org/10.13109/zptm.2021.67.oa10

Koch, S., Holland, R. W., Hengstler, M., & van Knippenberg, A. (2009). Body locomotion as regulatory process: Stepping backward enhances cognitive control. *Psychological Science, 20*(5), 549–550. https://doi.org/10.1111/j.1467-9280.2009.02342.x

Kohler, H. P., & Mencarini, L. (2016). The parenthood happiness puzzle: An introduction to special issue. *European Journal of Population, 32*(3), 327–338. https://doi.org/10.1007/s10680-016-9392-2

Köhler, W. (1969). *The task of Gestalt psychology.* Princeton University Press. (Original work published 1929)

Korte, J., Bohlmeijer, E. T., Cappeliez, P., Smit, F., & Westerhof, G. J. (2012). Life review therapy for older adults with moderate depressive symptomatology: A pragmatic randomized controlled trial. *Psychological Medicine, 42*(6), 1163–1173. https://doi.org/10.1017/S0033291711002042

Kramer, U. (Ed.). (2019). *Case formulation for personality disorders: Tailoring psychotherapy to the individual client.* Elsevier Academic Press.

Kramer, U., Kolly, S., Maillard, P., Pascual-Leone, A., Samson, A. C., Herpertz, S., Schmitt, R., Bernini, A., Allenback, G., Charbon, P., de Roten, Y., Conus, P., Despland, J.-N., & Draganski, B. (2017, June). *Emotional and sociocognitive change after a short-term treatment for borderline personality disorder: A neurobehavioral paradigm* [Paper presentation]. International Society for Emotion Focused Therapy, Toronto, ON, Canada.

Kramer, U., Kolly, S., Maillard, P., Pascual-Leone, A., Samson, A. C., Schmitt, R., Bernini, A., Allenbach, G., Charbon, P., de Roten, Y., Conus, P., Despland, J.-N., & Draganski, B. (2018). Change in emotional and theory of mind processing in borderline personality disorder: A pilot study. *Journal of Nervous and Mental Disease, 206*(12), 935–943. https://doi.org/10.1097/NMD.0000000000000905

Kramer, U., & Pascual-Leone, A. (2012, August 29). *Emotional processing across long-term psychotherapy in a patient presenting with borderline personality disorder: A case study* [Conference presentation]. Forty-Second European Association for Behavioral and Cognitive Therapy Congress, Geneva, Switzerland.

Kramer, U., & Pascual-Leone, A. (2016). The role of maladaptive anger in self-criticism: A quasi-experimental study on emotional processes. *Counselling Psychology Quarterly, 29*(3), 311–333. https://doi.org/10.1080/09515070.2015.1090395

Kramer, U., & Pascual-Leone, A. (2018). Self-knowledge in personality disorders: An emotion-focused perspective. *Journal of Personality Disorders, 32*(3), 329–350. https://doi.org/10.1521/pedi.2018.32.3.329

Kramer, U., Pascual-Leone, A., Berthoud, L., de Roten, Y., Marquet, P., Kolly, S., Despland, J.-N., & Page, D. (2016). Assertive anger mediates effects of dialectical behaviour-informed skills training for borderline personality disorder: A randomized controlled trial. *Clinical Psychology & Psychotherapy, 23*(3), 189–202. https://doi.org/10.1002/cpp.1956

Kramer, U., Pascual-Leone, A., Despland, J.-N., & de Roten, Y. (2015). One minute of grief: Emotional processing in short-term dynamic psychotherapy for adjustment disorder. *Journal of Consulting and Clinical Psychology, 83*(1), 187–198. https://doi.org/10.1037/a0037979

Kramer, U., Pascual-Leone, A., Rohde, K. B., & Sachse, R. (2016). Emotional processing, interaction process, and outcome in clarification-oriented psychotherapy for personality disorders: A process-outcome analysis. *Journal of Personality Disorders, 30*(3), 373–394. https://doi.org/10.1521/pedi_2015_29_204

Kramer, U., Pascual-Leone, A., Rohde, K. B., & Sachse, R. (2018). The role of shame and self-compassion in psychotherapy for narcissistic personality disorder: An exploratory study. *Clinical Psychology & Psychotherapy, 25*(2), 272–282. https://doi.org/10.1002/cpp.2160

Kramer, U., & Sachse, R. (2013). Early clarification processes in clients presenting with borderline personality disorder: Relations with symptom levels and change. *Person-Centered and Experiential Psychotherapies, 12*(2), 157–175. https://doi.org/10.1080/14779757.2013.804647

Kross, E., & Ayduk, Ö. (2011). Making meaning out of negative experiences by self-distancing. *Current Directions in Psychological Science, 20*(3), 187–191. https://doi.org/10.1177/0963721411408883

Kross, E., Bruehlman-Senecal, E., Park, J., Burson, A., Dougherty, A., Shablack, H., Bremner, R., Moser, J., & Ayduk, O. (2014). Self-talk as a regulatory mechanism: How you do it matters. *Journal of Personality and Social Psychology, 106*(2), 304–324. https://doi.org/10.1037/a0035173

Kross, E., Vickers, B. D., Orvell, A., Gainsburg, I., Moran, T. P., Boyer, M., Jonides, J., Moser, J., & Ayduk, O. (2017). Third-person self-talk reduces Ebola worry and risk perception by enhancing rational thinking. *Applied Psychology: Health and Well-Being, 9*(3), 387–409. https://doi.org/10.1111/aphw.12103

Krueger, K. R., Murphy, J. W., & Bink, A. B. (2017). Thera-prov: A pilot study of improv used to treat anxiety and depression. *Journal of Mental Health, 28*(6), 621–626. https://doi.org/10.1080/09638237.2017.1340629

Kruse, E., Chancellor, J., Ruberton, P. M., & Lyubomirsky, S. (2014). An upward spiral between gratitude and humility. *Social Psychological & Personality Science, 5*(7), 805–814. https://doi.org/10.1177/1948550614534700

Kübler-Ross, E. (1969). *On death and dying*. The Macmillan Company.

Kübler-Ross, E., & Kessler, D. (2005). *On grief and grieving: Finding the meaning of grief through the five stages of loss*. Simon & Schuster.

Kuburi, S., Di Passa, A.-M., Tassone, V. K., Mahmood, R., Lalovic, A., Ladha, K. S., Dunlop, K., Rizvi, S., Demchenko, I., & Bhat, V. (2022). Neuroimaging correlates of treatment response with psychedelics in major depressive disorder: A systematic review. *Chronic Stress, 6*. https://doi.org/10.1177/24705470221115342

Kucharski, B., Strating, M., Ahluwalia Cameron, A., & Pascual-Leone, A. (2018). Complexity of emotion regulation strategies in changing contexts: A study of varsity athletes. *Journal of Contextual Behavioral Science, 10*, 85–91. https://doi.org/10.1016/j.jcbs.2018.09.002

Kundera, M. (1997). *Slowness*. Harper Perennial.

LaBelle, O. P., & Edelstein, R. S. (2018). Gratitude, insecure attachment, and positive outcomes among 12-step recovery program participants. *Addiction Research and Theory, 26*(2), 123–132. https://doi.org/10.1080/16066359.2017.1333111

Laird, J. D., & Berglas, S. (1975). Individual differences in the effects of engaging in counter-attitudinal behavior. *Journal of Personality, 43*(2), 286–304. https://doi.org/10.1111/j.1467-6494.1975.tb00707.x

Laird, J. D., & Lacasse, K. (2014). Bodily influences on emotional feelings: Accumulating evidence and extensions of William James's theory of emotion. *Emotion Review, 6*(1), 27–34. https://doi.org/10.1177/1754073913494899

Lamers, S. M. A., Bohlmeijer, E. T., Korte, J., & Westerhof, G. J. (2015). The efficacy of life-review as online-guided self-help for adults: A randomized trial. *The Journals of Gerontology: Series B, 70*(1), 24–34. https://doi.org/10.1093/geronb/gbu030

Landin-Romero, R., Moreno-Alcazar, A., Pagani, M., & Amann, B. L. (2018). How does eye movement desensitization and reprocessing therapy work? A systematic review on suggested mechanisms of action. *Frontiers in Psychology, 9*, Article 1395. https://doi.org/10.3389/fpsyg.2018.01395

Lane, R. D. (2020). Alexithymia 3.0: Reimagining alexithymia from a medical perspective. *BioPsychoSocial Medicine, 14*, Article 21. https://doi.org/10.1186/s13030-020-00191-x

Lane, R. D., & Nadel, L. (Eds.). (2020). *Neuroscience of enduring change: Implications for psychotherapy*. Oxford University Press. https://doi.org/10.1093/oso/9780190881511.001.0001

Lane, R. D., Reiman, E. M., Axelrod, B., Yun, L. S., Holmes, A., & Schwartz, G. E. (1998). Neural correlates of levels of emotional awareness. Evidence of an interaction between emotion and attention in the anterior cingulate cortex. *Journal of Cognitive Neuroscience, 10*(4), 525–535. https://doi.org/10.1162/089892998562924

Lane, R. D., Ryan, L., Nadel, L., & Greenberg, L. (2015). Memory reconsolidation, emotional arousal, and the process of change in psychotherapy: New insights from brain science. *The Behavioral and Brain Sciences, 38,* Article e1. https://doi.org/10.1017/S0140525X14000041

Lane, R. D., & Schwartz, G. E. (1987). Levels of emotional awareness: A cognitive-developmental theory and its application to psychopathology. *The American Journal of Psychiatry, 144*(2), 133–143.

Lang, P. J., Melamed, B. G., & Hart, J. (1970). A psychophysiological analysis of fear modification using an automated desensitization procedure. *Journal of Abnormal Psychology, 76*(2), 220–234. https://doi.org/10.1037/h0029875

Laoide, A. Ó., Egan, J., & Osborn, K. (2017). What was once essential, may become detrimental: The mediating role of depersonalization in the relationship between childhood emotional maltreatment and psychological distress in adults. *Journal of Trauma & Dissociation, 19*(5), 514–534. https://doi.org/10.1080/15299732.2017.1402398

Lauriola, M., Iannattone, S., & Bottesi, G. (2023). Intolerance of uncertainty and emotional processing in adolescence: Separating between-person stability and within-person change. *Research on Child and Adolescent Psychopathology, 51*(6), 871–884. https://doi.org/10.1007/s10802-022-01020-1

Le, H.-N., Berenbaum, H., & Raghavan, C. (2002). Culture and alexithymia: Mean levels, correlates, and the role of parental socialization of emotions. *Emotion, 2*(4), 341–360. https://doi.org/10.1037/1528-3542.2.4.341

Leahy, F., Ridout, N., Mushtaq, F., & Holland, C. (2018). Improving specific autobiographical memory in older adults: Impacts on mood, social problem solving, and functional limitations. *Aging, Neuropsychology, and Cognition, 25*(5), 695–723. https://doi.org/10.1080/13825585.2017.1365815

LeDoux, J. E., Moscarello, J., Sears, R., & Campese, V. (2017). The birth, death and resurrection of avoidance: A reconceptualization of a troubled paradigm. *Molecular Psychiatry, 22*(1), 24–36. https://doi.org/10.1038/mp.2016.166

Lee, H., Jang, S., Lee, S., & Hwang, K. (2015). Effectiveness of dance/movement therapy on affect and psychotic symptoms in patients with schizophrenia. *The Arts in Psychotherapy, 45,* 64–68. https://doi.org/10.1016/j.aip.2015.07.003

Lemmens, L. H. J. M., Galindo-Garre, F., Arntz, A., Peeters, F., Hollon, S. D., DeRubeis, R. J., & Huibers, M. J. H. (2017). Exploring mechanisms of change in cognitive therapy and interpersonal psychotherapy for adult depression. *Behaviour Research and Therapy, 94,* 81–92. https://doi.org/10.1016/j.brat.2017.05.005

Levant, R. F., Hall, R. J., Williams, C. M., & Hasan, N. T. (2009). Gender differences in alexithymia. *Psychology of Men & Masculinity, 10*(3), 190–203. https://doi.org/10.1037/a0015652

Lewis, C., Lovatt, P., & Kirk, E. (2015). Many hands make light work: The facilitative role of gesture in verbal improvisation. *Thinking Skills and Creativity, 17,* 149–157. https://doi.org/10.1016/j.tsc.2015.06.001

Lewis, R. M. (2004). *The planning, design and reception of British home front propaganda posters of the Second World War* [Doctoral thesis, University of Southampton]. Manchester Metropolitan University's Research Repository. https://core.ac.uk/download/pdf/161892177.pdf

Libby, L. K., & Eibach, R. P. (2002). Looking back in time: Self-concept change affects visual perspective in autobiographical memory. *Journal of Personality and Social Psychology, 82*(2), 167–179. https://doi.org/10.1037/0022-3514.82.2.167

Libby, L. K., & Eibach, R. P. (2011). Self-enhancement or self-coherence? Why people shift visual perspective in mental images of the personal past and future. *Personality and Social Psychology Bulletin, 37*(5), 714–726. https://doi.org/10.1177/0146167211400207

Libby, L. K., Valenti, G., Hines, K. A., & Eibach, R. P. (2014). Using imagery perspective to access two distinct forms of self-knowledge: Associative evaluations versus propositional self-beliefs. *Journal of Experimental Psychology: General, 143*(2), 492–497. https://doi.org/10.1037/a0033705

Liberman, N., & Trope, Y. (2014). Traversing psychological distance. *Trends in Cognitive Sciences, 18*(7), 364–369. https://doi.org/10.1016/j.tics.2014.03.001

Lieberman, M. D., Eisenberger, N. I., Crockett, M. J., Tom, S. M., Pfeifer, J. H., & Way, B. M. (2007). Putting feelings into words: Affect labeling disrupts amygdala activity in response to affective stimuli. *Psychological Science, 18*(5), 421–428. https://doi.org/10.1111/j.1467-9280.2007.01916.x

Lifshitz, C., Tsvieli, N., Bar-Kalifa, E., Abbott, C., Diamond, G. S., Roger Kobak, R., & Diamond, G. M. (2021). Emotional processing in attachment-based family therapy for suicidal adolescents. *Psychotherapy Research, 31*(2), 267–279. https://doi.org/10.1080/10503307.2020.1745315

Lilgendahl, J. P., & McAdams, D. P. (2011). Constructing stories of self-growth: How individual differences in patterns of autobiographical reasoning relate to well-being in midlife. *Journal of Personality, 79*(2), 391–428. https://doi.org/10.1111/j.1467-6494.2010.00688.x

Lin, L. (2021). Longitudinal associations of meaning in life and psychosocial adjustment to the COVID-19 outbreak in China. *British Journal of Health Psychology, 26*(2), 525–534. https://doi.org/10.1111/bjhp.12492

Lindell, A. K. (2014). On the interrelation between reduced lateralization, schizotypy, and creativity. *Frontiers in Psychology, 5*, Article 813. https://doi.org/10.3389/fpsyg.2014.00813

Lindquist, K. A., Satpute, A. B., Wager, T. D., Weber, J., & Barrett, L. F. (2016). The brain basis of positive and negative affect: Evidence from a meta-analysis of the human neuroimaging literature. *Cerebral Cortex, 26*(5), 1910–1922. https://doi.org/10.1093/cercor/bhv001

Linehan, M. M. (2015). *DBT skills training manual* (2nd ed.). Guilford Press.

Lo, C. (2014). Cultural values and alexithymia. *SAGE Open, 4*(4). https://doi.org/10.1177/2158244014555117

Lømo, B., Haavind, H., & Tjersland, O. A. (2019). Finding a common ground: Therapist responsiveness to male clients who have acted violently against their female partner. *Journal of Interpersonal Violence, 36*(17–18), NP9930–NP9958. https://doi.org/10.1177/0886260519862271

Lotan, G., Tanay, G., & Bernstein, A. (2013). Mindfulness and distress tolerance: Relations in a mindfulness preventive intervention. *International Journal of Cognitive Therapy, 6*(4), 371–385. https://doi.org/10.1521/ijct.2013.6.4.371

Löwel, S., & Singer, W. (1992). Selection of intrinsic horizontal connections in the visual cortex by correlated neuronal activity. *Science, 255*(5041), 209–212. https://doi.org/10.1126/science.1372754

Lu, Q., & Stanton, A. L. (2010). How benefits of expressive writing vary as a function of writing instructions, ethnicity and ambivalence over emotional expression. *Psychology & Health, 25*(6), 669–684. https://doi.org/10.1080/08870440902883196

Luborsky, L., Barber, J. P., & Diguer, L. (1992). The meanings of narratives told during psychotherapy: The fruits of a new observational unit. *Psychotherapy Research, 2*(4), 277–290. https://doi.org/10.1080/10503309212331333034

Luborsky, L., Popp, C., Luborsky, E., & Mark, D. (1994). The core conflictual relationship theme. *Psychotherapy Research, 4*(3–4), 172–183. https://doi.org/10.1080/10503309412331334012

Lumley, M. A. (2004). Alexithymia, emotional disclosure, and health: A program of research. *Journal of Personality, 72*(6), 1271–1300. https://doi.org/10.1111/j.1467-6494.2004.00297.x

Lumley, M. A., Cohen, J. L., Borszcz, G. S., Cano, A., Radcliffe, A. M., Porter, L. S., Schubiner, H., & Keefe, F. J. (2011). Pain and emotion: A biopsychosocial review of recent research. *Journal of Clinical Psychology, 67*(9), 942–968. https://doi.org/10.1002/jclp.20816

Lumley, M. A., Gustavson, B. J., Partridge, R. T., & Labouvie-Vief, G. (2005). Assessing alexithymia and related emotional ability constructs using multiple methods: Inter-relationships among measures. *Emotion, 5*(3), 329–342. https://doi.org/10.1037/1528-3542.5.3.329

Lumley, M. A., Schubiner, H., Lockhart, N. A., Kidwell, K. M., Harte, S. E., Clauw, D. J., & Williams, D. A. (2017). Emotional awareness and expression therapy, cognitive behavioral therapy, and education for fibromyalgia: A cluster-randomized controlled trial. *Pain, 158*(12), 2354–2363. https://doi.org/10.1097/j.pain.0000000000001036

Lutz, J., & Krahé, B. (2018). Inducing sadness reduces anger-driven aggressive behavior: A situational approach to aggression control. *Psychology of Violence, 8*(3), 358–366. https://doi.org/10.1037/vio0000167

Lynch, T. R., Chapman, A. L., Rosenthal, M. Z., Kuo, J. R., & Linehan, M. M. (2006). Mechanisms of change in dialectical behavior therapy: Theoretical and empirical observations. *Journal of Clinical Psychology, 62*(4), 459–480. https://doi.org/10.1002/jclp.20243

Lyubomirsky, S., Dickerhoof, R., Boehm, J. K., & Sheldon, K. M. (2011). Becoming happier takes both a will and a proper way: An experimental longitudinal intervention to boost well-being. *Emotion, 11*(2), 391–402. https://doi.org/10.1037/a0022575

Macaulay, C. B., & Angus, L. E. (2019). Narrative-Emotion Process model: An integrative approach to working with complex posttraumatic stress. *Journal of Psychotherapy Integration, 29*(1), 42–53. https://doi.org/10.1037/int0000118

MacCormack, J. K., & Lindquist, K. A. (2019). Feeling hangry? When hunger is conceptualized as emotion. *Emotion, 19*(2), 301–319. https://doi.org/10.1037/emo0000422

Maciejewski, P. K., Zhang, B., Block, S. D., & Prigerson, H. G. (2007). An empirical examination of the stage theory of grief. *JAMA, 297*(7), 716–723. https://doi.org/10.1001/jama.297.7.716

Mackay, H. C., Barkham, M., Stiles, W. B., & Goldfried, M. R. (2002). Patterns of client emotion in helpful sessions of cognitive-behavioral and psychodynamic-interpersonal therapy. *Journal of Counseling Psychology, 49*(3), 376–380. https://doi.org/10.1037/0022-0167.49.3.376

Mackintosh, M.-A., Morland, L. A., Frueh, B. C., Greene, C. J., & Rosen, C. S. (2014). Peeking into the black box: Mechanisms of action for anger management treatment. *Journal of Anxiety Disorders, 28*(7), 687–695. https://doi.org/10.1016/j.janxdis.2014.07.001

Madore, K. P., & Schacter, D. L. (2014). An episodic specificity induction enhances means-end problem solving in young and older adults. *Psychology and Aging, 29*(4), 913–924. https://doi.org/10.1037/a0038209

Malan, D. H. (1979). *Individual psychotherapy and the science of psychodynamics.* Butterworth.

Malcolm, W., Warwar, S., & Greenberg, L. (2005). Facilitating forgiveness in individual therapy as an approach to resolving interpersonal injuries. In E. J. Worthington, Jr., (Ed.), *The handbook of forgiveness* (pp. 379–393). Routledge.

Manco, N., & Hamby, S. (2021). A meta-analytic review of interventions that promote meaning in life. *American Journal of Health Promotion, 35*(6), 866–873. https://doi.org/10.1177/0890117121995736

Manson, M. (2016). *The subtle art of not giving a f*ck: A counterintuitive approach to living a good life.* Harper Collins.

Margariti, A., Ktonas, P., Hondraki, P., Daskalopoulou, E., Kyriakopoulos, G., Economou, N. T., Tsekou, H., Paparrigopoulos, T., Barbousi, V., & Vaslamatzis, G. (2012). An application of the primitive expression form of dance therapy in a psychiatric population. *The Arts in Psychotherapy, 39*(2), 95–101. https://doi.org/10.1016/j.aip.2012.01.001

Marinary. (2013, September 15). *Fritz Perls: A session with college students* [Video]. YouTube. https://youtu.be/ZsZqJXf4vMI

Marks, E. H., Walker, R. S. W., Ojalehto, H., Bedard-Gilligan, M. A., & Zoellner, L. A. (2019). Affect labeling to facilitate inhibitory learning: Clinical considerations. *Cognitive and Behavioral Practice, 26*(1), 201–213. https://doi.org/10.1016/j.cscbpra.2018.05.001

Marshall, W. L., Marshall, L. E., Serran, G. A., & O'Brien, M. D. (Eds.). (2011). *Rehabilitating sexual offenders: A strength–based approach.* American Psychological Association. https://doi.org/10.1037/12310-000

Martin, J., Cummings, A. L., & Hallberg, E. T. (1992). Therapists' intentional use of metaphor: Memorability, clinical impact, and possible epistemic/motivational functions. *Journal of Consulting and Clinical Psychology, 60*(1), 143–145. https://doi.org/10.1037/0022-006X.60.1.143

Maruna, S. (2001). *Making good: How ex-convicts reform and rebuild their lives.* American Psychological Association. https://doi.org/10.1037/10430-000

Maruna, S., Wilson, L., & Curran, K. (2006). Why God is often found behind bars: Prison conversions and the crisis of self-narrative. *Research in Human Development, 3*(2–3), 161–184. https://doi.org/10.1080/15427609.2006.9683367

Mattingley, S., Youssef, G. J., Manning, V., Graeme, L., & Hall, K. (2022). Distress tolerance across substance use, eating, and borderline personality disorders: A meta-analysis. *Journal of Affective Disorders, 300,* 492–504. https://doi.org/10.1016/j.jad.2021.12.126

Maturana, H., & Varela, F. (1980). *Autopoesis and cognition: The realization of the living.* D. Reidel. https://doi.org/10.1007/978-94-009-8947-4

Mauss, I. B., & Robinson, M. D. (2009). Measures of emotion: A review. *Cognition and Emotion, 23*(2), 209–237. https://doi.org/10.1080/02699930802204677

Maxwell, K., Callahan, J. L., Holtz, P., Janis, B. M., Gerber, M. M., & Connor, D. R. (2016). Comparative study of group treatments for posttraumatic stress disorder. *Psychotherapy: Theory, Research, & Practice, 53*(4), 433–445. https://doi.org/10.1037/pst0000032

May, R. (1983). *The discovery of being: Writings in existential psychology.* W. W. Norton & Company.

May, R., & Yalom, I. D. (1989). Existential psychotherapy. In R. J. Corsini & D. Wedding (Eds.), *Current psychotherapies* (4th ed., pp. 363–402). F. E. Peacock Publishers.

Mayer, E. (2016). *The mind–gut connection: How the hidden conversation within our bodies impacts our mood, our choices, and our overall health.* Harper Collins.

Mazzoni, G., Scoboria, A., & Harvey, L. (2010). Nonbelieved memories. *Psychological Science, 21*(9), 1334–1340. https://doi.org/10.1177/0956797610379865

McAdams, D. P. (2019). Continuity and growth in the life story—Or is it stagnation and flux? *Qualitative Psychology, 6*(2), 206–214. https://doi.org/10.1037/qup0000151

McAdams, D. P., Bauer, J. J., Sakaeda, A. R., Anyidoho, N. A., Machado, M. A., Magrino-Failla, K., White, K. W., & Pals, J. L. (2006). Continuity and change in the life story: A longitudinal study of autobiographical memories in emerging adulthood. *Journal of Personality, 74*(5), 1371–1400. https://doi.org/10.1111/j.1467-6494.2006.00412.x

McAdams, D. P., Reynolds, J., Lewis, M., Patten, A., & Bowman, P. J. (2001). When bad things turn good and good things turn bad: Sequences of redemption and contamination in life narrative, and their relation to psychosocial adaptation in midlife adults and in students. *Personality and Social Psychology Bulletin, 27*(4), 474–483. https://doi.org/10.1177/0146167201274008

McCraty, R., Atkinson, M., Tiller, W. A., Rein, G., & Watkins, A. D. (1995). The effects of emotions on short-term power spectrum analysis of heart rate variability. *The American Journal of Cardiology, 76*(14), 1089–1093. https://doi.org/10.1016/S0002-9149(99)80309-9

McCullough, L., Kuhn, N., Andrews, S., Kaplan, A., Wolf, J., & Hurley, C. L. (2003). *Treating affect phobia: A manual for short-term dynamic psychotherapy.* Guilford Press.

McCullough, L., Larsen, A. E., Schanche, E., Andrews, S., & Kuhn, N. (2008). *Achievement of Therapeutic Objectives Scale: ATOS scale.* https://affectphobiatherapy.com/wp-content/uploads/2013/10/ATOS-scale-manual.pdf

McHugh, R. K., & Otto, M. W. (2012). Refining the measurement of distress intolerance. *Behavior Therapy, 43*(3), 641–651. https://doi.org/10.1016/j.beth.2011.12.001

McIsaac, H. K., & Eich, E. (2004). Vantage point in traumatic memory. *Psychological Science, 15*(4), 248–253. https://doi.org/10.1111/j.0956-7976.2004.00660.x

McLaughlin, K. A., Colich, N. L., Rodman, A. M., & Weissman, D. G. (2020). Mechanisms linking childhood trauma exposure and psychopathology: A transdiagnostic model of risk and resilience. *BMC Medicine, 18*(1), 96. https://doi.org/10.1186/s12916-020-01561-6

McLean, K. C., Lilgendahl, J. P., Fordham, C., Alpert, E., Marsden, E., Szymanowski, K., & McAdams, D. P. (2018). Identity development in cultural context: The role of deviating from master narratives. *Journal of Personality, 86*(4), 631–651. https://doi.org/10.1111/jopy.12341

McLean, K. C., Pasupathi, M., & Pals, J. L. (2007). Selves creating stories creating selves: A process model of self-development. *Personality and Social Psychology Review, 11*(3), 262–278. https://doi.org/10.1177/1088868307301034

McLean, K. C., & Pratt, M. W. (2006). Life's little (and big) lessons: Identity statuses and meaning-making in the turning point narratives of emerging adults. *Developmental Psychology, 42*(4), 714–722. https://doi.org/10.1037/0012-1649.42.4.714

McLean, K. C., Syed, M., Pasupathi, M., Adler, J. M., Dunlop, W. L., Drustrup, D., Fivush, R., Graci, M. E., Lilgendahl, J. P., Lodi-Smith, J., McAdams, D. P., & McCoy, T. P. (2020). The empirical structure of narrative identity: The initial big three. *Journal of Personality and Social Psychology, 119*(4), 920–944. https://doi.org/10.1037/pspp0000247

McMain, S. F., Goldman, R. N., & Greenberg, L. S. (1996). Resolving unfinished business: A program of study. In W. Dryden (Ed.), *Research in counselling and psychotherapy* (pp. 211–232). Sage. https://doi.org/10.4135/9781446279786.n9

McMain, S., Links, P. S., Guimond, T., Wnuk, S., Eynan, R., Bergmans, Y., & Warwar, S. (2013). An exploratory study of the relationship between changes in emotion and cognitive processes and treatment outcome in borderline personality disorder. *Psychotherapy Research, 23*(6), 658–673. https://doi.org/10.1080/10503307.2013.838653

McNally, S., Timulak, L., & Greenberg, L. S. (2014). Transforming emotion schemes in emotion focused therapy: A case study investigation. *Person-Centered and Experiential Psychotherapies, 13*(2), 128–149. https://doi.org/10.1080/14779757.2013.871573

McVea, C. S., Gow, K., & Lowe, R. (2011). Corrective interpersonal experience in psychodrama group therapy: A comprehensive process analysis of significant therapeutic events. *Psychotherapy Research, 21*(4), 416–429. https://doi.org/10.1080/10503307.2011.577823

Meisiek, S. (2004). Which catharsis do they mean? Aristotle, Moreno, Boal and organization theatre. *Organization Studies, 25*(5), 797–816. https://doi.org/10.1177/0170840604042415

Memarian, N., Torre, J. B., Haltom, K. E., Stanton, A. L., & Lieberman, M. D. (2017). Neural activity during affect labeling predicts expressive writing effects on well-being: GLM and SVM approaches. *Social Cognitive and Affective Neuroscience, 12*(9), 1437–1447. https://doi.org/10.1093/scan/nsx084

Memedovic, S., Grisham, J. R., Denson, T. F., & Moulds, M. L. (2010). The effects of trait reappraisal and suppression on anger and blood pressure in response to provocation. *Journal of Research in Personality, 44*(4), 540–543. https://doi.org/10.1016/j.jrp.2010.05.002

Meneses, C. W., & Greenberg, L. S. (2011). The construction of a model of the process of couples' forgiveness in emotion-focused therapy for couples. *Journal of Marital and Family Therapy, 37*(4), 491–502. https://doi.org/10.1111/j.1752-0606.2011.00234.x

Mergenthaler, E. (1996). Emotion-abstraction patterns in verbatim protocols: A new way of describing psychotherapeutic processes. *Journal of Consulting and Clinical Psychology, 64*(6), 1306–1315. https://doi.org/10.1037/0022-006X.64.6.1306

Messer, S. B., & McWilliams, N. (2006). Insight in psychodynamic therapy: Theory and assessment. In L. G. Castonguay & C. Hill (Eds.), *Insight in psychotherapy* (pp. 9–29). American Psychological Association. https://doi.org/10.1037/11532-001

Michalak, J., Mischnat, J., & Teismann, T. (2014). Sitting posture makes a difference— Embodiment effects on depressive memory bias. *Clinical Psychology & Psychotherapy, 21*(6), 519–524. https://doi.org/10.1002/cpp.1890

Michalak, J., Rohde, K., & Troje, N. F. (2015). How we walk affects what we remember: Gait modifications through biofeedback change negative affective memory bias. *Journal of Behavior Therapy and Experimental Psychiatry, 46,* 121–125. https://doi.org/10.1016/j.jbtep.2014.09.004

Miller, W. R., & Rollnick, S. (2013). *Motivational interviewing: Helping people change* (3rd ed.). Guilford Press.

Minuchin, S. (2012). *Families and family therapy* (2nd ed.). Routledge.

Missirlian, T. M., Toukmanian, S. G., Warwar, S. H., & Greenberg, L. S. (2005). Emotional arousal, client perceptual processing, and the working alliance in experiential psychotherapy for depression. *Journal of Consulting and Clinical Psychology, 73*(5), 861– 871. https://doi.org/10.1037/0022-006X.73.5.861

Mlotek, A. (2013). *The contribution of therapy empathy to client engagement and outcome in emotion-focused therapy for complex trauma* (Publication No. 4921) [Master's thesis, University of Windsor]. Electronic Theses and Dissertations.

Mlotek, A. (2018). *Contributions of emotional competence to the link between childhood maltreatment and adult attachment* (Publication No. 7649) [Doctoral dissertation, University of Windsor]. Electronic Theses and Dissertations.

Mohaupt, H., Duckert, F., & Askeland, I. R. (2020). How do men in treatment for intimate partner violence experience parenting their young child? A descriptive phenomenological analysis. *Journal of Family Violence, 35*(8), 863–875. https://doi.org/10.1007/s10896-019-00083-x

Mohr, D. C., Shoham-Salomon, V., Engle, D., & Beutler, L. E. (1991). The expression of anger in psychotherapy for depression: Its role and measurement. *Psychotherapy Research, 1*(2), 124–134. https://doi.org/10.1080/10503309112331335551

Moore, M. T., Lau, M. A., Haigh, E. A. P., Willett, B. R., Bosma, C. M., & Fresco, D. M. (2022). Association between decentering and reductions in relapse/recurrence in mindfulness-based cognitive therapy for depression in adults: A randomized controlled trial. *Journal of Consulting and Clinical Psychology, 90*(2), 137–147. https://doi.org/10.1037/ccp0000718

Moore, S. (1984). *The Stanislavski system.* Penguin.

Moormann, P. P., Bermond, B., Vorst, H. C. M., Bloemendaal, A. F. T., Teijn, S. M., & Rood, L. (2008). New avenues in alexithymia research: The creation of alexithymia types. In J. Denollet, A. J. M. Vingerhoets, & T. Nyklicek (Eds.), *Emotion regulation: Conceptual and clinical issues* (pp. 27–42). Springer. https://doi.org/10.1007/978-0-387-29986-0_3

Moreno, J. L. (1958). *Psychodrama* (Vol. 2). Beacon House.

Moreno, J. L. (Director). (1964). *Psychodrama of a marriage: A motion picture.* Radio and Television Center of France. https://youtu.be/zvgnOVfLn4k

Morris, C., Simpson, J., Sampson, M., & Beesley, F. (2014). Cultivating positive emotions: A useful adjunct when working with people who self-harm? *Clinical Psychology & Psychotherapy, 21*(4), 352–362. https://doi.org/10.1002/cpp.1836

Moscarello, J. M., & Hartley, C. A. (2017). Agency and the calibration of motivated behavior. *Trends in Cognitive Sciences, 21*(10), 725–735. https://doi.org/10.1016/j.tics.2017.06.008

Mundorf, E. S., & Paivio, S. C. (2011). Narrative quality and disturbance pre- and post-emotion-focused therapy for child abuse trauma. *Journal of Traumatic Stress, 24*(6), 643–650. https://doi.org/10.1002/jts.20707

Muntigl, P., Horvath, A. O., Chubak, L., & Angus, L. (2020). Getting to "yes": Client reluctance to engage in chairwork. *Frontiers in Psychology, 11,* Article 582856. https://doi.org/10.3389/fpsyg.2020.582856

Muran, J. C., Teachman, B., Aldao, A., Ehrenreich-May, J., Fonagy, P., Greenberg, L., Gross, J., Magnavita, J., Mayo-Wilson, E., McMain, S., Angel Soto, J., Bufka, L., Halfond, R., Kurtzman, H., & Marzalik, S. J. (2024). *Proposal to develop a clinical practice guideline on emotion regulation: Final report.* American Psychological Association.

Muschalla, B., & Schönborn, F. (2021). Induction of false beliefs and false memories in laboratory studies—A systematic review. *Clinical Psychology & Psychotherapy, 28*(5), 1194–1209. https://doi.org/10.1002/cpp.2567

Myung, H. S., Furrow, J. L., & Lee, N. A. (2022). Understanding the emotional landscape in the withdrawer re-engagement and blamer softening EFCT change events. *Journal of Marital and Family Therapy, 48*(3), 758–776. https://doi.org/10.1111/jmft.12583

Naragon-Gainey, K., & DeMarree, K. G. (2017). Structure and validity of measures of decentering and defusion. *Psychological Assessment, 29*(7), 935–954. https://doi.org/10.1037/pas0000405

Nardone, S., Baher, T., & Pascual-Leone, A. (2025). Changing emotion with emotion: The best sequence depends on the target concern. *Cognitive Therapy and Research.* Advance online publication. https://doi.org/10.1007/s10608-025-10590-5

Nardone, S., Pascual-Leone, A., & Kramer, U. (2022). "Strike while the iron is hot": Increased arousal anticipates unmet needs. *Counselling Psychology Quarterly, 35*(1), 110–128. https://doi.org/10.1080/09515070.2021.1955659

Nardone, S., Pascual-Leone, A., Kramer, U., Cristoffanini, F., Grandjean, L., Culina, I., & McMain, S. (2024). Emotions observed during sessions of dialectical behavior therapy predict outcome for borderline personality disorder. *Journal of Consulting and Clinical Psychology, 92*(9), 607–618. https://doi.org/10.1037/ccp0000903

Narkiss-Guez, T., Zichor, Y. E., Guez, J., & Diamond, G. M. (2015). Intensifying attachment-related sadness and decreasing anger intensity among individuals suffering from unresolved anger: The role of relational reframe followed by empty-chair interventions. *Counselling Psychology Quarterly, 28*(1), 44–56. https://doi.org/10.1080/09515070.2014.924480

Neacsiu, A. D., Rizvi, S. L., & Linehan, M. M. (2010). Dialectical behavior therapy skills use as a mediator and outcome of treatment for borderline personality disorder. *Behaviour Research and Therapy, 48*(9), 832–839. https://doi.org/10.1016/j.brat.2010.05.017

Neshat-Doost, H. T., Dalgleish, T., Yule, W., Kalantari, M., Ahmadi, S. J., Dyregrov, A., & Jobson, L. (2013). Enhancing autobiographical memory specificity through cognitive training: An intervention for depression translated from basic science. *Clinical Psychological Science, 1*(1), 84–92. https://doi.org/10.1177/2167702612454613

Neves, D., & Pinho, M. S. (2016). Specificity and emotional characteristics of the autobiographical memories of male and female criminal offenders. *Criminal Justice and Behavior, 43*(5), 670–690. https://doi.org/10.1177/0093854815613820

Nichols, M. P., & Efran, J. S. (1985). Catharsis in psychotherapy: A new perspective. *Psychotherapy: Theory, Research, & Practice, 22*(1), 46–58. https://doi.org/10.1037/h0088525

Niles, A. N., Byrne Haltom, K. E., Lieberman, M. D., Hur, C., & Stanton, A. L. (2016). Writing content predicts benefit from written expressive disclosure: Evidence for repeated exposure and self-affirmation. *Cognition and Emotion, 30*(2), 258–274. https://doi.org/10.1080/02699931.2014.995598

Niles, A. N., Craske, M. G., Lieberman, M. D., & Hur, C. (2015). Affect labeling enhances exposure effectiveness for public speaking anxiety. *Behaviour Research and Therapy, 68,* 27–36. https://doi.org/10.1016/j.brat.2015.03.004

Niles, A. N., Haltom, K. E., Mulvenna, C. M., Lieberman, M. D., & Stanton, A. L. (2014). Randomized controlled trial of expressive writing for psychological and physical health: The moderating role of emotional expressivity. *Anxiety, Stress, and Coping, 27*(1), 1–17. https://doi.org/10.1080/10615806.2013.802308

Noah, T., Schul, Y., & Mayo, R. (2018). When both the original study and its failed replication are correct: Feeling observed eliminates the facial-feedback effect. *Journal of Personality and Social Psychology, 114*(5), 657–664. https://doi.org/10.1037/pspa0000121

Nock, M. K., & Prinstein, M. J. (2004). A functional approach to the assessment of self-mutilative behavior. *Journal of Consulting and Clinical Psychology, 72*(5), 885–890. https://doi.org/10.1037/0022-006X.72.5.885

Nolen-Hoeksema, S. (1991). Responses to depression and their effects on the duration of depressive episodes. *Journal of Abnormal Psychology, 100*(4), 569–582. https://doi.org/10.1037/0021-843X.100.4.569

Nook, E. C., Sasse, S. F., Lambert, H. K., McLaughlin, K. A., & Somerville, L. H. (2018). The nonlinear development of emotion differentiation: Granular emotional experience is low in adolescence. *Psychological Science, 29*(8), 1346–1357. https://doi.org/10.1177/0956797618773357

Nord, C. L., Halahakoon, D. C., Limbachya, T., Charpentier, C., Lally, N., Walsh, V., Leibowitz, J., Pilling, S., & Roiser, J. P. (2019). Neural predictors of treatment response to brain stimulation and psychological therapy in depression: A double-blind randomized controlled trial. *Neuropsychopharmacology, 44*(9), 1613–1622. https://doi.org/10.1038/s41386-019-0401-0

Northoff, G., Heinzel, A., de Greck, M., Bermpohl, F., Dobrowolny, H., & Panksepp, J. (2006). Self-referential processing in our brain—A meta-analysis of imaging studies on the self. *NeuroImage, 31*(1), 440–457. https://doi.org/10.1016/j.neuroimage.2005.12.002

Nowlan, J. S., Wuthrich, V. M., Rapee, R. M., Kinsella, J. M., & Barker, G. (2016). A comparison of single-session positive reappraisal, cognitive restructuring and supportive counselling for older adults with Type 2 diabetes. *Cognitive Therapy and Research, 40*(2), 216–229. https://doi.org/10.1007/s10608-015-9737-x

Ogden, P., & Fisher, J. (2015). *Sensorimotor psychotherapy: Interventions for trauma and attachment.* W. W. Norton & Company.

Ogles, B. M. (2013). Measuring change in psychotherapy research. In M. J. Lambert (Ed.), *Bergin and Garfield's handbook of psychotherapy and behavior change* (6th ed., pp. 134–166). John Wiley & Sons.

Ogrodniczuk, J. S., Joyce, A. S., & Abbass, A. A. (2014). Childhood maltreatment and somatic complaints among adult psychiatric outpatients: Exploring the mediating role of alexithymia. *Psychotherapy and Psychosomatics, 83*(5), 322–324. https://doi.org/10.1159/000363769

Ogrodniczuk, J. S., Joyce, A. S., & Piper, W. E. (2013). Change in alexithymia in two dynamically informed individual psychotherapies. *Psychotherapy and Psychosomatics, 82*(1), 61–63. https://doi.org/10.1159/000341180

Ogrodniczuk, J. S., Kealy, D., Joyce, A. S., & Abbass, A. A. (2018). Body talk: Sex differences in the influence of alexithymia on physical complaints among psychiatric outpatients. *Psychiatry Research, 261*, 168–172. https://doi.org/10.1016/j.psychres.2017.12.072

Ogrodniczuk, J. S., Piper, W. E., & Joyce, A. S. (2011). Effect of alexithymia on the process and outcome of psychotherapy: A programmatic review. *Psychiatry Research, 190*(1), 43–48. https://doi.org/10.1016/j.psychres.2010.04.026

Orsillo, S. M., Roemer, L., Block Lerner, J., & Tull, M. T. (2004). Acceptance, mindfulness, and cognitive–behavioral therapy: Comparisons, contrasts, and application to anxiety. In S. C. Hayes, V. M. Follette, & M. M. Linehan (Eds.), *Mindfulness and acceptance: Expanding the cognitive–behavioral tradition* (pp. 66–95). Guilford Press.

Ortega y Gasset, J. (1914). *Meditaciones del Quixote* [Meditations on Don Quixote]. Residencia de Estudiantes.

Orvell, A., Vickers, B. D., Drake, B., Verduyn, P., Ayduk, O., Moser, J., Jonides, J., & Kross, E. (2021). Does distanced self-talk facilitate emotion regulation across a range of emotionally intense experiences? *Clinical Psychological Science, 9*(1), 68–78. https://doi.org/10.1177/2167702620951539

Osborn, K. A. R., Ulvenes, P. G., Wampold, B. E., & McCullough, L. (2015). Creating change through focusing on affect: Affect phobia therapy. In N. C. Thoma & D. McKay (Eds.), *Working with emotion in cognitive-behavioral therapy: Techniques for clinical practice* (pp. 146–171). Guilford Press.

Owen, J., Adelson, J., Budge, S., Wampold, B., Kopta, M., Minami, T., & Miller, S. (2015). Trajectories of change in psychotherapy. *Journal of Clinical Psychology, 71*(9), 817–827. https://doi.org/10.1002/jclp.22191

Paivio, S. C., Hall, I. E., Holowaty, K. A. M., Jellis, J. B., & Tran, N. (2001). Imaginal confrontation for resolving child abuse issues. *Psychotherapy Research, 11*(4), 433–453. https://doi.org/10.1093/ptr/11.4.433

Paivio, S. C., Holowaty, K. A. M., & Hall, I. E. (2004). The influence of therapist adherence and competence on client reprocessing of child abuse memories. *Psychotherapy: Theory, Research, & Practice, 41*(1), 56–68. https://doi.org/10.1037/0033-3204.41.1.56

Paivio, S. C., Jarry, J. L., Chagigiorgis, H., Hall, I., & Ralston, M. (2010). Efficacy of two versions of emotion-focused therapy for resolving child abuse trauma. *Psychotherapy Research, 20*(3), 353–366. https://doi.org/10.1080/10503300903505274

Paivio, S. C., & Laurent, C. (2001). Empathy and emotion regulation: Reprocessing memories of childhood abuse. *Journal of Clinical Psychology, 57*(2), 213–226. https://doi.org/b57n59

Paivio, S. C., & McCulloch, C. R. (2004). Alexithymia as a mediator between childhood trauma and self-injurious behaviors. *Child Abuse & Neglect, 28*(3), 339–354. https://doi.org/10.1016/j.chiabu.2003.11.018

Paivio, S. C., & Nieuwenhuis, J. A. (2001). Efficacy of emotion focused therapy for adult survivors of childhood abuse: A preliminary study. *Journal of Traumatic Stress, 14*(1), 115–133. https://doi.org/10.1023/A:1007891716593

Paivio, S. C., & Pascual-Leone, A. (2023). *Emotion focused therapy for complex trauma: An integrative approach* (2nd ed.). American Psychological Association. https://doi.org/10.1037/0000336-000

Pals, J. L. (2006a). Constructing the "springboard effect": Causal connections, self-making, and growth within the life story. In D. P. McAdams, R. Josselson, & A. Lieblich (Eds.), *Identity and story: Creating self in narrative* (pp. 175–199). American Psychological Association. https://doi.org/10.1037/11414-008

Pals, J. L. (2006b). Narrative identity processing of difficult life experiences: Pathways of personality development and positive self-transformation in adulthood. *Journal of Personality, 74*(4), 1079–1110. https://doi.org/10.1111/j.1467-6494.2006.00403.x

Panksepp, J. (2008). The affective brain and core consciousness: How does neural activity generate emotional feelings? In M. Lewis, J. M. Haviland-Jones, & L. F. Barrett (Eds.), *Handbook of emotions* (3rd ed., pp. 47–67). Guilford Press.

Park, J., Ayduk, Ö., & Kross, E. (2016). Stepping back to move forward: Expressive writing promotes self-distancing. *Emotion, 16*(3), 349–364. https://doi.org/10.1037/emo0000121

Parker, R. G. (1995). Reminiscence: A continuity theory framework. *The Gerontologist, 35*(4), 515–525. https://doi.org/10.1093/geront/35.4.515

Pascal, B. (1995). *Pensées* [Thoughts]. Penguin Classics. (Original work published 1669)

Pascual-Leone, A. (2009). Dynamic emotional processing in experiential therapy: Two steps forward, one step back. *Journal of Consulting and Clinical Psychology, 77*(1), 113–126. https://doi.org/10.1037/a0014488

Pascual-Leone, A. (2018). How clients "change emotion with emotion": A programme of research on emotional processing. *Psychotherapy Research, 28*(2), 165–182. https://doi.org/10.1080/10503307.2017.1349350

Pascual-Leone, A., & Baher, T. (2023). Chairwork. In C. E. Hill & J. C. Norcross (Eds.), *Psychotherapy skills and methods that work* (pp. 547–576). Oxford University Press. https://doi.org/10.1093/oso/9780197611012.003.0018

Pascual-Leone, A., Bierman, R., Arnold, R., & Stasiak, E. (2011). Emotion-focused therapy for incarcerated offenders of intimate partner violence: A 3-year outcome using a new whole-sample matching method. *Psychotherapy Research, 21*(3), 331–347. https://doi.org/10.1080/10503307.2011.572092

Pascual-Leone, A., Gilles, P., Singh, T., & Andreescu, C. (2013). Problem anger in psychotherapy: An emotion-focused perspective on hate, rage, and rejecting anger. *Journal of Contemporary Psychotherapy, 43*(2), 83–92. https://doi.org/10.1007/s10879-012-9214-8

Pascual-Leone, A., Gillespie, N. M., Orr, E. S., & Harrington, S. J. (2016). Measuring subtypes of emotion regulation: From broad behavioural skills to idiosyncratic meaning-making. *Clinical Psychology & Psychotherapy, 23*(3), 203–216. https://doi.org/10.1002/cpp.1947

Pascual-Leone, A., & Greenberg, L. S. (2007a). Emotional processing in experiential therapy: Why "the only way out is through." *Journal of Consulting and Clinical Psychology, 75*(6), 875–887. https://doi.org/10.1037/0022-006X.75.6.875

Pascual-Leone, A., & Greenberg, L. S. (2007b). Insight and awareness in experiential therapy. In L. G. Castonguay & C. E. Hill (Eds.), *Insight in psychotherapy* (pp. 31–56). American Psychological Association. https://doi.org/10.1037/11532-002

Pascual-Leone, A., & Greenberg, L. S. (2020). Emotion-focused therapy: Integrating neuroscience and practice. In R. D. Lane & L. Nadel (Eds.), *Neuroscience of enduring change: Implications for psychotherapy* (pp. 215–244). Oxford University Press.

Pascual-Leone, A., Herpertz, S. C., & Kramer, U. (2016). Experimental designs and the "emotion-stimulus critique": Hidden problems and potential solutions in the study of emotion. *Psychopathology, 49*(1), 60–68. https://doi.org/10.1159/000442294

Pascual-Leone, A., & Kramer, U. (2017). Developing emotion-based case formulations: A research-informed method. *Clinical Psychology & Psychotherapy, 24*(1), 212–225. https://doi.org/10.1002/cpp.1998

Pascual-Leone, A., & Kramer, U. (2019). How clients "change emotion with emotion": Sequences in emotional processing and their clinical implications. In L. S. Greenberg & R. N. Goldman (Eds.), *Handbook of emotion focused therapy* (pp. 147–170). American Psychological Association. https://doi.org/10.1037/0000112-007

Pascual-Leone, A., & Kramer, U. (2023). Advancing the assessment of emotional change: A matrix of processes by methods. *Journal of Psychotherapy Integration, 33*(4), 341–347. https://doi.org/10.1037/int0000312

Pascual-Leone, A., Metler, S., Singh, T., Harrington, S., Yeryomenko, N., Crozier, M. Sirois, F., Morrison, O., & Porter, L. (2012, August). *Experimental manipulation of emotion during a writing task: Implication for the practice of psychotherapy* [Conference presentation]. European Association for Behavioral and Cognitive Therapy, Geneva, Switzerland.

Pascual-Leone, A., Paivio, S., & Harrington, S. (2016). Emotion in psychotherapy: An experiential–humanistic perspective. In D. Cain, S. Rubin, & K. Keenan (Eds.), *Humanistic psychotherapies: Handbook of research and practice* (2nd ed., pp. 147–181). American Psychological Association. https://doi.org/10.1037/14775-006

Pascual-Leone, A., & Pascual-Leone, J. (2015). Memory reconsolidation keeps track of emotional changes, but what will explain the actual "processing"? *Behavioral and Brain Sciences, 38*, Article e20. https://doi.org/10.1017/S0140525X14000387

Pascual-Leone, A., Singh, T., Hanna, L., & Greenberg, L. S. (2025). Deepening the client's emotional process: What effective therapists focus on and when. *Counselling Psychology Quarterly*, 1–23. https://doi.org/10.1080/09515070.2025.2481848

Pascual-Leone, A., Yacoub, D., Abdullah, D., & Soucie, K. (2023). "I know what you're feeling": Narrative observations reveal underlying symptomatology. *Journal of Constructivist Psychology, 36*(1), 88–102. https://doi.org/10.1080/10720537.2021.1999351

Pascual-Leone, A., & Yeryomenko, N. (2016). The client "experiencing" scale as a predictor of treatment outcomes: A meta-analysis on psychotherapy process. *Psychotherapy Research, 27*(6), 653–665. https://doi.org/10.1080/10503307.2016.1152409

Pascual-Leone, A., Yeryomenko, N., Morrison, O.-P., Arnold, R., & Kramer, U. (2016). Does feeling bad, lead to feeling good? Arousal patterns during expressive writing. *Review of General Psychology, 20*(3), 336–347. https://doi.org/10.1037/gpr0000083

Pascual-Leone, A., Yeryomenko, N., Sawashima, T., & Warwar, S. (2017). Building emotional resilience over 14 sessions of emotion focused therapy: Micro-longitudinal analyses of productive emotional patterns. *Psychotherapy Research, 29*(2), 171–185. https://doi.org/10.1080/10503307.2017.1315779

Pascual-Leone, J., & Johnson, J. M. (2021). *The working mind: Meaning and mental attention in human development.* The MIT Press. https://doi.org/10.7551/mitpress/13474.001.0001

Pascual-Leone, J., Pascual-Leone, A., & Arsalidou, M. (2015). Commentary on Pessoa: Neuropsychology needs to model organismic processes "from within." *Behavioral and Brain Sciences, 38,* Article e83. https://doi.org/10.1017/S0140525X14000983

Pasricha, N. (2019). *You are awesome.* Simon & Schuster.

Pasupathi, M., & Hoyt, T. (2010). Silence and the shaping of memory: How distracted listeners affect speakers' subsequent recall of a computer game experience. *Memory, 18*(2), 159–169. https://doi.org/10.1080/09658210902992917

Pasupathi, M., Wainryb, C., Mansfield, C. D., & Bourne, S. (2017). The feeling of the story: Narrating to regulate anger and sadness. *Cognition and Emotion, 31*(3), 444–461. https://doi.org/10.1080/02699931.2015.1127214

Patihis, L., & Pendergrast, M. H. (2019). Reports of recovered memories of abuse in therapy in a large age-representative U.S. national sample: Therapy type and decade comparisons. *Clinical Psychological Science, 7*(1), 3–21. https://doi.org/10.1177/2167702618773315

Payne, H. (2017). *Essentials in dance movement psychotherapy: International perspectives of theory, research and practice.* Taylor & Francis. https://doi.org/10.4324/9781315452852

Peluso, P. R., & Freund, R. R. (2018). Therapist and client emotional expression and psychotherapy outcomes: A meta-analysis. *Psychotherapy: Theory, Research, & Practice, 55*(4), 461–472. https://doi.org/10.1037/pst0000165

Pennebaker, J. W., & Chung, C. K. (2007). Expressive writing, emotional upheavals, and health. In H. S. Friedman & R. C. Silver (Eds.), *Foundations of health psychology* (pp. 263–285). Oxford University Press.

Perera, T., George, M. S., Grammer, G., Janicak, P. G., Pascual-Leone, A., & Wirecki, T. S. (2016). The clinical TMS society consensus review and treatment recommendations for TMS therapy for major depressive disorder. *Brain Stimulation, 9*(3), 336–346. https://doi.org/10.1016/j.brs.2016.03.010

Perls, F. S. (1969). *Gestalt therapy verbatim.* Real People Press.

Perls, F. S., Hefferline, R. F., & Goodman, P. (1951). *Gestalt therapy.* Julian Press.

Pessoa, L. (2013). *The cognitive-emotional brain: From interactions to integration.* The MIT Press. https://doi.org/10.7551/mitpress/9780262019569.001.0001

Peters, J. R., Chester, D. S., Walsh, E. C., DeWall, C. N., & Baer, R. A. (2018). The rewarding nature of provocation-focused rumination in women with borderline personality disorder: A preliminary fMRI investigation. *Borderline Personality Disorder and Emotion Dysregulation, 5,* Article 1. https://doi.org/10.1186/s40479-018-0079-7

Peterson, C., Jesso, B., & McCabe, A. (1999). Encouraging narratives in preschoolers: An intervention study. *Journal of Child Language, 26*(1), 49–67. https://doi.org/10.1017/S0305000998003651

Philippe, F. L., Koestner, R., Beaulieu-Pelletier, G., & Lecours, S. (2011). The role of need satisfaction as a distinct and basic psychological component of autobiographical memories: A look at well-being. *Journal of Personality, 79*(5), 905–938. https://doi.org/10.1111/j.1467-6494.2010.00710.x

Philippot, P., Chapelle, G., & Blairy, S. (2002). Respiratory feedback in the generation of emotion. *Cognition and Emotion, 16*(5), 605–627. https://doi.org/10.1080/02699930143000392

Piccirilli, A. M., & Pos, A. E. (2023). Does emotional processing predict 18-month post-therapy outcomes in the experiential treatment of major depression? *Psychotherapy Research, 33*(2), 198–210. https://doi.org/10.1080/10503307.2022.2076628

Pinheiro, P., Gonçalves, M. M., Sousa, I., & Salgado, J. (2021). What is the effect of emotional processing on depression? A longitudinal study. *Psychotherapy Research, 31*(4), 507–519. https://doi.org/10.1080/10503307.2020.1781951

Pinquart, M., & Forstmeier, S. (2012). Effects of reminiscence interventions on psychosocial outcomes: A meta-analysis. *Aging & Mental Health, 16*(5), 541–558. https://doi.org/10.1080/13607863.2011.651434

Piolino, P., Coste, C., Martinelli, P., Macé, A. L., Quinette, P., Guillery-Girard, B., & Belleville, S. (2010). Reduced specificity of autobiographical memory and aging: Do the executive and feature binding functions of working memory have a role? *Neuropsychologia, 48*(2), 429–440. https://doi.org/10.1016/j.neuropsychologia.2009.09.035

Pollak, S. D., & Sinha, P. (2002). Effects of early experience on children's recognition of facial displays of emotion. *Developmental Psychology, 38*(5), 784–791. https://doi.org/10.1037/0012-1649.38.5.784

Poon, C. S., & Young, D. L. (2006). Nonassociative learning as gated neural integrator and differentiator in stimulus-response pathways. *Behavioral and Brain Functions, 2*(1), Article 29. https://doi.org/10.1186/1744-9081-2-29

Popper, C. W. (2014). Single-micronutrient and broad-spectrum micronutrient approaches for treating mood disorders in youth and adults. *Child and Adolescent Psychiatric Clinics of North America, 23*(3), 591–672. https://doi.org/10.1016/j.chc.2014.04.001

Porges, S. W. (2011). *The polyvagal theory: Neurophysiological foundations of emotions, attachment, communication, and self-regulation.* W. W. Norton & Company.

Pos, A. E., & Greenberg, L. S. (2012). Organizing awareness and increasing emotion regulation: Revising chair work in emotion-focused therapy for borderline personality disorder. *Journal of Personality Disorders, 26*(1), 84–107. https://doi.org/10.1521/pedi.2012.26.1.84

Pos, A. E., Greenberg, L. S., Goldman, R. N., & Korman, L. M. (2003). Emotional processing during experiential treatment of depression. *Journal of Consulting and Clinical Psychology, 71*(6), 1007–1016. https://doi.org/10.1037/0022-006X.71.6.1007

Pos, A. E., Paolone, D. A., Smith, C. E., & Warwar, S. H. (2017). How does client expressed emotional arousal relate to outcome in experiential therapy for depression? *Person-Centered and Experiential Psychotherapies, 16*(2), 173–190. https://doi.org/10.1080/14779757.2017.1323666

Power, M. J., & Fyvie, C. (2013). The role of emotion in PTSD: Two preliminary studies. *Behavioural and Cognitive Psychotherapy, 41*(2), 162–172. https://doi.org/10.1017/S1352465812000148

Power, N., Noble, L. A., Simmonds-Buckley, M., Kellett, S., Stockton, C., Firth, N., & Delgadillo, J. (2022). Associations between treatment adherence-competence-integrity (ACI) and adult psychotherapy outcomes: A systematic review and meta-analysis. *Journal of Consulting and Clinical Psychology, 90*(5), 427–445. https://doi.org/10.1037/ccp0000736

Powley, T. L., & Phillips, R. J. (2002). Musings on the wanderer: What's new in our understanding of vago-vagal reflexes? I. Morphology and topography of vagal afferents innervating the GI tract. *American Journal of Physiology: Gastrointestinal and Liver Physiology, 283*(6), G1217–G1225. https://doi.org/10.1152/ajpgi.00249.2002

Preschl, B., Maercker, A., Wagner, B., Forstmeier, S., Baños, R. M., Alcañiz, M., Castilla, D., & Botella, C. (2012). Life-review therapy with computer supplements for depression in the elderly: A randomized controlled trial. *Aging & Mental Health, 16*(8), 964–974. https://doi.org/10.1080/13607863.2012.702726

Proença Lopes, C., Allado, E., Poussel, M., Essadek, A., Hamroun, A., & Chenuel, B. (2022). Alexithymia and athletic performance: Beneficial or deleterious, both sides of the medal? A systematic review. *Healthcare, 10*(3), Article 511. https://doi.org/10.3390/healthcare10030511

Pugh, M. (2022). *Cognitive behavioural chairwork: Distinctive features.* Routledge.

Pugh, M., Bell, T., & Dixon, A. (2021). Delivering tele-chairwork: A qualitative survey of expert therapists. *Psychotherapy Research, 31*(7), 843–858. https://doi.org/10.1080/10503307.2020.1854486

Punkanen, M., Saarikallio, S., & Luck, G. (2014). Emotions in motion: Short-term group form dance/movement therapy in the treatment of depression: A pilot study. *The Arts in Psychotherapy, 41*(5), 493–497. https://doi.org/10.1016/j.aip.2014.07.001

Pylvänäinen, P. M., Muotka, J. S., & Lappalainen, R. (2015). A dance movement therapy group for depressed adult patients in a psychiatric outpatient clinic: Effects of the treatment. *Frontiers in Psychology, 6,* Article 980. https://doi.org/10.3389/fpsyg.2015.00980

Quigley, L., Dozois, D. J. A., Bagby, R. M., Lobo, D. S. S., Ravindran, L., & Quilty, L. C. (2019). Cognitive change in cognitive-behavioural therapy v. pharmacotherapy for adult depression: A longitudinal mediation analysis. *Psychological Medicine, 49*(15), 2626–2634. https://doi.org/10.1017/S0033291718003653

Raes, F., Hermans, D., Williams, J. M. G., Demyttenaere, K., Sabbe, B., Pieters, G., & Eelen, P. (2005). Reduced specificity of autobiographical memory: A mediator between rumination and ineffective social problem-solving in major depression? *Journal of Affective Disorders, 87*(2–3), 331–335. https://doi.org/10.1016/j.jad.2005.05.004

Raes, F., Verstraeten, K., Bijttebier, P., Vasey, M. W., & Dalgleish, T. (2010). Inhibitory control mediates the relationship between depressed mood and overgeneral memory recall in children. *Journal of Clinical Child and Adolescent Psychology, 39*(2), 276–281. https://doi.org/10.1080/15374410903532684

Raes, F., Williams, J. M. G., & Hermans, D. (2009). Reducing cognitive vulnerability to depression: A preliminary investigation of memory specificity training (MEST) in inpatients with depressive symptomatology. *Journal of Behavior Therapy and Experimental Psychiatry, 40*(1), 24–38. https://doi.org/10.1016/j.jbtep.2008.03.001

Raio, C. M., Orederu, T. A., Palazzolo, L., Shurick, A. A., & Phelps, E. A. (2013). Cognitive emotion regulation fails the stress test. *Proceedings of the National Academy of Sciences of the United States of America, 110*(37), 15139–15144. https://doi.org/10.1073/pnas.1305706110

Ralston, M. (2006). *Emotional arousal and depth of experiencing in imaginal confrontation versus evocative empathy* [Unpublished doctoral dissertation]. University of Windsor.

Range, L. M., & Jenkins, S. R. (2010). Who benefits from Pennebaker's expressive writing paradigm? Research recommendations from three gender theories. *Sex Roles, 63*(3–4), 149–164. https://doi.org/10.1007/s11199-010-9749-7

Reich, W. (1973). *Character analysis* (V. R. Carfagno, Trans.; 3rd ed.). WRM Press.

Renna, M. E., Quintero, J. M., Fresco, D. M., & Mennin, D. S. (2017). Emotion regulation therapy: A mechanism-targeted treatment for disorders of distress. *Frontiers in Psychology, 8,* Article 98. https://doi.org/10.3389/fpsyg.2017.00098

Rescorla, R. A., & Wagner, A. R. (1972). A theory of Pavlovian conditioning: Variations in the effectiveness of reinforcement and nonreinforcement. In A. H. Black & W. F. Prokasy (Eds.), *Classical conditioning: II. Current research and theory* (pp. 64–99). Appleton Century Crofts.

Ribeiro, A. P., Mendes, I., Stiles, W. B., Angus, L., Sousa, I., & Gonçalves, M. M. (2014). Ambivalence in emotion-focused therapy for depression: The maintenance of problematically dominant self-narratives. *Psychotherapy Research, 24*(6), 702–710. https://doi.org/10.1080/10503307.2013.879620

Ricarte, J. J., Hernández-Viadel, J. V., Latorre, J. M., & Ros, L. (2012). Effects of event-specific memory training on autobiographical memory retrieval and depressive symptoms in schizophrenic patients. *Journal of Behavior Therapy and Experimental Psychiatry, 43*(1, Suppl. 1), S12–S20. https://doi.org/10.1016/j.jbtep.2011.06.001

Rice, L. N., & Saperia, E. P. (1984). Task analysis and the resolution of problematic reactions. In L. N. Rice & L. S. Greenberg (Eds.), *Patterns of change* (pp. 29–66). Guilford Press.

Riggs, D. S., Dancu, C. V., Gershuny, B. S., Greenberg, D., & Foa, E. B. (1992). Anger and posttraumatic-stress-disorder in female crime victims. *Journal of Traumatic Stress, 5*(4), 613–625.

Rimé, B., Mesquita, B., Philippot, P., & Boca, S. (1991). Beyond the emotional event: Six studies on the social sharing of emotion. *Cognition and Emotion, 5*(5–6), 435–465. https://doi.org/10.1080/02699939108411052

Rizvi, S. L., Dimeff, L. A., Skutch, J., Carroll, D., & Linehan, M. M. (2011). A pilot study of the DBT coach: An interactive mobile phone application for individuals with borderline personality disorder and substance use disorder. *Behavior Therapy, 42*(4), 589–600. https://doi.org/10.1016/j.beth.2011.01.003

Rizvi, S. L., & Linehan, M. M. (2005). The treatment of maladaptive shame in borderline personality disorder: A pilot study of "opposite action." *Cognitive and Behavioral Practice, 12*(4), 437–447. https://doi.org/10.1016/S1077-7229(05)80071-9

Robinson, M. D., & Clore, G. L. (2002). Episodic and semantic knowledge in emotional self-report: Evidence for two judgment processes. *Journal of Personality and Social Psychology, 83*(1), 198–215. https://doi.org/10.1037/0022-3514.83.1.198

Rochman, D., & Diamond, G. M. (2008). From unresolved anger to sadness: Identifying physiological correlates. *Journal of Counseling Psychology, 55*(1), 96–105. https://doi.org/10.1037/0022-0167.55.1.96

Rohde, K. B., Caspar, F., Koenig, T., Pascual-Leone, A., & Stein, M. (2018). Neurophysiological traces of interpersonal pain: How emotional autobiographical memories affect event-related potentials. *Emotion, 18*(2), 290–303. https://doi.org/10.1037/emo0000356

Rohde, K. B., Stein, M., Pascual-Leone, A., & Caspar, F. (2016). Facilitating emotional processing: An experimental induction of psychotherapeutically relevant affective states. *Cognitive Therapy and Research, 30*(3), 373–394.

Röhricht, F., Papadopoulos, N., & Priebe, S. (2013). An exploratory randomized controlled trial of body psychotherapy for patients with chronic depression. *Journal of Affective Disorders, 151*(1), 85–91. https://doi.org/10.1016/j.jad.2013.05.056

Röhricht, F., & Priebe, S. (2006). Effect of body-oriented psychological therapy on negative symptoms in schizophrenia: A randomized controlled trial. *Psychological Medicine, 36*(5), 669–678. https://doi.org/10.1017/S0033291706007161

Rogers, C. R. (1959). The essence of psychotherapy: A client-centered view. *Annals of Psychotherapy, 1*, 51–57.

Ros, L., Ricarte, J. J., Serrano, J. P., Nieto, M., Aguilar, M. J., & Latorre, J. M. (2014). Overgeneral autobiographical memories: Gender differences in depression. *Applied Cognitive Psychology, 28*(4), 472–480. https://doi.org/10.1002/acp.3013

Rosen, G. M., & Davison, G. C. (2003). Psychology should list empirically supported principles of change (ESPs) and not credential trademarked therapies or other treatment packages. *Behavior Modification, 27*(3), 300–312. https://doi.org/10.1177/0145445503027003003

Rubin, D. C., & Umanath, S. (2015). Event memory: A theory of memory for laboratory, autobiographical, and fictional events. *Psychological Review, 122*(1), 1–23. https://doi.org/10.1037/a0037907

Rudge, S., Feigenbaum, J. D., & Fonagy, P. (2020). Mechanisms of change in dialectical behaviour therapy and cognitive behaviour therapy for borderline personality disorder: A critical review of the literature. *Journal of Mental Health, 29*(1), 92–102. https://doi.org/10.1080/09638237.2017.1322185

Rufer, M., Albrecht, R., Zaum, J., Schnyder, U., Mueller-Pfeiffer, C., Hand, I., & Schmidt, O. (2010). Impact of alexithymia on treatment outcome: A naturalistic study of short-term cognitive-behavioral group therapy for panic disorder. *Psychopathology, 43*(3), 170–179. https://doi.org/10.1159/000288639

Rukeyser, M. (2006). The speed of darkness. In J. Kaufman & A. Herzog (Eds.), *The collected poems of Muriel Rukeyser* (pp. 465–470). University of Pittsburgh Press. (Original work published 1968)

Ryder, A., Sunohara, M., Dere, J., & Chentsova-Dutton, Y. (2018). The cultural shaping of alexithymia. In O. Luminet, R. Bagby, & G. Taylor (Eds.), *Alexithymia: Advances in research, theory, and clinical practice* (pp. 33–48). Cambridge University Press. https://doi.org/10.1017/9781108241595.005

Ryff, C. D., & Keyes, C. L. M. (1995). The structure of psychological well-being revisited. *Journal of Personality and Social Psychology, 69*(4), 719–727. https://doi.org/10.1037/0022-3514.69.4.719

Safran, J. D. (2002). Brief relational psychoanalytic treatment. *Psychoanalytic Dialogues, 12*(2), 171–195. https://doi.org/10.1080/10481881209348661

Safran, J. D. (2003). *Psychoanalysis and Buddhism: An unfolding dialogue.* Simon and Schuster.

Safran, J. D., & Segal, Z. V. (1990). *Interpersonal process in cognitive therapy.* Jason Aronson.

Salsman, N. L., & Linehan, M. M. (2012). An investigation of the relationships among negative affect, difficulties in emotion regulation, and features of borderline personality disorder. *Journal of Psychopathology and Behavioral Assessment, 34*(2), 260–267. https://doi.org/10.1007/s10862-012-9275-8

Salter, J. E., Smith, S. D., & Ethans, K. D. (2013). Positive and negative affect in individuals with spinal cord injuries. *Spinal Cord, 51*(3), 252–256. https://doi.org/10.1038/sc.2012.105

Samson, A. C., & Gross, J. J. (2012). Humour as emotion regulation: The differential consequences of negative versus positive humour. *Cognition and Emotion, 26*(2), 375–384. https://doi.org/10.1080/02699931.2011.585069

Samur, D., Tops, M., Schlinkert, C., Quirin, M., Cuijpers, P., & Koole, S. L. (2013). Four decades of research on alexithymia: Moving toward clinical applications. *Frontiers in Psychology, 4,* Article 861. https://doi.org/10.3389/fpsyg.2013.00861

Sawashima, T. (2018). *How is shame resolved? An experimental study on the roles of anger and sadness* [Unpublished doctoral thesis]. University of Windsor.

Schachter, S., & Singer, J. E. (1962). Cognitive, social, and physiological determinants of emotional state. *Psychological Review, 69*(5), 379–399. https://doi.org/10.1037/h0046234

Schanche, E., Stiles, T. C., McCullough, L., Svartberg, M., & Nielsen, G. H. (2011). The relationship between activating affects, inhibitory affects, and self-compassion in patients with Cluster C personality disorders. *Psychotherapy: Theory, Research, & Practice, 48*(3), 293–303. https://doi.org/10.1037/a0022012

Schmais, C. (1985). Healing processes in group dance therapy. *American Journal of Dance Therapy, 8*(1), 17–36. https://doi.org/10.1007/BF02251439

Schmukle, S. C., Egloff, B., & Burns, L. R. (2002). The relationship between positive and negative affect in the Positive and Negative Affect Schedule (PANAS). *Journal of Research in Personality, 36*(5), 463–475. https://doi.org/10.1016/S0092-6566(02)00007-7

Schmutz, A. Stein, M., Fritsche, L., Rohde, K., Caspar, F., Pascual-Leone, A., & Koenig, T., (2025, January). EEG microstates of emotional processing during a psychotherapeutic intervention [Conference abstract presentation (T23)]. Alpine Brain Imaging Meeting (ABIM), Champery, Switzerland.

Schneider, K. J., & May, R. (1995). *The psychology of existence: An integrative, clinical perspective*. McGraw-Hill.

Schrauf, R. W., & Sanchez, J. (2004). The preponderance of negative emotion words in the emotion lexicon: A cross-generational and cross-linguistic study. *Journal of Multilingual and Multicultural Development, 25*(2–3), 266–284. https://doi.org/10.1080/01434630408666532

Scoboria, A., Boucher, C., & Mazzoni, G. (2015). Reasons for withdrawing belief in vivid autobiographical memories. *Memory, 23*(4), 545–562. https://doi.org/10.1080/09658211.2014.910530

Scoboria, A., Jackson, D. L., Talarico, J., Hanczakowski, M., Wysman, L., & Mazzoni, G. (2014). The role of belief in occurrence within autobiographical memory. *Journal of Experimental Psychology: General, 143*(3), 1242–1258. https://doi.org/10.1037/a0034110

Semerari, A., Carcione, A., Dimaggio, G., Nicolò, G., & Procacci, M. (2007). Understanding minds: Different functions and different disorders? The contribution of psychotherapy research. *Psychotherapy Research, 17*(1), 106–119. https://doi.org/10.1080/10503300500536953

Senior, J. (2010, July 2). All joy and no fun: Why parents hate parenting. *New York Magazine*. https://nymag.com/news/features/67024/

Serrano Selva, J. P., Latorre Postigo, J. M., Ros Segura, L., Navarro Bravo, B., Aguilar Córcoles, M. J., Nieto López, M., Ricarte Trives, J. J., & Gatz, M. (2012). Life review therapy using autobiographical retrieval practice for older adults with clinical depression. *Psicothema, 24*(2), 224–229.

Seuss. (1990). *Oh, the places you'll go!* Random House.

Shadmehr, R., & Ahmed, A. A. (2020). *Vigor: Neuroeconomics of movement control*. The MIT Press. https://doi.org/10.7551/mitpress/12940.001.0001

Shafir, T. (2016). Using movement to regulate emotion: Neurophysiological findings and their application in psychotherapy. *Frontiers in Psychology, 7*, Article 1451. https://doi.org/10.3389/fpsyg.2016.01451

Shafir, T., Tsachor, R. P., & Welch, K. B. (2016). Emotion regulation through movement: Unique sets of movement characteristics are associated with and enhance basic emotions. *Frontiers in Psychology, 6*, Article 2030. https://doi.org/10.3389/fpsyg.2015.02030

Shapiro, R., & Brown, L. S. (2019). Eye movement desensitization and reprocessing therapy and related treatments for trauma: An innovative, integrative trauma treatment. *Practice Innovations, 4*(3), 139–155. https://doi.org/10.1037/pri0000092

Shapiro, S. L., Carlson, L. E., Astin, J. A., & Freedman, B. (2006). Mechanisms of mindfulness. *Journal of Clinical Psychology, 62*(3), 373–386. https://doi.org/10.1002/jclp.20237

Sherman, D. K., Hartson, K. A., Binning, K. R., Purdie-Vaughns, V., Garcia, J., Taborsky-Barba, S., Tomassetti, S., Nussbaum, A. D., & Cohen, G. L. (2013). Deflecting the trajectory and changing the narrative: How self-affirmation affects academic performance and motivation under identity threat. *Journal of Personality and Social Psychology, 104*(4), 591–618. https://doi.org/10.1037/a0031495

Shevchuk, N. A. (2008). Adapted cold shower as a potential treatment for depression. *Medical Hypotheses, 70*(5), 995–1001. https://doi.org/10.1016/j.mehy.2007.04.052

Sicoli, L. A., & Hallberg, E. T. (1998). An analysis of client performance in the two-chair method. *Canadian Journal of Counselling, 32*(2), 151–162.

Siegel, D. (1999). *The developing mind: Toward a neurobiology of interpersonal experience*. Guilford Press.

Silverman, A., Logel, C., & Cohen, G. L. (2013). Self-affirmation as a deliberate coping strategy: The moderating role of choice. *Journal of Experimental Social Psychology, 49*(1), 93–98. https://doi.org/10.1016/j.jesp.2012.08.005

Simi, P., Blee, K., DeMichele, M., & Windisch, S. (2017). Addicted to hate: Identity residual among former White supremacists. *American Sociological Review, 82*(6), 1167–1187. https://doi.org/10.1177/0003122417728719

Singh, T., Pascual-Leone, A., Morrison, O. P., & Greenberg, L. (2021). Working with emotion predicts sudden gains during experiential therapy for depression. *Psychotherapy Research, 31*(7), 895–908. https://doi.org/10.1080/10503307.2020.1866784

Sirois, F., & Pychyl, T. (2013). Procrastination and the priority of short-term mood regulation: Consequences for future self. *Social and Personality Psychology Compass, 7*(2), 115–127. https://doi.org/10.1111/spc3.12011

Sletvold, J. (2011). "The reading of emotional expression": Wilhelm Reich and the history of embodied analysis. *Psychoanalytic Dialogues, 21*(4), 453–467. https://doi.org/10.1080/10481885.2011.595337

Sloan, D. M., Marx, B. P., Lee, D. J., & Resick, P. A. (2018). A brief exposure-based treatment vs. cognitive processing therapy for posttraumatic stress disorder: A randomized noninferiority clinical trial. *JAMA Psychiatry, 75*(3), 233–239. https://doi.org/10.1001/jamapsychiatry.2017.4249

Slotter, E. B., & Ward, D. E. (2015). Finding the silver lining: The relative roles of redemptive narratives and cognitive reappraisal in individuals' emotional distress after the end of a romantic relationship. *Journal of Social and Personal Relationships, 32*(6), 737–756. https://doi.org/10.1177/0265407514546978

Smallwood, J., & Schooler, J. W. (2015). The science of mind wandering: Empirically navigating the stream of consciousness. *Annual Review of Psychology, 66,* 487–518. https://doi.org/10.1146/annurev-psych-010814-015331

Snippe, E., Elmer, T., Ceulemans, E., Smit, A. C., Lutz, W., & Helmich, M. A. (2024). The temporal order of emotional, cognitive, and behavioral gains in daily life during treatment of depression. *Journal of Consulting and Clinical Psychology, 92*(8), 466–478. https://doi.org/10.1037/ccp0000890

Snyder, C. R., Lopez, S. J., Edwards, L. M., & Marques, S. C. (2021). *The Oxford handbook of positive psychology* (3rd ed.). Oxford University Press.

Snyder, S. (2018). *Love worth making: How to have ridiculously great sex in a long-lasting relationship.* St. Martin's Press.

Solbakken, O. A., Hansen, R. S., & Monsen, J. T. (2011). Affect integration and reflective function: Clarification of central conceptual issues. *Psychotherapy Research, 21*(4), 482–496. https://doi.org/10.1080/10503307.2011.583696

Sønderland, N. M., Solbakken, O. A., Eilertsen, D. E., Nordmo, M., & Monsen, J. T. (2024). Emotional changes and outcomes in psychotherapy: A systematic review and meta-analysis. *Journal of Consulting and Clinical Psychology, 92*(9), 654–670. https://doi.org/10.1037/ccp0000814

Sørensen, H. T., Mellemkjaer, L., & Olsen, J. H. (2001). Risk of suicide in users of β-adrenoceptor blockers, calcium channel blockers and angiotensin converting enzyme inhibitors. *British Journal of Clinical Pharmacology, 52*(3), 313–318. https://doi.org/10.1046/j.0306-5251.2001.01442.x

Spiegel, D. (1993). *Living beyond limits: New hope and help for facing life-threatening illness.* Random House.

Spiegler, M. D. (Ed.). (2015). *Contemporary behavior therapy* (6th ed.). Cengage Learning.

Spinhoven, P., Bamelis, L., Molendijk, M., Haringsma, R., & Arntz, A. (2009). Reduced specificity of autobiographical memory in Cluster C personality disorders and the role of depression, worry, and experiential avoidance. *Journal of Abnormal Psychology, 118*(3), 520–530. https://doi.org/10.1037/a0016393

Spinoza, B. (1967). *Ethics IV.* (Original work published 1677)

Stalikas, A., Fitzpatrick, M., Mistkidou, P., Boutri, A., & Seryianni, C. (2015). Positive emotions in psychotherapy: Conceptual propositions and research challenges. In O. C. G. Gelo, A. Pritz, & B. Rieken (Eds.), *Psychotherapy research: Foundations, process, and outcome* (pp. 331–349). Springer-Verlag Publishing. https://doi.org/10.1007/978-3-7091-1382-0_17

Stanton, A. L., Danoff-Burg, S., Cameron, C. L., Bishop, M., Collins, C. A., Kirk, S. B., Sworowski, L. A., & Twillman, R. (2000). Emotionally expressive coping predicts psychological and physical adjustment to breast cancer. *Journal of Consulting and Clinical Psychology, 68*(5), 875–882. https://doi.org/10.1037/0022-006X.68.5.875

Starr, L. R., Hershenberg, R., Shaw, Z. A., Li, Y. I., & Santee, A. C. (2020). The perils of murky emotions: Emotion differentiation moderates the prospective relationship between naturalistic stress exposure and adolescent depression. *Emotion, 20*(6), 927–938. https://doi.org/10.1037/emo0000630

Steger, M. F. (2022). Meaning in life is a fundamental protective factor in the context of psychopathology. *World Psychiatry, 21*(3), 389–390. https://doi.org/10.1002/wps.20916

Steinmann, R., Gat, I., Nir-Gottlieb, O., Shahar, B., & Diamond, G. M. (2017). Attachment-based family therapy and individual emotion-focused therapy for unresolved anger: Qualitative analysis of treatment outcomes and change processes. *Psychotherapy: Theory, Research, & Practice, 54*(3), 281–291. https://doi.org/10.1037/pst0000116

Stern, D. B. (1997). *Unformulated experience: From dissociation to imagination in psychoanalysis*. Analytic Press.

Stern, D. N. (2010). *Forms of vitality: Exploring dynamic experience in psychology, the arts, psychotherapy, and development*. Oxford University Press.

Sternbergh, A. (2006, October 6). Stephen Colbert has America by the ballots. *New York Magazine*. https://nymag.com/news/politics/22322/

Stevens, J. O. (1971). *Awareness: Exploring, experimenting, experiencing*. Real People Press.

Stiegler, J. R., Binder, P.-E., Hjeltnes, A., Stige, S. H., & Schanche, E. (2018). "It's heavy, intense, horrendous and nice": Clients' experiences in two-chair dialogues. *Person-Centered and Experiential Psychotherapies, 17*(2), 139–159. https://doi.org/10.1080/14779757.2018.1472138

Stiegler, J. R., Molde, H., & Schanche, E. (2018). Does an emotion-focused two-chair dialogue add to the therapeutic effect of the empathic attunement to affect? *Clinical Psychology & Psychotherapy, 25*(1), e86–e95. https://doi.org/10.1002/cpp.2144

Stiles, W. B. (1996). When more of a good thing is better: Reply to Hayes et al. (1996). *Journal of Consulting and Clinical Psychology, 64*(5), 915–918. https://doi.org/10.1037/0022-006X.64.5.915

Stiles, W. B. (2009). Responsiveness as an obstacle for psychotherapy outcome research: It's worse than you think. *Clinical Psychology: Science and Practice, 16*(1), 86–91. https://doi.org/10.1111/j.1468-2850.2009.01148.x

Stiles, W. B., Osatuke, K., Glick, M. J., & Mackay, H. C. (2004). Encounters between internal voices generate emotion: An elaboration of the assimilation model. In H. J. M. Hermans & G. Dimaggio (Eds.), *The dialogical self in psychotherapy* (pp. 91–107). Brunner-Routledge. https://doi.org/10.4324/9780203314616_chapter_6

St. Jacques, P. L. (2012). Functional neuroimaging of autobiographical memory. In D. Berntsen & D. C. Rubin (Eds.), *Understanding autobiographical memory: Theories and approaches* (pp. 114–138). Cambridge University Press. https://doi.org/10.1017/CBO9781139021937.010

St. Jacques, P. L., Conway, M. A., Lowder, M. W., & Cabeza, R. (2011). Watching my mind unfold versus yours: An fMRI study using a novel camera technology to examine neural differences in self-projection of self versus other perspectives. *Journal of Cognitive Neuroscience, 23*(6), 1275–1284. https://doi.org/10.1162/jocn.2010.21518

St. Jacques, P. L., Szpunar, K. K., & Schacter, D. L. (2017). Shifting visual perspective during retrieval shapes autobiographical memories. *NeuroImage, 148*, 103–114. https://doi.org/10.1016/j.neuroimage.2016.12.028

Stolovy, T., Lev-Wiesel, R., Doron, A., & Gelkopf, M. (2009). The meaning in life for hospitalized patients with schizophrenia. *Journal of Nervous and Mental Disease, 197*(2), 133–135. https://doi.org/10.1097/NMD.0b013e3181963ede

Stone, T. A. (1997). *Cure by crying: How to cure your own depression, nervousness, headaches, violent temper, insomnia, marital problems, addictions, by uncovering your repressed memories*. Cure By Crying.

Strachey, J. (1934). The nature of the therapeutic action of psychoanalysis. *The International Journal of Psycho-Analysis, 15*, 117–126.

Strack, F., Martin, L. L., & Stepper, S. (1988). Inhibiting and facilitating conditions of the human smile: A nonobtrusive test of the facial feedback hypothesis. *Journal of Personality and Social Psychology, 54*(5), 768–777. https://doi.org/10.1037/0022-3514.54.5.768

Strating, M. A., & Pascual-Leone, A. (2024). *Working through lingering anger following interpersonal grievances: Rumination, reappraisal, and identification of unmet needs* [Manuscript submitted for publication].

Suslow, T., & Junghanns, K. (2002). Impairments of emotion situation priming in alexithymia. *Personality and Individual Differences, 32*(3), 541–550. https://doi.org/10.1016/S0191-8869(01)00056-3

Swann, W. B., Jr., Griffin, J. J., Jr., Predmore, S. C., & Gaines, B. (1987). The cognitive-affective crossfire: When self-consistency confronts self-enhancement. *Journal of Personality and Social Psychology, 52*(5), 881–889. https://doi.org/10.1037/0022-3514.52.5.881

Talmi, D. (2013). Enhanced emotional memory: Cognitive and neural mechanisms. *Current Directions in Psychological Science, 22*(6), 430–436. https://doi.org/10.1177/0963721413498893

Tamminen, K. A., & Watson, J. C. (2022). Emotion focused therapy with injured athletes: Conceptualizing injury challenges and working with emotions. *Journal of Applied Sport Psychology, 34*(5), 958–982. https://doi.org/10.1080/10413200.2021.2024625

Tanner, B. A. (2012). Validity of global physical and emotional SUDS. *Applied Psychophysiology and Biofeedback, 37*(1), 31–34. https://doi.org/10.1007/s10484-011-9174-x

Tao, S., Li, J., Zhang, M., Zheng, P., Lau, E. Y. H., Sun, J., & Zhu, Y. (2021). The effects of mindfulness-based interventions on child and adolescent aggression: A systematic review and meta-analysis. *Mindfulness, 12*(6), 1301–1315. https://doi.org/10.1007/s12671-020-01570-9

Tarba, T. (2015). *Relating a model of resolution of arrested anger to outcome in emotion-focused therapy of depression* [Unpublished doctoral dissertation]. York University.

Taylor, G. J., & Bagby, R. M. (2013). Psychoanalysis and empirical research: The example of alexithymia. *Journal of the American Psychoanalytic Association, 61*(1), 99–133. https://doi.org/10.1177/0003065112474066

Taylor, G. J., Bagby, R. M., & Parker, J. D. (1997). *Disorders of affect regulation: Alexithymia in medical and psychiatric illness*. Cambridge University Press. https://doi.org/10.1017/CBO9780511526831

Teasdale, J. D., Moore, R. G., Hayhurst, H., Pope, M., Williams, S., & Segal, Z. V. (2002). Metacognitive awareness and prevention of relapse in depression: Empirical evidence. *Journal of Consulting and Clinical Psychology, 70*(2), 275–287. https://doi.org/10.1037/0022-006X.70.2.275

Tilley, D., & Palmer, G. (2013). Enactments in emotionally focused couple therapy: Shaping moments of contact and change. *Journal of Marital and Family Therapy, 39*(3), 299–313. https://doi.org/10.1111/j.1752-0606.2012.00305.x

Tillisch, K., Labus, J., Kilpatrick, L., Jiang, Z., Stains, J., Ebrat, B., Guyonnet, D., Legrain-Raspaud, S., Trotin, B., Naliboff, B., & Mayer, E. A. (2013). Consumption of fermented milk product with probiotic modulates brain activity. *Gastroenterology, 144*(7), 1394–1401.e4. https://doi.org/10.1053/j.gastro.2013.02.043

Timulak, L., & McElvaney, J. (2016). Emotion-focused therapy for generalized anxiety disorder: An overview of the model. *Journal of Contemporary Psychotherapy, 46*(1), 41–52. https://doi.org/10.1007/s10879-015-9310-7

Timulak, L., & Pascual-Leone, A. (2015). New developments for case conceptualization in emotion-focused therapy. *Clinical Psychology & Psychotherapy, 22*(6), 619–636. https://doi.org/10.1002/cpp.1922

Tolman, E. C., & Brunswik, E. (1935). The organism and the causal texture of the environment. *Psychological Review, 42*(1), 43–77. https://doi.org/10.1037/h0062156

Torre, J. B., & Lieberman, M. D. (2018). Putting feelings into words: Affect labeling as implicit emotion regulation. *Emotion Review, 10*(2), 116–124. https://doi.org/10.1177/1754073917742706

Town, J. M., Falkenström, F., Abbass, A., & Stride, C. (2022). The anger–depression mechanism in dynamic therapy: Experiencing previously avoided anger positively predicts reduction in depression via working alliance and insight. *Journal of Counseling Psychology, 69*(3), 326–336. https://doi.org/10.1037/cou0000581

Town, J. M., Hardy, G. E., McCullough, L., & Stride, C. (2011). Patient affect experiencing following therapist interventions in short-term dynamic psychotherapy. *Psychotherapy Research, 25,* 723–740.

Tracy, J. L., & Matsumoto, D. (2008). The spontaneous expression of pride and shame: evidence for biologically innate nonverbal displays. *Proceedings of the National Academy of Sciences of the United States of America, 105*(33), 11655–11660. https://doi.org/10.1073/pnas.0802686105

Trope, Y., & Liberman, N. (2010). Construal-level theory of psychological distance. *Psychological Review, 117*(2), 440–463. https://doi.org/10.1037/a0018963

Troy, A. S., Shallcross, A. J., Brunner, A., Friedman, R., & Jones, M. C. (2018). Cognitive reappraisal and acceptance: Effects on emotion, physiology, and perceived cognitive costs. *Emotion, 18*(1), 58–74. https://doi.org/10.1037/emo0000371

Tryon, W. W. (2005). Possible mechanisms for why desensitization and exposure therapy work. *Clinical Psychology Review, 25*(1), 67–95. https://doi.org/10.1016/j.cpr.2004.08.005

Tsvieli, N., Nir-Gottlieb, O., Lifshitz, C., Diamond, G. S., Kobak, R., & Diamond, G. M. (2020). Therapist interventions associated with productive emotional processing in the context of attachment-based family therapy for depressed and suicidal adolescents. *Family Process, 59*(2), 428–444. https://doi.org/10.1111/famp.12445

Tugade, M. M., & Fredrickson, B. L. (2004). Resilient individuals use positive emotions to bounce back from negative emotional experiences. *Journal of Personality and Social Psychology, 86*(2), 320–333. https://doi.org/10.1037/0022-3514.86.2.320

Twenge, J. M., Campbell, W. K., & Foster, C. A. (2003). Parenthood and marital satisfaction: A meta-analytic review. *Journal of Marriage and Family, 65*(3), 574–583. https://doi.org/10.1111/j.1741-3737.2003.00574.x

Ulberg, R., Amlo, S., Critchfield, K. L., Marble, A., & Høglend, P. (2014). Transference interventions and the process between therapist and patient. *Psychotherapy: Theory, Research, & Practice, 51*(2), 258–269. https://doi.org/10.1037/a0034708

van Agteren, J., Iasiello, M., Lo, L., Bartholomaeus, J., Kopsaftis, Z., Carey, M., & Kyrios, M. (2021). A systematic review and meta-analysis of psychological interventions to improve mental wellbeing. *Nature Human Behaviour, 5*(5), 631–652. https://doi.org/10.1038/s41562-021-01093-w

van Anders, S. M., Steiger, J., & Goldey, K. L. (2015). Effects of gendered behavior on testosterone in women and men. *Proceedings of the National Academy of Sciences of the United States of America, 112*(45), 13805–13810. https://doi.org/10.1073/pnas.1509591112

Van Boven, L., Kane, J., McGraw, A. P., & Dale, J. (2010). Feeling close: Emotional intensity reduces perceived psychological distance. *Journal of Personality and Social Psychology, 98*(6), 872–885. https://doi.org/10.1037/a0019262

Van Daele, T., Van den Bergh, O., Van Audenhove, C., Raes, F., & Hermans, D. (2013). Reduced memory specificity predicts the acquisition of problem solving skills in psychoeducation. *Journal of Behavior Therapy and Experimental Psychiatry, 44*(1), 135–140. https://doi.org/10.1016/j.jbtep.2011.12.005

Vandekerckhove, M., & Wang, Y. L. (2017). Emotion, emotion regulation and sleep: An intimate relationship. *AIMS Neuroscience, 5*(1), 1–17. https://doi.org/10.3934/Neuroscience.2018.1.1

van der Kaap-Deeder, J., Brenning, K., & Neyrinck, B. (2021). Emotion regulation and borderline personality features: The mediating role of basic psychological need frustration. *Personality and Individual Differences, 168,* Article 110365. https://doi.org/10.1016/j.paid.2020.110365

van der Kolk, B. A. (2014). *The body keeps the score: Brain, mind, and body in the healing of trauma.* Viking.

van der Velde, J., Gromann, P. M., Swart, M., Wiersma, D., de Haan, L., Bruggeman, R., Krabbendam, L., & Aleman, A. (2015). Alexithymia influences brain activation during emotion perception but not regulation. *Social Cognitive and Affective Neuroscience, 10*(2), 285–293. https://doi.org/10.1093/scan/nsu056

Van Oudenhove, L., McKie, S., Lassman, D., Uddin, B., Paine, P., Coen, S., Gregory, L., Tack, J., & Aziz, Q. (2011). Fatty acid-induced gut-brain signaling attenuates neural and behavioral effects of sad emotion in humans. *The Journal of Clinical Investigation, 121*(8), 3094–3099. https://doi.org/10.1172/JCI46380

Van Velsor, P., & Cox, D. L. (2001). Anger as a vehicle in the treatment of women who are sexual abuse survivors: Reattributing responsibility and accessing personal power. *Professional Psychology: Research and Practice, 32*(6), 618–625. https://doi.org/10.1037/0735-7028.32.6.618

Verhoeven, J. E., Han, L. K. M., Lever-van Milligen, B. A., Hu, M. X., Révész, D., Hoogendoorn, A. W., Batelaan, N. M., van Schaik, D. J. F., van Balkom, A. J. L. M., van Oppen, P., & Penninx, B. W. J. H. (2023). Antidepressants or running therapy: Comparing effects on mental and physical health in patients with depression and anxiety disorders. *Journal of Affective Disorders, 329,* 19–29. https://doi.org/10.1016/j.jad.2023.02.064

Vos, J., & Vitali, D. (2018). The effects of psychological meaning-centered therapies on quality of life and psychological stress: A metaanalysis. *Palliative & Supportive Care, 16*(5), 608–632. https://doi.org/10.1017/S1478951517000931

Wainryb, C., Pasupathi, M., Bourne, S., & Oldroyd, K. (2018). Stories for all ages: Narrating anger reduces distress across childhood and adolescence. *Developmental Psychology, 54*(6), 1072–1085. https://doi.org/10.1037/dev0000495

Wallace-Hadrill, S. M. A., & Kamboj, S. K. (2016). The impact of perspective change as a cognitive reappraisal strategy on affect: A systematic review. *Frontiers in Psychology, 7,* Article 1715. https://doi.org/10.3389/fpsyg.2016.01715

Wampold, B. E., & Imel, Z. I. (2015). *The great psychotherapy debate: The evidence for what makes psychotherapy work* (2nd ed.). Routledge.

Wang, Y., Vantieghem, I., Dong, D., Nemegeer, J., De Mey, J., Van Schuerbeek, P., Marinazzo, D., & Vandekerckhove, M. (2022). Approaching or decentering? Differential neural networks underlying experiential emotion regulation and cognitive defusion. *Brain Sciences, 12*(9), Article 1215. https://doi.org/10.3390/brainsci12091215

Warwar, S. (2024). The use of homework in emotion-focused therapy for depression. *Journal of Clinical Psychology, 80*(4), 744–761. https://doi.org/10.1002/jclp.23618

Warwar, S., Greenberg, L., & Perepeluk, D. (2003, June 25–29). *Reported in-session emotional experience in therapy* [Conference presentation]. Society for Psychotherapy Research, 34th International Annual Meeting, Weimar, Germany.

Waters, T. E. A., & Fivush, R. (2015). Relations between narrative coherence, identity, and psychological well-being in emerging adulthood. *Journal of Personality, 83*(4), 441–451. https://doi.org/10.1111/jopy.12120

Watkins, E., & Baracaia, S. (2001). Why do people ruminate in dysphoric moods? *Personality and Individual Differences, 30*(5), 723–734. https://doi.org/10.1016/S0191-8869(00)00053-2

Watkins, E., & Teasdale, J. D. (2001). Rumination and overgeneral memory in depression: Effects of self-focus and analytic thinking. *Journal of Abnormal Psychology, 110*(2), 353–357. https://doi.org/10.1037/0021-843X.110.2.333

Watkins, E., Teasdale, J. D., & Williams, R. M. (2000). Decentring and distraction reduce overgeneral autobiographical memory in depression. *Psychological Medicine, 30*(4), 911–920. https://doi.org/10.1017/S0033291799002263

Watson, J. C. (1996). The relationship between vivid description, emotional arousal, and in-session resolution of problematic reactions. *Journal of Consulting and Clinical Psychology, 64*(3), 459–464. https://doi.org/10.1037/0022-006X.64.3.459

Watson, J. C., & Bedard, D. L. (2006). Clients' emotional processing in psychotherapy: A comparison between cognitive-behavioral and process-experiential therapies. *Journal of Consulting and Clinical Psychology, 74*(1), 152–159. https://doi.org/10.1037/0022-006X.74.1.152

Watson, J. C., & Greenberg, L. S. (2017). *Emotion-focused therapy for generalized anxiety.* American Psychological Association. https://doi.org/10.1037/0000018-000

Watson, J. C., & Rennie, D. L. (1994). Qualitative analysis of clients' subjective experience of significant moments during the exploration of problematic reactions. *Journal of Counseling Psychology, 41*(4), 500–509. https://doi.org/10.1037/0022-0167.41.4.500

Watt, J. A., Goodarzi, Z., Veroniki, A. A., Nincic, V., Khan, P. A., Ghassemi, M., Thompson, Y., Tricco, A. C., & Straus, S. E. (2019). Comparative efficacy of interventions for aggressive and agitated behaviors in dementia: A systematic review and network meta-analysis. *Annals of Internal Medicine, 171*(9), 633–642. https://doi.org/10.7326/M19-0993

Watt, L., & Cappeliez, P. (2000). Integrative and instrumental reminiscence therapies for depression in older adults: Intervention strategies and treatment effectiveness. *Aging & Mental Health, 4*(2), 166–177. https://doi.org/10.1080/13607860050008691

Watters, C. A., Taylor, G. J., Quilty, L. C., & Bagby, R. M. (2016). An examination of the topology and measurement of the alexithymia construct using network analysis. *Journal of Personality Assessment, 98*(6), 649–659. https://doi.org/10.1080/00223891.2016.1172077

Webster, J. D., Bohlmeijer, E. T., & Westerhof, G. J. (2010). Mapping the future of reminiscence: A conceptual guide for research and practice. *Research on Aging, 32*(4), 527–564. https://doi.org/10.1177/0164027510364122

Wellenzohn, S., Proyer, R. T., & Ruch, W. (2018). Who benefits from humor-based positive psychology interventions? The moderating effects of personality traits and sense of humor. *Frontiers in Psychology, 9,* Article 821. https://doi.org/10.3389/fpsyg.2018.00821

Welling, H. (2012). Transformative emotional sequence: Towards a common principle of change. *Journal of Psychotherapy Integration, 22*(2), 109–136. https://doi.org/10.1037/a0027786

Wells, A. (2002). *Emotional disorders and metacognition: Innovative cognitive therapy.* John Wiley & Sons. https://doi.org/10.1002/9780470713662

Wells, A. (2005). The metacognitive model of GAD: Assessment of meta-worry and relationship with *DSM-IV* generalized anxiety disorder. *Cognitive Therapy and Research, 29*(1), 107–121. https://doi.org/10.1007/s10608-005-1652-0

Westerhof, G. J., Bohlmeijer, E., & Webster, J. D. (2010). Reminiscence and mental health: A review of recent progress in theory, research and interventions. *Ageing and Society, 30*(4), 697–721. https://doi.org/10.1017/S0144686X09990328

Westwood, M. J., McLean, H., Cave, D., Borgen, W., & Slakov, P. (2010). Coming home: A group-based approach for assisting military veterans in transition. *Journal for Specialists in Group Work, 35*(1), 44–68. https://doi.org/10.1080/01933920903466059

Whelton, W. J., & Greenberg, L. S. (2005). Emotion in self-criticism. *Personality and Individual Differences, 38*(7), 1583–1595. https://doi.org/10.1016/j.paid.2004.09.024

White, G. L., & Kight, T. D. (1984). Misattribution of arousal and attraction: Effects of salience of explanations for arousal. *Journal of Experimental Social Psychology, 20*(1), 55–64. https://doi.org/10.1016/0022-1031(84)90012-X

Wiebe, S. A., & Johnson, S. M. (2016). A review of the research in emotionally focused therapy for couples. *Family Process, 55*(3), 390–407. https://doi.org/10.1111/famp.12229

Wiley, A. R., Rose, A. J., Burger, L. K., & Miller, P. J. (1998). Constructing autonomous selves through narrative practices: A comparative study of working-class and middle-class families. *Child Development, 69*(3), 833–847. https://doi.org/10.2307/1132207

Wilkes, S. (2008). The use of bupropion SR in cigarette smoking cessation. *International Journal of Chronic Obstructive Pulmonary Disease, 3*(1), 45–53. https://doi.org/10.2147/COPD.S1121

Williams, J. M. G., Barnhofer, T., Crane, C., Herman, D., Raes, F., Watkins, E., & Dalgleish, T. (2007). Autobiographical memory specificity and emotional disorder. *Psychological Bulletin, 133*(1), 122–148. https://doi.org/10.1037/0033-2909.133.1.122

Willimann, L., Berthoud, L., Pascual-Leone, A., Grosse Holtforth, M., & Kramer, U. (2016, January). *Goodbye global distress—Hello what? Sequences of emotional processing in patients with borderline personality disorders* [Poster presentation]. Swiss National Science Foundation workshop, Lausanne, Switzerland.

Wilson, A. E., & Ross, M. (2003). The identity function of autobiographical memory: Time is on our side. *Memory, 11*(2), 137–149. https://doi.org/10.1080/741938210

Wilson, T. D., Centerbar, D. B., Kermer, D. A., & Gilbert, D. T. (2005). The pleasures of uncertainty: Prolonging positive moods in ways people do not anticipate. *Journal of Personality and Social Psychology, 88*(1), 5–21. https://doi.org/10.1037/0022-3514.88.1.5

Winnicott, D. W. (1971). *Playing and reality*. Tavistock Publications.

Witkin, H. A., & Goodenough, D. R. (1977). Field dependence and interpersonal behavior. *Psychological Bulletin, 84*(4), 661–689. https://doi.org/10.1037/0033-2909.84.4.661

Woike, B. A. (2008). A functional framework for the influence of implicit and explicit motives on autobiographical memory. *Personality and Social Psychology Review, 12*(2), 99–117. https://doi.org/10.1177/1088868308315701

Wolpe, J. (1958). *Psychotherapy by reciprocal inhibition*. Stanford University Press.

Woods, B., O'Philbin, L., Farrell, E. M., Spector, A. E., & Orrell, M. (2018). Reminiscence therapy for dementia. *Cochrane Database of Systematic Reviews, 2018*(3), Article CD001120. https://doi.org/10.1002/14651858.CD001120.pub3

Wotschack, C., & Klann-Delius, G. (2013). Alexithymia and the conceptualization of emotions: A study of language use and semantic knowledge. *Journal of Research in Personality, 47*(5), 514–523. https://doi.org/10.1016/j.jrp.2013.01.011

Wundt, W. (1998). *Outlines of psychology*. Thoemmes Press. (Original work published 1897)

Yalom, I. D. (1981). *Existential psychotherapy*. Basic Books.

Yasinski, C., Hayes, A. M., & Laurenceau, J.-P. (2016). Rumination in everyday life: The influence of distancing, immersion, and distraction. *Journal of Experimental Psychopathology, 7*(2), 225–245. https://doi.org/10.5127/jep.042714

Yerkes, R. M., & Dodson, J. D. (1908). The relation of strength of stimulus to rapidity of habit formation. *The Journal of Comparative Neurology and Psychology, 18*(5), 459–482. https://doi.org/10.1002/cne.920180503

Yonatan-Leus, R., Shefler, G., & Tishby, O. (2020). Changes in playfulness, creativity and honesty as possible outcomes of psychotherapy. *Psychotherapy Research, 30*(6), 788–799. https://doi.org/10.1080/10503307.2019.1649733

Yonatan-Leus, R., Tishby, O., Shefler, G., & Wiseman, H. (2018). Therapists' honesty, humor styles, playfulness, and creativity as outcome predictors: A retrospective study of the therapist effect. *Psychotherapy Research, 28*(5), 793–802. https://doi.org/10.1080/10503307.2017.1292067

Young, K. D., Bodurka, J., & Drevets, W. C. (2017). Functional neuroimaging of sex differences in autobiographical memory recall in depression. *Psychological Medicine, 47*(15), 2640–2652. https://doi.org/10.1017/S003329171700112X

Zeifman, R. J., Boritz, T., Barnhart, R., Labrish, C., & McMain, S. F. (2020). The independent roles of mindfulness and distress tolerance in treatment outcomes in dialectical behavior therapy skills training. *Personality Disorders, 11*(3), 181–190. https://doi.org/10.1037/per0000368

Zhan, J., Ren, J., Fan, J., & Luo, J. (2015). Distinctive effects of fear and sadness induction on anger and aggressive behavior. *Frontiers in Psychology, 6,* Article 725. https://doi.org/10.3389/fpsyg.2015.00725

Zhan, J., Tang, F., He, M., Fan, J., Xiao, J., Liu, C., & Luo, J. (2017). Regulating rumination by anger: Evidence for the mutual promotion and counteraction (MPMC) theory of emotionality. *Frontiers in Psychology, 8,* Article 1871. https://doi.org/10.3389/fpsyg.2017.01871

Zhan, J., Wu, X., Fan, J., Guo, J., Zhou, J., Ren, J., Liu, C., & Luo, J. (2017). Regulating anger under stress via cognitive reappraisal and sadness. *Frontiers in Psychology, 8,* Article 1372. https://doi.org/10.3389/fpsyg.2017.01372

Zilcha-Mano, S., Keefe, J. R., Fisher, H., Dolev-Amit, T., Veler-Poleg, N., & Barber, J. P. (2023). Is the use of interpretations associated with treatment outcome? A systematic review and meta-analytic answer. *Clinical Psychology: Science & Practice, 31*(1), 1–13. https://doi.org/10.1037/cps0000158

Zinner, L. R., Brodish, A. B., Devine, P. G., & Harmon-Jones, E. (2008). Anger and asymmetrical frontal cortical activity: Evidence for an anger-withdrawal relationship. *Cognition and Emotion, 22*(6), 1081–1093. https://doi.org/10.1080/02699930701622961

INDEX

E

ABOUT THE AUTHOR

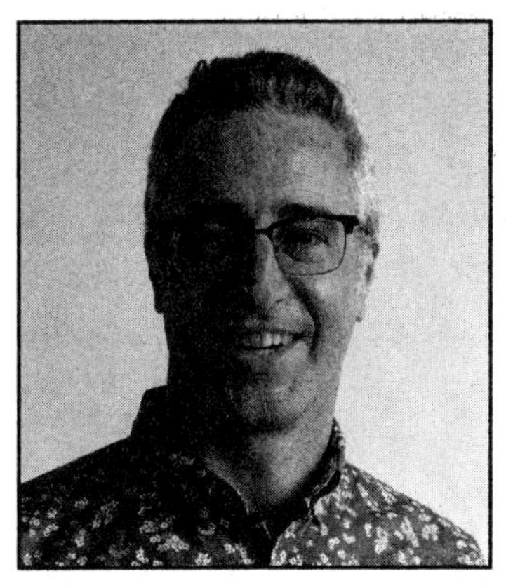

Antonio Pascual-Leone, PhD, is a clinician and professor of psychology at the University of Windsor, Canada and an honorary research professor of psychiatry at the University of Lausanne, Switzerland. Regarded as a world expert on emotion change, he has made seminal contributions to psychotherapy theory, research, and practice. His books include *Emotion Focused Therapy for Complex Trauma* (2nd ed., American Psychological Association [APA], 2023) and *Principles of Emotion Change* (APA, 2026). Dr. Pascual-Leone's work has been recognized with career awards from the Society for Psychotherapy Research (2014) and the Society for the Exploration of Psychotherapy Integration (2009), as well as several distinguished publication awards. A certified trainer in emotion-focused therapy, he has delivered workshops in over a dozen countries and received awards for his teaching and mentorship. His TEDx talk, "How to get over the end of a relationship," has been viewed over 6.3 million times.

Before focusing on psychology, Pascual-Leone studied theatre. Later, he earned a graduate degree in developmental psychology at the University of Toulouse in France. His PhD at York University, Canada was under the mentorship of Les Greenberg. His father, Juan Pascual-Leone (a developmental psychologist who worked with Jean Piaget), has also been a significant influence. Dr. Pascual-Leone maintains a private practice, seeing individuals and couples in Windsor, Canada, where he lives with his wife, Megan Thomas, and their sons, Jasper and Theodore.